Better Patient Care
Through Nursing Research

Third Edition

Better Patient Care Through Nursing Research

Third Edition

Faye G. Abdellah, R.N., Ed.D., Sc.D., F.A.A.N.
Deputy Surgeon General
Chief Nurse Officer, U.S. Public Health Service
Department of Health and Human Services
Washington, D.C.

Eugene Levine, Ph.D.
Consultant in Nursing Research
Washington, D.C.

with editorial assistance from

Barbara Stevenson Levine, B.A.
Formerly Editor and Information Specialist
Breast Cancer Task Force, National Cancer Institute
U.S. Public Health Service, Department of Health and Human Services, Washington, D.C.

Macmillan Publishing Company, Inc.
New York

Collier Macmillan Canada, Inc.
Toronto

Collier Macmillan Publishers
London

#12585314

Macmillan Publishing Company, Inc.
866 Third Avenue, New York, New York 10022

Collier Macmillan Canada, Inc.
Collier Macmillan Publishers • London

Library of Congress Cataloging-in-Publication Data

Abdellah, Faye G.
  Better patient care through nursing research.

  Bibliography: p.
  Includes index.
  1. Nursing—Research—Methodology.   I. Levine, Eugene.
II. Title.   [DNLM: 1. Nursing.   2. Research.
WY 20.5 A135b]
RT81.5.A25   1986   610.73′072   85-23051
ISBN 0-02-300080-5

    Printing: 1 2 3 4 5 6 7 8   Year: 6 7 8 9 0 1 2 3 4

Preface

In this the third edition of our book, we have undertaken a major revision of the material. First, the text has been rewritten to improve readability and clarify meaning. We have tried to avoid over-simplification and superficiality while making this research book accessible to nursing students.

Second, we have focused on the processes and techniques that are used in conducting nursing research. Previous editions of the book contained "Case Studies of Research" that were essentially descriptive and, to some readers, made our book a "reference" book rather than a "how-to" book. This material has been replaced by methodology oriented discussions such as the role of the computer in research.

Third, to help guide the reader, each chapter begins with a statement of objectives. The book has been redesigned to improve readability and highlight key points. Finally, all text, references, problems, and the glossary have been thoroughly updated.

Since the first edition of this book appeared in 1965 much has happened in nursing research. From what was a highly specialized activity undertaken by a small group of people, nursing research has become much more widespread. Courses in nursing research, originally taught only at the graduate level, are now given in most baccalaureate programs. The literature on nursing research has expanded enormously—there are at least a dozen books on methodology for nursing research and numerous journals specializing in research methods and applications. Undergraduate students are increasingly required to write research papers, and, of course, graduate-level theses and dissertations usually involve research methodology.

Practitioners of nursing, in the face of rapid scientific and technologic advances, need the ability to read and interpret reports and evaluate findings. Nursing researchers, a continuously growing body of experts, need guidance in the preparation of research proposals and in the execution of research projects. Nursing students need to learn the basic principles of evaluating and conducting research. This new edition of our book is intended to serve these three major audiences.

As in the previous editions we have attempted to avoid the "cookbook" approach. We present instead underlying meaning and rationale for various research designs, tools, and techniques within a practical, process-oriented framework. Our view is that research should be a thoughtful not mechanistic process.

Thus, our aim is to make our book more accessible, appealing, and useful, without over-simplifying. If we have achieved this goal, no small measure of our success is due to the thorough technical editing of Barbara Stevenson Levine who skillfully invigorated and clarified the language of the earlier editions.

Faye G. Abdellah
Eugene Levine

Contents

Preface   **v**

PART ONE   INTRODUCTION TO NURSING RESEARCH

Chapter 1   What is Nursing Research   **3**

Objectives   3
Definition of Nursing Research   4
Every Nurse as a Researcher: The Concept of Caring   4
Reasons for Doing Research   9
Research Aims   11
Methods for Conducting Research   13
Research Settings   17
Research Subjects   20
Who Does Research?   21
Substitutes for Research   21
When is Research Needed?   23
Summary   25
Problems and Suggestions for Further Study   27

Chapter 2   Evolution of Nursing Research   **28**

Objectives   28
Nursing Research—Its Roots   28
Nursing Research—Its Future   35
Problems and Suggestions for Further Study   36

Chapter 3   Nursing Science and the Research Process   **38**

Objectives   38
The Need for Research in Nursing   38
Technological Innovations in Nursing Education   39
Utilization of Research Findings   41
Strategies for Advancing Nursing Research by the Year 2000   42
The Impact of the Social Sciences on Nursing Research   45
Evolution of Nursing as a Science   46
Summary   47

Chapter 4   **Theoretical Basis of Nursing Research**   **50**

Objectives   50
The Role of Theory in Research   51
Nursing Practice Models   52
Summary   70

PART TWO   STEPS IN THE RESEARCH PROCESS

Chapter 5   **Overview of the Research Process**   **75**

Objectives   75
Topic Selection, Problem Formulation, and Literature Review   76
Theory, Hypothesis, and Variables   77
Research Design, Population, and Sampling   80
Data Collection, Processing, and Summarizing   82
Results Interpretation and Communication   83
Summary   84
Problems and Suggestions for Further Study   85

Chapter 6   **Select the Topic and Formulate the Problem**   **86**

Objectives   86
Sources of Research Topics   86
Stating the Problem   87
Assessing the Researchability of the Problem   89
Summary   93
Problems and Suggestions for Further Study   93

Chapter 7   **Review the Literature**   **94**

Objectives   94
Sources of Information   94
Computer-Assisted Information Retrieval   101
Questions to be Answered in Preparing a Literature Review   103
Guidelines for a Literature Review   104
Problems and Suggestions for Further Study   105

Chapter 8   **Formulate the Framework of Theory**   **106**

Objectives   106
Theories and Models   106
Summary   112
Problems and Suggestions for Further Study   112

Chapter 9   Formulate Hypotheses   **114**

    Objectives   114
    What are Hypotheses?   114
    Examples of Hypotheses   115
    Stating Hypotheses   121
    Summary   124
    Problems and Suggestions for Further Study   124

Chapter 10   Define and Quantify Variables   **125**

    Objectives   125
    How to Define Variables   125
    Quantification of Variables   128
    Scaling Techniques   131
    Types of Scales   132
    How to Select a Criterion Measure for a Study   147
    Criteria for Evaluating Sufficiency and Efficiency of Measures of
      Variables   148
    The Role of Criterion Measures in Research in Nursing   155
    Steps in Writing Outcome Criteria   159
    Summary   160
    Problems and Suggestions for Further Study   102

Chapter 11   Determine the Research Design   **164**

    Objectives   164
    Experimental Research   164
    Advantages and Disadvantages of the Experimental Design   168
    Advantages and Disadvantages of the Nonexperimental Design   170
    Types of Experimental Designs   176
    How to Conduct an Experiment   192
    Nonexperimental Designs   200
    How to Conduct Nonexperimental Research   207
    How to Choose Between an Experimental and Nonexperimental
      Design   208
    Summary   209
    Problems and Suggestions for Further Study   211

Chapter 12   Define the Study Population and Sample   **214**

    Objectives   214
    Selection of the Study Subjects   214
    Sampling   217
    Summary   228
    Problems and Suggestions for Further Study   229

Chapter 13 Collect the Data   **232**

Objectives   232
Methods of Collecting Data   232
How to Select a Data Collection Method   239
Precision in Data Collection   241
Summary   243
Problems and Suggestions for Further Study   243

Chapter 14 Process and Summarize the Data   **245**

Objectives   245
The Role of Computers in Research   245
Processing Data by Hand   249
Summarizing Research Data   250
Summary   259
Problems and Suggestions for Further Study   259

Chapter 15 Data Analysis   **261**

Objectives   261
Tests of Significance for Quantitative Variables   263
Tests of Significance for Qualitative Variables   269
Summary   277
Problems and Suggestions for Further Study   277

Chapter 16 Determine How to Interpret the Data   **279**

Objectives   279
The Meaning of Statistical Significance   279
The Null Hypothesis   281
Alternative Hypotheses   282
Common Errors   284
Interpreting Data in Statistical Tables   290
Problems and Suggestions for Further Study   296

Chapter 17 Communicating and Utilizing Results   **298**

Objectives   298
Research Utilization Process   298
Steps in Implementing Research Findings   299
Planning for Publication   299
Writing the Research Report   300
Evaluating Research   302
Problems and Suggestions for Further Study   305

**PART THREE   STRATEGIES AND FUTURE DIRECTIONS FOR NURSING
                RESEARCH**

Chapter 18   Research Tactics   **309**

Objectives   309
Securing Adequate Staff for the Research   310
Securing Facilities   314
The Rights of Human Subjects   314
Seeking Financial Support for Research   317
Roles of the Federal Government in Furthering Nursing Research   318
Peer Review of Federal Government Supported Research   322
Preparation of the Research Proposal in Applying for Financial
    Support   341
Writing a Research Proposal   343
Some Major Deterrents to Research   350
Summary   351
Problems and Suggestions for Further Study   353

Chapter 19   Future Directions of Research in Nursing   **355**

Objectives   355
Nursing Research Priorities   356
New Horizons in Nursing Research   361
Organization and Delivery of Nursing Services   362
Preventive Health Care   370
Research on Aging   372
Rural Health Services for the Long-term-care Patient/Resident   372
Health Care Systems Research   373
Technological Advances and Their Impact on Nursing Research   375

Glossary   **382**

Bibliography   **397**

Index   **407**

INTRODUCTION TO NURSING RESEARCH

CHAPTER

1

What Is Nursing Research

OBJECTIVES

- To understand the scope of nursing practice and to define nursing research.
- To identify the dimensions of nursing research.
- To identify the ideal attitudes of a nurse researcher.
- To understand the complexities of promoting research in practice-based settings.
- To understand the characteristics of practice-based research.

- To understand the scientific method as it relates to nursing research.
- To identify characteristics essential for developing a scientific base for practice.
- To understand the experimental and nonexperimental methods of conducting nursing research.
- To distinguish between basic and applied research.
- To learn how to use a typology of research

Before one can define nursing research, it is essential to have an agreed upon definition of *nursing*. In 1980, the American Nurses' Association published a comprehensive statement entitled *Nursing. A Social Policy Statement*,[1] which provides an historical orientation to a definition of nursing and to the influence of nursing theory as part of nursing's evolution.

Nightingale's *Notes on Nursing: What It Is and What It Is Not* defined nursing as "charge of the personal health of somebody . . . and what nursing has to do . . . is to put the patient in the best condition for nature to act upon him."[2] Henderson's classic definition stated that the purpose of nursing was "to assist the individual, sick or well, in the performance of those activities contributing to health or its recovery (or to a

peaceful death) that he would perform unaided if he had the necessary strength, will or knowledge. And to do this in such a way as to help him gain independence as rapidly as possible."[3]

Abdellah[4] defined nursing as a service to individuals and to families, and therefore, to society. It is based on an art and science that mold the attitudes, intellectual competencies, and technical skill of the individual nurse into the desire and ability to help people, sick or well, cope with their health needs. This service may involve recognizing health problems of the patient/client; deciding on appropriate courses of action; providing continuous care of the individual's total health needs; helping the individual to become more self-directing in attaining or maintaining a healthy state of mind and body; and carrying out continuous evaluation and research to improve nursing practice.

Thus, the definition of nursing has been evolutionary. It has evolved over a period of time as the concepts of nursing have been clarified and the horizons and responsibilities of the field broadened. The following definition of nursing is one supported by the profession:

KEY POINT

Nursing is the diagnosis and treatment of human responses to actual or potential health problems.[5]

The definition includes four distinct characteristics of nursing:

- *Phenomena:* of concern to nurses as human responses to actual or potential health problems.
- *Theory Application:* concepts, principles, processes to understand the phenomena within the domain of nursing practice.
- *Nursing Actions:* amelioration, improvement, or correction of conditions to which practices are directed, e.g., to prevent illness and to promote health.
- *Evaluation of Effects of Nursing Actions:* to determine if those actions have been effective in improving or resolving the conditions to which they were directed.

DEFINITION OF NURSING RESEARCH

Nursing research can be defined in two dimensions: (1) research conducted by nurses, and (2) research on nursing care.

KEY POINT

Research conducted by the nurse as principal investigator may be scientific inquiry concerning the causes, diagnoses and prevention of diseases, promotion of health in the processes of human growth and development, and the biological effects of environmental contaminants.

KEY POINT

Research on nursing care is research directed toward understanding the nursing care of individuals and groups and the biological, physiological, social, behavioral, and environmental mechanisms that influence health and disease relevant to nursing

care. Thus, nursing research develops (1) knowledge about health and the promotion of health over the life-span; (2) care of individuals with health problems and disabilities or dysfunctions; and, (3) nursing actions that can help individuals to respond effectively to actual or potential health problems.

Examples of human responses that provide a basis for research are self-care limitations; impaired functioning in any physiological area; pain and discomfort; behavioral problems related to illness; and dysfunctional perceptual orientation to health.

Research in nursing should lead to the generation and testing of theories directed toward the understanding of ways to promote a state of health in human beings.

EVERY NURSE AS A RESEARCHER: THE CONCEPT OF CARING

Caring is the heart of nursing. While there is a range of caring functions and activities that are procedural in nature, the basis for engaging in these efforts is an underlying feeling of benevolence and humanitarianism by one individual toward another. However simple, complex, or technical these activities are, they are based on a nurse's perception and judgment of a patient's need at a particular time.

The concept of caring in a nursing context refers to acts and related attitudes, predominantly the moral attitude of respect for the individual. Such caring acts have in common that they are all performed under the moral ethic of respecting the dignity and autonomy of another human being.[6] In addition to a knowledge base and skills, there are a number of ideal attitudes that every nurse researcher should have. Some of these are[7]:

- Creativity
- Curiosity
- Ability to question the status quo
- Ability to see a thing from a different perspective

- Open-mindedness
- Flexibility
- Imagination
- Conviction in self and work
- Ability to express self verbally and in writing
- Desire to learn
- Commitment and courage
- Patience
- Ability to reason effectively
- Ability to follow a line of reasoning to its conclusion
- Tenacity
- Appreciation of "mental" things
- Ability to pick out the problem from the mass of detail
- Enthusiasm
- Objectivity, as an aspect of detachment
- Ability to assess and judge impact of change on others
- Ability to accept responsibility for one's actions
- Ability to accept criticism
- Ability to assess one's own work objectively

Naturally, not every person will have all these characteristics, but an awareness of desirable characteristics will assist in conducting good research, most particularly when one is building a team. The characteristics that one team member lacks may be supplied and balanced by those of other members. A well-rounded team, in education, experience, and personality, is an enviable milieu in which to conduct research.

"Every nurse ought not just to do simple research tasks as part of her work but she also always ought to be a researcher."[8]

Promoting Practice-Based Research

Although most practicing nurses show little interest in nursing research, nurses do express concern about the state of professionalization of nursing. There is a link between research and professionalization. The latter cannot be achieved without a commitment to the former. The need to conduct research is related to the quality of practice in a direct cause-and-effect relationship. The greater the extent to which improved nursing practice is based on nurs-

KEY POINT

ing research, the higher the quality of practice. McClure points out that not much nursing research has been done in agencies where care is delivered, has not been done with recipients of care as subjects, and has had little impact on nursing practice.[9]

Research *can* form a basis for nursing practice. Good nursing practice reflects the results of good research. Such research ideally is precise and replicable and can produce predictable patient/client outcomes. "Research makes known the links between the parts of the nursing process —assessment, planning and intervention, and patient outcomes and evaluation."[10]

Climate for Conducting Research

How does one stress the importance of a positive attitude toward research by the working nurse? Nurses in practice settings, particularly nurse administrators, can demonstrate interest by committing time and resources and making available patients for nurse researchers on their staffs or those linked with a college of nursing. All those involved in the research—no matter how small the effort—must be shown the importance of that effort to the entire project. Commitment to the research can be encouraged by stressing the impact of each part on the whole and by acknowledging and showing appreciation for each person's efforts. A little cheerleading never hurts. The nurse administrator is in a key position to encourage nurse researchers to study practice-related problems. While much emphasis is on wellness and prevention of illness, there are still numerous sick patients who need the attention of researchers.

The appointment of a nurse researcher to the institution's staff can help to bring service and education together. Such an appointment states for all that scientific investigation is an integral part of the nursing profession. It is important that implementation follow research findings so that they will be accepted by the nurses who will bring about such changes in practice. Educators have the responsibility of trying to build into nursing education a foundational perspective that recognizes the educative aspects of caring as nurses prepare for the real world.[11]

The researcher usually is prepared through graduate education to the doctoral level by developing research skills through study and practical research experience either alone or in collaborating with other study team members. Of the two advanced degrees available, the more substantive and relevant they are to nursing science, nursing practice, or a pertinent science in general (e.g., physiology, anthropology, sociology, psychology), the firmer and sounder will be the basis for professional recognition. The collaborative role for the researcher is important and provides opportunities to learn and understand the investigative role. An important part of the nurse's education is the study of research design and methodology. Without a keen understanding and appreciation of these two aspects of research, one lacks totally the skills with which to even begin. Today's research is done, not by brilliant amateurs, but by trained professionals.[12]

Assessing the readiness for research is well worth the time and effort of the nurse researcher. The administrator of a clinical facility, the dean of a school of nursing, for example, must be willing to take a risk but must have assurance that the benefits to be derived to the patient/client or nursing staff warrant the risk. The organizational structure in which the research is to be conducted must include an efficient and effective means for reviewing research protocols, approving them for scientific merit and protection of human subjects, providing needed support services, and helping to communicate the research to others in a positive way.[13] Because implementation of research findings into practice rests heavily with the nurse administrator, gaining acceptance of the researcher by the nurse administrator depends on the inclusion of implications for nursing practice in any reports; making practical suggestions for introducing findings into the practice setting; extracting research-based knowledge that has validity and relevance for practice; and translating criteria for evaluating research findings into terms understandable to the practitioner.

Researchers themselves have a great deal of responsibility in fostering a positive attitude of the nurse administrator toward research. Researchers must interpret and present their findings in such a way that they can be implemented in the clinical setting. Nurses engaged primarily in patient care practice and who are not familiar with research are often unprepared to evaluate the quality of the research with which they must deal. Some nurses tend to see research as irrelevant to practice and may be overreliant on procedures learned in basic nursing practice, which may be outmoded and lacking a scientific basis. This attitude constitutes a real barrier to acceptance of and cooperation with the conduct of research and the subsequent implementation of research findings. It is up to the researcher to deal with the situation and find ways to overcome such attitudes, because the lack of acceptance within the profession magnifies itself when transferred to the broader world of medicine and the public in general.

Deterrents to nurse involvement in research in practical settings can be minimized by interpreting the research in such a way that its practical value is evident to the nursing and hospital administration, assuring cooperation from those people expected to implement or benefit from the research. Creditability of the nurse researcher and the appropriate use of consultants are also important to successful implementation.[14] If administrators and educators by their commitment to nursing research can help nurse researchers conduct research in practice settings, we will know that success has been achieved when nursing practice is perceived as both an art and a science.

Some Problems Associated with Studies

The question of how nursing research influences patient care has given rise to a large variety of studies using different approaches and concerned with different definitions of the question. Some studies have defined nursing care as size of nursing staff (average hours of care available per patient), while others have defined it as the method of organizing the nursing staff. Patient care can be defined as physiological phenomena such as blood pressure, psychological factors such as satisfaction with care, or in terms of the occurrence of certain events such as requests for sedatives, which are manifestations of physiological and psychological phenomena. There are also questions so difficult to answer that many different research studies, each building on the findings of previous studies, are required before a satisfactory answer is formulated.

An investigator may direct research to a question previously studied because of doubts about the validity of earlier findings, which may arise as a result of a perceived imperfection in the research design. The study is repeated with a new or corrected design. Many examples are available of faulty research designs leading to spurious findings later set straight by more properly conducted studies. The classic example is the research done at the Hawthorne Works of the Western Electric Company in the 1920s on the relationship between physical environment and worker productivity.[15] Because of improper research design (to be discussed later), sociopsychological responses were created in the subjects under study that were primarily due to their participation in the study itself and not to the factors (e.g., physical environment) being studied. This phenomenon became known as the "Hawthorne effect."

KEY POINT

Studies that are repetitions of previous studies and are directed toward the same question using the same methodology are called replication studies. Here the researcher is trying to confirm or deny the findings of earlier research. The earlier findings may be considered tentative. Only after the study has been repeated a number of times and equivalent findings obtained do we consider that the validity of the conclusion has been confirmed. Few individual studies, those primarily for a limited population and concerned with a narrow question, can produce definitive answers to any question. What is usually required, particularly when the research is directed toward questions affecting human health and well-being, is a series of studies, a research program, to provide well-documented conclusions. To illustrate: in clinical trials of drugs, in which the effect of the drug on patients is evaluated, precisely structured studies are independently carried out at the same time by different researchers among certain groups of patients in different hospitals. These are known as multiclinic trials.[16] Each trial is attempting to answer the same question: Is the drug beneficial? Each trial is considered research because it is part of a larger effort to either statistically validate or disprove earlier experimental data. Four problem areas to implementing research findings into practice include dissemination; access; assessment of the usability; and utilization.

KEY POINT

Beginning the Search for Scientific Knowledge

Nursing research has as its goal the improvement of nursing practice, to be achieved by providing a scientific basis for practice. Early on the researcher becomes aware of gaps in nursing knowledge, but can be comforted by the recognition that there are certainly gaps in all knowledge. In seeking to narrow this gap, the researcher must initiate a project. How to begin? Review of nursing and related literature and working with a collaborative team help the researcher identify problems for study. In selecting a problem several concerns must be borne in mind: How does the

KEY POINT research affect the patient/client? Can the study objective be met? How timely are the results? Is there any risk to the study subjects?[17]

The Scientific Way to Research

The research approach based on the scientific method is the accepted way to generate scientific knowledge. In pursuit of this knowledge, theories are constructed, and hypotheses are developed. Hypotheses and subhypotheses are examined by subjecting the ideas contained in them to testing in an organized and logical manner and are then either proved or disproved as a result of the testing.

KEY POINT A scientific research study is the systematic, controlled, empirical, and critical investigation of hypothetical propositions about presumed relations among phenomena.[18] Nursing science, as a part of scientific research, represents our understanding of human biology and behavior in health and illness, including the processes by which changes in health status are brought about, the patterns of behavior associated with normal and critical life events, and the principles and laws governing life states and processes.[19]

The Scientific Method

The launching of *Nursing Research* in 1952 stimulated nurses to undertake research during the three following decades. Where has this quest for new scientific knowledge taken us? Brown undertook an analysis of research in nursing from 1952 to 1980.[20] The analysis identified four characteristics essential for the development of a scientific base for a practice discipline. **KEY POINT** First, the research should be conducted mainly by members of the discipline itself. The research needs to be concerned with clinical problems. Second, the fact that nurses conduct research does not guarantee that the product will be relevant to practice. Third, scientific research must be based on a theoretical framework that is continuously refined and extended through replication. Unfortunately, replication, as a strategy to develop, extend, and refine theory, has not as yet been a characteristic of nursing research. Fourth is soundness of method. Although nurse researchers have become more sophisticated in their research designs, insufficient attention has been paid to the psychometric properties of their instruments.

In recent years, more nurses have prepared themselves to be researchers. There has been a marked increase (63 percent) in the number of clinical studies undertaken, and concurrently, there has also been a shift away from acute illness (from 56 percent to 20 percent) toward prevention and health promotion (from 13 percent to 35 percent). But the thrust toward clinical research should not negate the importance of research of nurse characteristics, nursing education, and nursing administration. A balance needs to be achieved. As, over the past three decades, the focus of nursing research has moved toward clinical issues, nursing research has become more theoretically oriented. There has also been a shift away from descriptive studies and an increase in explanatory studies. There is general agreement that those studies which use experimental designs will contribute most to changes in nursing practice, although the use of experimental designs may not always be feasible for ethical reasons, accessibility of patients for study, etc. In such situations correlational designs are still useful. A word needs to be said about the scarcity of methodological investigations; efforts must be directed toward developing useful instruments to measure phenomena important to nursing.[21]

It is recognized that nursing science is the base of knowledge underlying human behavior and social interaction under normal and stressful conditions across the lifespan. Nursing research (the systematic inquiry into problems associated with illness, health, and care) lends to and contributes to nursing science.[22] As nursing research moves toward more complex research designs, the researcher must be mindful that research should always be conducted in a meaningful and scholarly manner (no matter how small the study) in order to make a contribution to nursing science.

REASONS FOR DOING RESEARCH

Basic Research

Although all research stems from the desire to answer a question, it can serve various purposes. Research may be done to increase the state of knowledge in a certain area or for an accretion of general knowledge. The findings may be a collection of numerical data, as in a biological study of the weights of protein molecules, a lengthy narrative document, as in an anthropological study of some primitive society, or statements of propositions demonstrated to be true by the study, as in a psychological study of the effects of food deprivation on the behavior of rats. Studies such as these are sometimes called *basic* or *pure* research. The implication of this designation is that such research establishes fundamental verifiable information essential to the undertaking of further research. Findings from basic research are building blocks upon which further research and increments in knowledge are based. As defined in a governmental report, basic research is "that type of research which is directed toward increase of knowledge in science. It is research where the primary aim of the investigator is a fuller knowledge or understanding of the subject under study."[23]

All fields of endeavor advance in stages, each stage building on the knowledge gained in previous stages. Alexander Pope's famous quotation: "Not to go back is somewhat to advance and men must walk, at least, before they dance."[24] For instance, before a cure for cancer is found it will be necessary to obtain the answers to a host of important questions, perhaps including the fundamental question of what

life itself is. The stages that contribute to the advance in knowledge make up the process known as basic research. The research may not be directed toward an immediate or even a long-range practical purpose. It is knowledge for knowledge's sake.

Although their results have often not led to immediate action, the majority of nursing research studies can be classified as applied research, as many have been directed toward specific goals. Some of the goals have been:

- Improvement of patient/client care through identification of outcome measures
- Alleviation of the nursing shortage
- Enrichment of the curriculum in nursing education
- Increasing recruitment into nursing
- Optimizing the organization of nursing service

Because no single study can be expected to yield final answers to these global, multifaceted, and complex nursing problems, individual studies have not achieved these goals, but have provided new knowledge for their future attainment.

Applied Research

A sharp dividing line is often drawn between research whose end product is purely knowledge (basic research) and research that is directed toward so-called practical purposes (applied research). Both types are important to science and knowledge, and their contributions are of equal consequence. There is endless argument over whether "pure" or "applied" science is the "higher" calling. Archimedes, inventor of some of the most practical devices in history, e.g., the doctrine of levers and the threaded screw for raising water, refused to write about them because he was a "gentleman philosopher and a Greek!" Leonardo da Vinci, that giant of the early Renaissance, believed pure and practical research equally important, provided they both originated from experiment. An abstract thinker of great depth, he filled his diaries with ideas for practical inventions.

Nevertheless, applied research is conducted for practical reasons in order to

1. Solve a problem
2. Make a decision
3. Develop a new program, product, method, or procedure
4. Evaluate a program, product, method, or procedure

PROBLEM SOLVING

Most applied research studies are initiated to find solutions to existing problems. Examples are:

- How do premature infants respond to extra-uterine living?
- How can nursing action influence the response and well-being of premature infants?
- How does a child react to the mother who is rooming-in during the period of hospitalization?
- What are healthy children's conceptions of death? Of illness?
- How do chronic illnesses affect permanent life-style change?
- How can falls resulting in hip fracture in the elderly be prevented?

In problem solving the assumption is that there is some deficiency or shortcoming in present ways of doing things and that improvement can be achieved through research. Thus, improvement of specific situations is the objective in problem solving. Improvement, hopefully, will be accomplished by changes resulting from the research. The aim of the research is to provide appropriate facts on which to base the change.

DECISION MAKING

Decision making involves selecting a course of action from alternative courses. Examples of decision-making questions in nursing that could serve as bases for research are:

- How do DRGs affect the quality of patient care provided?
- Should computers be introduced to record nurses' notes?

- Which categories of nurses should receive direct reimbursement for nursing care?

The function of research in decision making is to yield facts upon which the selection of the course of action can most appropriately be made. While facts are not the only elements considered in decision making (other elements such as value judgments also influence the decision), to the extent that the decision question involves matters essentially factual in nature, research can play an important role.

DEVELOPMENTAL STUDIES

Research can be a valuable aid in the development of methods, procedures, and programs in nursing. For example, if it is desired to devise a CPR training program for nurses, factual data systematically gathered will assist in the design format, content, and scope of the program. If it is desired to create a new system of delivering medications to patients, a research approach can assist in developing an efficient and practical system.

Following is a list of just a few of the many programs, methods, procedures, and products in the field of nursing that require further development.

- A method for rating nursing performance
- Measuring instruments for assessing adequacy of patient care
- Procedures for forecasting patients' needs for nursing service
- Devices for electronic patient monitoring
- Procedures for effective matching of work load with staffing
- A method of assessing job satisfaction of nursing personnel

EVALUATIVE RESEARCH

Applied research is sometimes considered synonymous with evaluative research. In evaluative research a program, method, procedure, or product is tested to answer such questions as:

- Has a desirable change occurred?
- Is the product any good?

- Has the patient been helped?
- Has efficiency been increased?
- Have costs been reduced?
- Has service been improved?
- Have the students learned well?
- Can the patient take better care of himself/herself?

Evaluative research essentially looks backward to assess past achievement, whereas decision-making research looks to the future to suggest future effort. Evaluative research is pragmatic. The underlying question is, "Has it made any difference to do something one way as contrasted with another way?" This difference must be real, meaningful, and practically significant. . . .[25]

Examples of evaluative research abound. In the health fields the testing of drugs, known as clinical trials, is an important activity that has received much public attention in recent years. In the field of education evaluative studies are continuously made of curriculum, selection procedures, and teaching methods. In manufacturing quality control is used to check whether the finished product meets specifications. And in the field of market research much effort is devoted to consumer evaluation of a company's goods and services.

Many research studies classified as applied research cannot be fitted into one of the four categories just mentioned. Many such studies are multipurpose and may have features of all four categories. For example, in clinical drug trials the purpose is to evaluate the effectiveness of the drug. As a result of that evaluation a decision will be made also as to whether the drug will be marketed. In studies of the relationship between smoking and lung cancer, the major purpose is to find the causes of lung cancer. If the causes are isolated these studies may also shed light on what kinds of programs should be developed to combat the disease—a practical end.

Demonstrations

In the health field, particularly public health, the term "demonstration" is often used in connection with the process of research. Actually, demonstrations fall within the same area as developmental research but possess one feature that distinguishes them from true research. In developmental studies the aim is to develop a new procedure, program, or product, often without a specific application in mind but rather to be generally applicable to a variety of situations. By contrast, a demonstration takes a program, procedure, or product already developed and shows how it can be applied to a specific situation. A demonstration, then, can be considered the application phase of applied research and the research itself as the fact-finding and analysis stage.

Examples of demonstration projects in public health are:

- A referral system for patients discharged from hospitals
- Organization of a nursing care of the sick-at-home program
- A method of analyzing the activities of nursing personnel
- A system of forecasting patients' needs for nursing services
- Obtaining baseline data to prevent hip fractures

Why is it important to distinguish between demonstration and research? Often the two processes are confused. While a demonstration project may contain elements similar to those of a research project, such as study groups, statistical data, and an analysis of data, it merely presents the results of new work or information in a practical way for the education of a user group. The intent of a research project is to discover original or innovative information that may or may not have an immediate use.

RESEARCH AIMS

Research studies can be broadly divided into two categories according to whether they are primarily concerned with discovering new facts or assessing the relationship among facts. The former is sometimes called descriptive research, whereas the latter is termed explanatory research. In descriptive studies the research is primarily concerned with obtaining accurate and meaningful descriptions of the phenomena under study. In explanatory studies the primary interest is in investigating the *relationships* among the phenomena being studied—one phenomenon is compared with another in terms of effects on subjects (people, animals, inanimate objects). For example, medical research is often concerned with investigating the effects of different modes of treatment on patients. Explanation of how to treat disease can result from these studies. Kempthorne[26] suggests the use of the term "comparative" research as a synonym for explanatory studies.

Descriptive Research

Descriptive studies are concerned with a broad range of phenomena and the end product can take many forms. This can be a lengthy narrative statement, sometimes called a case study, as, for example, the anthropological studies of primitive societies in Margaret Mead's *The Coming of Age in Samoa* and the sociological studies of whole communities as in the Lynds' *Middletown*. Or the end result could be a collection of detailed statistical tabulations, exemplified by the reports of the U.S. Census Bureau in its descriptive surveys of the population of the United States and the monographs of the National Center for Health Statistics concerning the health of the American people. Another type of descriptive research is historical research.

Explanatory Research

In explanatory research the aim is to discover why a phenomenon occurred. It is not enough to say that something happens; the aim is to find out *why* it happens.

In a descriptive study the researcher observes certain phenomena, which can be labeled A and B. For his purposes, these phenomena are independent, discrete entities having no important relationship to each other. For example, assume that A represents the number of home visits to patients made by the staff of a public health agency during a certain period of time, and B represents the diagnoses of the patients who were visited. These facts are of interest by themselves as providing a description of the work of the agency. In other words, A can be examined independently of B and still provide meaningful facts.

In an explanatory study A would be studied in relation to B—that is, the number of visits would be related to the diagnoses of the patients. What is important in this type of study is not a description of A and B as isolated entities but, rather, the relationship between A and B. If we look at A and B separately we answer the questions: "How many visits are made by the staff of the agency?" "What kinds of patients compose the case load of the agency?" If we study the relationship between A and B, we can answer the question: "How many home visits are made to patients in different diagnostic categories?" Expressed as a *rate* of visits, the data might show that certain diagnostic categories receive considerably more visits than patients in other categories. Such a relationship goes much further in explaining the work load of the agency than does a study that regards visits and diagnoses as unrelated entities.

Explanatory studies are concerned with discovering how the phenomena under study are related. Does A influence B, or vice versa? Or are A and B affected by a third factor, C? In essence then, explanatory studies are predictive studies in which the behavior of one phenomenon is investigated in relation to the behavior of another phenomenon. Since if we are able to predict we may also control, explanatory research offers a powerful tool in harnessing some of the forces of nature and making technological advances.

Most studies classified as applied research are predictive or explanatory. In a problem-solving study, for example, we seek to isolate all the relevant factors associated with the problem, so that by explaining these relationships we can predict how these factors will behave in the future. Thus, in investigating the problem of why hospital costs are rising, such factors as poor administrative organization and inefficient physical layout might be isolated as important contributors to costs. By controlling these factors we can influence hospital costs, thereby exerting control over this important problem.

Evaluative studies, for the most part explanatory rather than descriptive, try to determine whether certain procedures, methods, products, or processes achieve better results than other ones. Thus, a study of whether thoroughly informing a patient about the nature of his illness favorably affects his rate of recovery can supply valuable facts for improving patient care. And a study of consumer preferences for the same product wrapped in different packages can result in increased sales.

As in most classification systems, many studies cannot be rigidly classified as either descriptive or explanatory but have attributes of both categories. Descriptive research may generate theories about the relationship among the various phenomena studied, which may then be tested in an explanatory study. Nursing science is advanced by both research and utilization, which are interdependent processes. Research identifies and refines solutions to problems through the generation of new knowledge. Research utilization employs new solutions for the improvement of nursing practice. Nursing must find ways to achieve both purposes.[27]

METHODS FOR CONDUCTING RESEARCH

There are two methods for conducting research: experimental and nonexperimental, either of which can be used to conduct applied or basic research. Both can serve the purposes of either descriptive or explanatory research.

The simplest and perhaps the most useful distinction between experimental and nonexperimental research has been provided by Stuart Chapin in his valuable book *Experimental Designs in Sociological Research*. Chapin says that "an experiment is simply observation under controlled conditions."[28] It follows, then, that nonexperimental research is observation without controlled conditions. Now what does this rather stark definition mean? The key words are "controlled conditions" because the critical distinction between experimental and nonexperimental research is that in experiments the researcher consciously manipulates (controls) the conditions—he interferes with "nature." In nonexperimental research "nature" is uncontrolled.

Let us say we are interested in the problem of job turnover of nursing personnel in hospitals. From descriptive studies we see that turnover is very high, so high that it undoubtedly adversely affects patient care. How can this high turnover be reduced? If we raise the salaries of nursing personnel, will it be reduced? This latter question possesses the ingredients for a research study. It is an important question the solution of which could be valuable to hospital administration. Moreover, it could feasibly serve as the basis for a study, since it poses a question that is researchable. Methodologically, the basic question is, shall we conduct this research experimentally or nonexperimentally?

At the risk of oversimplification, but to illustrate the distinction between the two major methods of research, this study could be conducted experimentally as follows. In one type of design (not by any means the best design, as will be made clear in a later chapter), nursing personnel working in two hospitals with identical rates of personnel turnover could be selected as the study population. Then, the salaries of the personnel in one hospital would be raised a

KEY POINT

KEY POINT

substantial amount, 20 percent, while the salaries in the other hospital would be kept at the same level. After a period of time the rates of job turnover would be measured in the two hospitals and a comparison made. If the turnover rate in the higher-paying hospital is considerably lower than in the other hospital, we have evidence that a solution to the problem of high personnel turnover has been found—the payment of higher salaries.

In the nonexperimental approach two similar hospitals, with differences in their salary levels, could be chosen as the study population. The turnover rates in the two hospitals would be compared. If the hospital with the higher salaries had significantly lower turnover rates, we might infer that turnover could be reduced by increasing salaries.

It is obvious that the main difference between these two study designs is that in the experimental approach "nature" is consciously interfered with—the salaries of the personnel in one hospital are raised. In the nonexperimental approach the salary levels are not interfered with, but are taken in their "natural state"—that is, as they have been established prior to the study. In this approach the salary difference is indirectly controlled by *selection* of hospitals that have different salary levels.

KEY POINT The *time, order,* and *manner* in which study conditions are created—in the example given, the difference in salary levels between the two hospitals—are the characteristics that really distinguish experimental from nonexperimental research. In the former the conditions are created by the researchers; in the latter the conditions are in effect *prior* to the study. Only by the selection of study subjects do the researchers exert "control" over them.

Because of the time order of the establishment of the conditions for the study, experimental studies are sometimes called prospective or "carry-forward" studies, whereas nonexperimental studies are called retrospective, "carry-back," or ex post

facto studies. The main advantages of the experimental approach, because it is prospective in nature, are: (1) In explanatory experimental studies it is possible to come closer to establishing cause and effect relationships among the phenomena studied than in nonexperimental explanatory studies. (2) In experimental descriptive studies it is possible to achieve greater purity of description than in nonexperimental descriptive studies because of the greater control over study conditions.

In explanatory experimental research, the kind of research fundamental to the advancement of knowledge, the time sequence of the occurrence of the phenomena under study is controlled by the researcher. In the example cited the salary differential, called A, is established by the researcher. After a period of time elapses, he observes the turnover differential, if any, called B. If B is significantly large, then the researcher can say—subject to the limitations imposed by study design and probabilistic inferences, discussed in later chapters—that A caused B.

In nonexperimental research the time sequence of the occurrence of the phenomena under study is *not* controlled by the researcher. The researcher attempts to trace a causal relationship between B and A, although there is danger in studies like these that another factor, called C, not considered by the researcher, may actually be responsible for B instead of A, which he was supposed to control by selecting subjects who differed in the amount of salary they received. For example, in the nonexperimental study of the relationship between salaries and turnover it was found that the hospital with higher salaries had much less turnover than the hospital with lower salaries. We might infer that low salaries cause high turnover. However, we could be quite wrong in this inference. We must consider the fact that the salary differential between the hospitals existed prior to the initiation of the study and may have been a long-standing phenomenon. Thus, salary difference is not a stimulus in this study design in the same way it is in the experimental approach, where the salary is dramatically changed in one hospital.

Not subjected to the stimulus of a sudden change in salary, as are the personnel in the experimental study, the reactions of the nursing personnel in the nonexperimental study to salary differentials may not be at all comparable to those in the experimental group. For one thing, some personnel in the nonexperimental study may have taken the job in the hospital with lower salary with full knowledge and acceptance they were being underpaid because other features of the job were desirable—its convenient location to home. For these personnel the lower salary would have no effect at all on turnover behavior. Conversely, some personnel in the hospital paying higher salaries might be predisposed to leave for factors totally unrelated to salary. In other words, a multitude of uncontrolled factors besides salaries can influence turnover. Besides the personal factors numerous social factors can affect turnover behavior. Perhaps the administrative climate in the lower-paying hospital is friendlier, more permissive, more productive in fostering altruistic motives, than in the hospital that pays more. The presence of these characteristics can promote greater job stability even in the face of lower salaries.

It must be borne in mind that unlike the rather simple, mechanistic means-ends situation illustrated by Pavlov's animal experiments on conditioned reflexes, every social situation involving human beings has interwoven and interacting with the phenomena isolated for study many other individual and social factors that can influence the study results. This is as true for experimental as for nonexperimental research. The problem for research design, therefore, is to sort out and control the effects of extraneous factors so that we can draw valid and accurate inferences from the study. It is this problem to which the next part of this book is addressed.

Barriers to Experimentation

The major advantage of experimental research is that it permits greater control over the phenomena under study, enabling the drawing of more valid inferences of causal relationships among the phenomena studied. However, because nature is interfered with in experiments, we often run into more practical difficulties in conducting these studies than in nonexperimental studies, particularly in studies involving human beings. Some of the changes that might have to be made in conducting certain experiments could interfere so radically with the natural course of events as to be impossible. Other changes could offer hazards to health or even life. Still others may be too costly.

In the illustration of the relationship between salaries and turnover, in the experimental design we are faced with the administrative problem of actually changing the salary level. In the "natural setting" of the nonexperimental design we do not change salaries but take them as they have been established outside the study by "natural" forces. In other experiments we may have to introduce rather drastic changes into the existing situation, as seen by the following examples:

1. In a study of the effects of different kinds of leadership on employee productivity, some employees may react negatively to the introduction of certain types of leadership, and may even quit the organization.
2. An experiment concerned with testing the impact of the structure of physical facilities on patient care might involve expensive renovations in the existing plant which may have to be scrapped at a later date.
3. A study of the effects of different amounts of nursing care on patient satisfaction with care might require some patients to receive such inadequate nursing care as to endanger their health and well-being.
4. Experimentation with various methods of organizing nursing homes should drastically disrupt the ongoing services provided to patients.

5. A study of lengthening the course of training for practical nurses from one year to two years may result in a drastic rise in the dropout rates from these schools during the course of the experiment.
6. Experimentation with different methods of recording home visits made by public health nurses might result in a loss of valuable information that would normally have been kept.

Of course, if we develop a new system, method, or product, one whose use cannot be found in existing situations, there is no alternative to experimentation if we want to conduct an evaluation. The nonexperimental approach can be used only where the phenomenon we are interested in studying already exists and is available for study. Thus, the evaluation of a new drug is generally conducted as an experimental study, because before the drug is released for general use it must be given a thorough clinical trial under rigid research conditions. If a drug is released to the general public without such study, as in the case of thalidomide, the consequences as discovered in a retrospective evaluation could be very unfortunate.

On the other hand, many questions do not lend themselves to experimentation and can only be investigated through a nonexperimental case study approach. These are questions, generally in the area of descriptive research, that because of the uniqueness of the phenomena under study, experimentation is not only impractical but foolish. Moreover, because this uniqueness is the reason for the study it should be described as naturally as possible. In such fields as anthropology, geology, astronomy, archeology, and sociology, the purpose of the study is often to describe the existing situation in its natural state as accurately as possible. Any kind of control over the research conditions, other than over the accuracy of the observations, could actually destroy the study.

In certain kinds of comparative studies experimentation is also out of the question. Consider a study directed to the question:

"Does the system of nursing in Great Britain provide better patient care than the system of nursing in the United States?" Essentially this a descriptive study in which observations would be made of actual nursing care provided in the two countries in their natural settings. However, on closer inspection the question actually goes beyond pure description and moves into the realm of explanatory research directed toward the relationship between two different systems of nursing and the quality of care. If the descriptions of the systems can be generalized to broader concepts that provide abstractions of the empirical facts of nursing in Great Britain and the United States, it is possible to conceive of an experimental approach to this study. That is, if nursing in Great Britain can be characterized as, say, authoritarian, stable, personalized, while that in the United States as permissive, mobile, depersonalized, it may well be possible to create these conditions in an experimental setting. Many areas of research exhibit just such an evolutionary development, progressing from a descriptive, nonexperimental study of a specific situation to a testing of general constructs through an experimental design.

Another disadvantage of the experimental method is the length of time it can take to carry out such a study. Nowadays, answers to research questions are wanted in a hurry. It is sometimes impractical to consider conducting an experiment if another approach could get an answer more quickly even though the answer may not be as definitive. The following example illustrates this difference in time requirements.

Suppose someone wanted to answer the question: Is a graduate of a degree program more proficient as a bedside nurse in a general hospital than a graduate of a basic diploma program? If the study were conducted experimentally, a group of high school graduates could be selected and assigned to either a diploma program or a degree program, and followed up after they had graduated from nursing school and been employed as graduate nurses in hospitals. Then, their proficiency as nurses would be measured to see whether there were a difference in proficiency between the graduates of the two types of programs. If the study were conducted nonexperimentally a sample of graduate nurses in hospitals would be selected, their proficiency as bedside nurses would be measured, a determination made of whether they had attended a degree program or a diploma program, and an analysis performed to evaluate the difference in proficiency scores between graduates of the two types of programs. The study, if carried out experimentally, might take a minimum of five years and require much money and effort. If carried out nonexperimentally, it could possibly be done in about a year and with considerably less expense.[29]

Still another deficiency of experiments is their artificiality. Many experiments are constructed of such unnatural elements that they have little real-life applicability. One such unnatural element may be the setting. Special facilities are sometimes set up which permit little applicability of findings beyond the study setting. Also, the subjects of the study may be atypical. Because they are a captive audience, students are frequently used in experimental work and their reactions to the phenomena under study may be quite different from those of other persons. Sometimes animal studies are pursued, particularly in psychology and medicine, as analogues of human studies. Finally, even the phenomena under study in experiments are sometimes too artificial to have any practical meaning and extrapolation of animal data to human beings is difficult, to say the least.

Because of the various difficulties in conducting experimental research in fields of study dealing with human populations —time, cost, administrative difficulties, possible artificiality— it often becomes necessary to restrict the scope of an experiment, to narrow the problem. Great care should be taken not to reduce the scope of experiments to the point where they become little more than sterile academic exercises. Experiments offer the surest way of explaining causality and as such can make a valuable contribution to scientific knowledge in nursing.

RESEARCH SETTINGS

Highly Controlled Settings

Research can be performed in a variety of settings. At one end of this spectrum is the highly controlled, specially devised setting called a laboratory, experimental center, research center, or test unit set up outside the actual life situation for the sole purposes of conducting research. Usually the kind of research carried out in these settings is experimental in methodology and for the most part explanatory in purpose although descriptive research is also conducted.

Although specialized, highly controlled settings enhance the purity of research observations, they suffer from the drawback of artificiality, which can be particularly bothersome in studies involving human beings. When a study proposes to put human beings in a special test unit, several things can happen. First, it may be difficult to obtain cooperation from the people because of negative reaction to a strange environment. Second, if people do agree to cooperate, they may then behave in completely unpredictable and unnatural ways. The famous Hawthorne effect describes the way people in a research setting respond to study conditions because they know they are participating in something special and therefore fail to exhibit their normal behavior, which biases the study findings and leads to spurious conclusions. Such behavior consists of exaggeration and distortion in responding to research questions, reacting favorably to a "treatment" when none or a placebo was given, and behaving more productively and energetically in the experimental situation than normally.

Another aspect of artificiality of research settings is that the settings may have small resemblance to the real-life situation they are supposed to represent so that it becomes difficult to apply the study findings to the real world. In social psychology, for example, among the studies done in rigidly controlled settings are those concerned with how people behave in small groups. Many of these studies attempt to create in a laboratory setting an analogue of the real-life situation. Thus, in studies of responses to different styles of leadership behavior, a group of individuals may be subjected to a variety of artificially created administrative situations. Care must be taken when translating the findings of these studies to the situations of actual working conditions.

With all the limitations of the use of specialized, highly controlled settings in research, there is much to be said in their favor. Removal from normal day-to-day activities can "purify" the study situation. And, most important, in specialized research settings it is possible to modify the environment, to manipulate the study conditions, and, in short, to conduct a proper experiment with all the scientific virtues that the method possesses.

Natural Settings

At the other extreme of research settings are natural settings, also called uncontrolled settings, field settings, or real-life situations, characterized by an absence of control over the environment. The setting is studied just as it is, the only direct "controls" exerted by the researcher being mainly in relation to such matters as the selection of study subjects and data collection and analysis. By definition, only nonexperimental studies can be conducted in natural settings. Although both descriptive and explanatory purposes can be served by studies in uncontrolled settings, explanatory research is less likely to be found in such settings.

The terms "field surveys" and "case studies" describe particular types of natural setting research. A field survey usually gathers statistical data on a particular subject through questions asked of people in their natural habitat, either directly by interview or indirectly in a mailed questionnaire.

A case study is a detailed, intensive, factual description of individuals, groups of individuals, institutions, communities, whole societies, incidents, situations, inanimate objects, or animals. Such studies are characterized by lengthy narrative statements that describe in depth the subjects under study in their natural settings. The studies may delve into past history as well as report a current situation, include statistical data as well as verbal description, and contain explanatory and evaluative statements as well as descriptive data. In the field of patient care, illustrations of case studies abound. A study of the sociology of a hospital, entitled *The Give and Take in Hospitals,* is one example of the case study approach.[30] Particularly good examples of case studies are anthropological investigations of primitive societies. By definition, these types of studies, anthropological and sociological case studies, must be conducted in uncontrolled settings. In other studies the advantages of the use of natural settings include the following: they are generally less expensive than specialized research settings, they are more factually descriptive of the existing situation, the problem of obtaining cooperation of study subjects is less formidable, and the artificiality of the controlled situation is eliminated, permitting more direct applicability of findings.

However, natural settings do offer certain disadvantages to the researcher. For one, the questions for which answers are being sought may not be easily approached, if at all, through a study conducted in a setting completely uncontrolled by the researcher. If, for example, we are interested in finding out whether certain types of patients receive better care in an intensive nursing unit than in a conventional unit, we will probably have to interfere with the natural situation to some extent, such as moving some patients into the intensive care unit who ordinarily would not be placed there. Moreover, in the evaluation of a new method, procedure, or product, it will be necessary to change existing conditions by introducing it into the natural settings. In addition, uncontrolled settings often pose formidable problems in delimiting the scope of the study. But the major disadvantage of research in natural settings is the great difficulty in establishing causal relationships because of the presence of intervening and disturbing factors.

Partially Controlled Settings

It is probably correct to say that the majority of studies involving human beings as subjects are conducted in settings not totally controlled. In explanatory studies conducted outside a laboratory or test unit the researcher manipulates the environment only partially. Studies in this category are labeled experimental field studies. Thus, in studies of the reactions of people to health education programs the researcher introduces the educational material into the community and observes the effect on behavior—say, the rate at which people go for health examinations. The "unnatural" element is the introduction of the educational program into the community. However, no other aspects of the settings are tampered with; hopefully, they remain the same as before the study.

If this study were conducted in a highly controlled setting, a group of subjects would be placed in a laboratory or a test room, exposed to the educational material, and their responses measured by a written evaluation on a questionnaire.

Finally, if the study were done in a completely uncontrolled setting, it would be necessary to locate an existing community in which the educational program to be studied was already in operation—if such a community could be found. Another community, similar in composition but without the health education program, would serve as a basis for comparison of the rates at which the members of the two communities took health exams.

Of the three approaches the last would be most subject to spurious relationships. In this uncontrolled situation differences in rates of seeking physical exams could well be due to factors other than the presence or absence of the health education program. The second approach, that of a completely controlled setting, could yield meaningful causal relationships, but such relationships may be valid only within the study setting itself and not be applicable to the population at large.

The partially controlled setting is undoubtedly the most satisfactory compromise and can probably yield results that give a more valid evaluation of the health education program. Moreover, findings from the partially controlled study would be applicable to a much wider population than the laboratory experiment. Thus, for many research questions a field experiment can offer the best of two worlds. It can yield data for predictive purposes, and it can apply to large populations. For these reasons field experiments have proven to be a popular approach to the conduct of research.

As a summary of the varieties of settings in which research can be done the following listing provides illustrations of actual studies in patient care conducted in different settings:

Highly Controlled Settings

1. In an experimental unit a study was made of the response to group psychotherapy of psychiatric patients.
2. Observations were made in a special nursery of the weight gain of infants fed different formulas.
3. Detailed records of the life-span of the various strains of laboratory mice have been useful in studies concerned with cancer control.
4. Several hospitals in this country are devoted completely to research. One of these, the Public Health Service's Clinical Center in Bethesda, Maryland, has over 1000 research inpatients.

Partially Controlled Settings

1. One group of nurses making home visits interviewed the patients using tape recorders,

the other group made notes after the visit was over, and the effectiveness of the two systems was later evaluated.

2. Disposable syringes were introduced into clinics. The attitudes of the physicians and nurses toward the syringes were recorded on a questionnaire.

3. The nursing school curriculum was altered to include a course in interpersonal relations given to the junior class. After completing the course the students' ability to talk to patients was evaluated when they took their clinical practice to see if they scored higher than students from schools that did not offer such a course.

4. One unit of the hospital was converted to an "experimental" unit staffed completely by registered nurses. Two weeks after the patients on these units were discharged, they were asked to rate the adequacy of the care they received. Their ratings were compared with ratings by patients who have been assigned to units that were staffed with practical nurses and nursing aides as well as registered nurses.

5. In one group, every patient visiting the maternity clinic was told about the desirability of practicing weight control. In another group, literature on weight control was provided, without oral communication. The third group received the information both orally and through the written material. At time of delivery the weights of the patients in the three groups were recorded and a comparison made of the differences among the groups.

Uncontrolled Settings

1. A study was made of the number of times the patients rang the call bell. It was found that female patients called the nurses 50 percent more often then did male patients.

2. The National Health Survey found that chronic and disabling conditions were prevalent among a high proportion of persons aged 65 years or over.

3. The study showed that during the first year after graduation from a diploma school of nursing 20 percent of the nurses had married. During the same period of time 35 percent of the graduates of a collegiate school had married.

4. The curriculum of the school of nursing for the past seventy-five years was analyzed. It was found that less than a fifth of the course content had not changed over the years.

5. The death records of nearly ten thousand men were reviewed. The occupations of those dying from coronary artery disease were compared with the occupations of those dying from other causes.

RESEARCH SUBJECTS

Just as research settings do vary, so do research subjects. In fact, the variety of possible research subjects is staggering. Research can focus on, for example, humans, animals, plants, or inanimate objects. Research can also be concerned with parts of people, such as the effect of fluoridation on teeth or the condition of feet among older persons, or research with human traits, attributes, or functions, which may be physiological, psychological, sociological, political, economic, and so on.

Some research can have as its study population, not a concrete physical object, human or otherwise, but ideas, theories, or formulations. Mathematical research is an example of such studies.

In the health field the primary subjects of most research studies are human beings. However, only a few studies may be concerned with the whole person. Many are directed toward some selected aspect or trait. Specific traits as subjects are found in the following brief list:

1. A study of private duty nurses who have left the profession

2. A comparison of the personalities of medical and surgical nurses

3. The relationship between myocardial infarctions among older men and the amount of physical exercise they pursue

4. Absenteeism among nursing aides in general hospitals

5. Educational goals of staff-level public health nurses in state health departments

6. Nursing care of mentally retarded children

The delimitation and definition of study subjects are dictated by the purpose and problem of the study. The methods for selecting the individual members to participate in a research study involve such concepts as the universe, sample, randomization, and allocation, to be discussed later.

WHO DOES RESEARCH?

Another way in which research can be classified is in terms of who conducts the research. The doers of research can be classified into several categories. There are the people who work full time on research in organizations devoted almost entirely to research activities. Lazarsfeld calls these organizations research institutes.[31] Several schools of nursing have established their own nursing research institutes.

Others working in an operating organization such as a hospital or public health agency may occasionally engage in research in order to satisfy a specific objective connected with operating responsibilities. Usually such research is conducted to solve some current problem, to make a decision, or to evaluate a procedure or program. Thus, a director of nursing in a hospital may undertake a study of the utilization of personnel because of a heavy work load and insufficient staff.

Between these extremes are a great variety of research doers. In an operating organization such as a hospital, a special research office may be set up with full time staff. An example of this was the Operations Research Division of Johns Hopkins Hospital, established to carry out hospital research.[32] And in the Division of Nursing, U.S. Public Health Service, which has a number of responsibilities besides research, several branches are engaged exclusively in research activities.[33] In addition, professional organizations, such as the National League for Nursing, American Nurses' Association, and American Hospital Association, have components concerned with research.

Another type of research is that found in educational institutions. Faculty members often engage in research on a part-time basis while they maintain teaching responsibilities. Some faculty members pursue research on a full-time basis and are relieved of all teaching responsibilities. Students frequently engage in research as part of their academic requirements. In nursing many excellent studies have been conducted as master's theses and doctoral dissertations.

The closer the researcher is related to an ongoing operating situation, the more likely the research will be applied rather than basic. Conversely, when research is conducted by personnel who are not administratively connected with an operating organization, the research is more likely to be of the basic variety. Moreover, the more separated the researcher is from the work situation, the greater the possibility that the research can yield findings that have applicability beyond the immediate research setting. The less separated the researcher is from the operating situation, the more difficult it becomes to classify his activity as research rather than demonstration, management improvement, methods analysis, or just plain troubleshooting. One of the values in creating specialized settings in which to conduct research is the freedom these settings provide from the day-to-day work environment.[34]

SUBSTITUTES FOR RESEARCH

Among the purposes of research are the following:

1. To obtain new knowledge
2. To solve a stated problem
3. To make a decision
4. To develop a program, procedure, or product
5. To evaluate a program, procedure, or product

Research can achieve these purposes with accuracy and validity by a systematic, planned approach according to established principles of research design. Discussion of these principles forms the basis for much of the material in this book. Research is not a simple, easily accomplished activity but requires great effort, mental as well as physical, and demands considerable time, money, and patience. In view of these difficulties the question can be raised as to whether there are substitutes for the undertaking of formal research that make fewer demands on human and economic resources. It is obvious there are. Every day, millions of decisions are made—in personal affairs, in business activities, in government. Few are based on formalized research. Moreover, in all of areas of life, problems are solved without recourse to formalized research.

The numerous substitutes to research that can yield new knowledge, solve problems, and assist in decision making are:

1. Trial and error
2. Experience
3. Empirical evidence
4. Common sense
5. Faith, custom, precedent, habit

Trial and Error

Much knowledge has been accumulated through the ages by the simple technique of trial and error. Try something, and if it does not work, try something else. Keep trying until the problem is solved. The history of medicine is full of examples of the trial and error approach. Different treatments were used on patients until one was found that worked.

In a sense the method of trial and error is analogous to a poorly controlled experiment that lacks theoretical underpinning. Suppose an administrator is concerned with the rising costs of operating his hospital. He decides to take steps to reduce them. He makes a change in the situation, perhaps not filling vacant positions. This does not have an appreciable effect on costs, so he makes another change: he replaces some of his R.N. positions with aides. This does not appear to reduce costs much either, so he cuts down on the amount of annual leave grated to new personnel, and so on. Finally, the financial statement shows a reduction in the operating costs of the hospital. At this point he stops making changes and is con-

vinced that he has found a solution to his problem.

There are several things wrong with this helter skelter approach. First, he cannot be sure which change, if any, was responsible for the reduction in costs. It probably was not the last change he made, because the effect of all the changes may be cumulative and interactive, and only the combination of changes may have produced the lowered costs. On the other hand, he cannot be sure that some factor he did not control and of which he was unaware was operating while he was making changes. It could well have been this factor that was actually responsible for lowering costs. This outside factor could have been, for example, greater bed utilization during the period of trial and error, which could have resulted in an increase in the hospital's income.

Trial and error often produces an unstable solution with only a short run effect on the problem it is supposed to solve. Moreover, a solution based on a trial and error approach usually has only local applicability, lacking one of the major virtues of a well-designed research study—the generalization of findings. Finally, trial and error suffers from being conducted outside of the framework of theory. Without a theoretical framework as a guide to point out negative consequences that could result from certain actions, solutions to problems obtained by trial and error may not be real solutions at all. In the example just cited, by reducing professional nursing care the administrator may reduce some salary costs, but this saving could be more than offset by a drop in the quality of nursing care provided to patients.

Experience

One of the definitions of a good, experienced administrator is that he be able to solve problems, make decisions, and evaluate programs off the top of his head, so to speak. This may well be true for the majority of situations he is confronted with, which are uncomplicated and straightforward. However, complex problems and decisions may demand considerably more data for their solution than the experiential background of the administrator can provide. As society advances, as knowledge in all fields multiplies, as problems become thornier, the need for research in this area to be conducted outside the rough and tumble atmosphere of the ongoing administrative process becomes greater.

Empirical Evidence

Many problems, many decisions, many needs to develop new programs or procedures, can be met by recourse to existing facts. "How many nurses do I need to staff my obstetrics unit?" is an example of a specific problem question. Study of available empirical data on existing patterns in large numbers of hospitals can serve as a guideline, rough as it is, for the staffing of a specific nursing unit. Research may not be needed for a whole class of problems such as these which can be served adequately by existing data. On the other hand, there is danger in overreliance on using old data to solve current problems. Data representing the average situation in a large population may hide important differences that exist among individual members of the target population. Moreover, data describing an existing situation tell only what was then and not what should be. They are not norms or standards and should not be reagrded as such.

Common Sense

One of the attributes of a "common-sense" approach to problem solving, decision making, or evaluating is that it operates from a heterogeneous and rather superficial collection of facts rather than an orderly and systematic arrangement of knowledge and theories. While the common-sense approach is quite workable in many situations and can serve as a practical substitute for formal research, in other situations—those that are complex and many-faceted—it has the same deficiencies as do trial and error and reliance on existing

empirical data. Foremost among the deficiencies of these methods is their superficiality, which can result in "solutions" that are transitory and insubstantial. Moreover, common-sense knowledge, like that acquired by trial and error, may even turn out to be dangerous. For example, the common-sense "solutions" to the treatment of certain illnesses that medical historians so often describe have sometimes had undesirable consequences to health.

Faith, Tradition, Habit

Decisions are made, programs are launched, procedures and methods are carried out, that primarily depend on what can be called faith, or reliance on custom, habit, or ritualism. To illustrate: for the past fifty years hundreds of hospitals have been built following the design of previously built hospitals, with rigid compartmentalization of patients according to factors such as major category of illness (medical, surgical, etc.) and sex. Studies, such as those concerned with the system of hospital organization known as progressive patient care, have shown that other ways of organizing patients, e.g., according to their nursing care needs, could well prove to be more efficient and economical. How many of the routine nursing procedures, such as TPRs, for example, are ritualistic and serve little purpose?

Reliance on faith, tradition, and routine can perpetuate inefficient performance. An important attribute of research is that it raises pertinent questions about the value of customary ways of doing things.

WHEN IS RESEARCH NEEDED?

There are many substitutes to formal research that can often serve as useful guides to making decisions, solving problems, or developing or evaluating programs, procedures, and methods. However, when the situation becomes too complex the homely devices of trial and error, common sense, empirical evidence, and reliance on past behavior can prove to be inadequate. At this point the need for formal research becomes apparent.

The decision to actually engage in research probably depends on one critical factor—the importance of the problem. Because research usually requires a large expenditure of human and economic resources, the decision to pursue a research study cannot be taken lightly. The importance of the problem must be demonstrated, and, in many cases, can be evaluated in terms of three criteria: the frequency with which the problem arises; the amount of money affected by the existence of problem; and the degree to which human health and safety are influenced by the problem.

In addition, two other criteria are important in deciding to undertake research. These are a genuine interest of a researcher to conduct the research, and the capability of expressing the problem in terms that can be researched.

In the problem of the shortage of nurses all the criteria just mentioned were present. The shortage of nurses was spread throughout the country and nursing fields. Moreover, it can easily be demonstrated that large sums of money were affected by this shortage. The possible harm to human health and safety by not having enough nurses to give adequate nursing care was an important consideration. Finally, many researchers had strong interests in solving the problem, and the problem was researchable.

The extent to which the problem of the shortage of nurses met all the criteria for deciding when to undertake research helps to explain why so many studies were focused on this problem in recent years. However, a problem need not meet all the criteria to show a need for research.

Typology of Research

There are several useful typologies or classifications of research studies that provide guides for nursing researchers. One of the most useful developed by Simmons and Henderson, uses ten categories:[35]

1. *Historical, philosophical, and cultural studies:* movements, trends, themes, or patterns extending over specific periods; history of particular institutions, agencies, organizations; specialized types of nursing to meet particular needs; influence of outstanding individuals on nursing.
2. *Occupational orientation and career dynamics:* needs and resources surveys; employment; economic studies; legal aspects of nursing practice; psychosocial and ethical aspects—protection of human subjects; image of nursing profession.
3. *Specialties in nursing:* by position; clinical specialties; employment.
4. *Nursing organizations and organizations including nursing:* studies of structure, policies, programs, operations, and relationships.
5. *Administration of nursing services in hospitals, clinics, and public health and other agencies:* organizational patterns of authority, responsibility, and communication.
6. *Nursing care:* in homes, schools, industries, health agencies, or institutions; nursing care focused on certain patient states or conditions, and without reference to a particular disease; studies in evaluation of nursing care (e.g., criteria, quality and quantity, continuity of care).
7. *Patient's reactions and adjustments to identifiable variables related to their illnesses:* physical conditions under which the patient acquired or developed the illness; social forces affecting the patient in the community; physical surroundings and equipment within any therapeutic setting; patients' reactions to medical and nursing ministrations.
8. *Interaction patterns:* between nurse, patient, patients' family, other nurses, physicians, and other members of the health team.
9. *Nursing education:* studies of all types of schools and programs.
10. *Conducting research—facilities, personnel, support, and methods:* conferences on nursing research; definitions of nursing research; facilities and tools; history or

development of research; research
methods and types including devices and
techniques.

SUMMARY

The purpose of this chapter was to
provide some idea of what research is—the
purposes of research, the methods for conducting research, the types of research settings, the kinds of subjects upon whom
research is focused, and finally some criteria for determining when research is
needed. In this chapter, research has been
shown to be an activity directed toward
finding answers to questions. More definitively, research can be defined as a planned
and systematic activity directed at the discovery of new facts and/or the identification of relationships among facts.

REFERENCES

1. American Nurses' Association, *Nursing. A Social Policy Statement.* Kansas City, MO, American Nurses' Association, 1980.
2. Florence Nightingale, *Notes on Nursing: What It Is and What It Is Not.* London, Harrison and Sons, 1859.
3. Virginia Henderson, *Basic Principles of Nursing Care.* London, International Council of Nurses, 1961, p. 42.
4. Faye G. Abdellah, *et al., Patient-Centered Approaches to Nursing.* New York, Macmillan Publishing Co., Inc., 1960, pp. 24–25.
5. American Nurses' Association, *op. cit.,* pp. 9–13.
6. Anne P. Griffin, "Philosophy and Nursing." *J. Advanced Nursing,* **5**:261–272, 1980.
7. Fannie M. Rettio, "Ideal Attitudes of a Nurse Researcher." *AORN J.,* **32**:63–65, July 1980.
8. David L. Evans, "Every Nurse as a Researcher: An Argumentative Critique of Principles and Practice of Nursing." *Nursing Forum,* **19**, (4):347, 1980.
9. Margaret L. McClure, "Promoting Practice-Based Research: A Critical Need," in T. Audean Duespohl, *Nursing in Transition.* Rockville, MD., Aspen Systems Corp., 1983, pp. 25–26.
10. Jo Anne Horsley and Joyce Crane, *Using Research To Improve Nursing Practice: A Guide.* New York, Grune & Stratton, Inc., 1983, p. 1.
11. Anne P. Griffin, "A Philosophical Analysis of Caring in Nursing." *J. Advanced Nursing,* **8**(4):289–295, July 1983.
12. Sylvia R. Lelean, "The Implementation of Research Findings into Nursing Practice." *Int. J. Nursing Stud.,* **19**(4):223–230, 1982.
13. Ellen C. Egan *et al.* "Practice-Based Research: Assessing Your Department's Readiness." *J. Nursing Administration,* **11**(10):26–32, October 1981.
14. Elizabeth A. Hefferin *et al.,* "Promoting Research-Based Nursing: The Nurse Administrator's Role," *J. Nursing Administration,* **12**(5): 34–41, May 1982.
15. Fritz J. Roethlisberger and William J. Dickson, *Management and the Worker.* Cambridge, Harvard University Press, 1939.
16. Bernard G. Greenberg, "Conduct of Cooperative Field and Clinical Trials." *Am. Statistician,* **13**:13–17, 28, June 1959.
17. Reuben B. Bowie, "The Nurse Researcher's Roles and Responsibilities." *AORN J.,* **31**(4): 609–611, March 1980.
18. Rosanne Wille, "An Introduction to Nursing Research," *J. of Neurosurg. Nursing,* **13**(5): 265–266, October 1981.
19. Susan R. Gortner, "Nursing Science in Transition." *Nursing Res.,* **29**(3):180–183, May-June 1980.
20. Julia S. Brown *et al.,* "Nursing's Search for Scientific Knowledge." *Nursing Res.,* **33**(1):26–32, January/February, 1984.
21. Julia S. Brown, *op. cit.*
22. Gortner, *op. cit.,* 180–183.
23. Naval Research Advisory Committee, *Basic Research in the Navy* (Volume 1 of a Report to the Secretary of the Navy on Basic Research in the Navy, June 1, 1959), p. 2.
24. Alexander Pope, *Epistle I.* Book 1.
25. Elizabeth Herzog, *Some Guidelines for Evaluative Research.* Childrens Bureau Publication No. 375, 1959. Washington, D.C., U.S. Department of Health, Education, and Welfare, 1959, pp. 15–26.
26. Oscar Kempthorne, *The Design and Analysis of Experiments.* New York, Robert E. Krieger Publishing Co., Inc., 1973.
27. Jo Anne Horsley and Joyce Crane, *Using Research to Improve Nursing Practice: A Guide,* New York, Grune & Stratton, Inc., 1983, pp. 1–2.
28. F. Stuart Chapin, *Experimental Designs in Sociological Research,* Westport, CT, Greenwood Press, Inc., 1974, p. 1.
29. Eugene Levine, "Experimental Design in Nursing Research." *Nursing Res.,* **9**:203–212, fall 1960.
30. Temple Burling, Edith M. Lentz, and Robert N. Wilson, *The Give and Take in Hospitals.* New York, G. P. Putnam's Sons, 1956.
31. Paul F. Lazarsfeld, "The Sociology of Empirical Social Research." *Am. Sociol. Rev.,* **27**:757–767, December 1962.

32. Charles D. Flagle, "Operational Research in the Health Sciences," in L. M. Schuman (ed.)., "Research Methodology and Potential in Community Health and Preventive Medicine." *Ann. NY Acad. Sci.*, **107**:748–759, May 22, 1963.

33. Dorothy G. Sutherland, "Nursing's New Look in the Public Health Service." *Nursing Outlook*, **8**:571–572, 1962.

34. Jack C. Haldeman and Faye G. Abdellah, "Concepts of Progressive Patient Care." *Hospitals*, **33**:38–42, 142–144, May 16, 1959.

35. Leo W. Simmons and Virginia Henderson, *Nursing Research. A Survey and Assessment.* New York, Appleton-Century-Crofts, 1964, pp. 71–81.

PROBLEMS AND SUGGESTIONS FOR FURTHER STUDY

1. Various definitions of research given in this chapter have used the term "facts." What are facts? Are there different types of facts?

2. List ten questions that could serve as the starting point for a research study. Briefly indicate whether each question would initiate basic or applied research. Are the questions as you have stated them researchable?

3. List some of the pros and cons of experimental versus nonexperimental research. Why can nonexperimental studies usually have greater breadth in terms of range of problems studied, number of study subjects included, and so on, than can experimental studies?

4. Can you think of any new procedures or products that should be developed in your area of work? List some of these and indicate briefly how you think a research study could help in the development of these procedures or products.

5. How does trial and error really differ from a research approach? What are some of the dangers in using a trial and error approach in patient care? Can you think of some examples of the use of trial and error in your personal life, your work?

6. Review some recent issues of the nursing and hospital journals (e.g., *Nursing Research*) to see if you can find any examples of reports of research studies. Select three of these, and using the typology of research given in the end of this chapter, indicate into which categories under each major heading the research study you have selected would fall. Did you find any reports of experimental studies conducted in highly controlled settings?

7. Describe the kinds of problems, administrative and otherwise, you might run into if you wanted to undertake the following research studies:
   a. Testing a new way of controlling incontinence in elderly patients.
   b. Designing a new plan to introduce primary care.
   c. Investigating the question: How do DRGs affect quality care?
   d. A study of the quality of nursing care provided in nursing homes
   e. A study of physicians' attitudes toward higher education among nurses
   f. Investigating the causes of drop-outs from a baccalaureate program of nursing education

8. Discuss what is meant by explanation in the use of the term "explanatory" research. What is meant by the statement, if we can explain we can also predict? Is this always true?

9. Give some examples of "common sense" knowledge in nursing. How does common-sense knowledge differ from scientific knowledge? What are the limitations of common-sense knowledge, and what are its advantages?

10. Describe a study of the relationship between nurse staffing and adequacy of patient care that is in a partially controlled setting. A highly controlled setting.

11. Can you conceive of studies involving animals in nursing research? How could the findings of such studies be applied to human beings? What are the advantages of using animals as subjects in research studies?

12. What are the disadvantages of conducting explanatory surveys in completely uncontrolled settings? Can cause and effect relationships be isloated in natural settings or can they be studied only in a laboratory?

13. Give three examples of existing data (e.g., such as the data in *Facts about Nursing* published by the American Nurses' Association), that could be used in solving problems or making decisions in specific nursing situations. A hint: how could the data on nursing salaries in *Facts* be used in a specific situation?

14. Do the criteria for determining when research is needed, given in this chapter, apply to basic research as well as to applied research? Can you think of other criteria that could be used to determine when research is needed?

15. Discuss the kinds of basic research that could be done in your field of interest. In what sense would these projects be considered as basic research?

16. Can you think of examples of research that is being done that could have been stimulated by the frequency with which the problem being studied occurred? Can you think of examples where the research was probably stimulated by the amount of money involved in the problem? By the health and welfare of human beings?

17. Which of the following activities can be defined as research and which cannot? If you do not feel they are research, what kind of activity or process are they (e.g., demonstration, common sense, etc.)?

    a. Analyzing results of public opinion polls
    b. Writing a history of nursing
    c. Conducting a cost analysis of a school of nursing
    d. Developing the architectural plans for a new health center
    e. Administering intelligence tests to a group of applicants for a job
    f. Conducting a census of unemployment in a large city

18. There is a current trend toward the use of the term "evaluation research." What does this term mean? How does it differ from other kinds of research? Examples of evaluation research can be found in Gene V. Glass (ed.), *Evaluation Studies Review Annual,* Vol. I. Beverly Hills, Sage Publications, 1976.

CHAPTER 2

Evolution of Nursing Research

OBJECTIVES

- To understand the "roots" of nursing research

- To identify significant milestone contributions that have furthered nursing research.

Nursing research may be thought to be a systematic, detailed attempt to discover or confirm the facts that relate to a specific problem or problems. It has as its goal the provision of scientific knowledge. The use of the scientific method and a scientific attitude is indicative of progress in research.

NURSING RESEARCH—ITS ROOTS

The tremendous growth and interest in nursing research in the United States are remarkable when one considers that the first organized and continuing effort to do studies of nursing problems on a national basis was in 1949 when the Division of Nursing Resources of the U.S. Public Health Service was established to carry out

research and consultation in nursing.[1]* In spite of Florence Nightingale's pioneering efforts to do research in the health field, professional nurses did not pursue research of nursing practice to any great extent during the quarter century after her death (1910–1935). Nurses have been preoccupied with pressures of hospital expansion, development of health agencies, and increasing demands for nursing services. The nursing profession's organized efforts were toward the improvement of the nurse practitioner and nurse educator and not in the preparation of the nurse scholar nor the nurse investigator in research. The study of

*The Division of Nursing was organized in 1960 and combined the Division of Nursing Resources and the Division of Public Health Nursing. The Division encompasses both intramural and extramural research programs.

nursing practice itself and the study of the art and science underlying the practice of nursing are only beginning to be recognized as "musts" for the profession.

The lack of a formal mechanism by the professional organizations for carrying out research during this period, such as the American Nurses' Foundation, later established in 1955,[2] did not deter individual nurses from carrying out projects of their own in which they sought new knowledge about nursing.

The National League for Nursing has had a notable history in initiating and conducting studies in nursing since 1952. The former National League for Nursing Education through its study unit established in 1930 ". . . developed record forms for basic schools of nursing, a comprehensive record system, a national testing service, a method for collecting and dissemination of basic school data, and established criteria for both a hospital nursing service and schools of nursing."[3]

Since 1912, the then National Organization for Public Health Nursing kept census data about the distribution and preparation of public health nurses by official and nonofficial public health agencies. This was later continued by the United States Public Health Service. Analyzing cost of service and education in public health nursing agencies was one of the first methodological studies to be developed in nursing.

To seek out the roots of nursing research one would need to study the time period spanning the years 1900–1985. The great nurse scholar and historian Mary M. Roberts in her major contribution to the profession, *American Nursing, History and Interpretation,* has depicted a dramatic period in nursing, particularly in nursing research.[4] It is not the purpose of the authors to make an assessment of nursing research during this period, but one cannot discuss current research without looking at some of the major milestones and pioneering efforts in nursing research. Only a few

of these major contributions have been highlighted in the following paragraphs:

KEY POINT

1920   A comprehensive hospital and health survey was carried out by Josephine Goldmark under the direction of Dr. Haven Emerson.[5] This study identified the many inadequacies of housing for student nurses and the paucity of instructional facilities.

1922   The first recorded time study of institutional nursing was released by the New York Academy of Medicine.[6] This was a report of the nursing section's survey of New York hospitals. Significant findings of the survey indicated wide discrepancies in practice such as physicians writing multiple orders for patients beyond a point that they could be carried out effectively by adequate nursing personnel. Likewise, at the time of the study there were fifty two schools of nursing in the New York area for which no evidence could be shown regarding the cost of nursing education and nursing service. During this same year, at an annual meeting of the National League of Nursing Education an initial effort was made to look at the cost of nursing education.[7]

1923   A milestone in nursing education was reached by a comprehensive study of nursing education made by the Committee for the Study of Nursing Education.[8] This was a classic study in nursing research in that it was the first representative study of schools of nursing and public health agencies with firsthand observation of nurses at work as public health nurses, as teachers, and as administrators. Many of the recommendations of this committee are still to be achieved. A major recommendation was that the hospital should be so supported that it is independent of the school for its permanent nursing staff, and the school in turn must be able to maintain an independent education program. This study provided a method for carrying out large-scale representative studies which was subsequently used in carrying out national nursing surveys. The final report, entitled *Nursing and*

Nursing Education in the United States, was published in 1923.

1923   The Yale University School of Nursing, established in 1923, was to grant its first bachelor's degrees to two graduates of the school three years later.[9] University education was thus forging the way to prepare nursing leaders who were scientifically and culturally prepared. Vanderbilt University School of Nursing (1925) and the Western Reserve University School of Nursing (1923), also endowed institutions, were to poineer in many experiments in nursing education. These three programs carried on the pioneering efforts initiated in 1899 when the first step toward university recognition of the nurse's need for higher education was undertaken by Teachers College, Columbia University, and later in 1910 when the University of Minnesota established the first basic school of nursing to become a part of a university system.

1926   The Committee on the Grading of Nursing Schools appointed May Ayres Burgess to direct a monumental study extending over an eight-year period.[10,11] The broad function of the committee was to study ways and means for insuring an ample supply of nursing service at a level essential for the adequate care of the patient. The study encompassed three major projects. The first was directed at the supply and demand for nursing service; the second a job analysis; and the third the grading of nursing schools. The first project was reported in the now classic publication *Nurses, Patients, and Pocketbooks.*[12] The findings are still meaningful today in that in spite of more nurses in practice there are still few qualified to meet the many demands.

1934   The second project of the Committee on the Grading of Nursing Schools was reported in the publication *An Activity Analysis of Nursing.*[13]

The third project, the grading of nursing schools, utilized a survey approach in which each participating school was graded on each item, in relation to all other schools in 1929 and in 1932.[14]

Statistically this project was sound, but the interpretation of the data required a great deal of additional review and study. Consequently, the schools were not classified. This was not to become a realization until 1950 with the establishment of the National Nursing Accrediting Service.

1935   ANA first published *Some Facts About Nursing: A Handbook for Speakers and Others,* which contained yearly compilations of statistical data about registered nurses.

1938   Economic security was under scrutiny by the American Nurses' Association, which conducted a study of incomes, salaries, and employment conditions of nurses (exclusive of public health nurses).

1940   A major breakthrough in providing basic information about the cost of nursing service and nursing education was made by Pfefferkorn and Rovetta.[15] An earlier study by the Committee on the Costs of Medical Care provided a series of factual reports on the overall costs of medical care, including nursing service.[16]

1941   The United States Public Health Service conducted a national census of nursing resources in cooperation with state nurses' associations.

1943   The National Organization of Public Health Nursing made a survey of needs and resources for home care in sixteen communities. This was reported in *Public Health Nursing Care of the Sick.*

1948   The Brown report, scholarly and objective, brought to a focal point many of the issues facing nursing education and nursing services for the past half century.[17] The recommendations put forth in this report spearheaded many of the research studies that were to be carried out in the next ten years. Studies of inservice education, nursing functions, nursing teams, practical nurses, role and attitude studies, the nurse technician, nurse-patient relationships, hospital environment, economic security, are examples of the studies that were to find their roots in the recommendations of the Brown report.

Nursing Schools at Mid-Century, a report of the National Committee for the Improvement of Nursing Services, was a direct effort on the part of the committee to implement some of the recommendations of the Brown report.[18] An Interim Classification of schools of Nursing Offering Basic Progams (1949) was prepared, which classified the schools in Class I, II, III, according to criteria for judging a good school. *Nursing Schools at Mid-Century* provided a factual report of the basic nursing schools. The National Nursing Accrediting Service (1950) under Dr. Helen Nahm's able direction was to take on the major task of establishing a sound system for accrediting schools of nursing.

1948   The Division of Nursing Resources (now the Division of Nursing), U.S. Public Health Service, pioneered in carrying out statewide surveys and developing manuals and tools for nursing research.[19]

1949   ANA conducted its first national inventory of Professional Registered Nurses in the United States and the territories of Alaska, Hawaii, and Puerto Rico.

1952   The professional organization's first official journal for the reporting of studies related to nursing and health research was published in June 1952. The journal was named *Nursing Research* and pioneered in reporting studies to furthering nursing research. One of its main functions was to provide a means for the investigator to communicate ongoing research.

1953   Under the leadership of a social anthropologist, Dr. Leo Simmons, and a renowned expert nurse teacher and practitioner, Virginia Henderson, a survey and assessment of nursing research was initiated by the National Committee for the Improvement of Nursing Serivces, under the auspices of Yale University. A major purpose of the Yale survey was to find, classify, and evaluate the research in nursing during the past decade.[20]

The establishment of the Institute of Research and Service in Nursing Education, Teachers College, Columbia University, under the able leadership of its first director, Dr. Helen Bunge, marked another major milestone for nursing research. This was the first formalized mechanism within a university to carry out nursing research. The institute had three main purposes, aimed at strengthening and improving education for nursing through research by: (1) conducting research on selected problems in nursing and nursing education; (2) disseminating the results of the research undertaken by the institute; and (3) assisting in the preparation of nurses for the conduct of research in nursing.

1954   ANA Committee on Research and Studies established to plan, promote, and guide research and studies relating to the functions of the Association. It existed for sixteen years and published the *ANA Blueprint for Research in Nursing* (1962), and *The Nurse in Research: ANA Guidelines in Ethical Values* (1968).

1955   The American Nurses' Foundation, a center for research, supported mainly by the American Nurses' Association was established. It serves as a receiver and administrator of funds and as a donor of grants for research in nursing. The foundation also conducts its own programs of research in nursing and provides its own consultation services to nursing students, research facilities, and other engaged in nursing research.[21]

Studies sponsored by the American Nurses' Foundation and the American Nurses' Association (1950-1957) appeared in *Twenty Thousand Nurses Tell Their Story.*[22] This, too, was a milestone for nursing research in reporting thirty four studies in such areas as nursing functions, job satisfaction, role, and attitude. Several of the recommendations of the Brown report (1948) were achieved by the completion and reporting of these studies.

In 1961, ANF assumed the responsibility for an Abstracting Service, and from 1962 to 1974 the service was a part of the Foundation's program. Susan D. Taylor developed the system and made use of volunteer abstractors. The abstracts were designed to make information about the results of research readily available.

1955 The Nursing Research Grants and Fellowship Programs of the Division of Nursing of the U.S. Public Health Service were established to stimulate and provide financial support for research investigators and research training in nursing. The PHS act authorizing the extramural grant and award programs provides that the Surgeon General of the PHS shall encourage and render assistance to appropriate public authorities, scientific institutions, and scientists in the conduct and coordination of research related to the cause, diagnosis, treatment, control, and prevention of physical and mental diseases.[23]

1957 Nursing research gained still greater impetus by the establishment of the Department of Nursing in the Walter Reed Army Institute of Research. The institute supported a program of military nursing research projects that were patient care oriented, and implemented a program to develop a small core of competent nurse practitioner-researchers.[24]

1957 The Western Interstate Commission for Higher Education (WICHE) sponsored the Western Council on Higher Education for Nursing (WCHEN) with Faye G. Abdellah as the first consulting director and Jo Eleanor Elliott who became its permanent director in July 1957. The Council was established to improve the quality of higher education for nursing in the West with an early focus on the preparation of nurses for research, the development of new scientific knowledge, and the communication of research findings. Since 1968 WCHEN sponsored several research conferences. The Southern Regional Education Board (SREB) and the New England Board of Higher Education (NEBHE) were regional counterparts to WICHE.[25] Midwest Alliance in Nursing (MAIN) and the Mid-Atlantic Regional Nurses Association (MARNA) are the most recent regional compact groups to be formed.

1959 NLN Research and Studies Department created (name changed to Division of Research). Examples of functions include conducting research studies, providing consultations to NLN staff, and maintaining information about NLN research projects. Publications include *NLN Nurse Career Pattern Study (1975)*, and *The Open Curriculum Study* (1974, 1975, 1976).

1959 Abstracts of Studies in Public Health Nursing, 1924-1957 by Hortense Hilbert published in *Nursing Research,* 1959.

1963 The Surgeon General's Consultant Group on Nursing issued a report on its study of the nursing situation in the United States. Among its many findings and recommendations the group found that "the potential contributions of nursing research to better patient care are so impressive that universities, hospitals, and other health agencies should receive all possible encouragement to conduct appropriate studies." (p. 53).[26] The group recommended a substantial increase in federal government support for research in nursing and for the training of researchers.

Nursing Studies Index, Volume IV, 1957-1959, by Virginia Henderson, completed. The remaining three volumes have been published. The Index provides a valuable guide to the analytical and historical aspects of the literature on nursing published in English from 1900 to 1959.[27] Volume I, 1900-1929 (published 1972); Volume II, 1930- 1949 (published 1970); Volume III, 1950- 1956 (published 1966).

1964 *Nursing Research, A Survey and Assessment,* was completed by Leo W. Simmons and Virginia Henderson. It provides a review and assessment of research in the areas of occupational orientation, or career dynamics, and nursing care.[28]

1965 ANA Nursing Research Conferences (1965-1973) were sponsored by the U.S. Public Health Service. The first of nine conferences was held in New York. These conferences provided a forum for critiquing nursing research and for providing opportunities for nurse researchers to examine critical issues.

1966   *International Nursing Index* established. Lucille E. Notter was its first editor.

1970   ANA Commission on Nursing Research officially formed. The Commission was the first to prepare position papers on human rights in research and participated in the dissemination of research. Papers of the Commission included *Human Rights Guidelines for Nurses in Clinical and Other Research* (1974), *Research in Nursing: Toward A Science of Health Care* (1976), *Preparation of Nurses for Participation in Research* (1976), and *Priorities for Nursing Research* (1976).

1970   *An Abstract for Action* by Jerome P. Lysaught. The purpose of this report was to identify recommendations for change in nursing in terms of increased research into practice, improved educational systems, clarification of roles and practice, and increased financial support for nurses and nursing.[29]

1970   *Overview of Nursing Research 1955-1968* by Faye G. Abdellah. A comprehensive overview of nursing research projects supported in part by the Department of Health, Education, and Welfare to provide a "state of the art" assessment of nursing research, the knowledge available, and the gaps and needed research.[30]

1971   ANA Council of Nurse Researchers established by the ANA Commission on Nursing Research. The Council was formed to advance research activities, provide for the exchange of ideas, and recognize excellence in research. The Council published *Issues in Research: Social, Professional, and Methodological* (1973).

1971   *Extending the Scope of Nursing Practice.* A report of the Secretary's Committee to study Extended Roles for Nurses. A position paper of the health professions supporting the expansion of the functions and responsibilities of the nurse practitioner.[31]

1973   The American Academy of Nursing established under the aegis of the Ameri-

can Nurses' Association with thirty six charter fellows. The purposes of the Academy are to advance new concepts in nursing and health care; to identify and explore issues in health, in the profession, and in society as they affect and are affected by nurses and nursing; examine the dynamics within nursing; and identify and propose resolutions to issues and problems confronting nursing and health, including alternative plans for implementation.

1977   *Nursing Research* celebrates twenty-fifth anniversary year. Dr. Helen L. Bunge, first volunteer editor, helped *Nursing Research* grow as a scientific periodical. Hortense Hilbert and Barbara Tate served as part-time editors until Lucille E. Notter became the first full-time editor in 1961. *Nursing Research* became the first nursing journal to be included in MEDLINE, the computerized information retrieval service.

1977   "An Overview of Nursing Research in the United States" by Susan R. Gortner and Helen Nahm. Provides a historical perspective of the development of nursing research in education, practice, and traced research resources.[32]

1977   "U.S. Public Health Service's Contribution to Nursing Research—Past, Present, Future" by Faye G. Abdellah traces the role of the PHS in the development of nursing research.[33]

1979   "Defining the Clinical Content of Nursing" by S. Donalsond, in *Proceedings of the Forum on Doctoral Education in Nursing*. San Francisco, University of California at San Francisco.

1979   *Healthy People.* The Surgeon General's resort on health promotion and disease prevention. DHEW, PHS Publication No. 79-55071. Washington, D.C., U.S. Government Printing Office.

1980   *Promoting Health Preventing Disease: Objectives for the Nation.* DHHS, PHS. Washington, D.C., U.S. Government Printing Office.

1980   American Nurses' Association publishes *A Social Policy Statement.* The profession defined the nature and scope of nursing practice and characteristics of specialization in nursing. This statement is a fundamental delineation that provides a foundation that promotes unity in nursing in a basic and common approach to practice.[34]

1981 Department of Health and Human Services publishes *Report of Graduate Medical Education National Advisory Committee* (GMENAC). A report to the Secretary, DHHS with recommendations to achieve a balance between supply and requirements of physicians in the 1990s and nonphysician health care providers.[35]

1981 American Hospital Association publishes *Report and Recommendations of National Commission on Nursing.* A multidisciplinary effort to address current nursing-related problems in the U.S. health care system and to develop and implement action plans for the future.[36]

1981 DHHS, *Strategies for Promoting Health for Specific Populations.* DHHS, PHS. Washington, D.C., U.S. Government Printing Office.

1982 *Hospital Prospective Payment for Medicare*—Report to the Congress by Richard S. Schweiker. DHHS, Washington, D.C. Major changes in which services are provided and reimbursed.

1983 The 1981 *White House Conference on Aging: Executive Summary of Technical Committee on Health Maintenance and Health Promotion.* Washington, D.C., U.S. Government Printing Office. Also published in 1983: *Report of the Mini Conference on Long-Term Care; Report of the Technical Committee on Health Services.*

1983 Institute of Medicine, NAS, *Nursing and Nursing Education: Public Policies and Private Actions.* Particular reference is made to appendix 8, which provides definition and directions of nursing research.[37]

1983 American Academy of Nursing, *Magnet Hospitals. Attraction and Retention of Professional Nurses.* Report of Task Force on Nursing Practice in Hospitals.[38]

1983 Legislation passed to establish new reimbursement policies for hospitals

based on prospective payment using a system of diagnostis related groups (DRGs) to determine flat amount paid for each Medicare patient discharged.[39]

1984 American Nurses' Association establishes ANA Council on Computer Applications in Nursing to focus on computer technology pertinent to nursing practice, education, administration, and research.

1984 House and Senate of Ninety-Eighth Congress passed legislation to establish a National Institute of Nursing to conduct and support basic and clinical research, training, and related programs in nursing. The Institute would focus on the study and investigation of the prevention of disease, health promotion, and the nursing care of individuals with, and the families of individuals with, acute and chronic illnesses. The Institute was also intended to provide a focal point for promoting the growth and quality of nursing research.[40]

President Reagan vetoed legislation creating the new Institute (October 30, 1984) because it was too expensive.[41]

1984 American Nurses' Association, Cabinet on Nursing Research. *Directions for Nursing Research: Toward the Twenty-First Century.*[42]

1985 A new Center for Nursing Research was established in the U.S. Public Health Service on January 14, 1985. The Center's programs will be designed to enlarge the body of scientific knowledge that underlies nursing practice, nursing services administration, and nursing education. The Center provides national leadership for both nursing research and development of nurse scientists and ensures close coordination between research and other federal programs in nursing education and practice. The Center is located in the Division of Nursing, Bureau of Health Professions, Health Resources and Services Administration. The National Advisory Council on Nurse Training will provide overall policy direction for the center's activities and make recommendations to the secretary regarding support of projects.

1985 On November 21, 1985 congress overrode a Presidential veto and established a National Center of Nursing Research at NIH to conduct, support, and disseminate information respective to basic and clinical nursing research, training and other programs in patient care research.

NURSING RESEARCH—ITS FUTURE

We believe that nursing is a service to individuals and to families, therefore to society. It is based upon an art and science that mold the attitudes, intellectual competencies, and technical skills of the individual nurse into the desire and ability to help people, sick or well, cope with their health needs.

The primary task of nursing research is the development and refinement of nursing theories which serve as guides to nursing practice and which can be organized into a body of scientific nursing knowledge. A concomitant task of nursing research is the discovery and development of valid means of measuring the extent to which nursing action attains its goal—these to be stated in terms of patient behavior.[43]

The purpose of this book is to provide a framework from which nursing research can develop, one which places the ultimate test of the significance of the research on the patient/client.

REFERENCES

1. E. M. Vreeland, "The Nursing Research Grant and Fellowship Program in the Public Health Service." *Am. J. Nursing,* 58:1700–1702, December 1958. See also "Nursing Research Programs of the Public Health Service." *Nursing Res.,* 13:148–158, spring 1964.
2. The American Nurses' Foundation, "Research—Pathway to Future Progress in Nursing Care." *Nursing Res.,* 9:4–7, winter 1960.
3. National League for Nursing, Research and Studies Service, "The National League for Nursing—Its Role in Nursing Research." *Nursing Res.,* 9:190–195, fall 1960.
4. Mary M. Roberts, *American Nursing, History and Interpretation.* New York, Macmillan Publishing Co., Inc., 1954.
5. Haven Emerson and Josephine Goldmark, *Cleveland Hospital and Health Survey,* "Nursing," Part IX. Cleveland. Cleveland Hospital Council, 1920.
6. E. H. Lewinski-Corwin, "The Hospital Nursing Situation." *Am. J. Nursing,* 22:603, 1922.
7. "Sub-Committee Report on the Cost of Nursing Education." Twenty-Eighth Annual Report of the National League of Nursing Education, 1922, p. 93.
8. *Nursing and Nursing Education in the United States.* Report of the Committee for the Study of Nursing Education and a Report of a Survey, by Josephine Goldmark. New York, Macmillan Publishing Co., Inc., 1923.
9. Annie W. Goodrich, *The Social and Ethical Significance of Nursing.* "A Description of the Yale University School of Nursing." New York, Macmillan Publishing Co., Inc., 1923.
10. May Ayres Burgess, *A Five-Year Program for the Committee on the Grading of Nursing Schools.* Committee on the Grading of Nursing Schools, New York, 1926.
11. *Nursing Schools Today and Tomorrow.* Final Report of the Committee on Grading of Nursing Schools, New York, 1934.
12. May Ayres Burgess, *Nursing, Patients, and Pocketbooks.* Report of a Study of the Economics of Nursing conducted by the Committee on the Grading of Nursing Schools, New York, 1928.
13. Ethel Johns and Blanche Pfefferkorn, *An Activity Analysis of Nursing.* Committee on the Grading of Nursing Schools, New York, 1934.
14. S. P. Capen, "A Member of the Grading Committee Speaks." *Am. J. Nursing,* 32:307–311, 1932.
15. Blanche Pfefferkorn and Charles A. Rovetta, *Administrative Cost Analysis for Nursing Service and Nursing Education.* New York, National League for Nursing Education, 1940.
16. *Medical Care for the American People.* Final Report, No. 28 of the Publications of the Committee on the Costs of Medical Care. Chicago, University of Chicago Press, 1932.
17. Esther Lucile Brown, *Nursing for the Future.* A report prepared for the National Nursing Council. New York, Russell Sage Foundation, 1948.
18. Margaret West and Christy Hawkins, *Nursing Schools at Mid-Century.* A report of the Subcommittee on School Data Analysis for National Committee for the Improvement of Nursing Services. New York, National League for Nursing, 1950.
19. Faye G. Abdellah, "State Nursing Surveys and Community Action." *Pub. Health Rep.,* 67:554–560, 1952.
20. Virginia Henderson (editorial), "Research in

Nursing Practice—When?" *Nursing Res.,* **4**:99, February 1956.

21. American Nurses' Foundation, Inc., *The First Three Years.* New York, American Nurses' Foundation, Inc., 1958.

22. Everett C. Hughes, Helen Hughes, and Irwin Deutscher, *Twenty Thousand Nurses Tell Their Story.* Philadelphia, J.B. Lippincott Co., 1958.

23. E.M. Vreeland, *op. cit.*

24. Harriet Werley, "Promoting the Research Dimension in the Practice of Nursing Through the Establishment and Development of a Department of Nursing in an Institue of Research." *Military Med.,* **127**:219–231, March 1962.

25. Jo E. Elliott, *Communicating Nursing Research 1967–1974.* (Final Report, USPHS Research Grant No. NU-00289.) Boulder, CO, Western Interstate Commission for Higher Education, 1974.

26. *Toward Quality in Nursing: Needs and Goals.* Report of the Surgeon General's Consultant Group on Nursing. U.S. Public Health Service Publication No. 992, Washington, Government Printing Office, February 1963.

27. Virginia Henderson, *Nursing Studies Index,* Vol. IV, 1957–1959. Philadelphia, J. B. Lippincott Co., 1963.

28. Leo W. Simmons and Virginia Henderson, *Nursing Research: A Survey and Assessment.* New York, Appleton-Century-Crofts, 1964.

29. Jerome P. Lysaught, *An Abstract for Action.* New York, McGraw-Hill Book Co., 1970; *An Abstract for Action: Appendices,* 1971.

30. Faye G. Abdellah, "Overview of Nursing Research." *Nursing Res.,* Part I, **19**:6–17, January–February 1970; Part II, **19**:151–162, March–April 1970; Part III, **19**:239–252, May–June 1970.

31. Department of Health, Education, and Welfare, *Extending the Scope of Nursing Practice.* A Report of the Secretary's Committee to Study Extended Roles for Nurses. Washington, D.C., Government Printing Office, November 1971.

32. Susan R. Gortner and Helen Nahm, "An Overview of Nursing Research in the United States." *Nursing Res.,* **26**:1:10–33, January–February 1977.

33. Faye G. Abdellah, "U.S. Public Health Service's Contribution to Nursing Research—Past, Present, Future." *Nursing Res.,* **26**:244–249, July–August 1977.

34. American Nurses' Association, *Nursing. A Social Policy Statement.* Kansas City, MO, American Nurses' Association, 1980.

35. DHHS, *Summary Report of the Graduate Medical Education National Advisory Committee to the Secretary, Department of Health and Human Services.* Sept. 30, 1980. Washington, D.C., U.S. Government Printing Office, DHHS Publication No. (HRA) 81-651, April 1981.

36. The Hospital Research and Educational Trust, *National Commission on Nursing. Initial Report and Preliminary Recommendations.* Chicago, The Hospital Research and Educational Trust, 1981.

37. Institute of Medicine (Division of Health Care Services). *Nursing and Nursing Education: Public Policies and Private Actions,* Washington, D.C., 1983.

38. American Academy of Nursing (Task Force on Nursing Practice in Hospitals), *Magnet Hospitals. Attraction and Retention of Professional Nurses.* Kansas City, MO, American Nurses' Association, 1983.

39. Eugene Levine and Faye G. Abdellah, "DRGs: A Recent Refinement to an Old Method." *Inquiry,* **21**:105–112, summer 1984.

40. American Nurses' Association, "Capitol Update." **2**:9, October 1984.

41. Margaret Shapiro, "Reagan Signs Trade Measure, Vetoes Bill for Youth Jobs." *The Washington Post,* October 30, 1984.

42. American Nurses' Association, Cabinet on Nursing Research, *Directions for Nursing Research: Toward the Twenty-First Century.* Kansas City, MO, ANA, 1984.

43. Rozella M. Schlotfeldt, Reflections on Nursing Research. *Am. J. Nursing,* **60**:492–494, April 1960, p. 494.

PROBLEMS AND SUGGESTIONS FOR FURTHER STUDY

1. Review the life of Florence Nightingale, and cite specific incidents in which she undertook pioneering efforts to do research in the health field.

2. What were some of the studies developed by the former National League for Nursing Education? Select one of these studies, and show what influence it had in our present-day approach to problems.

3. Describe the first recorded time study of institutional nursing conducted in 1922. What methods used in this study would be useful in present-day studies of what nurses do with their time?

4. Compare the organizational structure of the following and describe the goals of each:
   Division of Nursing, U. S. Public Health Service
   Institute of Research and Service in Nursing Education, Teachers College, Columbia University
   The American Nurses' Foundation
   The Walter Reed Army Institute of Research

Division of Public Policy and Research, National League for Nursing

5. Evaluate the comment that prior to 1950 most of the research studies in nursing were directed toward nursing education rather than nursing service.
6. Discuss the various ways in which nurses have participated in research activities.
7. Read Ellwynne M. Vreeland's article, "Nursing Research Programs of the Public Health Service" (*Nursing Res.*, 13:148–158, spring 1964), and parallel significant developments in nursing with those events important to the development of nursing research.

8. Considering the concern with the rising costs of health care, discuss the ways in which nursing research could be helpful in containing these costs. For suggestions see, Franklin A. Shaffer, ed., *Costing Out Nursing: Pricing Our Product.* New York, NLN, 1985.
9. Read Rozella M. Schlotfeldt's article "Nursing Research: Reflection of Values" (*Nursing Res.*, 26:4–9, January–February 1977). Discuss the author's conclusion that commitment to research is a key prediction of nursing's fulfillment of its potential.

3

Nursing Science and the Research Process

THE NEED FOR RESEARCH IN NURSING

The turbulence found in nursing research today is the result of the ever-increasing number and sophistication of medical and technological advances becoming available to general practice. But other significant factors have an impact on the nursing profession and, perhaps more than anything else, focus the need for research on nursing practice.

Many medical and nursing leaders believe that there is a thirty-year gap between existing knowledge directly affecting nursing and its application. This gap exists in both nursing education and nursing service. Much research is needed to test this fairly ancient knowledge to see if it is still valid in light of emerging concepts affecting patient care. Let us examine these concepts and

view them in terms of needed research that should be undertaken or subjected further to scientific inquiry. Attention should be given to these emerging concepts lest nursing fail to find a justifiable role among the health professions.

The Patient as a Person

No single concept has greater significance for nursing research than that of appreciating the patient as a person. The social sciences challenge our ritualistic preoccupation with the merely physical care of the patient. If the latter focused upon the basic health needs of patients such as hygienic care, maintaining nutritional needs of patients, elimination, this form of preoccupation might be viewed as essential nursing care. But as we are well aware, meeting the basic health needs of patients

KEY POINT

has long since been delegated to the non-professional worker. Today, nursing's preoccupation is with the technical aspects of nursing care, the highest status symbols being attributed to those tasks formerly carried out by the physician such as administering intravenous solutions. What then is the nurse's role?

As the professional student becomes more proficient in the technical aspects of nursing, she builds an ever-increasing gap between herself as caregiver and her patients. Machines may precisely record certain physical measurements, but in the ordinary course of events instruments cannot replace skilled and knowledgeable observation, interpretation, and judgment. A human eye, hand, and mind are required to catch the clues, both physical and psychological, that make the nursing determinations necessary for the patient's welfare. Few patients spend much time hooked up to the array of electronic equipment available. The major responsibility for the patient's day-to-day welfare still rests with the nurse, and this idea must not be submerged in the vast sea of electronic and other technological devices. The concept of "patient as a person" must remain in the forefront of nursing consciousness, lest the very purpose and end of nursing philosophy be lost.

The responsibilities of the nurse practitioner are similar to those of the clinical nurse specialist and differ only in degree and depth. In general, nurse practitioners assess patients'/clients' needs; carry out patient care, including the use of specialized equipment for monitoring or therapeutic purposes; make decisions for carrying out appropriate nurse actions; assist in the development of patient care plans; and initiate preventive measures to protect the patient from complications.[2]

Patients' Common Medical and Nursing Needs

The concept of common medical and nursing needs as related to patient care challenges several ritualistic patterns in nursing service and nursing education.[3] If patients have recognizable common medical and nursing needs, segregation by diagnosis, sex, and age becomes unrealistic.

It has been demonstrated that it costs a hospital much more a year to staff each bed by the traditional pattern than by grouping patients by their common medical and nursing needs.[4] The saving is based upon better utilization of medical and nursing personnel, a significant factor in a period when many feel we are faced with nurse shortages which may well be the result of poor utilization of available skills rather than an actual numerical shortage.

Identifying of patients' needs and then grouping these patients by their common medical and nursing needs is the heart of the now widely accepted Progressive Patient Care program.[5] If one accepts this concept as it is related to nursing education and nursing service, ritualistic systems in both education and service need to be studied to determine which are useful and which are not.

Liberalization of Nursing Education

The work of Russell[6] has pointed out that "... professional practice today calls for individuals who have a wide range of knowledge, keen intellect, and clarity of vision concerning human values." This demands that the nursing curriculum include a major portion, possibly two years, of study in the humanities: history, philosophy, and political science. The objective is to help the student develop a strong desire for continual self-education long after she has graduated. Much study and research need to be undertaken to develop a common core curriculum that provides a generic base for all the health professions.

TECHNOLOGICAL INNOVATIONS IN NURSING EDUCATION

The development of microcomputers and the interactive videodisk has transformed   **KEY POINT** the concept of computer-aided learning and provided the nurse educator with unprecedented capabilities for interactive and visual presentation of educational material. The door is open for new educational designs and new theoretical approaches to the process of education. The new technology will be used to implement problem-based patient-related learning strategies in all phases of nursing education. (See Virginia Saba and Kathleen McCormick, *Essentials of Computers in Nursing,* Lippincott, 1986, for suggested strategies.[7])

Nursing as a Science

This is one of the most controversial concepts today, centering around the interpretation of the profession of nursing as a practice and/or a science. In its development thus far as a profession, nursing is more easily defined as a practice rather than as a science. However, the fact that the latter is unclear does not mean that a nursing science does not exist. Many nursing leaders feel that a nursing science will emerge.[8] This can be furthered by a series of studies that can test the physiological and anatomical basis of nursing practices.

Self-Care as a Form of Extending the Patient's Therapy

A broader concept of patient care has emerged.

> The nurse today must teach patients to care for themselves. She must assume greater responsibility in the whole process of therapy. She must divide her responsibilities with other hospital workers and cooperate with other specialties in the health field. These changed responsibilities require the nurse practitioner to have a deep knowledge of people and to possess keen judgment, in addition to having a grasp of the basic sciences that underlie health.[9]

The self-care unit is a part of a "P.P.C." program and provides an opportunity for the professional nurse to teach patients to care for themselves by learning to take their own medications, simple treatments, and when indicated to prepare a special diet. Self-care thus provides a way of extending the physician's therapy for the patient while he is still under hospital supervision.

Research needs to be undertaken to find out how this concept can be applied and how nursing personnel and professional nursing students can make full utilization of this area.

The Hospital as a Community Health Center

This concept is placed last as it is a long-range goal to be achieved. The professional nurse who functions within a community health center will use all of her professional skills. In such an environment, the hospital is only one element. Community health agencies, nursing homes, and other long-term facilities are also part of the health center.

The nurse's competencies must extend beyond the hospital walls. She must be as concerned about the chronically ill patient in the community as she is about the acutely ill in the hospital. To function in a community health center environment demands full knowledge of total health needs of patients as well as the resources within the community. Identification or diagnosis of the patients' total needs in either setting becomes paramount.

These concepts have been presented to point up much needed research to be undertaken to help the professional nurse better understand her changing role as a member of the health team and the changing environment in which she must function.

The Clinical Nurse as Researcher

An ideal goal is for clinical nurses to accept research as an integral part of their professional role. However, how does one get started? The clinical nurse must first evaluate her own research skills and availability of time to conduct research. Serving as a research subject is an excellent way of learning about the skills and time required. Such an experience can help one understand the nature of the procedure to be followed and the importance of adhering to essential procedures and responding to directions and provide opportunities to observe investigators in carrying out their methodologies.

Another approach is for the clinical nurse to provide supportive care to the subject(s) being studied. This requires learning about the study being conducted so that patient needs can be anticipated and learning any variations in procedures that must be taught. The clinical nurse can become much more knowledgeable and comfortable in the research role by assuming and experiencing a variety of roles.[10]

Initiating a Research Program

Initiating a research program in a hospital or community setting requires thoughtful planning and a commitment of resources and time. Each setting to be used needs to meet three crucial tests: The attitude of the administrator toward research must be positive; there must be an environment that is conducive to the use and acceptance of research findings; and the values of the administrative and nursing departments must be in harmony. It is also helpful to enlist the support of the dean of the college of nursing. Such support could be financial support of a portion of the project or the assignment of staff to the project.

In some settings, particularly one that is university affiliated, it is desirable to consider establishing a research section that might later become a nursing research center. The goals of such a section should be clearly identified, e.g.:

- To investigate factors basic to the delivery of quality of nursing care to provide data essential for administrative decisions.
- To investigate clinical questions and problems confronting patients and nursing staff to provide data on which to base patient outcome measures.
- To provide for staff involvement in the investigation of clinical problems.
- To evaluate the effectiveness of clinical management and staff development programs.

- To promote the utilization of research findings to improve nursing practice.[11]

Collaborative Research

The health problems patients/clients encounter are usually complex requiring a collaborative effort in dealing with the multiple problems. Two collaborative research models have gained wide acceptance. One is a university-based research model in which research is initiated and designed by faculty and students, conducted in laboratories or health care agencies and reported in research journals. The other is the agency-based model, which might involve hiring a researcher to conduct studies and affords an opportunity for clinical nurses to be actively involved in the research. The limiting feature of this model is that the findings are applicable to that agency and cannot be generalized to other settings.

An innovative approach developed by the staff of the CURN project (Conduct and Utilization of Research in Nursing) combines the benefits of both models. The collaborative research development model is one in which university-based researchers and agency-based clinicians, as equal contributors, collaborate at each stage of the research process and have common research goals.[12] The collaborative research model can be an effective approach in producing more practical and relevant clinical nursing research that practicing nurses can use to improve patient care.

UTILIZATION OF RESEARCH FINDINGS

For three decades the primary concern of nursing research focused on the effort to get it carried on in the first place. It is therefore vitally important to assure that valid and reliable research question are raised:

1. Are relevant nursing research findings available?
2. Do the findings provide useful changes in nursing practice?

3. Will the findings be used by nurse practitioners?

The CURN project found only ten areas in which sufficient research information was available to provide valid and reliable indicators for practice. Therefore, many areas of nursing practice remain available for serious investigation.

Once research findings are determined, it is important to consider replicating the findings with different populations and in different settings.[13] The nurse researcher early on has the responsibility to publish methodologies and instruments with sufficient information to permit other researchers to replicate the research. However, not all research should be replicated. Stetler and Marram provide a useful model with which to evaluate the usefulness of research findings and help one decide whether a study should be replicated. The model has three phases: validation, comparative evaluation, and decision making. In addition, one needs to ask the following questions:

- How similiar is your clinical setting and population to the study's setting and population?
- Is there sufficient evidence to support the conclusions?
- Has the researcher provided a conceptual framework?
- Are the study's recommendations feasible and applicable to your practice setting?[14]

STRATEGIES FOR ADVANCING NURSING RESEARCH BY THE YEAR 2000

The Cabinet on Nursing Research of the American Nurses' Association has proposed several directions and strategies for advancing nursing research by the year 2000.[15] It is an accepted principle that nursing focuses on the entire spectrum of human responses to actual and potential health problems across the life-span. Nurse researchers are viewed as emphasizing the study of whole human beings in interaction with their environment. Thus, human biology, the environment, and behavior interact one with the other. Placed within the context of nursing research, knowledge is generated about health and health promotion in individuals and families and about the influence of social and physical environments on health.[16]

What kinds of new knowledge need to be generated?

Prevention Research

Prevention research includes that research designed to yield results directly applicable to interventions to prevent occurrence of disease or disability, or the progression of detectable but asymptomatic disease.

Preintervention
- Identification of risk factors for disease or disability
- Development of methods for identification of disease controllable in the asymptomatic stage
- Refinement of methodological and statistical procedures for quantitatively assessing risk and measuring the effects of preventive interventions

Intervention
- Development of biological interventions to prevent occurrence of disease or disability, or progression of asymptomatic disease
- Development of environmental interventions to prevent occurrence of disease or disability, or progression of asymptomatic disease
- Development of behavioral interventions to prevent occurrence of disease or disability, or progression of asymptomatic disease
- Conduct of clinical and community trials and demonstrations to assess preventive interventions and to encourage their adoption

Some interventions may be applicable to primary prevention as well as to disease treatment (e.g., diet and exercise as components of rehabilitation for coronary heart disease). Research into such interventions is considered prevention research.

Prevention-Relevant Research

More broadly defined, prevention research also includes that research which

KEY POINT

KEY POINT

has a high probability of yielding results that will likely be applicable to disease prevention. Included are studies aimed at elucidating the chain of causation—the etiology and mechanisms—of acute and chronic diseases. Such basic research efforts generate the fundamental knowledge that contributes to the development of future preventive interventions.

- New health technologies and their use in dealing with acute and chronic health problems.
- Identification and classification of outcome measures related to nursing practice phenomena.
- Development of integrative methodologies for the holistic study of human beings.
- Design and evaluation of alternative models for delivering and administering health care services.
- Evaluation of the effectiveness of alternative approaches to nursing education for practice.
- Analysis of historical and contemporary influences on the profession and impact on health policy.

KEY POINT The Cabinet on Nursing Research of the ANA suggests the following strategies to achieve goals for nursing research:[17]

- An increase in the proportion of doctorally prepared nurses to the total nurse population (0.5–1.0 percent). Parallel to this effort increased attention needs to be given to the preparation of nurse scientists (postdoctoral level).
- Establishment of a visible and viable entity within the federal government such as a nursing research institute for the conduct, support, and dissemination of basic and clinical research and training. (This is an attainable goal within five to ten years provided there is financial support with a base of $50–75 million per year; a cadre of postdoctoral fellows; and high-priority nursing research projects ready to be funded.)
- Establishment of a national nursing research retrieval system for unpublished research that would be available to national and international nurse researchers.
- Support of laboratories and research facilities with equipment essential for nursing investigations.

Use of Concepts from the Physical Sciences

Circulating blood is a means of transporting substances to and from the cells, and the volume and pressure must be maintained within certain limits to meet changing demands of various organs.[18] The basic principles related to this concept become important in caring for patients where there is apt to be postsurgical hemorrhage or where hemorrhage is imminent, such as in a patient with a bleeding gastric or duodenal ulcer.

The application of dressings, bandages, casts, or traction may be constricting, and close observation is essential to avoid any interference with circulation. Knowledge of the circulatory system provides the nurse with basic principles to apply in emergency situations.

Instruments, such as a sphygmomanometer, provide useful diagnostic data about the patient's changing condition which help both the physician and nurse make valid decisions regarding the patient's care. The nurse must be able to take an accurate blood pressure reading, and she must also be able to interpret this reading and make judgments about the systolic and diastolic readings.

The concepts of physics applied to nursing have wide application. For example, the principle that fluids flow from an area of higher pressure to one of lower pressure comes into play in the withdrawal and administering of fluids whether by means of an irrigating tube, an intravenous infusion, or a suction machine.

Maintaining a constant supply of oxygen to all body cells is a physiological concept upon which the survival of the organism depends. The nurse must have knowledge of the factors influencing the maintenance of this supply.[19]

1. An adequate supply of oxygen
2. A clear airway
3. An intact thoracic cage
4. An adequate diffusing surface in the lung
5. An adequate system of transportation

To make an intelligent decision about the

appropriate nursing practices, the nurse must recognize which factor is interfering with providing a constant supply of oxygen. For example, lack of oxygen in the environment is the interfering factor in patients undergoing an anesthetic. The same difficulties would be experienced by those individuals at high altitudes.

Maintaining a clear airway is vital for postoperative patients in chest surgery, for the asthmatic, and for the unconscious patient. The lack of an intact thoracic cage may be the interfering factor in chest injuries such as stab wounds or crushing injuries. The patient with pneumonia, pulmonary edema, or congestive heart failure does not receive sufficient oxygen because of an inadequate diffusing surface. The circulatory system of an anemic patient, or the patient with carbon monoxide poisoning, is unable to transport oxygen because of insufficient red blood cells.

Use of Social Science Concepts

The application of social science concepts to nursing practices is as important as applying the physical and biological concepts. However, because there is no immediate association of these concepts with survival there are less urgency and commitment on the part of nurses to utilize them. Lately there has been a greater understanding by many nursing leaders of the importance of giving increased attention to these principles.[20]

The general issues studied by the behavioral scientist are critically important to medical and health research. The scientific study of behavior is just beginning to be developed and dates back less than a century.

The research methods used by the behavioral scientist are no different from those used by any other scientist—namely, observation, instrumentation, field and laboratory experiments, construction of models and theories, and application of statistical processes to analyze data.

Increased support for research in the behavioral sciences has been given by the Public Health Service's National Institutes of Health, which already support major basic research in neurophysiology and psychology. The National Science Foundation has also given increased recognition to the behavioral sciences by the establishment of a Division of Social Science.

Examples of large-scale studies in the behavioral sciences include studies of mass communications, personality development, effects of sensory deprivation, and how injury to the brain affects speech, memory, and problem solving. The anthropologist is concerned with changes in primitive societies, sociological research with communication, and psychological research with perception and problem solving.[21]

Significant to nursing research is that all the fundamental research tools used by the physical scientist are also used by the behavioral scientist. Observation, experimentation, and the development of working hypotheses are tools for both, although the observations of the physical scientist are often more readily accessible than those made by the behavioral scientist.

The concept, "to identify and accept positive and negative expressions, feelings, and reactions," is particularly important in dealing with patients with psychoneuroses, psychoses, geriatric patients, and physical diseases that threaten physical appearance and/or vital functions.[22] Recognition of the importance of this concept helps the nurse to create an atmosphere in which the patient can express his positive and negative feelings and emotions.

Another social science concept vital to nursing care is, "to facilitate awareness of self as an individual with varying physical, emotional, and development needs."[23] This concept is applicable to all patients in varying degrees. The nurse is challenged to plan a program of care directed at the relief of the problems and needs of the whole individual. It means making provision for the combination of allied health services that can be directed toward helping the patient to a full and meaningful life.

THE IMPACT OF THE SOCIAL SCIENCES ON NURSING RESEARCH

The social sciences have had a twofold impact on nursing research. The first has been in the formulation of research problems. A review of completed research in nursing will quickly reveal the extent to which so many studies are formulated in terms of theories, models, and concepts derived from the field of social sciences. Second, the social sciences have had an important impact on the methods used in the design of nursing research. Many nursing studies have depended heavily on the logical approaches for conducting research, the instruments for data collection, and the techniques of data analyses that have been developed in the social sciences.

The importance of the social sciences is underscored by the high proportion of social scientists involved in nursing studies. In a review of 460 studies in nursing, Hilbert and Hildebrand have pointed out that about 22 percent of all investigators have been social scientists.[24] Only two groups—nurses (31 percent) and physicians (30 percent) had a higher percentage of investigators. Moreover, these data show that social scientists rank next to nurses in the number of times they appear as authors or coauthors of research articles reported in the journal *Nursing Research*.[25] Many studies directed by nurse researchers employ social scientists as consultants in the design and execution of the studies.

In order to analyze the impact of the social sciences on nursing research it is necessary to delineate what these sciences include. In her work *Social Science in Nursing,* Macgregor has pointed out the difficulties in arriving at a definition of the social sciences.[26] Recognizing that disciplines such as political science, economics, and law can be classified as social sciences, Macgregor limits her discussion to those social sciences she terms the behavioral sciences: "All those intellectual activities that contribute more or less directly to the scientific understanding of problems of individual behavior and human relations."[27] In the behavioral sciences she includes sociology, social psychology, and cultural anthropology. For the purpose of the discussion that follows, the social sciences will be defined as including the basic disciplines of sociology, psychology, and anthropology, and all mixtures of these disciplines, such as social psychology.

Formulation of Research Problems

It is not surprising to find that much nursing research that has been undertaken is dependent to some extent on the social sciences. Nursing is essentially a social activity in that much of what a nurse does takes place within a framework of interpersonal relationships. From the basic relationship between a nurse and a patient to the complex system of relationships present in the organized structure of a total nursing service department, it is possible to identify a multitude of social activities in which the nurse takes part. We find studies in nursing at all levels of these social activities. At the nurse-patient level Whiting studied the perception of nursing personnel and patients of the relative importance of various facets of the nurse-patient relationship.[28] At another level of interpersonal relationships, Bennis and others investigated the organizational loyalty of groups of nursing personnel in outpatient departments.[29] At the highest level of complexity of interpersonal relationships, Burling and others studied the total social system of six hospitals.[30]

These studies and many others applied theories and concepts from the social sciences to the study of nursing problems. Role theory, small group theory, leadership, informal organization, status, communication, and job satisfaction are among the many social science ideas used to investigate such problems as:

1. The sociopsychological causes of turnover of nursing personnel
2. Barriers to communication among nurses and patients

3. Causes of attrition among student nurses
4. Authoritarian versus democratic leadership in nursing
5. The consequences of the formation of informal groups in nursing service organizations
6. Definition and delineation of the role of the professional nurse

In addition to studies concerned with the interpersonal relations in nursing, some research, using theories and techniques from the field of psychology, has dealt with the psychological aspects of nurses and nursing, concerned with such factors as personality, abilities, needs, perceptions, and attitudes of nursing personnel and students. For example, Navran and Stauffacher studied the comparative personality structure of psychiatric and nonpsychiatric nurses,[31] and Lentz and Michaels compared the personality of medical and surgical nurses.[32] Boyle investigated the ability of student nurses to perceive patient needs.[33]

Research Methodology

The use of methods developed in the social sciences has been widespread in nursing research, for example, techniques for collecting and analyzing data such as psychological tests, sociometric measurements, scaling techniques, and quantitative analysis of data such as factor analysis and correlation of attributes. The following are brief descriptions of four of these techniques as used in nursing studies:

1. In sociometric measurements, using a device called a sociogram, members of a group may be asked to identify a small number of people who occupy extreme positions on certain characteristics such as the most liked, most disliked, most respected, least respected, and so on.[34] Sociograms are also used to identify groupings of individuals according to such factors as whom they find most congenial or with whom they would like most to engage in a particular activity. With the sociometric technique, a study was made of forty patients in a Montreal Hospital in which the patients drew sociograms twice each day for a one-month period.[35] It was found that such factors as age, sex, and language similarities had important influences on congenial groupings.
2. The Q-sort is a device for sorting into a few categories a large number of statements concerning the topic being studied (e.g., satisfaction with nursing care).[36] The sorter is instructed to place each statement into one of the categories according to some evaluative criterion. The number of statements that can be placed in each category is established in advance. An example of the use of the Q-sort technique is found in a study of attitudes toward psychiatric nursing care. In this study, hospital personnel and patients sorted fifty statements describing activities concerning psychiatric nursing care according to a scale of importance.[37]
3. Role analysis—a sociological technique—is based on the concept of a role as a patterned sequence of learned actions or deeds performed by a person in an interaction situation.[38] In nursing research a role analysis led to the classification of the roles of nurses as professionalizer, traditionalizer, and utilizer.[39]
4. A Guttman-type scale is one in which the different items composing the scale have a cumulative property so that a person who responds a certain way to, say, the third item on the scale is almost certain to have responded the same way to the preceding two items.[40] In a study of nursing in Israel, a Guttman-type scale was developed to measure interest in nursing as a career among high school girls.[41]

In a later chapter of this book, discussing measurement in research, other research methods from the social sciences having applicability in nursing studies will be described.

EVOLUTION OF NURSING AS A SCIENCE

The nursing profession is in agreement that nurses are to be autonomous. To

KEY POINT

achieve this goal, nurses must achieve status as scientific professionals. Research is one way to achieve this goal.[42] Education to acquire needed technical research skills is essential, and must be taught at all levels. By the year 2000 research will be an integral part of every nurse's workload. Nurse researchers and clinical nurses will work together to identify potential research projects. All professional nurses committed to achieving the goal of autonomy need to become involved in some aspect of research.

The scientific method is the most common and rewarding model used in nursing research. The concept of the holistic view of man is part of almost every nursing philosophy.[43] The nurse thus becomes the advocate of the individual's autonomy and acts to safeguard the patient's/client's rights. The scientific method is accepted as the one of choice as it has been found to be the most effective way of determining relationships between variables, enabling understanding, prediction, and some control. The scientific method is a process, each step contributing to a better understanding of the problem. Most important, the scientist learns to choose a measurable part and sets limits of selected variables, chooses a conceptual framework, selects the treatment modality (or the effect variable), and sets the parameters of the research. Finally, the researcher interprets the data and makes recommendations.

Nursing will emerge as a science when a highly organized and specialized field of knowledge in nursing is based upon a consistent system of concepts that organize logically a given area of phenomena.[44] Nursing science is thus systematic, logical organization of phenomena. Some steps already have been made in organizing a substantive body of knowledge to serve as an initial basis for such a science.[45]

The professional disciplines in general represent applied rather than basic sciences. They are committed to the task of utilizing knowledge to achieve some well-defined social goal.

They draw heavily upon the basic sciences to derive their bodies of knowledge. They are sciences, however, and are concerned with the systematization of knowledge and with its expansion. These characteristics have very direct implications for the development of a science of nursing.[46]

Crucial to the development of a nursing science is the nurse's ability to make a nursing diagnosis and prescribe nursing actions that will result in specific responses in the patient. Nursing diagnosis is a determination of the nature and extent of nursing problems presented by individual patients or families receiving nursing care. It is an independent function of the professional nurse to make a nursing diagnosis and to decide upon a course of action to be followed for the solution of the problem.

Research can help to clarify underlying theories and concepts related to nursing, each step leading toward an identification of a nursing science.

SUMMARY

The turbulent atmosphere that surrounds nursing research today has been brought about by many medical and technical advances. Specific concepts such as viewing the patient as a person, the clinical nurse specialist and nursing diagnosis, and grouping patients by their common medical and nursing needs must be given consideration if nursing is to find a justifiable role among the health professions.

The contributions of the sciences have become recognized as increasingly important to nursing research. In research, scientific inquiry begins with observations of seemingly unrelated phenomena, which are then organized into intelligible systems that show the relationships among the phenomena. The research methodologies of the physical, biological, and social scientist are basically very similar; observation, experimentation, and working hypotheses are crucial tools of all researchers.

REFERENCES

1. Rena E. Boyle, *A Study of Student Nurse Perception of Patient Attitudes.* U.S. Public Health Service Publication No. 769, Washington, D.C., Government Printing Office, 1960.
2. Department of Health, Education, and Welfare, *Extending the Scope of Nursing Practice.* A Report of the Secretary's committee to study Extended Roles for Nurses, Washington, D.C., Government Printing Office, November, 1971.
3. Faye G. Abdellah *et al., Patient-Centered Approaches to Nursing.* New York, Macmillan Publishing Co., Inc., 1960, p. 9.
4. Charles D. Flagle, *The Problem of Organization for Hospital Inpatient Care.* New York, Pergamon Press, Reprint No. 55, 1959.
5. Jack C. Haldeman and Faye G. Abdellah, "Concepts of Progressive Patient Care." *Hospitals,* **33:**38–42, 142, 41–46, May 16 and June 1, 1959.
6. Charles H. Russell, ". . . on a Liberal Education." *Am. J. Nursing,* **60:** 1485–1487, October 1960.
7. Virginia Saba and Kathleen McCormick, *Essentials of Computers in Nursing.* Philadelphia, J. B. Lippincott Co., 1986.
8. Dorothy E. Johnson, "The Nature of a Science of Nursing." *Nursing Outlook,* **7:**291–294, May 1959.
9. Russell, *op. cit.,* p. 1486.
10. Reuben B. Bowie, "Research Responsibilities of the Clinical Nurse." *AORN Journal,* **31:**2:238–241, February 1980.
11. Helen C. Chance and Ada Sue Hinshaw, "Strategies for Initiating a Research Program." *J. Nursing Administration,* **10**(3):32–39, March 1980.
12. Maxine E. Loomis and Kathleen P. Krone, "Collaborative Research Development." *J. Nursing Administration,* **10**(12):32–35, December 1980.
13. Jennifer Hunt, "Indicators for Nursing Practice: The Use of Research Findings." *J. Advanced Nursing,* **6**(3):189–194, May 1981.
14. Fannie M. Rettig, "Assessing Research for Clinical Use." *AORN J.,* **33**(5):873–881, April 1981.
15. American Nurses' Association Cabinet on Nursing Research, *Directions for Nursing Research: Toward the Twenty-First Century.* Kansas City, MO, American Nurses' Association, May 1984.
16. *Ibid.,* p. 2.
17. *Ibid.,* p. 9.
18. Madelyn Titus Nordmark and Anne W. Rohroeder, *Science Principles Applied to Nursing.* Philadelphia, J. B. Lippincott Co., 1959.
19. Faye G. Abdellah *et al., Patient-Centered Approaches to Nursing, op. cit.,* pp. 168–170.
20. Frances Cooke Macgregor, *Social Science in Nursing.* New York, Russell Sage Foundation, 1960.
21. "Strengthening the Behavioral Sciences." *Science,* **136:**233–241, April 20, 1962.
22. Faye G. Abdellah *et al., Patient-Centered Approaches to Nursing, op. cit.,* p. 195.
23. *Ibid.,* p. 199.
24. Hortense Hilbert and Edna M. Hildebrand, "Studies in Nursing—Notes and Observations." *Nursing Outlook,* **10:**44–46, January 1962.
25. *Ibid.,* p. 46.
26. Frances Cooke Macgregor, *op. cit.,* p. 36.
27. The Ford Foundation, Behavioral Sciences Division, *Report,* 1953, p. 13.
28. Frank J. Whiting, *The Nurse-Patient Relationship and the Healing Process.* Pittsburgh, Pittsburgh Veterans Administration Hospital, 1958.
29. W. G. Bennis, N. Berkowitz, M. Affinito, and M. Malone, "Reference Group and Loyalties in the Outpatient Department." *Admin. Sc. Quart.,* **2:**481–500, March 1958.
30. Temple Burling, Edith M. Lentz, and Robert N. Wilson, *The Give and Take in Hospitals.* New York, G. P. Putnam's Sons, 1956.
31. Leslie Navran and James C. Stauffacher, "A Comparative Analysis of the Personality Structure of Psychiatric and Nonpsychiatric Nurses." *Nursing Res.,* **7:**64–67, June 1958.
32. Edith M. Lentz and Robert W. Michaels, "Comparisons Between Medical and Surgical Nurses." *Nursing Res.,* **8:**192–197, fall 1959.
33. Rena E. Boyle, *op. cit.*
34. Benjamin Wright and Mary Sue Evitts, "Direct Factor Analysis in Sociometry." *Sociometry,* **24:**82–98, March 1961.
35. B. Harvey and R. Mark, "Sociogramatic Study of Spontaneous Patient Groupings." *Canad. Nurse,* **54:**924–928, October 1958.
36. W. Stephenson, *The Study of Behavior: Q-Technique and Its Methodology.* Chicago, University of Chicago Press, 1953.
37. Donald R. Gorham, "An Evaluation of Attitudes Toward Psychiatric Nursing Care." *Nursing Res.,* **7:**71–76, June 1958.
38. Theodore R. Sarben, "Role Theory," in G. Lindzey (ed.), *Handbook of Social Psychology.* Reading MA, Addison-Wesley Publishing Co., 1954, Vol. 1, pp. 223–258.
39. Robert A. Habenstein and Edwin A. Christ, *Professionalizer, Traditionalizer, and Utilizer.* Columbia, MO, University of Missouri Press, 1965.
40. Louis Guttman, "Measurement and Prediction," *Am. Sociol. Rev.,* **9:**139–150, 1944.
41. Judith T. Shuval, "Perceived Role Components of Nursing in Israel." *Am. Sociol. Rev.,* **28:**37–46, February 1963.
42. Patricia A. Rittenmeyer, "The Evolution of Nursing Research." *Western J. Nursing Res.,* **4**(2):223–225, spring 1982.
43. Patricia L. Munhall, "Nursing Philosophy and Nursing Research: In Apposition or Opposition." *Nursing Res.,* **31**(3):176–177, 181, May/June 1982.

44. Faye G. Abdellah *et al., Patient-Centered Approaches to Nursing, op. cit.,* p. 21.
45. *Ibid.*
46. Dorothy E. Johnson, "The Nature of a Science of Nursing." *Nursing Outlook,* **7:**292, May 1959.

SUGGESTIONS FOR FURTHER READING

1. Plato. "The Dialogues of Plato. The Republic Bk VII," *Great Books of the Western World.* Chicago, Encyclopaedia Britannica, Inc., 1952, Vol. 7, pp. 391–398.
2. Galilei, Galileo. "Dialogues Concerning the Two New Sciences," *Great Books of the Western World.* Chicago, Encyclopaedia Britannica, Inc., 1952, Vol. 28, pp. 131–260.
3. Harvey, William. "An Anatomical Disquisition on the Motion of the Heart and Blood in Animals," *Great Books of the Western World.* Chicago, Encyclopaedia Britannica, Inc., 1952, Vol. 28, pp. 267–496.
4. Aristotle, "The Works of Aristotle," *Great Books of the Western World.* Chicago, Encyclopaedia Britannica, Inc., 1952, Vol. 8, pp. 119–137.
5. Bacon, Francis. "Advancement of Learning," *Great Books of the Western World.* Chicago, Encyclopaedia Britannica, Inc., 1952, pp. 43–48.
6. Kant, Immanuel. "The Critique of Pure Reason," *Great Books of the Western World.* Chicago, Encyclopaedia Britannica, Inc., 1952, Vol. 42, pp. 93–115.
7. Einstein, Albert. *Relativity: The Special and the General Theory.* New York, Holt, 1920.
8. Huxley, J. S. *Science and Social Needs.* New York, Harper and Row, 1935.
9. Newman, James R. (ed.). *What Is Science?* New York, Washington Square Press, Inc., 1955.
10. Conant, James B. *On Understanding Science,* New York, Mentor Book, The New American Library of World Literature, Inc., 1951.
11. Sheldon, Eleanor B. "The Use of Behavioral Sciences in Nursing: An Opinion." *Nursing Res.,* **12:**150–152, summer 1963.
12 Berthold, Jeanne T. "Nurses and Behavioral Scientists: An Alternate Assessment." *Nursing Res.,* **12:**153–156, summer 1963.
13. "Nurse Practitioner Research and Evaluation," *Nursing Outlook* (entire issue), **23:**147–177, March 1975.
14. Bates, Barbara. "Doctor and Nurse: Changing Roles and Relations." *N. Eng. J. Med.,* **283:**129–134, July 6, 1970.
15. Bates, Barbara. *A Guide to Physical Examination.* Philadelphia, J. B. Lippincott Co., 1974.
16. Bloch, Doris, "Some Crucial Terms in Nursing. What Do They Really Mean?" *Nursing Outlook,* **22:**689–694, November 1974.

CHAPTER

4

Theoretical Basis
of Nursing Research

OBJECTIVES

- To clarify and define the uniqueness of nursing through the role of theory development.
- To understand the process of theory development, evaluation, and utilization.
- To understand how the practice of nursing is directly related to the development and revision of nursing theory.
- To learn about nursing theorists and identify their contributions to the practice of nursing.

- To understand the relevance of theory for explaining and predicting human experiences within the nursing framework.
- To understand the importance of theory to reserach.
- To identify the components of a theory.
- To examine nursing practice models.
- To understand the relationship between theories and models.

In nursing research, much emphasis has been placed on finding solutions to operational problems rather than using scientific inquiry to discover the fundamental cause(s) of a problem. It is often more difficult to find and to formulate a problem than to find its solution. One difficulty in putting nursing research on a scientific basis lies in posing the appropriate questions that can be answered by a formal research study.

In science, the questions that matter are of a particular kind. They are so formulated that the answers to them will confirm, amplify, or variously revise some part of what is currently taken as knowledge in the field.[1] Every problem in science involves a question(s), but not every question qualifies as a scientific problem. Much emphasis has been placed on the John Dewey process of

problem solving but little on the process of "problem finding."

What is "problem finding"? Where does it begin? Unfortunately, there is no set formula to follow. One approach is to begin by challenging existing facts and questioning the evidence at hand. In research, facts are often included in generalizations that relate one fact to another. The facts may be correct, but the deductions about the relationships may be wrong. One might also begin by examining the facts to see if their application in current situations is still relevant. Examples can be found by examining current nursing practices that have become ritualistic rather than being based on sound physiological principles. Such practices may have served useful purposes in the past, but situations change, and current practices must be examined in light of changing situations. Merton summarizes the process of "problem finding" in the three following steps:[2]

1. Originate the question. State what it is you want to know.
2. Specify the rationale or conceptual framework (to be described later). State why you want to have this particular question answered.
3. State the questions that point toward the possible answers to the originating questions in terms that satisfy the rationale for having raised the question.

The process of nursing involves a problem-solving mode of action in which the nurse has to make informed clinical judgments.[3] Why theory development? Criteria are needed to assess the quality of nursing practice in relation to personal growth, nursing science, and societal health. Developing a method of assessing the impact of nursing practice on the health status of patients/clients is a critical step in theory development.[4] The fragmented nature of research efforts is a major deterrent to the development of a cohesive body of nursing knowledge. The development and use of theoretical models can help in the organization of curricula or practice, but because of the lack of cohesiveness they have not generated the testing of theory. Theory generation must show how abstract perspectives can be empirically specified.[5]

THE ROLE OF THEORY IN RESEARCH

A review of current studies in nursing research points to a major limitation of these studies—namely, the need for systematic knowledge founded on a broad base. This lack means that any inferences drawn from the findings usually have to be limited to the specific situation in which the research has been conducted. The development of a theory is the most direct way of systematizing knowledge founded on a broad base. The proof of the theory, which is a general statement that seeks to explain certain phenomena or events, is the reason to conduct the research.

Theory attempts to summarize existing knowledge, provide an explanation for facts and their relationships, and predict the occurrence of future events and relationships.[6] Braithwaite[7] defines a theory as a set of hypotheses that form a deductive system that is arranged in such a logical pattern that some of the hypotheses become premises of other hypotheses. These in turn become premises of still other hypotheses, thus forming a system of scientifically derived knowledge.

A scientific theory is composed of three parts. These are:

1. *Definitions:* Operationally defined terms of words or phrases used in the statement of the problem. Whenever possible they should be expressed in observable and quantifiable terms.

2. *Postulates:* Concepts or abstract ideas of universal significance later may be translated into principles and laws. Each must be documented from the literature or from previous research.

It is necessary to distinguish laws from postulates. Laws originate as postulates that eventually may become laws when the hypotheses tested are proven to be true. Peirce[8] refers to laws as generalizations from observation of facts that are representative of outward conditions. A law must not be based upon a chance coincidence among the observations from which it is derived.

The validity of postulates is determined by testing deductions that derive from them. Deductions thus comprise the third part of a scientific theory.[9]

3. *Deductions:* These are commonly referred to as hypotheses. Deductions are conclusions reached by logically proceeding from a clarification of definitions to acceptable postulates (concepts) and then to hypotheses that can be tested in research.

The testing of the hypothesis either serves to confirm the validity of the theory or leads to a modification of the postulates upon which the theory was based. The usefulness of a theory is dependent upon the deductions that can be made from it.

The degree to which the nursing profession succeeds in defining a scientific body of knowledge that is uniquely nursing will be dependent upon research that will provide a body of facts from which generalizations and laws can be developed and applied to the solution of nursing problems. Exhibit 4–1 summarizes major nursing theories; a bibliography listed as the "Definitive Works of Theorists" appears in the reference section at the end of this chapter (p. 72). Theories are not "ivory-tower" phenomena but have great importance in developing research.[10] A theory serves as the basis for the exploration of phenomena and testing of hypotheses.[11] Theories are guides for the direction of research by pointing to areas likely to be productive of meaningful relationships among phenomena. The more research is guided by scientific methods, the more likely are its results to contribute directly to a scientific body of knowledge in nursing.

More nurses are engaged in research today than ever before, but systematic investigation into a range of practice, educational, and administrative issues is still needed. Systematic inquiry designed to evaluate the extent to which practice strategies are effective in improving the quality of patient care will help to identify deficiencies in knowledge, practice, and technology.[12] Improved health care will result from better decision making founded on practice-based research that is translated into improved practice. The most realistic model that is linking education and practice through research is collaborative research in which university-based researchers and agency-based clinicians are equal contributors and collaborators at each stage of the research process.

NURSING PRACTICE MODELS

What are nursing practice models? Models are useful to solve both simple and complex problems in that they concentrate attention on a portion or a key feature rather than the entire problem. "Model" is often used as a synonym for "theory". Theories represent aspects of real-world phenomena that could be considered models. Models, however, are not theories, because not all models have the requisites of theoretical construction. To be considered theory, the phenomena under consideration must be precise and limited, and the concepts clearly defined.[13] Theories also have the capability to predict and control.

The purpose of theory is to increase scientific understanding through a systematized structure capable of both explaining and predicting phenomena.[14]

Models provide a useful mechanism for depicting relationships that exist among the variables of the theory. Theories and models are essential if nursing is to build a base of knowledge. To apply to the practice of nursing, they must be capable of translation into a form where they can be tested.

The challenge is now to develop theories which are logically related to fundamental issues around which practice is actually organized, that is around single core concepts which themselves represent specific areas of practice currently being carried out.[15]

Nursing Practice—Theory Development

Approaches to nursing theory development range from a scientific to a practice approach and are essential to the establishment of a theoretical body of knowledge unique to nursing as a science. Furthermore, it must be integrated with nursing practice.[16]

Four stages in theory construction:

1. Describe phenomena related to field of inquiry.
2. Specify, define, and classify the concepts relating to corresponding empirical entities.
3. Develop statements that propose how concepts are interrelated.
4. State how the statements relate to each other in a systematic and logical way.[17]

KEY POIN

There is a need for a practice theory in

nursing that will set out the kinds of knowledge utilized in nursing practice.[18]

Use of Models to Evaluate Clinical Practice

How do you determine the effectiveness of your nursing practice? Would your answer be: the patient gets better; you, the nurse, feel satisfied; you, the student, please the instructor; the physician is happy with patient progress; and/or the patient's family is content with the care given? In other words, from what perspective do you, as a nurse, evaluate the effectiveness of your nursing actions?[19]

Nursing models claim to provide you with a blueprint for objectively and directly evaluating your nursing actions. Use of nursing models to guide practice is a relatively new concept being proposed for use in daily practice. Such a proposal implies a need to change. How can a model of nursing be used to directly and objectively assist you in determining the effectiveness of your nursing actions? What is necessary to clarify how a nursing model can be applied to situations in daily nursing practice that will culminate in a scientific and valid evaluation of nursing interventions?

Description of a Model

A model defines your nursing goal, the patient or appropriate recipient of your nursing care, your role (or roles) in delivering that care, the difficulty indicating the need for nursing, the relevant database, the focus and mode, and the consequences (intended and unintended) of your nursing interventions. These elements are present in all fully developed models, although the specific content defining these elements differs from model to model. The content defining the model elements provides you with a particular view of the patient, yourself, and your approach in planning, implementing, and evaluating nursing care.

Although you may never have thought of your own nursing practice in these terms, you do have a model (or framework) from which you function. Underlying all you do

is your basic philosophy arising from your beliefs about people and life. In the same way, each model of nursing is based on a specific philosophy. This philosophy arises from the beliefs of the particular model theorist and is reflected in the model's supporting assumptions and values. In order to make a knowledgeable choice regarding a working model of nursing for yourself, your own philosophy must be congruent with the philosophy of the model. For example, what is your view of the patient? Do you believe the patient is a holistic being with multidimensional needs (i.e., physical, psychological, sociological, spiritual, and cultural) or a system-segmented being (i.e., digestive, reproductive, respiratory, etc.)? What is your belief regarding the patient's right to accept or refuse care? What is your belief regarding the impact of environmental forces on patient care outcomes? Do you believe the patient is an acute, accountable participant in his/her own health care? Do you believe motivation is internally or externally regulated (i.e., the nurse motivates the patient or the patient motivates himself)? What is your focus of care—preventive or curative? Do you believe your nursing role is one of physical care provider, teacher, counselor, problem solver, assessor, collaborator, or a combination of these roles? Thus, the caring model versus the medical curing model comes into play.

Once these questions have been answered, you are ready to compare and contrast a model's stated assumptions and values with your own. When this process has been completed, you will be able to evaluate whether your own philosophy and that of the model are congruent.

Mrs. Jones, aged 52, enters the rural health care clinic for a routine physical examination. She is a self-care agent with no known self-care deficits. As Mrs. Jones's nurse practitioner, you conduct your routine screening tests and make the differential diagnosis of diabetes mellitus. As nurse practitioner you identify self-care deficits for Mrs. Jones. You assess a certain lack of knowledge, orientation, and skill on the part of Mrs. Jones to be

EXHIBIT 4–1.
Comparison of Nurse Theorists' Views of
Patient/Client, Nursing, Society/Environment, and Health

NURSE THEORIST	PATIENT/CLIENT	NURSING	SOCIETY/ENVIRONMENT	HEALTH
Florence Nightingale 1860	All disease viewed as a reparative process; an effort of nature to remedy a process of poisoning or of decay.	Noncurative process dependent upon reparative process which nature has instituted. Nursing signifies proper use of fresh air, light, warmth, cleanliness, quiet, proper diet.	Stress on environment as contributing factors to disease.	Laws of health and nursing viewed as the same.
Hildegard Peplau 1952	Patient and nurse viewed as a continuum—two individuals with separate goals and interests and working together to solve a presenting difficulty.	Nursing is a function—one of many functions of a professional health team. It is an interpersonal process and a therapeutic one. Nurses participate with other professional workers in the organization of conditions that facilitate forward movement of personality and other ongoing human processes in the direction of creative, constructive, productive, personal and community living.	Human processes that are of social origin (e.g., education, nursing, medicine) have their origins in human insights and desires to influence progress in meeting human needs.	Not clearly defined. Implies forward movement of personality and other ongoing human processes in the direction of creative, constructive, productive, personal, and community living. Health dependent upon physiological demands of human organism and interpersonal conditions that are individual and social.
Faye G. Abdellah 1960	Patient/client presents nursing problem which is a condition faced by the patient or family which the nurse can assist him or them to meet through the performance of professional functions. The problem can either be overt or covert. (1984—Dr. Abdellah recognizes the shift from nursing problems to patient/client outcomes).	Based on an art and science which mold the attitudes, intellectual competencies, and technical skills of the individual nurse into the desire and ability to help people sick or well, cope with their health needs. Nursing problems classified into a typology of 21 nursing problems: physical, sociological, and emotional needs; interpersonal relations between nurse and patient; and common elements of patient care. Typology served as a basis for developing a scien-	Societal and environmental needs recognized as contributing factors to actual and/or anticipated impairments. Problems presented by patient/client not limited to the hospital but also include the home and community.	Movement toward care model and away from medical model. Concept of self-help stressed. Self-help ability developed and maintained at a level at which need satisfaction can take place without assistance. (1984—Dr. Abdellah would place importance upon prevention and rehabilitation with "wellness" as a lifetime goal. The holistic approach to patient/client need to be considered).

	Nursing	Person/Patient	Environment	Health
Ida Jean Orlando 1961	tific body of knowledge unique to nursing. Nursing diagnosis defined as the determination of the nature and extent of nursing problems presented by individual patients or families. Nurse acts to alleviate distress due to: physical limitations (either temporary or permanent); adverse reactions to the setting; and inability to communicate. Patient behavior, nurse reactions, and nurse actions comprise a nursing situation. Overall goal of nursing is to meet needs.	Patient/client individual with a need, a requirement if supplied, diminishes distress, increases adequacy, or enhances well-being.	Adverse reactions to the setting can cause unmet need.	Primary concern with sustaining the patient in his/her immediate need. Needs are generated by physical limitations; setting; or inability to communicate.
Ernestine Wiedenbach 1964	Nursing is concerned with patients' need for help. Clinical nursing has four components —philosophy, purpose, practice, and art. Nursing practice includes identification of perceived need for help: ministration of help needed. Validation that help is given needed; and coordination of help and resources for help. Clinical goal is to meet needs for help, integrating practice and process of nursing.	Patient/client individual under treatment or care who experiences needs. Needs are defined as measures or actions required and desired which potentially restore or extend ability to cope with situational demands.	Environment viewed as one of the situational demands.	Greater professional goals include conservation of life and promotion of health.
Lydia E. Hall 1966	Nursing made up of three interlocking circles: core—therapeutic use of self to help patient; cure circle—carrying out medical, surgical and rehabilitative services; and care—professional nurse function. Nursing's goal is to help patient/client to learn.	Patient/client made up of a person (core aspect), a pathology and treatment (cure aspect), and a body (care aspect).	Care occurs in setting where patient/client is free to learn.	Overall goals for patient/client is rehabilitation and a greater measure of self-actualization and self love.

EXHIBIT 4-1.
Comparison of Nurse Theorists' Views of
Patient/Client, Nursing, Society/Environment, and Health (cont.)

NURSE THEORIST	PATIENT/CLIENT	NURSING	SOCIETY/ENVIRONMENT	HEALTH
Virginia Henderson 1966	Patient individual who requires help toward independence.	Professional nursing means the performance for compensation of any act in the observation, care, and counsel of the ill, injured, or infirm, or in the maintenance of health or prevention of illness of others. Fourteen components of basic nursing care are identified such as helping the patient to breathe normally; eat and drink adequately etc.	Defined within the components of basic nursing: "Avoid dangers in the environment and avoid injuring others."	Defined within the 14 components of basic nursing: "Learn, discover, or satisfy the curiosity that leads to 'normal' development and health."
Myra E. Levine 1967	Patient/client viewed as a holistic being who exists in an environment—a unity who is to remain conserved and integral.	Nurse receives and interprets messages and intervenes supportively or therapeutically. Intervention guided by four principles of conservation—conservation of energy and structural, personal, and social integrity. Conservation is based on assessment of man's adaptive needs. Goal for nursing is the wholeness of the patient brought about by conservation in the four areas.	Society comprises total environment of the patient/client including family and nurse.	Restoration of wholeness of the patient/client is the health goal.
Martha E. Rogers 1970	Man is viewed as an energy field coextensive with the universe. Humans are perceived in their wholeness, acting in the midst of a field of dynamic forces.	Nursing is a science that will guide nursing practice based on principles of homeo dynamics: reciprocy, synchrony, helicy, and resonancy.	Man and environment are energy fields that are coextensive with the universe.	Goal is maximum health potential for unitary man achievable by applying emerging science based on the principles of homeodynamics. Rogers focuses on the human life process, how to maintain it, and how to encourage its evolution.

56

	Person/Patient-Client	Nursing	Environment	Health/Goal
Dorothea E. Orem 1971	Patients/clients have self-care needs for which they perform learned self-care behaviors.	Nursing viewed as providing therapeutic self-care in persons with deficits in self-care ability and demands for care. Nursing goal is optimal wellness. Self-care needs include: universal, developmental, and health deviation. Self-care to meet these needs focus on: life process support; maintenance of normal human structure and function; support and development consistent with potential; prevention of injury; cure and regulation of pathologic processes; and cure and regulation of their effects.	Environment makes up the elements external to the person interacting with the individual to achieve a state of wholeness.	Goal is to maintain persons in or return them to a state where their therapeutic self-care abilities achieve a state of wholeness.
Imogene M. King 1971	Patient/client viewed as a composite of mind and body. Individual reacts as a total organism to experiences which are viewed as a flow of events in time. Transactions that occur in human interactions are an exchange of energy and information within the persons involved (intrapersonal) and between the individual and the environment (interpersonal).	Nursing is an interpersonal process of action, reaction, interaction and transaction. The process provides assistance to patient/client in meeting basic activities of daily living and ability to cope with health and illness. The goal of nursing process interaction is transaction that leads to attainment of goals set in relation to health promotion, maintenance, and recovery from illness.	Action results from factors in the situation and in the individual at any point in time. Societal systems and environmental systems constantly interact with the individual. The patient/client is a personal system within the environment who coexists with other personal systems.	Health is a constant flowing dynamic state in the individual's life cycle requiring adaptation to stress in the environment to achieve the goal of maximum potential for daily living or die with dignity.
Sr. Callista Roy 1976	Patient/client viewed as biopsychosocial being who must be considered as a whole and exists within an environment. Stimuli impact on the individual and create needs in one or more four interrelated adaption models: physiologic needs, self-con-	Nursing involves assessing behavior, assessing stimuli as factors influencing needs, problem identification, goal setting, intervention, and evaluation.	Individual interacts with the environment. Man's environment and man's self are sources of stimuli (focal, residual, and contextual).	Individual adapts to environment to restore a norm based integrity by solving adaptation problems.

EXHIBIT 4–1.
Comparison of Nurse Theorists' Views of
Patient/Client, Nursing, Society/Environment, and Health (cont.)

NURSE THEORIST	PATIENT/CLIENT	NURSING	SOCIETY/ENVIRONMENT	HEALTH
	cept, role function, and inter-dependence. The individual adapts through two adaptive mechanisms—the regulator and the cognator.			
J.G. Patterson and L.T. Zderad 1976	Patient/client is unique with ability to make choices based on awareness and knowledge.	Nursing is a response to human need and can build a humanistic nursing science. Humanistic nursing—response of one human in need to another.	Total commitment to value of humanistic nursing.	Health-illness quality of human condition.
M. M. Leininger 1978	Patient/client part of a universal phenomenon in which every nursing situation has transcultural nursing care elements.	Nursing viewed as caring which includes assistive, supportive, and facilitative acts toward or for another individual or a group with evident or anticipated needs.	Caring improves human conditions and lifeways.	Scientific and humanistic modes of helping or enabling receipt of personalized service to maintain a favorably healthy condition for life or death.
J. Watson 1979	Patient/client viewed as requiring holistic care that promotes humanism, health, and quality of living.	Nursing viewed as promoting health, preventing illness, caring for the sick, and restoring health. Caring is practice interpersonally. Ten carative factors structure science of caring basic	Caring environment offers choices, assists environmental coping.	Emphasis on promoting health and restoring health through holistic care.

	Patient/Client	Nursing	Environment	Health
		to nursing practice, e.g., cultivation sensitivity to self and others.		
M. A. Newman 1979	Patient/client part of a greater whole and multiple system levels in space.	Nursing embodied in movement—time and space, to change any system level and help patient/client move toward health.	Environment one of multiple system levels in space.	Health encompasses pathology and illness, and is an expansion of consciousness.
Dorothy E. Johnson 1980	Patient/client viewed as a behavioral system comprised of subsystems.	Nursing viewed as behavioral system and subsystems. The four structural elements in each subsystem are drive stimulated; set or predispositioned to act in a certain way; choices; and behavior. Subsystems include attachment, dependency, ingestive, eliminative, sexual, aggressive and achievement. Nursing problems arise when subsystems are not stable and not functioning at optimal level.	Behavioral systems tie individual to environment.	Health achieved when behavior modifications are used to reestablish balance of subsystems.
R. R. Parse 1980	Patient/client viewed as an individvisible energy field who interacts with the environment while cocreating health capable of making own choices.	Implications for nursing practice:	Individual evolves with the environment—connecting and separating.	Health co-created in open energy exchange with the environment.

an effective self-care agent in the management of her diabetes. Because self-care deficits exist for Mrs. Jones, there is a need for nursing. In collaboration with the rural clinic physician, Mrs. Jones's treatment regimen is planned.

As nurse practitioner you then enter into the educative-developmental role with Mrs. Jones. Over the next several weeks you teach her the physiological aspects of her diabetes, how to test for glucose levels, how to do self-injection of insulin, how to determine need for insulin adjustments, how to prepare food and eat within the dietary restrictions necssitated by her diabetes, and when, or if, self-care is appropriate. Depending on Mrs. Jones's self-care action abilities and limitations in the management of her diabetes, she may move toward increasing independence in self-care. As Mrs. Jones's primary health care provider, you continue to see her monthly, monitoring her progress and supporting and guiding her self-care actions.

Evaluation

The elements of the model that enable you to evaluate, both objectively and directly, are the goals of action and consequences (intended and unintended). According to Orem's model, the goals of action are: patient self-care is accomplished; the patient moves toward responsible action in matters of self-care; and members of the patient's family become increasingly competent in making decisions relative to the patient's continuing daily personalized care.

This same evaluative process done with the Orem model can also be done with any other fully developed model of nursing. It is the process that guides you in the evaluation of your practice via a nursing model.

Models of Clinical Practice (Important Components)

In structuring a model of nurse practitioner clinical practice, one of the first components to consider is the scope of practice.

What are the N.P.'s responsibilities? How many patients are seen? What is the range of diagnoses presented? How complex is the demand for care?

Another component of the model involves the practitioner's degree of responsibility. What is the nature of the practitioner's relationship with other health care providers? Is collaborative practice possible? Are referrals readily accepted by other team members or community health care workers? Is there sufficient legal definition of the expanded nursing role to allow full implementation of the position? Is there adequate backup and advisory help available?

A third area of concern is working conditions. These include: work hours, rotation, on-call requirements, provision of working space and equipment, scheduling of patients, provision for follow-up and access to typewriters, dictation equipment, etc. You might not think of these as being important, but you will soon learn that they are.

Fourth, the nurse practitioner model contains a focus on power and authority. Where does the nurse practitioner fit in the organization scheme? How much control does the N.P. have over his or her personal schedule? How many layers of authority does the N.P. have to go through to get to the top? Does the N.P. have enough authority to implement changes or policies to allow role expansion and development?

Fifth, how much creativity is possible in this setting? Is the practice stable and well structured with traditional roles assigned to all caregivers, or is there room for innovation? Is the setting itself open to modification and change? How much tolerance will there be for implementation of different ways of doing things?

Finally, how is the incentive structure defined? Salary range and benefits such as insurance, organizational share holding, vacation time, educational, and/or pregnancy leave should all be included in this component.[20]

Inquiry belongs to all fields not just nursing. But who does research in nursing? The

KEY
POIN

broad conceptualization of nursing research does not require that the researcher be a nurse. Likewise, nursing research has no distinctive setting. It can take place in a hospital, community, home, or school. Those criteria that distinguish nursing research are associated with identifying nursing phenomena—the actions and the theories that make up nursing practice. Phenomena in nursing are man-made—artificial rather than natural phenomena. They are shaped and determined by normative judgments (rules, ideas that govern the profession).

There is need for emphasis on studies that provide a conceptual basis shaping the theory of nursing. It is here that the case study is so important. By examining the total one can see and evaluate the normative judgments taken. One must discover the sets of values operating; they cannot be separated from research. A few attempts have been made to develop conceptual models for nursing research. A conceptual model must be defined as a diagrammatic representation of a postulate or concept.[21] A brief description of some of these models follows.

A Reaction Model

Hayes and Leik[22] envisioned developing a reaction model that might be used to predict behaviors related to interpersonal relationships. The investigators raised the question: Why are there such differences in reaction to essentially the same situations among several persons or in the same person over time? Basic to a model is the theory upon which it is built. The dimensions of the reaction model are "relevance" and "value", which affect all situations such as interpersonal relationships, nurse-patient interactions, nurse actions taken that affect the patient (e.g., nurse action and pain).

Following is an interpretation of the way in which Hayes and Leik[23] conceived the theoretical structure basic to their model.

Relevance

- *Operational definition:* Relevance is considered an omnipresent dimension of all situations to which one is exposed. The dimension or degree of relevance may range from low to high.
- *Postulates (concepts):*
  1. Experience and imagination help to establish the relevance of a situation.
  2. High levels of satisfaction or deprivation substantially modify one's reaction to many situations.
  3. What we believe to be the relevance of essentially the same situation may undergo substantial change as a product of our experiences with it.
- *Deduction (hypothesis):* The more relevant we perceive a situation to be for us, the stronger will our reaction be.

Value

- *Operational definition:* Value refers to the individual's evaluation of the positive, neutral, or negative character of an object, someone's behavior, or a situation. The value dimension is bipolar—it has two high points, positive and negative, and one low point, neutral.
- *Postulate (concept):* Experience contributes heavily to producing the standards of judgment in deciding whether a situation is primarily positive, neutral, or negative.
- *Deduction (hypothesis):* Reaction strength increases as our judgment of values moves from neutral to either the positive or negative pole.

To illustrate, a situation test may be used to measure the degree of relevance and value placed upon a situation. Following is a test that might be used. The situation is first described. The person must then select *one* choice that would be the appropriate course of action where value and relevance may both be high.

A professional nurse is assigned to ambulance duty in a hospital situation where there is an acute shortage of interns. A call comes in to proceed to a nearby lake where a child has been rescued. She arrives on the scene ten minutes after the child has been taken from the water. The parents are with the child. No one has attempted to resuscitate the child. The nurse knows that if she should be successful in resuscitating the child, the child would more than likely suffer considerable brain damage due to lack of oxygen. If you were in this situation which one of the following courses of action would you follow?

1. Attempt to resuscitate the child and hope that brain damage would be minimal.
2. Explain the alternatives to the parents and let them decide.
3. Do not attempt to resuscitate the child, knowing that brain damage might be extensive.
4. Place the child in the ambulance and take her to the hospital.

The situation is then repeated. Everything is exactly the same with one exception—the child is the niece of the nurse on ambulance duty. You are asked to choose once again from the above choices.

Since all choices are possible there is no right or wrong answer. However, the choice the respondent makes does provide information as to the dimensions of relevance and value. The choice of these dimensions in repeated situation tests can help to predict types of behavior and provide clues to possible answers to the original question posed by Hayes and Leik—namely, why are there such differences in reactions to the same situation among several persons?

A Nursing Care Model

From the beginning of organized nursing practice on the battlefield, in the home, and in the hospital there has been a need to predict nurse staffing patterns. Several attempts[24] have been made to study the nurse at work and then to plan staffing patterns based on empirical knowledge. This tends to perpetuate ritualistic nursing practices no longer useful; it also fosters staffing patterns organized to meet the needs of the health agency or hospital rather than those of the patient.

In an attempt to derive nurse staffing pat-

terns based on patient needs, the following nursing care model was developed.

In developing a conceptual framework from which a nursing care model[25] might evolve, the first step was to define the terms from which the derivation of nurse staffing patterns might be traced.

TERM	DEFINITION
Nursing care	1. Assistance is provided a patient when, for some reason, he cannot provide for the satisfaction of his own needs. 2. It is commensurate with the abilities and skills of the person providing the assistance. 3. It is derived from a study of the patient's requirements for nursing care. 4. It is directed toward making the patient better able to help himself.

TERM	DEFINITION
Personal need	A considerable variety of optimal conditions such as air, water, food, temperature, and intactness of body tissue is required for survival. When, for some reason, any of these necessities departs from the optimum, *a state of need* can be said to exist.
Self-help ability (SHA)	An ability of the person to provide for the satisfaction of his own needs.
Impaired state	An impairment to the body or person that limits the individual's ability to satisfy his needs and results from injury, disease, malformations, or maldevelopment.

Once these definitions were spelled out the next step was to spell out the postulates and deductions related to nursing care requirements (see Figure 4-1 for an application of the model to a coronary patient).

Nursing Care Requirements

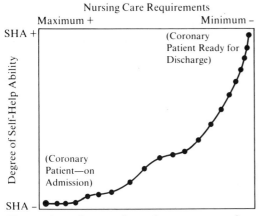

Figure 4–1 Progression of coronary patient during three weeks of hospitalization according to self-help ability and nursing care requirements.

NURSING CARE REQUIREMENTS

Postulate	As long as self-help ability is developed and maintained at a level in which need satisfaction can take place without assistance, nursing care will not be required. Need satisfaction will then be a function of SHA etc.
Deduction	Need satisfaction will then be a function of self-help ability and nursing care.

NEED FOR IMPAIRMENT CARE

Postulate	When, as a result of an impaired state, self-help ability is reduced to a minus state and certain personal needs cannot be satisfied, a need for impairment care will arise.
Deduction	Impairment care is a function of the need for sustenal care, for remedial care, and for restorative care.

NEED FOR SUSTENAL CARE

Postulate	When self-help ability is diminished as a result of an impaired state and the patient cannot of his own accord provide for the satisfaction of his personal needs, care must be administered to augment

self-help ability to the extent that the personal needs can be satisfied.

Deduction   The need for sustenal care will be a function of the reduced state of self-help ability and unsatisfied personal needs.

$$N\ CaSus = f\ [(SHA\ -) \times (Np)]$$

(The need for care, sustenal, is a function of self-help ability minus, multiplied by the patient's personal needs.)

The development of the postulates (concepts) to explain the effect(s) of the application of the stimulus and a rational presentation of what is taking place are often called theoretical research.

If an investigator does not provide a conceptual framework for his research, he is in danger of basing his research on an isolated postulate or hypothesis that does not tie in with other knowledge. A postulate is significant only if it occurs together with others in statements of law that we have reason to believe are true. A conceptual framework can state functional relationships between qualitative phenomena and is not limited to statistical relationships. [26]

A concept frightening to some is patient-centered care. One hears, "Isn't this what we have always been doing?" Is this just another cliché for "total patient care," "comprehensive care," "nursing the whole patient? Theoretical concepts must be defined precisely and unambiguously.

The concept of patient-centered care can be clarified only by presenting the facts about the concepts. What words translate it into meaningful terms? Operationally one might agree that patient-centered care is assistance provided a patient in meeting his individual requirements for nursing care when he cannot provide for his own needs.

The concept can be clarified if criteria are spelled out that can be used to identify its implementation—that is, if patient-centered care were being provided in a patient care situation, one might use the following criteria to determine if the objectives were being met:

1. The patient is able to provide for his own needs.
2. The nursing care plan makes provision to meet four needs—sustenal care, remedial care, restorative care, and preventive care.
3. The care plan extends beyond the patient's hospitalization and makes provision for continuation of the care at home.
4. The level of nursing skills provided vary with the individual patient care requirements.
5. The entire care plan is directed at having the patient help himself.
6. The care plan makes provision for involvement of members of the family throughout the hospitalization and after discharge.

Any concept not defined clearly in terms that are universally acceptable will create confusion and withdrawal from its use. One must continue to question each concept to determine how it fits into a theoretical framework. The danger is in withdrawing from the concept and saying, "That's beyond me." An investigator who takes time to spell out a sound conceptual framework is more likely to base the research on facts rather than conjecture. The following might serve as a conceptual framework from which a nursing care model might evolve.

Model for the Study of Pain

The physical sciences provide the physiological basis of nursing practices. Following is a theoretical framework developed by two nurse research students in studying the problem of the frequency with which pain accompanies intramuscular injections ad-

List of 21 Specific Needs Presented by Patients at Different Stages of Illness[27]

	1. To maintain good hygiene and physical comfort
	2. To promote optimal activity: exercise, rest, and sleep
Basic to all patients	3. To promote safety through prevention of accident, injury, or other trauma and through the prevention of the spread of infection
	4. To maintain good body mechanics and prevent and correct deformities
	5. To facilitate the maintenance of a supply of oxygen to all body cells
	6. To facilitate the maintenance of nutrition to all body cells
Sustenal care needs	7. To facilitate the maintenance of elimination
	8. To facilitate the maintenance of fluid and electrolyte balance
	9. To recognize the physiological responses of the body to disease conditions—pathological, physiological, and compensatory
	10. To facilitate the maintenance of regulatory mechanisms and functions
	11. To facilitate the maintenance of sensory function
	12. To identify and accept positive and negative expressions, feelings, and reactions
	13. To identify and accept the interrelatedness of emotions and organic illness
Remedial care needs	14. To facilitate the maintenance of effective verbal and nonverbal communication
	15. To promote the development of productive interpersonal relationships
	16. To facilitate progress toward achievement of personal and spiritual goals
	17. To create and/or maintain a therapeutic environment
	18. To facilitate awareness of self as an individual with varying physical, emotional, and developmental needs
Restorative care needs	19. To accept the optimum possible goals in the light of limitations, physical and emotional
	20. To use community resources as an aid in resolving problems arising from illness
	21. To understand the role of social problems as influencing factors in the cause of illness

ministered in two selected sites.[28] The two sites selected for study were the gluteus maximus muscle and the vastus lateralis muscle.

Definition

Pain is seen as a specific sensation with a special and separate mechanism for the detection and transmission of pain impulses. A distinct feeling state accompanies the sensation. The sensation and the feeling state together constitute the pain experience.

The investigators make an intensive review of the literature and were able to identify the following postulates (concepts) that had bearing on their research.

Postulates

1. Each structure such as skin, subcutaneous tissue, fascia, muscle, periosteum, bone, and blood vessels has a characteristic pain sensation.
2. Each structural category demonstrates specific variations within its group which are consistent from individual to individual.
3. Pain threshold does not vary markedly from person to person, but there are certain localized conditions that will modify it in the individual.
4. Diseases of the nervous system modify the cutaneous sensitivity.
5. Muscles differ in their relative sensitiveness in the same individual. Deep muscle pain can modify the cutaneous pain threshold purely by reason of the fact that in certain instances both may be served by the same set of nerves.

A patient's previous experience with pain will have a decided effect upon the patient's response.

The investigators hypothesized the following deductions:

Deductions[29]

There is no difference in the frequency with which pain occurs concomitant to an initial injection of a given medication into the inner aspect of the upper outer quadrant of the gluteus maximus muscle as compared with the frequency with which it occurs during a simi-

lar injection into the longitudinal midpoint of the vastus lateralis muscle as reported by the patient.

There is no difference in the frequency with which pain occurs concomitant to an initial injection of a given medication into the inner aspects of the upper outer quadrant of the gluteus maximus muscle at 6:00 A.M. as compared with the frequency with which it occurs during a similar injection given at 6:00 P.M. in the same site as reported by patients.

There is no difference in the frequency with which pain occurs concomitant to an initial injection of a given medication into the longitudinal midpoint of the vastus lateralis muscle at 6:00 A.M. as compared with the frequency with which it occurs during a similar injection given at 6:00 P.M. in the same site as reported by patients.

Model for Study of Aggression

As in the physical sciences, questions essential for formulating the problems of the social sciences have greater relevancy if they stem from a sound theoretical framework. A nurse investigator majoring in anthropology was interested in the problem of aggression, specifically the way in which it is controlled in primitive societies.[30] Understanding this would hopefully give her a better understanding of the ways in which patients suppress and repress drives and needs. A review of the literature showed that although aggression in these societies is rigidly controlled in interpersonal relations, the drive or need remains. Since aggression cannot be expressed freely in interpersonal relations, it must be expressed indirectly, symbolically, and in disguised forms. She further rationalized that religious systems provide for such expressions by the mechanisms of projection, displacement, and rationalization.

A further spelling out of the rationale or theoretical framework led the investigator to formulate the following hypothesis: The greater the control over the expression of aggression in interpersonal relations by the member in societies, the greater the expression of aggression in religious practices and beliefs.

Religion was defined as a set of beliefs and practices with respect to supernaturals that the members of a society report and/or that the investigator observes.

Model for Study of Emotional Stress

Another example of formulating a theoretical framework for a problem utilizing social science concepts was a study of patients undergoing major surgery in a general hospital to determine the level of emotional tension preoperatively and postoperatively.[31] The investigator hoped to differentiate levels of emotional tension in patients undergoing major surgery.

Examples of definitions used in the investigator's framework were:

1. *Anxiety:* An apprehension of threat or danger
2. *Emotional Tension:* Behavioral and physiological reaction to a stress situation.
3. *Stress:* Type of stimuli most likely to arouse anxiety in most individuals.
4. *Stress situation:* A circumstance in which adjustment is difficult or impossible, but in which motivation is very strong.

Postulates were also stated that helped to show the derivation of such concepts as: Surgery is almost uniformly a source of stress depending on how the patient perceives it.

Individuals react differently to stress. Most patients are fearful of surgery although they may not express this fear.

All human behavior is purposeful and goal seeking; it is energized by tension and anxiety; it is designed wittingly or unwittingly in terms of how an individual perceives himself in relation to others and in terms of skills and abilities that he brings into play when his personality is threatened and requires that he defend himself. These behaviors require transformation of energy derived from tension and/or anxiety.[32]

This led to the deduction that "it is possible to differentiate levels of emotional ten-

sion in preoperative and postoperative patients."

Conceptual Framework for Study of the Role of the Public Health Nurse

Faced with the problem of evaluating the readiness of a student to assume the role of a practicing public health nurse, investigators first divided the role into components and then developed a means of assessing these components.[33] To develop a framework for the study of the role of the public health nurse required a definition of the role.

An expectations file was developed to provide a picture of the complexity of the role of the public health nurse. A coding system was developed to use the information in the expectations file. The approach used by the investigators in searching for criteria for evaluation could form the basis for a research of the public health nurse and nursing.

Framework for the Study of the Role of the Public Health Nurse

I. Counter Position Holding Expectation

A. Staff public health nurse.
B. Public health nurse director, consultant, or supervisor.
C. Nurse educator.
D. Professional nursing organizations (when the organization, rather than an identifiable counter position within the organization, expresses an expectation) and nurses other than public health nurses.
E. Community service agencies —including Department of Welfare, Tuberculosis Association, Cancer Society, Family Service Society, Mental Health Association, Crippled Children's Society, Urban League, and Health Department personnel exclusive of nurses and health officers.
F. Health officers.
G. Physicians, other than health officers.

H. Principals or teachers (public schools).
I. Patients.
J. Families of patients and other members of household.
K. Other consumers, including community groups and community leaders.
L. Members of allied professions not mentioned above, such as psychologists, sociologists, and anthropologists.
M. Miscellaneous, including USPHS and State Board of Health when the specific counter position cannot be identified.

II. Statement of Expectation or Behavior
  A. The *types* of expectation or behavior are:
    1. Nursing service for particular patients or family. (Examples: Talk to patients about low calorie diet. Give skilled nursing care to arthritic patients.)
    2. Nursing service or general nursing procedures transcending individual cases. (Examples: Interpret local health regulations. Take an active part in classroom teaching.)
    3. Policies relating the public health nurse to other professionals and community workers in ways neither directly concerned with patient or family care nor to general nursing procedures. Anything concerned with smooth, organized functioning of interdisciplinary and interprofessional groups. (Examples: Interpret to appropriate groups the health and welfare needs of the community. Hold meetings to discuss work of teachers and nurses in order to obtain closer working relationship.)
    4. Activities of public health nurses not directly related to patient or family care, and not primarily concerned with interprofessional relationships. Activities that are related to intraprofessional affairs, civic affairs, research or professional development of individ-

ual nurse. (Examples: Work through professional organizations for the advancement and improvement of public health nursing. Study and evaluate own job performance.)
    5. Knowledge and attributes assumed to be necessary for action in above categories and miscellaneous expectations. (Examples: Should be able to recognize deviations from normal growth and development. Should have the ability to help others help themselves.)
  B. The *sorts of skills* primarily involved are:
    1. Technical nursing skills. (Examples: Visit tuberculosis patients in the home to demonstrate and supervise care. Visit the chronically ill at home to give injections.)
    2. Skill in motivating an individual or face-to-face group to adopt a course of action. (Examples: Encourage arthritic to do as much for himself as possible. Plan, with patient, ways of meeting long-term medical needs.)
    3. Skill in convincing a large group to adopt a course of action, by such means as lectures, written communiques, etc. (Examples: Make a talk to the whole school on accident prevention. Take every opportunity to influence public opinion against taking mental patients to jail pending hospitalization.)
    4. Skill in applying medical or other scientific knowledge in a situation that is primarily noninstructional, such as ability to discuss patient's health problems with M.D. or others, or ability to refer to M.D. or others, when basic aim is not to motivate a course of action. (Examples: Work with teachers on psychological problems of pupils. Observe, evaluate, and report to the physician patient's reaction to drugs and treatment.)
    5. Skill in giving instruction when the primary purpose is to increase

knowledge or understanding rather than to motivate a course of action. (Examples: Explain hospital admission procedures, rules, and regulations to family of hospitalized mental patient. Interpret public health nursing to the community.)

6. Skill in gathering information—active or passive —regardless of its purpose. (Examples: Take histories on psychiatric patients. Find out why patient is reluctant to attend clinic.)

7. Other skills whose nature cannot be determined from the statement. (Examples: Establish rapport with the patient. Work with the patient, not for him.)

8. Any combination of the above when one skill does not seem predominant.

C. The *values* that underlie the expectations and behaviors are:

1. Direct service to particular patients or families. (Example: Explain dietary regulations to diabetic patient. Give family health counseling.)

2. Deemphasis of individual health problems or emphasis on community health. (Examples: Apply measures for prevention and control of communicable diseases. Cooperate with professional groups in analyzing community health needs.)

3. Service to the nursing profession, and professional development of the individual nurse. (Examples: Work through professional organizations for advancement and improvement of nursing. Keep in touch with the newest developments in medicine and nursing.)

4. Advancement of the healing arts and improvement of health and welfare services. (Examples: Participate in developing methods for coordinating nursing service. Plan with other health personnel in order to secure completeness and continuity of service to families and individuals.)

5. Other, including any combination of the above.

D. The expectation or behavior refers to patients of the age group:
1. Premature.
2. Infant.
3. Preschool.
4. School.
5. Adult.
6. Old age.
7. All ages.

E. The expectation or behavior refers to the patient's condition or situation of:
1. Venereal disease.
2. Tuberculosis.
3. Communicable disease (other than above).
4. AP and PP.
5. Chronic disease, including cancer.
6. Orthopedics.
7. Mental health.
8. Disaster.
9. Accident prevention and safety education.
10. General health.
11. Vision, speech, and hearing.
12. Dental health.

III. Counter Position with which Nurse Interacts in Fulfilling Expectation

Same counter positions as listed under I.

IV. How Expectations are Transmitted to Nurse

A. By face-to-face interaction between nurse and counter position holding expectation. (Example: A teacher tells the public health nurse of some expectation she—the teacher—holds.)

B. Directly from the counter position holding the expectation via literature or lecture. (Example: A nurse educator writes of her expectations for public health nurses.)

C. Indirectly, via another counter position in face-to-face interaction. (Example: The supervisor tells a staff

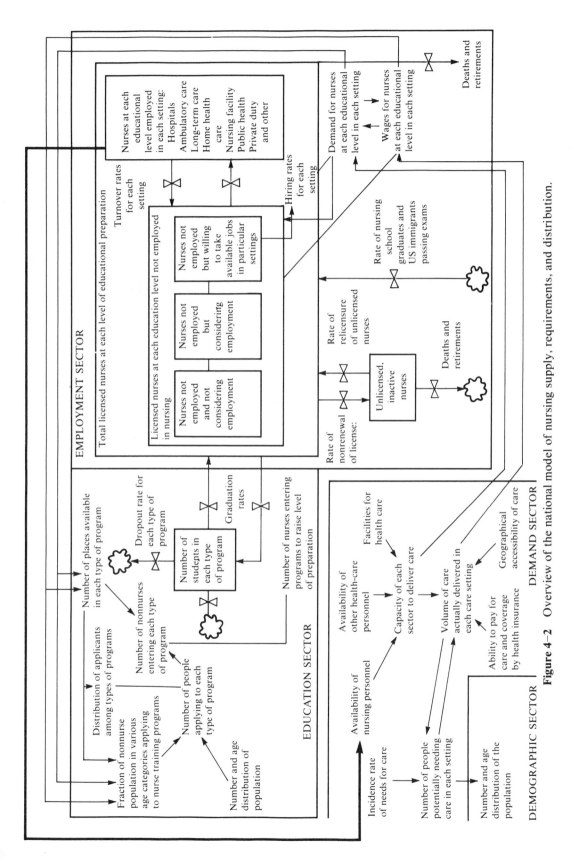

Figure 4-2 Overview of the national model of nursing supply, requirements, and distribution.

EMPLOYMENT SECTOR

Total licensed nurses at each level of educational preparation

Nurses at each educational level employed in each setting:
Hospitals
Ambulatory care
Long-term care
Home health care
Nursing facility
Public health
Private duty and other

Turnover rates for each setting

Demand for nurses at each educational level in each setting

Wages for nurses at each educational level in each setting

Deaths and retirements

Hiring rates for each setting

Rate of nursing school graduates and US immigrants passing exams

Licensed nurses at each education level not employed in nursing

Nurses not employed but willing to take available jobs in particular settings

Nurses not employed but considering employment

Nurses not employed and not considering employment

Rate of relicensure of unlicensed nurses

Rate of nonrenewal of license:

Unlicensed, inactive nurses

Deaths and retirements

EDUCATION SECTOR

Number of places available in each type of program

Dropout rate for each type of program

Graduation rates

Distribution of applicants among types of programs

Number of nonnurses entering each type

Number of students in each type of program

Number of nurses entering programs to raise level of preparation

Fraction of nonnurse population in various age categories applying to nurse training programs

Number of people applying to each type of program

Number and age distribution of population

DEMAND SECTOR

Facilities for health care

Availability of other health-care personnel

Capacity of each sector to deliver care

Volume of care actually delivered in each care setting

Geographical accessibility of care

Availability of nursing personnel

Ability to pay for care and coverage by health insurance

Incidence rate of needs for care

Number of people potentially needing care in each setting

Number and age distribution of the population

DEMOGRAPHIC SECTOR

69

nurse of some expectation of the health officer.)

D. Indirectly, via another counter person, through literature or lecture. (Example: An article by a sociologist regarding the expectations social workers hold for the public health nurse.)

E. Self-expectation of the nurse.

A Model of Nursing Supply, Requirements, and Distribution

In an ambitious attempt to construct a comprehensive model of nursing supply and requirements, the technique of "system dynamics" was applied to the important variables impacting on nursing manpower and likely to impact in the future.[34] A major use of such a model is to analyze the effect of changes in these variables on the supply, demand, and distribution of nursing personnel and services. With the current emphasis on health planning, such analysis can help in the formulation of policy decisions concerning nursing manpower. (See Figure 4–2.)

The model's relationships are grouped into four main sectors:

- *Nursing education:* Representing the factors affecting the number of students in each major type of educational program and the graduation rates from these programs.
- *Nursing employment:* Representing the factors affecting the number of nurses employed in each setting and various characteristics of employment in each setting such as nurses' wages and nurses' roles.
- *Demand:* Representing the health care provided in each sector of the health-care-delivery system, nursing needs, and nursing jobs available in each employment setting.
- *Demographic:* Representing key demographic characteristics of the total population that impact on other sectors of the model, principally the demand sector.

The model is useful for the United States as a whole, although it could, with further development, be made applicable for smaller geographic areas. Such a model with a vast database and a complex computing program requires sophisticated computer resources. In fact, this model is an excellent example of a family of models (this one based on a technique known as simulation) made possible by the development of high-speed electronic computers.

SUMMARY

A major deterrent to nursing research is the lack of a conceptual framework for the proposed research. The development of a theory for nursing research is the most direct way of systematizing knowledge founded on a broad base.

A scientific theory is composed of operational definitions, postulates, and deductions. A few direct attempts have been made to develop theoretical models in the health field, but, much still needs to be done.

The building of a scientific theory for nursing research will directly affect the degree to which the nursing profession progresses in defining a scientific body of knowledge that is uniquely nursing.

REFERENCES

1. Robert K. Merton, Leonard Broom, and Leonard S. Cottrell, Jr. (eds.), *Sociology Today.* New York, Basic Books, Inc., 1959, p. ix.
2. *Ibid.*, p. xiii.
3. Faye G. Abdellah *et al., Patient Centered Approaches to Nursing,* New York, Macmillan Publishing Co., Inc., 1960.
4. Joan Scialli Bilitski, "Nursing Science and the Laws of Health: The Test of Substance as a Step in the Process of Theory Development." *Advances Nursing Sci.,* 4(1): 15–29, October 1981.
5. Florence S. Downs, (Editorial) "Dig We Must." *Nursing Res.,* 33(5): 254, September/October 1984.
6. Claire Selltiz, Marie Jahoda, Morton Deutsch, and Stuart W. Cook, *Research Methods in Social Relations.* New York, Holt, Rinehart and Winston, Inc., 1962, p. 481.
7. R. B. Braithwaite, *Scientific Explanation: A Study of the Functions of Theory, Probability and Law in Science.* Cambridge, England, Cambridge University, 1955.

8. C. S. Peirce, *Selected Writings of Charles S. Peirce,* "Values in a Universe of Chance," edited by Philip Wiener. New York, Doubleday and Co., Inc., 1958.

9. Robert M. W. Travers, *An Introduction to Educational Research.* New York, Macmillan Publishing Co., Inc., 1958.

10. *Ibid.,* p. 22.

11. Florence S. Wald and Robert C. Leonard, "Towards Development of Nursing Practice Theory." *Nursing Res.,* 13:309–313, fall 1964.

12. Jeanette Lancaster, "Bonding of Nursing Practice and Education Through Research." *Nursing and Health Care,* 5(7):379–382, September 1984.

13. Wade Lancaster and Jeanette Lancaster, "Models and Model Building in Nursing." *Nursing Education: Practice Methods and Models,* Rockville, Md., Aspen Press, 1980, pp. 37–48.

14. *Ibid.,* p. 39.

15. Rosemary Crow, "Frontiers of Nursing in the Twenty-First Century: Development of Models and Theories on the Concept of Nursing." *J. Advanced Nursing,* 7(2):115. March 1982.

16. Susan L. Craig, "Theory Development and Its Relevance for Nursing." *J. Advanced Nursing,* 5(4):341–355, July 1980.

17. *Ibid.,* p. 351.

18. Rosemarie J. Collins and John H. Fielder, "Beckstrand's Concept of Practice Theory: A Critique." *Res. in Nursing and Health,* 4(3):517–521, September 1981.

19. Susan E. Runtz and J. G. Urtel, "Evaluating Your Practice Via a Nursing Model." *Nurse Practitioner,* 8(3):30–32, 37–40, March 1983.

20. Marilyn Edmunds, "Models of Clinical Practice." *Nurse Practitioner,* 8(9):59–64, October 1983.

21. Horace B. English and Ava Champney English, *A Comprehensive Dictionary of Psychological and Psychoanalytical Terms.* New York, Longmans, Green and Co., 1958, p. 326.

22. Donald P. Hayes and Robert K. Leik, "A Reaction Model." University of Washington (unpublished paper), 1962.

23. *Ibid.*

24. Everett C. Hughes, Helen Hughes, and Irwin Deutscher, *Twenty-Thousand Nurses Tell Their Story.* Philadelphia, J. B. Lippincott Co., 1958.

25. Faye G. Abdellah, "Criterion Measures in Nursing." *Nursing Res.,* 10:21–26, winter 1961.

26. Robert M. W. Travers, *op. cit.,* p. 27.

27. Faye G. Abdellah *et al., Patient-Centered Approaches to Nursing,* New York, Macmillan Publishing Co., Inc., 1960.

28. Marie Haddad and Vivian Holdsworth, "A Proposed Research Design." A project submitted in partial fulfillment of the course requirements of *Nursing 570a,* University of Washington, 1960.

29. *Ibid.,* pp. 1–2.

30. Lorraine Phillips, "Aggression and Religious Beliefs and Practices—A Proposed Research Design." A project submitt of the course requirements versity of Washington, 19

31. Marie L. Sadlick, "A Stud ing Major Surgery in a Ge mine the Level of Emo Post-operatively." A proj project submitted in partial ... course requirements of *Nursing 570a,* University of Washington, 1960.

32. Hildegard E. Peplau, *Interpersonal Relations in Nursing.* New York, G. P. Putnam's Sons, 1952, p. 132.

33. Ann C. Hansen and Harry S. Upshaw. "Evaluation Within the Context of Role Analysis." *Nursing Res.,* 11:144–150, summer 1962.

34. Tom Bergan and Gary Hirsch, "A National Model of Supply, Demand and Distribution." Summary Report. Boulder, CO, The Western Interstate Commision on Higher Education, 1976.

SUGGESTIONS FOR FURTHER READING

1. Myrtle Irene Brown, "Research in the Development of Nursing Theory." *Nursing Res.,* 13:109–112, spring 1964.

2. John Dewey, *How We Think.* New York, D. C. Heath Co., 1910.

3. Jean Baptiste Joseph Fourier, "Analytical Theory of Heat," *Great Books of the Western World,* Vol. 45. Chicago, Encyclopaedia Britannica, Inc., 1952, pp. 169–172.

4. David J. Fox, "A Proposed Model for Identifying Research Areas in Nursing." *Nursing Res.,* 13:29–36, winter 1964.

5. C. G. Hempel, "Fundamentals of Concept Formation in Empirical Science." *International Encyclopaedia of the Unified Science,* Vol. 2, No. 7. Chicago, University of Chicago Press, 1952.

6. Ada Jacox, "Theory Construction in Nursing: An Overview." *Nursing Res.,* 23:4–13, January–February 1974.

7. Dorothy E. Johnson, "Development of Theory: A Requisite for Nursing as a Primary Health Profession." *Nursing Res.,* 23:372–377, September–October 1974.

8. Immanuel Kant, "The Critique of Pure Reason," *Great Books of the Western World,* Vol. 42. Chicago, Encyclopaedia Britannica, Inc., 1952, pp. 68–69, 179–182.

9. Sir Isaac Newton, "Mathematical Principles of Natural Philosophy," *Great Books of the Western World,* Vol. 34. Chicago, Encyclopaedia Britannica, Inc., 1952, pp. 5–24.

10. Ida Jean Orlando, *The Dynamic Nurse-Patient Relationship. Function, Process and Principles.* New York, G. P. Putnam's Sons, 1961.

11. Hildegard E. Peplau, *Basic Principles of Patient*

Counseling. Philadelphia, Smith, Kline and French Laboratories, 1964.

12. Walter R. Reitman, "Information-Processing Models in Psychology." *Science,* **144:**1192–1198, 1963.

13. P. D. Reynolds, *A Primer in Theory Construction.* Indianapolis, Bobbs-Merrill, 1971.

14. Joan P. Riehl and Sister Callista Roy, *Conceptual Models for Nursing Practice.* New York, Appleton-Century-Crofts, 1974.

Definitive Works of Theorists

1. Florence Nightingale, *Notes on Nursing: What It Is and What It is Not.* Boston, William Carter, 1860.

2. Hildegard E. Peplau, *Interpersonal Relations in Nursing.* New York, G. P. Putnam's Sons, 1952.

3. Faye G. Abdellah *et al., Patient Centered Approaches to Nursing.* New York, Macmillan Publishing Co., Inc., 1960.

4. Faye G. Abdellah and Eugene Levine, *Effect of Nurse Staffing on Satisfaction with Nursing Care.* Hospital monograph series, No. 4, Chicago, American Hospital Association, 1958.

5. Faye G. Abdellah *et al., New Directions in Patient-Centered Nursing: Guidelines for Systems of Service, Education, and Research.* New York, Macmillan Publishing Co., Inc., 1973.

6. Ida Jean Orlando, *The Dynamic Nurse-Patient Relationship: Function, Process, and Principles.* New York, G. P. Putnam's Sons, 1961.

7. Ida Jean Orlando, *The Discipline and Teaching of Nursing Process: An Evaluation Study.* New York, G. P. Putnam's Sons, 1972.

8. Ernestine Wiedenbach, *Clinical Nursing: A Helping Art.* New York, Springer Publishing Co., Inc., 1964.

9. Lydia E. Hall, "Another View of Nursing Care and Quality," in K. M. Straub and K. S. Parker (eds.), *Continuity of Patient Care: The Role of Nursing.* Washington, D.C., Catholic University Press, 1966, pp. 47–60.

10. Virginia Henderson, *The Nature of Nursing, a Definition and Its Implications for Practice, Research, and Education.* New York, Macmillan Publishing Co., Inc., 1966.

11. Myra E. Levine, "Adaptation and Assessment: A Rationale for Nursing Intervention." *Am. J. Nursing,* **66**(11):2450–2453, November 1966.

12. Myra E. Levine, "The Four Conservation Principles of Nursing." *Nursing Forum,* **6**(1):45–59, January 1967.

13. Myra E. Levine, "The Pursuit of Wholeness." *Am. J. Nursing,* **69**(1):93–98, January 1969.

14. Martha E. Rogers, *An Introduction to the Theoretical Basis of Nursing.* Philadelphia, F. A. Davis Co., 1970.

15. Martha E. Rogers, "Nursing: A Science of Unitary Man," in J. P. Riehl and Sr. C. Roy (eds.), *Conceptual Models for Nursing Practice* (2nd ed.). New York, Appleton-Century-Crofts, 1980, pp. 329–337.

16. Dorethea E. Orem, *Nursing: Concepts of Practice.* New York, McGraw-Hill Book Co., Inc., 1971; 2nd ed., 1980.

17. Imogene M. King, *Toward A Theory for Nursing: General Concepts of Human Behavior.* New York, John Wiley and Sons, Inc., 1971.

18. Imogene M. King, *A Theory for Nursing: Systems, Concepts, Process.* New York, John Wiley and Sons, Inc., 1981.

19. Sister Callista Roy, *Introduction to Nursing: An Adaptation Model.* Englewood Cliffs, NJ, Prentice-Hall, Inc., 1976.

20. Sister Callista Roy, "An Adaptation Model," in J. P. Riehl and Sr. C. Roy (eds.), *Conventional Models for Nursing Practice* (2nd ed.). New York, Appleton-Century Crofts, 1980, pp. 179–188.

21. Sister Callista Roy and S. Roberts, *Theory Construction in Nursing: An Adaptation Model.* Englewood Cliffs, NJ, Prentice-Hall, Inc., 1981.

22. J. G. Paterson and L. T. Zderad, *Humanistic Nursing.* New York, John Wiley and Sons, 1976.

23. M. M. Leininger, *Transcultural Nursing: Concepts, Theories, and Practices.* New York, John Wiley and Sons, Inc., 1978.

24. J. Watson, *Nursing: The Philosophy and Science of Caring.* Boston, Little, Brown and Co., 1979.

TWO

STEPS IN THE RESEARCH PROCESS

CHAPTER

5

Overview of the Research Process

There are a variety of research purposes, aims, settings, and subjects just as there are a variety of ways of conducting a study. Although there is no one right way to pursue a study, there is a definite sequence of recognizable steps that most researchers take in conducting projects. Because research is a planned and systematic activity, these steps must be thought out before launching the study. The steps must be described in a document that will serve as the plan for guiding the research activity. A written research plan, called a research proposal, is mandatory when applying for a financial grant to do research or in fulfilling the requirements for a doctoral degree and it is a valuable document to have in all instances where research is undertaken. By spelling out the research plan in advance, it can be evaluated and improved before the project is launched.

This chapter presents the various elements to be considered in developing the research plan. Once determined, these elements become the specifications by which the study is carried out.

Not every research project requires consideration of all the steps in the research process. In methodological and descriptive studies, certain steps need not be taken.

The twelve major steps are listed in order of the logical development of a project:

1. Select the topic and formulate the problem.
2. Review the literature.
3. Formulate the framework of theory.
4. Formulate hypotheses.
5. Define the variables and determine how they will be quantified.
6. Develop the research design.
7. Define the study population and sample.
8. Determine how to collect the data.

KEY POINT

9. Determine how to process and summarize data.
10. Formulate data analysis.
11. Formulate interpretation of data.
12. Determine the method of communicating results.

In developing the research plan, it is not an absolute rule that each section must be fully complete before moving to the next. It is reasonable to expect that ideas developed in one part may lead to changes and improvements in another. One must always be alert to the impact of new information and have the flexibility to change currently held ideas, recognizing that resolution of the interplay of ideas is part of the developmental process. While all steps are not applicable to all types of research, such processes as formulating the problem, reviewing the literature, and defining the variables must occur in all studies.

Equal time and effort need not be devoted to each step. In some studies the major part of the research effort may be necessary in the early stages—the intellectual process of formulating and defining the problem, the framework of theory, the hypotheses, and the variables. In others most of the time is spent on the more active processes of collecting and analyzing the data. Explanatory studies often fall into the first category, whereas descriptive studies are more likely to be of the second kind. In some descriptive studies, particularly nonexperimental field surveys, as much as 90 per cent of the total research effort may be devoted to collection and analysis of data.

In developing the research plan all the steps must be carefully thought out; the success of the research project heavily depends on the quality of the plan. Development of the plan is a process of continuous refinement of various elements of the study. First, the researcher outlines the specifications of the steps. These are then thoroughly analyzed, expanded, and rewritten. When the plan is developed as far as the researcher can take it without actually trying out all or parts of the plan, the *pretest* stage is reached. Here the methodology for collecting data is tested using the same types of research subjects and creating the same kind of environment as in the study. The results of the pretest are carefully examined against the elements of the plan, revised if necessary, and final polishing is done. When the researcher is satisfied that he has gone about as far as he can in perfecting the plan, the study is ready to be launched.

The development of a research plan is a process of moving back and forth through the different steps and continuously refining until no further improvement is possible. The plan may not be ideal; in such research areas as nursing and patient care compromises often have to be made in order to conduct the project. For example, if the ideal research plan requires one thousand patients with a certain disease as study subjects, and if it would take ten years to accumulate data on such a large population, it would be practical to reduce the number of subjects, even if it meant sacrificing accuracy in results.

It is understandable that there is often an urge to complete the passive phase of developing the plan as quickly as possible. However, it cannot be stressed too strongly that time spent on constructing an efficient and workable research plan contributes significantly to the success of the project. A project hastily conceived and poorly designed defeats the entire effort.

The remainder of this chapter will briefly discuss each of the major steps in conducting a research study. In the next part of this book the steps will be more fully discussed in separate chapters.

TOPIC SELECTION, PROBLEM FORMULATION, AND LITERATURE REVIEW

Select a Topic

The first step in the research process: select a topic. Topics for research arise in various ways. For the student a topic may be suggested by his instructor. Professional researchers who conduct research on request, either as paid employees of the agency initiating the research or as members of a research institute, also perform studies on topics selected by others.

Most research is conducted on topics selected by the researcher, although the general area of the research may be suggested by the knowledge of pressing problems.

Some believe that dictated research—the topic is selected by others—weakens an important characteristic of research—intellectual curiosity. If the content of the research is dictated by others, curiosity and interest may be replaced by the drive to get the job done.

Formulate the Problem

Many research topics are so complex and present so many difficulties in design and execution that they cannot be successfully carried out as a solo activity or in a piecemeal fashion. It becomes necessary for a research team to pursue the topic. As a member of a team, the individual may have little influence on the selection of the topic or on other important decisions made in formulating the plan. This is a far cry from the appealing picture often evoked of the lone worker who not only selects his own topic, formulates the problem, and establishes the theoretical framework, but collects, tabulates, analyzes his own data, and, of course, astounds the world with a remarkable discovery.

In small, well-circumscribed studies, it is still possible to pursue research as a solo effort. Doctoral dissertations represent one example, but even here some studies are done as a group activity. A team approach is often necessary, particularly where the research deals with complex phenomena, cuts across several intellectual disciplines, requires large amounts of data, and has potential application in a number of fields. Interest of the team member must be generated and sustained by means different from the satisfactions accruing to the lone worker. How to motivate the efforts of a research team will be discussed in a later chapter.

Review the Literature

Review of the literature is essential to the development of a research project for several reasons. First, it reveals previous work in the problem area, relieving the researcher of the necessity of repeating those aspects of the research where sufficient knowledge already exists. Of course, if the knowledge from prior research is tentative, equivocal, or incomplete, there is justification in repeating the study in its entirety, called *replication*. Second, review of the literature should show whether it is feasible to do the planned research by revealing difficulties encountered by previous researchers. Third, review of other research designs can uncover promising methodological tools, shed light on ways to improve efficiency of data collection, and provide useful advice on how to increase effectiveness of data analysis. Fourth, but certainly not least, literature review can be the link between findings of previous research and postulated results of the proposed study. Only by relating the findings from one study to the next can we hope to establish a comprehensive body of scientific knowledge in a professional discipline from which valid and pertinent theories might be established.

The objectives of the literature review in the total process should always be kept in mind. Essentially, the objectives are to see what previous researchers in the same area have discovered and to find out which kinds of methodology have proved useful. Consideration of extraneous material, as interesting as it may be, can be wasteful and can retard the development and execution of the project.

THEORY, HYPOTHESIS, AND VARIABLES

Formulate the Framework of Theory

The formulation of a theoretical basis or framework for a study is frequently not given adequate consideration. In many studies reported in the literature only passing reference is made to underlying theory. One of the reasons for this situation in nursing studies is the relative newness of the research effort and the recency of attempts to place the discipline of nursing on a scientific footing. Much of what composes the body of knowledge known as nursing is a collection of unrelated empirical facts, practical advice, and material from the fields of medicine, physiology, and psychology. As nursing matures intellectually, so will theories of nursing.

What is a theory and how does it assist the research project? A theory is a general statement, formulated from the observation of relationships among phenomena, that explains or summarizes those relationships in a verifiable way.

A theory is not a hypothesis, a speculation, or a guess. A theory must be proved to be correct, either by formal research or by some other form of systematic observation.

Many years ago a theory was considered to be final and immutable. Now, all scientific theories, even the theory of relativity, are subject to revision as new knowledge emerges. Theories in the social sciences are especially subject to change. One of the functions of research is to revise or reformulate existing theory, which often has not provided satisfactory explanation of phenomena, by producing new knowledge.

To be truly useful theories must correspond meaningfully to that aspect of the real world which they describe. An important test of the adequacy of a theory is its relevance. Often theories in the natural sciences can be tested in terms of how well they work when practically applied. In the social sciences such empirical validation is sometimes not possible. Without validation, theory construction can degenerate into an intellectual exercise that consists of playing with words.

Formulate Hypotheses

The design of a study begins with the formulation of hypotheses, which provide guidance for the investigator as to kinds of data needed as well as the method for analyzing the data. The previous stages of the process—that is, selecting the topic, formulating the problem, reviewing the literature, and establishing the framework of theory—provide the background. These are, of course, essential steps in the process, but they have less direct impact on the data than do the hypotheses.

Hypotheses can be defined as *statements of the expected relationship(s) among the phenomena being studied.* In the language of research these phenomena are called variables. A variable can be defined as a *quality, property or characteristic of the persons or things being studied that can be quantitatively measured or enumerated.* Hypotheses then are speculations on how the variables in the study behave. The object of the study is to find out whether this speculation is correct. The purpose of the study is to test the hypotheses. Once tested and proven true, a hypothesis may then be incorporated into a theory. In most science the corroboration of many studies may be needed to verify the status of a hypothesis. Moreover, many hypotheses tested in research represent only a piece of a whole theory. All parts of the theory must be tested to provide a composite meaningful whole.

Define the Variables and Determine How They Will be Quantified

In explanatory studies, the hypotheses contain statements of the dependent and independent variables, known as the explanatory variables. In descriptive studies, in the absence of explicit hypotheses, the research plan should clearly state the variables to be investigated. In many studies, descriptive as well as explanatory, data are often collected for variables that are not really explanatory variables, but nevertheless are of interest to the researcher. There are organismic variables—age, sex, marital status, education, occupation, and so on. In reporting the findings of a study, data on these variables provide background information on the composition of the study group and are helpful in interpreting the findings on the main explanatory variables.

As part of the plan, skeleton outlines of statistical tables for the data must be prepared. Such table outlines, called dummy tables, show the different variables for which data will be collected. Variables appearing in these tables must be carefully defined.

KEY POINT The definition of variables has to be completed before any data are collected. Defining variables is a process of making them meaningful, concrete, and unambiguous in order to achieve an operational definition. An operational definition is a series of words which clearly designate performable and observable actions that can be verified by others.

The term "patient welfare" by itself is not an operational definition of a variable because it does not represent an observable act that can be verified by independent observers. One operational definition of patient welfare might be the number of times a day the patient rings his call-bell. Here, it is possible to make reliable observations. However, the question may be raised as to whether this is a *meaningful* definition of patient welfare. A low frequency of ringing the call-bell might not necessarily be indicative of good patient welfare, nor would a high frequency of ringing mean that the level of patient welfare was low. Many other definitions of patient welfare are possible; some are physiological, others psychological, and still others sociological. Ways of determining the most valid, reliable and meaningful definitions of variables are found in Chapter 10. The importance of this step cannot be stressed too much, since the way the variables are defined determines how they will be measured and how data concerning them will be collected.

Because much research in nursing deals with quantitative observations of variables, it is necessary to define variables in a way that they can be measured according to a numerical scale. By definition, every variable has a theoretical underlying scale of value, ranging from one extreme to another. The example of an operational definition of patient welfare—the number of times a day the call-bell is rung—is in quantitative form. The scale could range from zero times a day to an upper limit of, say, 100.

The value of quantifying data in research is self-evident. One value is the ability to apply meaningful tools of statistical analysis when the data are in numerical form. Not all research deals with quantified data. Anthropological research as well as some types of sociological studies often have no numerical data, instead depending on verbal descriptions and other types of narrative data. Case studies, whether of people, institutions, communities, or whole societies, are largely composed of anecdotal data.

Quantification of the variables can vary from a simple procedure, demanding little or no technical skill, to a highly involved process of measurement requiring specialized technicians. At its simplest, quantification of variables is merely a matter of recording the number of times something occurs according to a straightforward classification scale. In the example of the use of the call-bell as an indication of patient welfare, the classification scale counts each time the bell is rung. At the end of the day the total occurrences of bell ringing are determined for each patient.

At the other extreme, patient welfare can be operationally defined as a complex psychological phenomenon requiring measurement through a battery of tests. Such measurement might require the skills of specialized psychometricians, particularly if the tests did not already exist.

For many variables a scale of measurement already exists and, if found to be applicable to the study, can be used by the researcher even though not developed especially for it. Where the scale of measurement is a classification of variables into discrete categories in which the frequency of occurrence of each class is measured by counting, the scale classes are often established through traditional use and are similar in study after study. Thus, the variable *sex* has two classes: male, female; the variable *marital status,* four classes: single, married, widowed, divorced or separated; the variable *hair color,* four classes: black, brown, blond, red; and so on. But even if prior studies have not established the classification scale, some variables are so obviously defined for quantification purposes that little difficulty is presented. Thus, if patient welfare is defined in terms of how many times a patient uses tranquilizing or pain-killing drugs, an expert in measurement is not needed.

RESEARCH DESIGN, POPULATION, AND SAMPLING

Develop the Research Design

Defining variables and determining how they will be quantified is another stage in refining the research problem. When the variables have been defined as precisely as possible, and the methods of quantification determined, the researcher can consider the type of research design he will use although this does not mean that definition of variables is complete. The goal of the development of a valid and workable plan can be attained only by carefully polishing the steps until no further improvement can be envisioned. Definition of variables and determination of how to quantify them will be influenced by later stages of the process and will be modified by decisions made during them.

KEY POINT Determination of the research design is an important decision because the type of design employed affects each step of the total process. Determination of the research design involves choosing the method by which the study subjects shall be selected, controlled, and, in experimental studies, assigned to the various experimental groups. Two main types of research design are: experimental and nonexperimental. In the experimental method the researcher controls all the conditions of the study. In nonexperimental research, called "surveys," the researcher has considerably less control over subjects and setting. Experimental research at its most controlled is conducted in a specialized research setting—laboratory, experimental unit, or research center. Nonexperimental research is frequently conducted in a natural setting—school, public health agency, hospital, or patient's home. The major benefit of the use of a tightly controlled experimental design is the possibility of establishing causal relationships.

There are many kinds of nonexperimental research designs. In one type the main elements of experimental and nonexperimental research are combined and are called *partial or quasi experiments.* Partial experiments may be of the kind where a natural setting is used, e.g., a nursing unit in a hospital, but the researcher exercises some control in the assignment of study subject to study group. Completely nonexperimental designs can be of several types—cross-sectional, retrospective, or prospective. In the *cross-sectional design,* the research dips into the study setting at a given point in time and obtains data on events occurring at that time. A *cross-sectional study* can be made of the amounts of nursing care that patients actually receive during a day according to a classification of their needs for nursing care. In a *retrospective study,* data are collected on past events—before the study design was completed. A retrospective study could be made of what happened to patients discharged from the hospital during the past year. In a *prospective* study, the events upon which data are collected occur after the study design is completed, and the data collection continues over a relatively long period of time and not briefly as in the cross-sectional type of study.

A prospective nonexperimental study could be made of patients discharged from the hospital during the next year. These studies, called *follow-up cohort studies,* are most useful in studying the relationship among independent and dependent variables where the effects of the independent variable may be long-term.

Completely nonexperimental designs can be either descriptive or explanatory. *Historical research* and *case studies* are primarily descriptive and retrospective nonexperimental studies. The term survey is usually applied to a descriptive cross-sectional study but can also be explanatory. *Evaluative research,* a term commonly applied to studies that assess the performance of a product, program, or organization, can be either prospective or retrospective, or a combination of both.

Prospective and retrospective studies are also called *longitudinal studies* because they can extend over a relatively long period of time in contrast to a cross-sectional study, where the time period is of relatively short duration. Since in retrospective studies the events have occurred prior to the study and in some types of retrospective studies the data concerning the events have also already been collected, such studies are often simply a matter of bringing together the data either by means of questionnaires or existing records. It is possible to collect longitudinal data reflecting a patient's medical history spanning many years of his life in the one or two hours that it takes for him to fill out the questionnaire. Likewise the personnel office of a health agency contains data in personnel records that may be useful in research covering a number of years of an employee's work experiences.

By definition, all experimental studies are prospective. Among the advantages of prospective studies is the capability of manipulating variables and observing effects. In the retrospective study of what happened to patients after discharge from the hospital, there was no control by the researcher over the activities of the patient. In the prospective study, the patient's activities can be influenced by establishing, as part of the research, a referral system which may be the independent variable being tested.

Another limitation of retrospective stud-

ies is that the researcher has less control over the definition and measurement of the variables. In a retrospective study of patients' needs for nursing services using existing records and the hospital's own classification of needs, the investigator must accept the definition established by the hospital, which could present serious limitations to the research. Moreover, retrospective studies are limited by availability of data. We could not conduct a retrospective study of patients' needs if the hospital had not already recorded data on this variable. Similarly, we are limited in questioning the job or health history of a person by the recall ability of the respondent.

Research design is concerned with controlling and eliminating the many biases that produce fallacious data. Among these biases are those attributable to extraneous variables. In studies on human beings such variables are especially abundant. One way to control the influences of these variables is by randomization, a key element in experimental design. Much technical writing has been devoted to methods of achieving randomization. These methods will be discussed as well as ways of controlling other sources of possible bias.

The decision to use one type of research design or another is often not a matter of choice for the researcher. Certain kinds of research problems cannot easily be approached through the experimental process. Also the time and effort required to conduct a true experiment are often considerably greater than for a nonexperimental approach. The advantage of the experimental approach is the possibility of being able to establish causal relationships.

Define the Study Population and Sample

A research study must establish a population, or "universe," to which its findings are applicable. This target population may consist of human beings; parts of human beings, such as limbs, teeth, hair; or human characteristics, such as personality, job activities, education; inanimate objects such as refrigerators, schools, or hospitals; abstract concepts such as community attitudes, professional ethics, forms of government; and so on. Moreover, a study population can consist of animals, plants, or other living matter. The individual members of a population are called "sampling units." Each unit must be a discrete entity and independent of all other units. A study usually is done on only a fraction of all the sampling units in the population, and this fraction is called the *sample*. The process of selecting the sample is called *sampling*.

Delineating the target population is another step in narrowing and tightening the research problem. By focusing on the composition of the target population the researcher is forced to analyze the extent to which findings of the study can be extrapolated beyond the sampling units. Does the study refer to all patients in the United States? To all patients in one state? To all patients in one hospital? To only male patients in one hospital? And so on.

The concept of target population is elusive. Even if we were to study all patients in the United States, or in the world, we could do so only during a specific time period. Although the findings of a study today may hold true tomorrow, next year, and even for the next ten years, we must be aware of the limitations imposed by the time specificity of the research in interpreting the results of the study.

KEY POINT

We must recognize that the findings of a single study are restricted by the fact that we have included a limited study population and conducted the study in a particular geographical location and at a particular time in history.

DATA COLLECTION, PROCESSING, AND SUMMARIZING

Determine How to Collect the Data

The next step, after delineating the target population, is to decide how to collect the data. This requires two important decisions. The first: how the study population (sampling units) will be selected. The second: how the data will be collected.

Selection of the study population is done by *sampling*, a technical procedure that is the subject of numerous books and articles in the field of statistical methodology. Unfortunately, in many studies no distinction is drawn between target and study population, so that sampling is not considered in the development of the research plan. What occurs in these studies is that the target population is not clearly defined, and the study population represents a "chunk" of an ill-defined larger population.

The aim in selecting a sample is to obtain a study population that is as *representative* of the total population as possible. The more representative the study population, the greater the accuracy of generalizations made from sample to total population.

A number of techniques are available to the researcher for data collection. Choice of the technique to use in a study depends on the nature of the problem, the kinds of variables, the type of research design, and the type and number of sampling units. Since, in the conduct of a study, collection of data is often the most expensive and time-consuming of all the steps, it is essential that decisions concerning this step be carefully made well in advance. Even if all other steps in the process were carried out perfectly, imperfections in the data-collecting instruments would invalidate the findings.

Determine How to Process and Summarize Data

After the data are collected they must be processed in a way that permits a valid analysis of their meaning. In small studies processing data can be a simple task of combining by hand the data of each sampling unit with the data from all other sampling units. In larger studies, where the number of sampling units is large, or where the number of variables upon which data have been collected are many, or where complete statistical analyses are planned electronic computers must be used for data processing.

It is essential that the method by which the data are to be processed be decided in advance of data collection, since this influences the way in which the data are to be collected. For example, if the data are to be electronically processed, the data-collecting form could be set up to facilitate the transference of data from form to computer tape.

Summarizing data consists of converting raw data into an orderly and "digestible" body of knowledge that can be interpreted meaningfully. It includes a variety of techniques such as summarization of data in tables and charts and computation of summary measures of central tendency and variation of the data.

KEY POINT Statistical analysis of the data after they are collected and summarized is an important part of the research process. This essentially involves the application of statistical techniques to draw inferences from study data to target population. These can be descriptive inferences in which individual characteristics of the population are estimated. Or the inferences can be explanatory, describing the relationship between two or more characteristics (variables).

A broad array of statistical methods are available to the researcher, based upon the *general linear hypothesis,* to analyze relationships among variables. The advent of computers and highly sophisticated "software" has made the most complex analyses possible even on modest "personal" computers. A deep understanding of the theory and computational procedures involved in the calculation of such advanced techniques as multiple regression, multivariate analysis of variance, and path analysis is no longer essential to applying the techniques to research data through the computer.

Sometimes researchers become preoccupied with the computerized statistical analysis of data. Overanalysis may result. After all, it is understanding the meaning of the data that is important, not the joys of manipulating it with marvelous and ingenious programs.

RESULTS INTERPRETATION AND COMMUNICATION

Determine How Results Will Be Interpreted

Interpretation of data consists of relating the findings of the study to the problem, the hypotheses, if appropriate, and the theoretical framework for the study. If the study is descriptive, concerned with the problem of describing the characteristics of patients in nursing homes, for example, interpretation may proceed from a series of questions. What can we conclude from the data collected about the age of patients, their economic status, the reasons they are in nursing homes, and other pertinent facts that will contribute to understanding the problem?

If the study is a test of the hypothesis that seriously ill cardiac patients placed in intensive care units have a lower mortality rate than patients in conventional units, what is the statistical significance of the difference in the rates found? What is the practical significance of the difference? To what extent can we generalize the findings to the target population? To other target populations? To what extent can we generalize our findings into the future? Is there need for additional tests of the same hypothesis to support our findings or disprove them?

Interpretation of data, then, consists of drawing meaning from data. In interpreting data the researcher takes a stand on what **KEY POINT** he feels the data say, their significance and their importance. In interpreting data the investigator can refer to other research and can relate his findings to existing theories and hypotheses. An important function of interpretation is to link the findings of the study to the mainstream of scientific knowledge. Proper and objective assessment of the significance and limitations of his findings will suggest gaps in knowledge that require additional research. This step requires the greatest intellectual activity in order to assure that the value and meaning of findings are maximized.

Determine Method of Communicating Results

The end product of a research study is the report of the findings. It may be a brief paper that contains the main findings, or it may be a publication that reports in great detail.

Unfortunately, much research is never written up or published. One reason is that many otherwise highly competent researchers feel unequal to the task of writing a report and having other researchers challenge their findings. Obviously, a research study can have no impact if results are not communicated to members of the professional field. Communication should take the form of at least one published article in a professional or scientific journal reporting the highlights of the study as well as a complete report available to all interested persons.

KEY POINT

Another reason that some researchers find preparation of the final report so burdensome is that the entire writing task has been left to the end, a time when a great deal of energy has already been expended and interest in the project may have waned. One way to avoid writing the entire report at the end is to prepare intermediate reports —working papers—at the conclusion of each major stage of the project. For example, a working paper could be prepared on the research problem, another on the literature review, another on the research design. Working papers can serve a dual purpose with some of the material becoming part of the final report. Also, working papers can serve as a vehicle for critically reviewing the stages of the development of the project, thereby improving the whole project. Sometimes, individual working papers such as those concerned with reviewing the literature or developing a conceptual framework are of such value that

they may find their way into the published literature prior to completion of the study.

Another reason for a lack of enthusiasm for reporting on a research project is that the study may have produced findings contrary to the researcher's expectations. It should be stressed that any findings from a study should be communicated to the members of the professional field. By permitting the study to be scrutinized by others, we are more likely to obtain constructive criticisms necessary to professional growth.

Indeed, a researcher has an obligation to communicate to the members of his professional field on the methodology and findings of the study. Only through such communication and the resultant accumulation of facts, ideas, interpretations, and analyses can a body of scientific knowledge and theories in nursing be developed.

SUMMARY

The twelve major steps in the research process have been discussed. Although the development of a research project usually proceeds in chronological order from the first step—selection of a topic and formulation of the problem—to the last—writing the final report—there is a great deal of back and forth through the steps as the plan is tightened, polished, and formalized. Not all types of studies include all the stages of the process. For example, descriptive studies may not include hypotheses. Methodological studies may omit certain phases of data collection.

SUGGESTIONS FOR FURTHER READING

There are numerous overviews of the research process. With rare exceptions, all include the twelve steps discussed in this chapter. References to these overviews are contained in the bibliography.

PROBLEMS AND SUGGESTIONS FOR FURTHER STUDY

1. Why is it important to develop a written plan before conducting a research project? Can such a plan be revised during the course of the project?
2. Obtain a copy of a federal research grant application (e.g., Public Health Service Form 398). How do the twelve steps in the research process fit into the various sections and parts of the application?
3. In developing a research plan, explain why some of the initial steps in the process (e.g., review the literature) should be accomplished prior to data collection.
4. What other elements need to be considered in preparing a research proposal in addition to the twelve steps outlined in this chapter?
5. On page 93 of his *The Practice of Social Research* (Belmont, CA, Wadsworth, 1983), Earl Babbie discusses the dangers of "cookbook research." What are these dangers? How can they be avoided?

6

Select the Topic
and Formulate the Problem

OBJECTIVES

- To describe sources of research ideas and topics.
- To describe how a problem becomes a topic.
- To explain how to formulate research problems.
- To provide guidelines for assessing a problem's researchability.

The initial step in research is, of course, to select the topic. This chapter will discuss sources of research topics and how a topic becomes the problem—the basis of the research. The chapter concludes with guidelines to assess the applicability of a problem to research.

SOURCES OF RESEARCH TOPICS

Research topics can be suggested by a variety of sources. A main source is the literature review, particularly that dealing with other research. The stimulus for pursuing a study can be provided by learning what other researchers have found as well as suggestions for further research. So-called "landmark" studies often trigger a large number of studies, some of which may be repetitions of the original study, called *replications,* having identical research designs and for the purpose of either confirming or denying the earlier findings. In nursing, in the early 1950s, stimulated by the financial support of the American Nurses' Association and the findings of surveys related to shortages of nursing personnel, a number of studies on a similar topical area (but often different in purpose and methodology) were undertaken. These were concerned with the job activities of nursing personnel and became known as "function" studies, many of which are summarized in *Twenty Thousand Nurses Tell Their Story.*[1]

Another source of research topics is the researcher's own background and experiences. For example, Hasselmeyer's previous experience included work in the care of premature infants before she undertook her study of the effects on such infants of diaper roll support;[2] Fitzwater was a supervisor in an operating room when she conducted her investigation of the use of surgical instruments;[3] and Belcher was a faculty member of a school of nursing when she became a member of the study team concerned with curriculum research.[4]

Still another source of research topics is that provided by theory and models. In the social sciences, theories pertaining to learning, personality, behavior of small groups, social and occupational roles, perception, and so on, have formed the basis for many studies. The purpose of these studies has been either to test the theory for workability or to apply it to a new situation among different study populations or settings. A "stress-transactional" framework played an important part in the research conducted by Magilvy on hearing-impaired older women.[5] And some of the studies directed by Flagle at Johns Hopkins have employed linear programming and other statistical and mathematical models from the field of operations research.[6]

Subject matter areas for research topics in nursing and patient care are vast. Moreover, there are many ways of classifying these areas. These classification schemes could be useful in suggesting topics for research. One type of classification scheme could categorize research in nursing and patient care according to the professional and technical discipline primarily concerned with the problem to be studied: sociological, psychological, anthropological, biological, and so on. Another classification could be by the facility in which nursing care is provided: hospital or other type of inpatient facility, outpatient department, physician's office, home. Still another categorization of research topics could place major emphasis on the patient characteristics: pediatric, obstetrical, surgical, psychiatric, etc. Another could be procedure-oriented: teaching, observing, physical care, emotional support, and so on. Finally, a simple classification of research topics consists of only three categories: nursing practice, nursing administration, and nursing education. The first area includes all activities that provide direct and indirect patient care—the physical work of the organization. Nursing administration is concerned with activities that maintain the organization in operation: staffing, directing, budgeting, coordinating, and so on. Nursing education includes all activities related to the undergraduate and graduate training of students as well as the continuing education of practitioners.

STATING THE PROBLEM

Once a research topic is selected the research problem is formulated as specifically as possible. Mere selection of a topic does not provide sufficient basis for developing a research plan. To state that a study is to be done on nursing practice or on the provision of emotional support to patients with myocardial infarction is not an adequate statement of the research problem, since it does not provide specific direction to the research effort. The statement of the problem should serve as the cornerstone on which the plan is based. A problem should concern some sitiuation in need of solution, improvement, modification, or change. A problem may be geared to a practical, real-life situation and initiate what has been described as applied research. Or it may concern a theoretical situation the solution of which may not have immediate practical consequences, and this would be termed basic research.

KEY POINT

In nursing there are a host of problems that could serve as the basis for research. A persistent problem has been the apparent shortage of nursing personnel. In its broadest sense, this problem can be stated, "Why is there a shortage of nursing personnel?" Stated this way it is questionable whether a research project could be developed. First, the question is much too broad. It implies that a shortage exists in all fields of nursing, all areas of the country, and all levels of nursing. Review of the literature will quickly reveal that a shortage is not universal. If study of the nursing shortage is to be successful, the scope of inquiry must be narrowed.

Second, what is meant by shortage? If defined as the number of vacant positions in institutions employing nurses, it could lead to a different type of study than if the concept of "shortage" is defined in a qualitative sense. Third, the problem as stated assumes that a shortage exists—i.e., that the existence of a shortage has been proved. But this may not necessarily be the case. Perhaps the problem should be restated as, "Is there a shortage of nurses?"

Note that formulating a problem for research is essentially defining concepts and terms, narrowing a broadly stated problem area into one more restricted in scope, and relating it to findings already obtained.

A broad topical area when narrowed into a manageable problem can stimulate other research studies. Some may aim to add to general knowledge (basic research) whereas others may have practical aims, such as the improvement of practice, administration, or education (applied research). Moreover, some of the studies from the same problem area may be experimental in methodology while others may be designed as field surveys or employ another type of nonexperimental approach.

One way in which a broadly stated problem can be more precisely stated is by formulating a significant question, such as "Why is there a shortage of nurses?" A series of relevant questions can then be posed to mold into a meaningful basis for research:

- What is the extent of the shortage?
- Is the shortage spread uniformly through all fields and levels of nursing?
- Is the shortage related to insufficient numbers of entrants into the field?
- Is the shortage related to the inefficient use of nursing time?
- Can the shortage be alleviated by improving working conditions for nurses?

- Is the shortage related to lack of adequate numbers of personnel or a deficiency in the quality of services provided, or both?
- Does the use of practical nurses and aides contribute to the relief of the nursing shortage?

From questions such as these it is possible to describe the problem specifically, as, "Does the quantity of nursing care available influence the condition of the patient?" This question, with additional refinement, definition of terms, and restatement as a hypothesis, has formed the basis for numerous studies in nursing. Some are explanatory studies the purpose of which is to determine optimum staffing patterns for providing patient care. Other studies developed from such questions are more descriptive in nature. The previously mentioned function studies, supported by the American Nurses' Association, are examples.

The selection of a research problem or question is of prime importance:

It is the difficulty or problem which guides our search for some order among the facts, in terms of which the difficulty is to be removed. We could not possibly discover the reasons for the inundation of the Nile unless we first recognize in the inundation a problem demanding solution.[7]

As Merton said, "... the experience of scientists is summed up in the adage that it is often more difficult to find and formulate a problem than to solve it."[8] This truism has relevance in that although much highly sophisticated methodology is available for conducting research, choosing and developing the problem must be left to the individual.

For no rule can be given by means of which men can learn to ask significant questions. It is a mark of scientific genius to be sensitive to difficulties where less gifted people pass by untroubled with doubt.[9]

Guidelines do exist to help decide whether it would be worthwhile to develop a problem into a formal research project. These guidelines can be applied to situations where some difficulty is felt and the question arises as to how best can the difficulty be solved—i.e., through research or some other means? In Chapter 1 it was pointed out that there are several widely used substitutes for research. These include problem solving by logical reasoning, use of judgment, experience, expert advice, and trial and error. But in many instances these substitutes are not satisfactory. Conversely, there are situations where formal research may not be appropriate. By asking the following questions about a problem it is possible to decide whether it should be pursued through formal research or other means:

ASSESSING THE RESEARCHABILITY OF A PROBLEM

Is it Feasible to Conduct Research on the Problem?

It is not always practical to try to turn a problem into a research project. For one thing, appropriate methodology may not be available. Many problem areas cannot now be adequately studied because appropriate tools do not exist, although this may only be temporary. Even a casual look at new tools for everyday life, not to mention the more exotic advances in heart, lung, and liver replacements in medicine, and the machinery for recovery of lost space satellites, will show what marvelous things are in store for the future.

A second obstacle is that the study may require so large a number of subjects and so much time to complete that the findings will be out of date. Thus, if we are concerned with the effect of certain nursing procedures on patients with rare conditions, it will probably take years to accumulate sufficient cases to yield valid findings. In the meantime the procedures being studied may become obsolete. Obsoleteness is a distinct possibility in these times when changes occur frequently in the care of patients.

Another obstacle to the pursuit of a research problem is the possibility of harming the health of the study subjects. Many drugs, for example, cannot be tested because they are too toxic in humans. Certain kinds of psychological or sociological research cannot be done because of possible detrimental effects on the emotions and attitudes of subjects.

Still another obstacle to the pursuit of a research problem is the project cost. Some problems would cost so much to solve that the results would not be worth the effort.

In brief, then, feasibility of pursuing a research problem can be evaluated by the following criteria:

• Availability of methodology
• Time needed to complete the study
• Danger to life or physical and mental well-being of subjects
• Cost of the research

Is the Problem of Sufficient Importance?

Because the conduct of research may involve large expenditures of time, effort, and money, the decision to launch a study must balance the expected value of the findings against the expenditures. If the project can be done inexpensively, we can be satisfied with modest results. If the study will require large amounts of time and money, the importance of results should certainly be commensurate with resources expended. A strenuous research effort that costs much and produces little is to be avoided, not least because the investigator may wish to do another study in the future.

The importance of a research problem can be evaluated in terms of various criteria, one of which is the economic effect of the findings. If a problem requires large sums of money, there is incentive for undertaking research to reduce this expenditure. Market research illustrates this point. Before manufacturers spend large sums of money in developing a new product, they must test its acceptability on a sample of potential users. Another example is found in hospitals, where research on the application of automatic data processing to the reporting of data on patients is motivated by the amount of time and money expended on such systems. And justification for studies of nursing personnel turnover is based on the huge economic cost of high job turnover.

Another criterion of the importance of a research problem is the possible effect of application of the findings on the health and welfare of people. Much of the justification for employing research to solve problems in the nursing field can be related to the intimate connection between nursing care and patient welfare. In medicine, the impetus for subjecting new drugs to carefully controlled clinical trials is their vital effect on the health of individuals. The impact of research on peoples' health overrides any other criterion in determining whether a problem should be pursued as a formal research study.

A third measure of the importance of a research problem is the frequency of occurrence. For example, if a public health agency finds it has an excessive number of broken appointments, it may well be best to formally investigate the problem rather than accept the assessments of clinic supervisors, especially if the judgments conflict with each other. Another example: interest in the relationship between smoking and lung cancer precipitated a great deal of research after there were dramatic increases in the number of deaths from lung cancer. Of course, wide occurrence of a problem is not a necessary condition for undertaking research. A problem that is not widespread may often possess justification for a research project if other criteria of importance are present.

To What Extent Can the Findings of the Study of the Problem Be Generalized?

Sometimes research is evaluated according to the extent to which its findings can be applied to situations other than the research setting. This criterion has greatest relevancy to explanatory research where the purpose is either to confirm or reject an hypothesis. There usually is more justification to support a research project if its findings have broad implications. Many investigators dream of an ideal research problem that would lead to "earth-shaking" findings. The danger here, of course, is that the desire to make an impact can lead to the neglect of important research problems that do not have such glamour.

What Need Will Solution of the Research Problem Meet?

To fully evaluate whether a problem merits the effort of a formal study, the need the solution of the problem will meet should be clearly described, that is, defining the purpose of the study. If the purpose cannot be defined, the problem is clearly not researchable. By definition, research is a purposeful activity. This purpose may be to add to knowledge in the field or to attain some more immediately practical objective as in applied research, such as developing a new procedure, method, or product. Sometimes the same problem can lead to different research purposes. For example, the problem of how best to train professional nurses could be developed into a descriptive study to provide data on the characteristics of graduates of various kinds of educational programs. Or it could lead to an experimental study that would compare the effectiveness of different kinds of educational programs. But whatever purpose is formulated it should meet a real need.

To the extent that the hypothesis concerning a problem is carefully and completely formulated, both long- and short-range objectives become clear. To illustrate, assume that the research problem was concerned with the reasons why recent graduates from schools of professional nursing withdrew from nursing at a high rate. The short-range need to be served by the research may be to point out ways of reducing this attrition, such as offering economic or other types of incentives for the young graduate to remain at work. The long-range need may be the shedding of light on the possibility of changing the emphasis on the type of individual recruited to a nursing school, or revising the curriculum. These objectives are long-range because they may take years to achieve. Once achieved, however, the effect on solving the problem of attrition would undoubtedly be more substantial than in meeting the short-range need.

Another illustration of the ways in which research can meet both long- and short-range needs is that while research findings can serve an immediate specific need in solving a practical problem, they can also contribute, perhaps modestly, to the development of a theory, principle, or other generalized knowledge. For example, studies concerned with the determination of optimum staffing patterns for providing patient care may provide information that is immediately useful to administrators of patient care. At the same time, they can contribute to the development of a generalized theory of the relationship between nursing care and patient welfare.

In developing a research problem, therefore, the following question should be continuously raised: What are the long- and short-range needs to be met by this study? The answers to this question should influence the study during its entire course.

Is the Problem of Interest to the Researcher?

An important criterion in selecting problems for research is that they be of interest to the researcher. This criterion may appear to be so self-evident as not to warrant any discussion at all, but many studies are conducted by people who do not have a real interest in the research problem. Often these studies become bogged down and end without attaining their purposes, or else produce findings that may be trivial, irrelevant, or invalid. Lack of interest on the part of the researcher may stem from the fact that the research problem was chosen not because of intellectual curiosity, but because it was appealing to a grant-giving agency or to the employing organization or faculty committee.

Interest in the problem can only be a strong motivation for the researcher to pursue the project to its conclusion, energetically, creatively, and with intellectual honesty. Interest and dedication can sustain the researcher through the arid stretches when nothing much seems to be happening or through those difficult, arduous, or boring phases that sometimes occur.

Does the Researcher Have Competence to Pursue the Research Problem?

Just as interest in the problem is an important and rather obvious characteristic of the researcher, so is his level of competence in the area of the research. Obviously, a researcher cannot expect to possess all skills demanded by all research, particularly in projects so large and complex that a team approach is required. For example, a researcher concerned with a problem related to the emotional needs of patients does not need to be an accomplished psychometrician, psychoanalyst, or statistician, if such skills are required. But he should be sufficiently knowledgeable to make appropriate decisions as to when such expertise shall be called upon either as consultants to the project or members of the team.

The qualities that make up a competent researcher are difficult to define. Research as a completely independent activity does not exist. It must be related to some subject matter discipline—medicine, psychology, nursing, and so on. One can specialize in certain aspects of research methodology, such as psychometrics, sociometrics, or statistics, but being expert in one of these areas does not automatically qualify one as a competent researcher. These qualities, although difficult to define, are quite real. They sometimes exhibit themselves in rather subtle ways. One characteristic of the accomplished researcher is the sophistication of the formulation of the problem. Although research courses can enhance the skills of a researcher, the most important way in which research competencies are developed is through experience. It is ironic that research, always formally described as a rational and systematic approach to the solution of problems, can probably best be learned by a firsthand experience similar to the process of trial and error. This is because there is not one way to tackle a research problem, but many. Moreover, in the course of a project there are numerous places where decisions must be made that can significantly affect the total effort. In making many of these decisions there are no firm rules to tell the researcher which alternative to select, but only guidelines based on experience acquired in the execution of previous research. These guidelines allow appreciable room for the exercise of the researcher's own judgment.

KEY POINT It appears, then, that a competent researcher should possess some technical skill in research methodology, some knowledge of the subject matter, the ability to know how to use technical experts, good judgment in coping with the many decisions to be made, and last, but indeed not least, sufficient imagination to take advantage of the many opportunities that present themselves during the research to "try something a little different," which could lead to an unexpectedly rich payoff, called "serendipity."

To recapitulate, in formulating a research problem the researcher should raise the following six questions:

1. Is it feasible to conduct research on the problem?
2. Is the problem important?
3. To what extent might the findings of the research be generalized?
4. What need will be met by solution of the problem?
5. Is the researcher really interested in the problem?
6. Does the researcher have adequate competence to pursue the problem through research?

A final word on formulating research

problems concerns a topic that could well have been discussed first: How do research problems arise and where are research problems found? They are found in all areas of human activity. In nursing, research problems arise from activities involving giving care to patients, administering this care, or teaching people to give the care—the three content areas of nursing practice, nursing administration, and nursing education. These problems can arise in many ways—from an actual work situation, for example, problems confronting administrators of nursing service when they try to adequately staff their units. Or from hypothetical situations, such as what would happen if acutely ill patients were discharged earlier from hospitals. Research problems may also be suggested by experiences encountered in one's personal life. For example, some psychological studies dealing with the problems of children were suggested to a researcher by observation of the behavior of his own children or those of neighbors. And, of course, there is the famous but somewhat dubious anecdote of how the falling apple started Newton on the road toward the establishment of the laws of gravity.

Whether arising from real or hypothetical considerations, research problems in nursing can also crop up in any setting in which nursing takes place. Problems related to the provision of nursing care can arise in a hospital, public health agency, physician's office, or the home. Problems concerned with the education of nurses can arise not only in schools, but in work situations as well as in off-duty, leisure time. "Does the after-hours reading of nursing journals really serve the educational purpose of keeping nurses informed about the latest developments in the field?" is an example of the latter type of research question. Finally, researchable administrative problems are especially plentiful, since they can be found in any situation where two or more people are working together toward the same goal or just working in close proximity.

Indeed, the range of problems that can

serve as the basis for research in nursing and patient care is potentially limitless. There is a great need for people with the ability to perceive these problems, to evaluate them, and to develop them into research projects that would make significant contributions to knowledge.

SUMMARY

The research process begins with a selection of a topic for study. This signifies the content area and suggests in a general way the nature of the problem. The next step is to formulate the problem. This expresses in concrete terms a situation in need of solution. To determine whether the problem should be approached through formal research, such criteria as feasibility, importance, extensiveness of the problem, as well as interest and competence of the researcher can be applied. At this stage the purpose of the research evolving from the problem should also be crystallized.

Once the problem is formulated, the next step is review of the literature. However, the process of formulating the problem cannot be complete until the total research design is developed, since it is subject to redefinition, revision, restatement, and reformulation.

REFERENCES

1. Everett C. Hughes, Helen MacGill Hughes, and Irwin Deutscher, *Twenty Thousand Nurses Tell Their Story*. Philadelphia, J. B. Lippincott Co., 1958.
2. Eileen G. Hasselmeyer, *Behavior Patterns of Premature Infants*. U.S. Public Health Service Publication No. 840, Washington, D.C., Government Printing Office, 1961.
3. Janet Fitzwater, "The Selection of Instruments for Major Operations." *Nursing Res.*, 9:129–136, summer 1960.
4. Mary S. Tschudin, Helen C. Belcher, and Leo Nedelsky, *Evaluation in Basic Nursing Education*. New York, G. P. Putnam's Sons, 1958.
5. Joan K. Magilvy, "Quality of Life of Hearing Impaired Older Women." *Nursing Res.* 34:140–144, May/June 1985.
6. Charles D. Flagle, *The Problem of Organization for Hospital Inpatient Care*. Reprint No. 55 of a paper presented at the 6th Annual International Meeting of the Institute of Management Sciences, September 1959.
7. Morris R. Cohen and Ernest Nagel, *An Introduction to Logic and Scientific Method*. New York, Harcourt, Brace and Co., 1934, p. 199. Note: Darby Books, Darby, PA, issued a reprint of this book in 1982.
8. Robert K. Merton, "Notes on Problem Finding in Sociology," in Robert K. Merton *et al.* (eds.), *Sociology Today*. New York, Basic Books, 1959, p. ix.
9. Cohen and Nagel, *op. cit.*, p. 200.

PROBLEMS AND SUGGESTIONS FOR FURTHER STUDY

1. Make a list of ten topics that might be fruitful to develop into research problems. Apply the guidelines for assessing the researchability of a problem to the topics and determine the extent to which they meet the criteria of the guidelines.

2. Review recent issues of nursing journals to see if they suggest topics for possible research projects. The article "Nursing Careers in the Emerging Systems," by John R. Coleman, Elizabeth C. Dayani, and Elsie Simms (*Nursing Manage.* 15:19–27, January 1984) contains numerous ideas for research topics.

3. What makes a problem important enough to carry out research? Can a problem that initially seems to be unimportant turn out to be important?

4. What is the difference between the research problem and the research purpose? Why is it important to state the purpose of a study?

5. Read Chapter 5 in *Annual Review of Nursing*, Harriet H. Werley and Joyce J. Fitzpatrick (eds.) (New York, Springer, 1984), "Nursing Research on Death, Dying and Terminal Illness: Development, Present State, and Prospects," by Jeanne Quint Benoliel. What are some of the research problems that are suggested by the review? Evaluate the researchability of some of these topics.

CHAPTER

7

Review the Literature

OBJECTIVES

• To become familiar with computerized literature retrieval services.
• To be able to identify main reference sources
for a literature review.

• To be able to carry out a literature review of a
study.

Literature review is an important part of any research project because its purpose is to reveal what is already known about a problem. A literature review, properly conducted, can suggest ideas for research projects and, after a topic is selected and the problem formulated, help in designing an efficient research plan. The review can also assist in not "reinventing the same wheel" and in avoiding pitfalls that have frustrated earlier researchers. This chapter will delineate the major bibliographic developments affecting nursing. The important literature sources for nursing research will be described. Guidelines are provided for assessing the adequacy of the literature review.

SOURCES OF INFORMATION

The greater involvement of nurses in research and increased investigations of nursing problems have influenced the bibliographic developments affecting nursing. The U.S. Public Health Service's Division of Nursing regarded the need for access to the literature important and supported two bibliographic projects—a survey and assessment of nursing research by investigators at Yale University and the abstracting of reports and studies in nursing by the Institute of Research and Service in Nursing Education, Teachers College, Columbia University. The Yale survey led to the development of two annotated bibliographies: *Nursing Studies Index*[1] (1900–1959) in four volumes and *Nursing Research—A Survey and Assessment*.[2] The project on abstracting resulted in two special issues to *Nursing Research*. The abstracting service is now a permanent program of the American Nurses' Foundation and is a regular feature of *Nursing Research*.

The Interagency Council on Library

Tools was established in 1960 to exchange information on problems and needs of the nursing literature. The name was changed later to the Interagency Council on Library Resources for Nursing.[3] Membership includes the American Hospital Association, American Nurses' Association, American Nurses' Foundation, Catholic Library Association, Medical Library Association, National League for Nursing, Yale Nursing Survey Project, and the U.S. Public Health Service.

The Interagency Council on Library Tools, a brain child of Miss Virginia Henderson, came into being because of her vision. Miss Henderson, a nursing scholar and teacher, has devoted her life to achieving quality nursing practice through her teaching, writings, and pioneering efforts in developing the first comprehensive *Nursing Studies Index.*[4]

As far as original research reports are concerned, rich sources are the technical reports of government-sponsored research. It is possible to obtain reports of many of these projects by writing to the investigator who conducted the research. Many of these reports are published and are identified by title, author, and research grant number, for example: Gerald J. Griffin and Robert E. Kinsinger, *Teaching Clinical Nursing by Closed Circuit TV*—A Demonstration Project of the Department of Nursing, Bronx Community College at Montefiore Hospital in New York City, supported by Research Grant Number NU 00116 from the Division of Nursing, Public Health Service.

It is sometimes difficult to locate reports of government-sponsored research, particularly in fields where the research deals with classified information. An important source of information about reports on government-sponsored research is the National Technical Information Service of the U.S. Department of Commerce located at 5285 Port Royal Road, Springfield, Virginia 22161. Announcements of new reports are made biweekly in the publication *Government Reports.* Since 1964 over one-half

million reports of research have been compiled by N.T.I.S., copies of which can be purchased from the Service.

In the health field, the Division of Research Grants of the National Institutes of Health publishes a *Research Grants Index* that describes current research projects supported by the Public Health Service. These are listed three ways: by subject matter, name and address of principal investigator (including publications produced on the research project), and institute or division through which the grant was awarded. The Bureau of Health Professions, of which the Division of Nursing is a part, annually publishes a *Directory of Grants, Awards and Loans.* Projects are listed by state and city of location of grantee, institution name, area of support, and amount awarded. There is a several years' lag between issuance of the directory and the time period of the data. The Division of Nursing issues abstracts of the research grants it has supported.

In 1962, the American Nurses' Association published a series of monographs containing clinical papers presented during its 1962 convention. Similar monographs entitled *ANA Clinical Sessions* and containing about fifty papers each, have been published for subsequent conventions.

In 1965 the American Nurses' Association began a series of research conferences funded by the U.S. Public Health Service's Division of Nursing. These were held in different cities and included presentations on a variety of research topics. Papers presented at the conferences were put together by the Association in a single volume presented to the Division of Nursing and some were later published in journals. The last conference, held in 1973 in San Antonio, Texas, presented over twenty research papers.

Beginning in 1968, in Salt Lake City, Utah, the Western Interstate Commission on Higher Education in Nursing sponsored a series of annual research conferences, initially funded by the Division of Nursing. Each conference had a particular theme.

The theme at the 1978 conference in Portland, Oregon was "New Approaches to Communicating Nursing Research." Reports on all the conferences have been published by WICHEN.

Another compilation of papers, some of which deal with research topics, is *The Nursing Clinics of North America,* published quarterly by W. B. Saunders Company. Although not exclusively oriented to reports of research, the material can be of value to those interested in clinical research in nursing.

The Health Planning and Resources Development Act of 1974 (P.L. 93-641) established an information system known as the National Health Planning Information Center (NHPIC). The Center's primary objective is to provide access to current information on health planning methodology as well as information to be used in the analysis of issues and problems in health planning.[5] The U.S. Public Health Service's Division of Nursing has provided support to the center in order to establish a central source of information on nurse manpower planning. Services available from the center include announcements of relevant documents. The National Technical Information Service publishes reference and referral services and issues monographs and bibliographies on subjects relevant to nursing research.

In the education field the U.S. Education Resources Information Center (ERIC) disseminates educational research results, research-related material, and other resource information. Since 1966 the Center has published *Research in Education* on a monthly basis, with annual accumulations. Available from the U.S. Government Printing Office, it is a rich source of education research information on nursing education.

Interagency Conference on Nursing Statistics (ICONS)[6]

ICONS serves a coordinating role in developing nursing statistics and serves to stimulate the collection and dissemination of data on nurses in their practice settings. ICONS is an association of statisticians composed of organizations directly concerned with compiling and analyzing statistics on nursing. Begun in 1953 by ANA and the Division of Nursing Resources, PHS, it was formally named the Interagency Conference on Nursing Statistics in 1955 and expanded to include the National League for Nursing and the American Hospital Association. Other organizations and agencies are invited to attend meetings. *Nursing Related Data Sources 1984* is prepared and published by ICONS.

Literature Searches

MEDLARS—produced and individualized bibliographies are available from the National Library of Medicine without charge. A complete list appears each month in *Index Medicus* and *Abridged Index Medicus.* For single copies write to Literature Search Program, Reference Section, National Library of Medicine, 8600 Rockville Pike, Bethesda, Maryland 20209. Enclose name and address on a gummed label.

Examples of searches:

- 82–1 Nursing Diagnosis
- 82–21 Audiovisual Aids, Computer-Assisted Instruction, and Programmed Instruction in Patient Education
- 83–12 Sleep Apnea
- 83–15 Anorexia Nervosa and Bulimia
- 84-3 Osteoporosis
- 84-7 DRGs and Prospective Pricing

Consensus Development Conference Summaries

The Consensus Development Program sponsored by the U.S. Public Health Service, National Institutes of Health, provides a process through the Consensus Development Conferences held at NIH to improve the process of transferring technology from laboratory to health care system. Copies of published volumes and individual conference summaries are available from the office of Medical Applications of Research, Building 1, Room 216, National Institutes of Health, PHS, Bethesda, Maryland 20205.

The main reference sources for a literature review consist of the following:

- Journals*
- Abstract journals
- Indexes
- Bibliographies and book lists
- Computerized and bibliographic databases
- Guides and directories
- Statistical reports

The Interagency Council on Library Resources for Nursing has compiled the following reference sources for nursing:[7]

Abstract Journals

Abstracts of Health Care Management Studies (formerly *Abstracts of Hospital Management Studies*). University of Michigan School of Public Health, Cooperative Information Center for Health Care Management Studies, 1021 E. Huron, Ann Arbor, MI 48109. Annual.

Abstracts of Studies in Nursing, 1949-1952: in *American Journal of Nursing,* indexed under Research and Studies; 1953-April 1954: in *Nursing Outlook* indexed under Research and Studies; 1954-1959: in *Nursing Research* 9:53-106, Spring 1960, index 9:107-117, Spring 1960; also in *Cumulative Index to Nursing Research,* 1952-1963.

Abstracts of Studies in Public Health Nursing, 1924-1957: in *Nursing Research* 8:45-115, Spring 1959.

Nursing Abstracts. P.O. Box 295, Forest Hills, NY 11375. Quarterly. Other abstract journals of interest are *Abstracts for Social Workers, Biological Abstracts, Chemical Abstracts, Dissertation Abstracts International, Excerpta Medica, Medical Care Reviews, Nutrition Abstracts and Reviews, Psychological Abstracts, Resources in Vocational Education,* and *Sociological Abstracts.*

Audiovisuals

Audio-Visual Equipment Directory, 1983-84. 28th ed. Ed. by S. Herickes. National Audio-Visual Association, Fairfax, VA, 1983.

Audiovisual Market Place 1983: A Multimedia Guide with Names & Numbers. 13th ed. R. R. Bowker Co., New York, NY.

Abbott Laboratories, Professional Relations. Abbott Park D-383. North Chicago, IL 60064. $^3/_4''$ video cassette programs for patient education.

American Journal of Nursing Company, Educational Services Division. Multimedia Materials, Publications, Audio Visuals, 555 West 57th Street, New York, NY 10019 (212-582-8820). Catalogue of audio cassettes, films, filmstrips, slides, and videotapes on nursing for purchase or rental.

Audio-Visual Materials. In appendices of *Cumulated Index to Nursing and Allied Health Literature.* Glendale Adventist Medical Center, Box 871, Glendale, CA 91209.

Audiovisual Resources in Food and Nutrition. Compiled from data provided by the National Agricultural Library. Oryx Press, Phoenix, 1979.

AVLINE (Audiovisuals on Line), one of the MEDLARS online interactive (described under Databases online) data bases of the National Library of Medicine, contains citations to audiovisuals that have been cataloged by the library for use in health sciences education.

Concept Media, P.O. Box 19542, Irvine, CA 92714 (714-833-3347). Filmstrip series of 5-8 programs related to nursing.

The Educational Film Locator of the Consortium of University Film Centers and R.R. Bowker Company. 2nd ed. R.R. Bowker Co., New York, 1980.

Educators Guide to Free Health, Physical Education and Recreation Materials. 15th ed. Ed. by F. A. Horkheimer. Educators Progress Service, Inc., Randolph, WI, 1982.

Guide to Audiovisual Resources for the Health Care Field. Medical Media Publishers, a division of Medical Planning and Consultants, Inc., 160 N. Craig St., Pittsburgh, PA 15213, 1981.

*DHHS, PHS: National Library of Medicine. *List of Journals Indexed in Index Medicus 1984,* Bethesda, MD. National Library of Medicine, NIH Publication No. 84-267.

Instructional Resources: Video Cassette, Slide/Tape. University of Michigan Media Library, University of Michigan Medical Center, Ann Arbor, MI 48109.

Media Resources Catalogue, 1983-1984, Western Psychiatric Institute and Clinic Library, Benedum Audiovisual Center, Western Psychiatric Institute and Clinic Library, Pittsburgh, 1982.

National Library of Medicine Audiovisuals Catalog. U.S. Government Printing Office, Washington, DC, quarterly.

The Nursing Audiovisual Resource List, 1981-1982. Subject/Title Index. 2 vol. Ed. by Lorna Wright and Malcolm H. Brantz. University of Connecticut Health Center, Farmington, CT, 1981.

NICEM. Index to Health and Safety Education, Multimedia. 2 vol. 4th ed. National Center for Educational Media, Los Angeles, 1980.

Patient and Health Education Audiovisual Resource List, 1983. National Library of Medicine, Bethesda, MD, 1983. (free)

Robert J. Brady Co., Bowie, MD 20715 (800-638-0220). Extensive list of nursing and allied health multimedia instructional materials.

Trainex Corporation Video Library Catalog, P.O. Box 116, Garden Grove, CA 92642 (800-854-2485). Multimedia health training aids.

The Video Source Book. 2nd ed. The National Video Clearinghouse, Inc., Syosset, NY, 1980.

Bibliographies and Book Lists

Binger, J. L., and Jensen, L. M. Lippincott's Guide to Nursing: A Handbook for Students, Writers, and Researchers. J. B. Lippincott Co., Philadelphia, 1980.

Books of the Year. In each January issue of the *American Journal of Nursing.*

Brandon, A. N., and Hill, D. R. "Selected List of Books and Journals for the Small Medical Library." 10th rev. *Bulletin of the Medical Library Association.* 71:147-175, April 1983. Reprints available from the Medical Library Association.

————. "Selected List of Nursing Books and Journals." 3rd rev. *Nursing Outlook* 32:92-101, March/April 1984.

Ewens, W. A., and others, comps. Bibliography of Nursing Monographs, 1970-1978. Georgetown University Medical Center, Dahlgren Memorial Library, Washington, DC, 1978.

A Major Report. Published quarterly by Majors Scientific Books, Inc., 2221 Walnut Hill Lane, Irving, TX 75061. Free. Updates the Brandon/Hill lists and annotates important new nursing books.

Medical Books and Serials in Print. R. R. Bowker Co., New York, annual.

Medical Media Corporation. Medical Books '84. Flemington, NJ: The Corporation, 1984. Available free from various medical book distributors.

Medical Reference Works, 1679-1966:Selected Bibliography. Ed. by J. B. Blake and C. Roos. Medical Library Association, Chicago, 1967. Suppl. I (1967-1968), 1970, out of print; Suppl. II (1969-1972), 1973; Suppl. III (1973-1974), 1975.

Nursing Text Book List of All Publishers '84-'85. Majors Scientific Books, Inc., 2221 Walnut Hill Lane, Irving, TX 75061. Annual. (free)

Strauch, K. P., and Brundage, D. J. Guide to Library Resources for Nursing. Appleton-Century-Crofts, New York, 1980.

World Health Organization. Catalogue of Publications, 1947-1979. Suppl. 1980-1983; 1983-1984. Available free from the United Nations Bookshop, UN Plaza, New York, NY 10017.

Drug Lists and Pharmacologies

Albanese, Joseph. Nurses' Drug Reference. 2nd ed. McGraw-Hill Book Co., New York, 1982. *1982 Drug Update.* McGraw-Hill Book Co., New York, 1983.

American Drug Index. 26th ed. Ed. by Norman Billups. J. B. Lippincott, Philadelphia, 1982.

American Hospital Formulary Service. 2 vols. American Society of Hospital Pharmacists, Washington, DC, 1981. Loose-leaf set. Yearly Suppls.

AMA Drug Evaluations. 5th ed. American Medical Association, Chicago, 1983.

Drugs in Current Use and New Drugs. 30th ed. Ed. by Walter Modell. Springer, New York, 1984.

Drugs of Choice, 1984-85. Ed. by Walter Modell, C. V. Mosby Co., St. Louis, 1984.

Facts and Comparisons. Annual. Order from 111 West Port Plaza, Suite 423, St. Louis, MO, 63141. Loose-leaf edition with monthly updates.

Falconer's Current Drug Handbook, 1982-84. W. B. Saunders, Philadelphia, 1982.

Goodman and Gilman's. The Pharmacological Basis of Therapeutics. 6th ed. Macmillan, New York, 1980.

Handbook of Nonprescription Drugs. 7th ed. American Pharmaceutical Association, Washington, DC, 1982.

Loebl, Suzanne, and Spratto, George. The Nurse's Drug Handbook. 3rd ed. John Wiley & Sons, New York, 1983.

Merck Index: An Encyclopedia of Chemicals and Drugs. 10th ed. Ed. by Martha Windholz. Merck & Co., Rahway, NJ, 1976. Revised every 8 years.

Merck Manual of Diagnosis and Therapy. Ed. by Robert Berkow. Merck & Co., Rahway, NJ, 1982.

Modern Drug Encyclopedia and Therapeutic Index. 16th (final) ed. Ed. by G. D. Gonzales and A. L. Lewis. Yorke Medical Books, New York, 1981.

Nursing Drug Handbook. Intermed Communication, Inc., Horsham, PA, 1984. Annual.

Physicians' Desk Reference. Medical Economics, Oradell, NJ. Annual with updates.

Health Services

The Use of Health Services: Indices and Correlates—A Research Bibliography. 1981 by Cheryl A. Maurana; Robert L. Eichorn; and Lynne E. Lonnquist, Purdue University. Available from NTIS, PB 82-24422. Links research findings to specific trends and factors influencing health services use.

Histories

Abel-Smith, Brian. A History of the Nursing Profession. Heinemann Educational Books, London, 1976.

Austin, A. L. History of Nursing Source Book. G. P. Putnam's Sons, New York, 1957.

Bullough, Vern and Bullough, Bonnie. The Care of the Sick: The Emergency of Modern Nursing. Neale Watson, New York, 1978.

Bullough, Bonnie, et al. Nursing: A Historical Bibliography. Garland Publishing, New York, 1981.

Davies, Celia, ed. Rewriting Nursing History. Croom Helm, London, 1980.

Deloughery, G. L., and Griffin, G. J. History and Trends of Professional Nursing. 8th ed. C. V. Mosby Co., St. Louis, 1977.

Dolan, J., Fitzpatrick, M., and Herrmann, E. Nursing in Society: An Historical Perspective. W. B. Saunders Co., Philadelphia, 1983.

Fitzpatrick, M. L., ed. Historical Studies in Nursing: Papers Presented at the 15th Annual Stewart Conference on Research in Nursing, March 1977. Teachers College Press, New York, 1978.

Fitzpatrick, M. L. Prologue to Professionalism: Topics in Nursing History. Brady, Bowie, MD, 1983.

Flanagan, Lyndia, comp. One Strong Voice: The Story of the American Nurses' Association. American Nurses' Association, Kansas City, MO, 1976.

Fondiller, S. The Entry Dilemma: The National League for Nursing and the Higher Education Movement, 1952-1972. NLN, New York, 1983.

Goostray, Stella. Memoirs: Half a Century in Nursing. Nursing Archives, Boston University Mugar Memorial Library, Boston, 1969.

Jamieson, Elizabeth M., Sewell, Mary F., and Suhrie, Eleanor B. Tends in Nursing History: Their Social, International, and Ethical Relationships. W. B. Saunders Co., Philadelphia, 1966.

Kalisch, P. A., and Kalisch, B. J. The Advance of American Nursing. Brown and Co., Boston, 1978.

Lagemann, E., ed. Nursing History: New Perspectives, New Possibilities. Teaching College Press, New York, 1983. (Essays originally prepared for a conference held in May 1981, sponsored by Rockefeller Archives Center.)

Melosh, Barbara. The Physician's Hand: Work Culture and Conflict in American Nursing. Temple University Press, Philadelphia, 1982.

Noel, N., ed. The History of American Nursing Conference Proceeding. Nursing Archives, Boston University Mugar Memorial Library, Boston, 1983.

Nutting, M. A., and Dock, L. L. History of Nursing. 4 vols. G. P. Putnam's Sons, New York, 1907-1912.

Reverby, S., ed. The History of American Nurs-

ing. Garland, New York. 32-volumes facsimile series.

Roberts, M. M. *American Nursing: History and Interpretation.* Macmillan, New York, 1954.

Sellew, Gladys, and Ebel, Sister M. E. *A History of Nursing.* C. V. Mosby Co., St. Louis, 1955.

Stewart, I. M., and Austin, A. L., eds. *History of Nursing,* 5th ed. G. P. Putnam's Sons, New York, 1962. First four editions by L. L. Dock and I. M. Stewart under the title *Short History of Nursing.*

Shyryock, R. H. *The History of Nursing: An Interpretation of the Social and Medical Factors Involved.* W. B. Saunders, Philadelphia, 1959.

The History of Nursing: Essential Resources to Support Nursing Studies. University Microfilms International, Ann Arbor. Includes Adelaide Nutting Historical Nursing Collection and the Archives of the Department of Nursing Education at Teachers College, Columbia University, on microfiche.

Yesterday: *"History in the Nursing Curriculum." Perspectives in Nursing 1983-1985.* NLN, New York 1983. (Six papers presented at the NLN's 16th Biennial Convention, 1983.)

Indexes

Abridged Index Medicus. U.S. Government Printing Office, Washington, DC, monthly. Each issue contains citations to articles in 117 English language journals. *Cumulative Abridged Index Medicus.* 1970-1975, out of print.

American Journal of Nursing Cumulative Indexes. New York: American Journal of Nursing Co. 1971-1975; 1966-1970; 1956-1960; 1951-1955. Earlier cumulative indexes, dating from 1900, are now out of print.

Cumulative Index to Nursing and Allied Health Literature (formerly, *Cumulative Index to Nursing Literature*). Glendale Adventist Medical Center, Box 871, Glendale, CA 91209. Bimonthly with annual cumulations.

Earlier cumulations, 1956-60, available from University Microfilms, Ann Arbor, MI.

Nursing Subject Headings have been included in annual cumulations since 1971.

An author-subject index to English-language periodical literature in nursing and paramedical fields.

Hospital Literature Index. American Hospital Association, Chicago, quarterly, with annual cumulations.

Hospital Literature Subject Headings. 1977.

Cumulative Index of Hospital Literature. 1945-1949. 1960-1964, out of print.

Index Medicus. Compiled by the U.S. National Library of Medicine. U.S. Government Printing Office, Washington, DC, monthly; annual *Cumulated Index Medicus.*

Subject and author index to articles selected from more than 2,600 biomedical journals. Includes bibliography of medical reviews.

Index to Public Health Nursing Magazine. 1909-1952. National League for Nursing, New York, 1974.

International Nursing Index. 1966-present. American Journal of Nursing Co., New York, quarterly, with annual cumulations.

Indexes over 200 nursing journals, U.S. and foreign, and includes nursing articles indexed from nonnursing journal for Index Medicus.

International Nursing Index, Nursing Thesaurus. American Journal of Nursing Company. Included in first issue INI each year. Reprint available from the INI editor.

Nursing Outlook Cumulative Indexes. American Journal of Nursing Co., New York. 1958-1962 out of print. 1953-57 available.

Nursing Studies Index. 4 vols. Virginia Henderson and the Yale University Index staff. J. B. Lippincott Co., Philadelphia, 1963–1972. Out of print.

An annotated guide to reported studies, research in progress, research methods, and historical materials in periodicals, books, and pamphlets published in English.

U.S. National Library of Medicine. Medical Subject Headings. U.S. Government Printing Office, Washington, DC, annual as #1, Pt. 2, of January issue of *Index Medicus.*

See Also annual indexes to various nursing journal, e.g., *American Journal of Nursing* (index published separately) and *Nursing Outlook,* usually found in final issue of each volume. Other indexes of interest are: *Education*

Index, Humanities Index, and *Social Sciences Index.*

Legal Guides

Creighton, Helen. *Law Every Nurse Should Know.* 4th ed. W. B. Saunders, Philadelphia, 1981.

Fiesta, Janine. *Law and Liability: A Guide for Nurses.* John Wiley & Sons, New York, 1983.

Murchison, Irene, et. al. *Legal Accountability in the Nursing Process.* 2nd ed. C. V. Mosby & Co., St. Louis, 1982.

Pavalon, Eugene I. *Human Rights and Health Care Law.* American Journal of Nursing Co., New York, 1980.

Rocereto, LaVerne R., and Maleski, Cynthia M. *Legal Dimensions of Nursing Practice.* Springer Publications Co., New York, 1982.

Research and Statistical Sources

For statistics compiled by the Federal government consult the *Monthly Catalog of U.S. Government Publications* and the publication lists of the U.S. Census Bureau and the U.S. Public Health Service, especially those of the National Center for Health Statistics, and the Bureau of Health Manpower.

Facts About Nursing. American Nurses' Association, Kansas City, MO, biannual.

LPNs: 1974 Inventory of Licensed Practical Nurses. Prepared by A. V. Roth and G. T. Schmittling. (Publ. No. D-59) American Nurses' Association, Kansas City, MO, 1977.

Inventory of Registered Nurses. 1977-1978. Prepared by Duane C. Schulte. (Publ. No. D-70). American Nurses' Association, Kansas City, MO, 1981.

NLN Nursing Data Book: Statistical Information on Nursing Education and Newly Licensed Nurses. National League for Nursing, New York, annual.

The National Referral Center for Science and Technology of the Library of Congress publishes a number of directories periodically. These selected directories are available from the Superintendent of Documents. U.S. Government Printing Office, Washington, DC 20402.

COMPUTER-ASSISTED INFORMATION RETRIEVAL

The nurse researcher must know how to access the professional literature using a computerized system know as MEDLARS (Medical Literature Analysis and Retrieval System). The system is based at the U.S. Public Health Service's National Library of Medicine (NLM) in Bethesda, Maryland and is available through a nationwide network of centers at more than 1,900 universities, hospitals, government agencies, and commercial organizations. At many online centers the librarian will do the search; at others, requesters must do their own search. The charge for a search varies among centers. Some absorb all or most of the costs; others charge a modest fee. MEDLARS contains more than six million references to journal articles and books in the health sciences published after 1965. Following are the databases online in the MEDLARS Network:

Databases Online Network

Medline contains references to biomedical journal articles published in the current and three preceding years. An English abstract is frequently included. The articles are from journals published in the U.S. and foreign countries. Medline can also be used to update a search periodically.

Toxline (Toxicology Information Online) is a bibliographic database covering the pharmacological, biochemical, physiological, environmental, and toxicological effects of drugs and other chemicals. Almost all references in Toxline have abstracts and/or indexing terms and Chemical Abstracts Service (CAS) Registry Numbers.

Chemline is an online chemical dictionary containing chemical names, synonyms, CAS registry numbers, molecular formulas, NLM file locators, and limited ring information. Chemline assists the user in searching the other MEDLARS databases by providing synonyms and CAS registry numbers.

RTECS is an online, interactive version of the National Institute of Occupational Safety and Health (NIOSH) publication *Registry of Toxic Effects of Chemical Substances.* It contains basic acute and chronic toxicity data for potentially toxic chemicals. Records include toxicity data, chemical identifiers, exposure standards, and status under various federal regulations and programs.

TDB (Toxicology Data Bank) is composed of peer-reviewed chemical records. It contains toxicological, pharmacological, environmental, occupational, manufacturing, and use information, as well as chemical and physical properties.

Catline (Catalog Online) contains references to books and serials cataloged at NLM. Catline gives libraries in the network immediate access to authoritative cataloging information, thus reducing the need for these libraries to do their own original cataloging.

Serline (Serials Online) contains bibliographic information for serial titles, including all journals on order or cataloged for the NLM collection. For many of these, Serline has locator information for the user to determine which U.S. libraries own a particular journal.

Avline (Audiovisuals Online) contains citations to audiovisual teaching packages covering a wide range of subject areas in the health sciences. In some cases, review data such as rating, audience levels, instructional design, specialties, and abstracts are included. Procurement information on titles is provided.

Health Planning & Admin (Health Planning and Administration) is produced cooperatively by NLM and the American Hospital Association. It contains references to literature on health planning, organization, financing, management, manpower, and related subjects. The references are from journals indexed for Medline and *Hospital Literature Index,* selected for their emphasis on health care matters.

Histline (History of Medicine Online) has citations to monographs, journal articles, symposia, congresses, and similar composite publications for the NLM's *Bibliography of the History of Medicine.* The scope includes the history of medicine and related sciences, professions, individuals, institutions, drugs, and diseases of given chronological periods and geographical areas.

Cancerlit (Cancer Literature) is sponsored by NIH's National Cancer Institute (NCI) and contains references dealing with various aspects of cancer. All references have English abstracts. U.S. and foreign journals, as well as books, reports, and meeting abstracts are abstracted for inclusion in Cancerlit.

Clinprot (Clinical Cancer Protocols) is another NCI database designed primarily as a reference tool for clinical oncologists, but it is also useful to other clinicians interested in new cancer treatment methods. Clinprot contains summaries of clinical investigations of new anticancer agents and treatment modalities. The protocol descriptions are provided by NCI and by major U.S. cancer centers and sources outside the United States.

PDQ (Protocol Data Query), sponsored by NCI, contains active, NCI-sponsored protocols from the *CLINPROT* file. To each of these research protocol descriptions, NCI has added a list of the institutions at which the protocol is being used to treat patients and the name of an oncologist to contact at each institution for information.

Bioethicsline contains citations to documents that discuss ethical questions arising in health care or biomedical research. It is a comprehensive, cross-disciplinary collection of references to print and nonprint materials on bioethical topics. Among the publication types included in the databases are journal and newspaper articles, monographs, analytics, court decisions, and audiovisual materials. Citations in Bioethicsline appear also in the *Bibliography of Bioethics,* an annual publication of the

Center for Bioethics, Kennedy Institute of Ethics, Georgetown University.

Popline (Population Information Online) provides bibliographic citations to the worldwide literature on population and family planning. Popline is produced in co-operation with the Population Information Program of Johns Hopkins University, the Center for Population and Family Health of Columbia University, and Population Index, Office of Population Research, Princeton University. Popline contains citations and abstracts to a variety of materials including journal and newspaper articles, monographs, technical reports, and unpublished works.

Two subsidiary online files that support the bibliographic databases are the Name Authority File (an authority list of personal names, corporate names, and decisions on how monographic series are classed) and the MeSH Vocabulary File (information on medical subject headings and chemical substances) used for indexing and retrieving references.

Dirline (Director of Information Resources Online) is the National Library of Medicine's (NLM) online, interactive directory, which refers users to organizations providing information in specific subject areas, e.g., venereal diseases, herpes simplex virus, public health, medical research, and professional associations. Records come from the Library of Congress's National Referral Center (NRC) database and the National Health Information Clearing house (NHIC) database. *Dirline* is updated quarterly. *Dirline* can be accessed by a variety of terminals connected to the central computer facility at the NLM. *Dirline* can be searched by organization name to find the scope of coverage and/or services provided by a particular resource center.

Other Online Databases

CINAHL Online. The database equivalent of the *Cumulative Index to Nursing and Allied Health Literature* became available for online searching in spring 1984. It covers articles from all English language nursing journals as well as from selected journals in allied health, including health sciences librarianship. ANA and NLN pamphlets are included. Subject access is provided by the *CINAHL List of Subject Headings*.

Psycinfo. Produced by the American Psychological Association, this database is the online equivalent to *Psychological Abstracts*. Subject access is provided by the *Thesaurus of Psychological Index Terms*. Includes abstracts 1967+.

CDA (Comprehensive Dissertation Abstracts). Contains citations to virtually all American dissertations accepted at accredited institutions since 1861 and to selected master's theses (including nursing) since 1962. Subject access by discipline only. Includes abstracts 1861+.

Social Sciresearch database prepared for Scientific Information and established in 1963. Extensive coverage is provided for references in social sciences.

Databases are available through the major commercial vendors. For information on additional databases or to find out how to run your own computer searches, contact: Bibliographic Retrieval Services, 702 Corporation Park, Scotia, New York 12302; DIALOG Information Retrieval Service, 3460 Hillview Avenue, Palo Alto, California 94304; SDC Search Service, 2500 Colorado Avenue, Santa Monica, California 90406; Institute for Scientific Information, 325 Chestnut Street, Philadelphia, Pennsylvania 19106.

QUESTIONS TO BE ANSWERED IN PREPARING A LITERATURE REVIEW

The preparation of a literature review follows no prescribed pattern. It should be directed toward answering the following questions:

- What has been done in the past to address the problem?
- Has the problem been addressed successfully?

- Have any reasons why the problem has not been addressed successfully been reported?
- Does the literature suggest any new ways to address the problem?
- Are there inconsistencies among the research findings reported?
- Who are the main researchers and what are their affiliations in the research area of interest?

There are many examples of literature reviews. Most research proposals and reports of completed research contain reviews. These are usually succinctly stated in a few pages, in which the findings from pertinent studies are synthesized and evaluated and a bibliography (not abstracts) appended. Sometimes literature reviews stand alone as journal articles.[8]

Other reviews are large scale, of monograph or book length, and include abstracts of studies as well as summarizations and syntheses of findings. Such large-scale reviews may include references to material other than research reports—philosophical, anecdotal, statistical, for example.

Role of the Literature Review in a Study

The material gathered in the literature review must be treated as an integral part of the research data, since what is found in the literature not only can have an important influence on the formulation of the problem and the design of the research but also can provide useful comparative material when the data collected in the research are analyzed. In many research reports the literature review occupies an important place, usually in the section where the background of the problem is discussed.

It is easy for a researcher to become bogged down in the literature review, especially if the area is one where much previous research work has been done. In fact some research never gets beyond this stage, and the reviewing itself becomes the end product. A hard-and-fast rule as to the proportion of time that should be spent on literature review is difficult to state. In a project budgeted for a period of, say, two years, certainly two months should be more than adequate for the review—in many cases a lesser time should be sufficient. With the use of indexes, abstracts, and computerized information retrieval systems the process can be considerably hastened. Also, personnel might be especially assigned to the research project to assist in the literature search and the preparation of abstracts.

The objectives of the literature review in the total process of research should always be kept in mind so as not to allow this step to get out of hand. Essentially, the objectives are to see what previous researchers in the same area of study have discovered and to find out which kinds of methodology have proved useful. Consideration of extraneous material, as interesting as it may be, can be wasteful and can retard the development and execution of the project.

GUIDELINES FOR A LITERATURE REVIEW

In preparing a literature review or reading a review prepared by others, the following questions can be helpful:

1. What is the purpose of the review? Is it to support an entire research plan or is it directed toward a specific step in the research process such as the conceptual framework, the data collection instruments, or the method of analysis?
2. What time period does the review cover? Shall only the most recent literature be included or shall the review go back many years?
3. What kinds of journals are the articles included in the review taken from? Are the journals referenced? Is the journal noted for publishing authoritative material?
4. Is there a comparability of research design among the studies reviewed? Do differences in design affect the interpretation of study results?
5. To what population do the study results refer? What kinds of samples are used, if any? Can the findings from the samples be generalized to a larger population? How

different are the samples/populations in the studies reviewed from the study you are proposing to do?

6. What is the significance of the findings of the reviewed study? Has the study definitively addressed the research problem so that the study you are proposing would be redundant?

7. What guidance do the studies reviewed provide for future studies? In what ways will the proposed study build on previous studies?

8. Are provisions made for continuously updating the literature review as the proposed study is carried out? Are there plans to incorporate the original and updated literature review in the final report on the proposed study?

REFERENCES

1. Virginia Henderson, *Nursing Studies Index,* Vol. IV. Philadelphia, J. B. Lippincott Co., 1963, subsequent volumes are Vol. III (1950–1956) published 1966; Vol. II (1930–1949); Vol. I (1900–1929), published 1972.
2. Leo Simmons and Virginia Henderson, *Nursing Research—A Survey and Assessment.* New York, Appleton-Century-Crofts, 1964.
3. Interagency Council on Library Resources for Nursing, "Reference Sources for Nursing." *Nursing Outlook,* **32**(5):273–277, September/October 1984.
4. Virginia Henderson, *op. cit.*
5. Division of Nursing, *The National Health Planning Information Center.* DHEW Publication No. (HRA) 76-33. Washington, DC, Health Resources Administration, 1976.
6. Interagency Council on Library Resources for Nursing, *op. cit.*
7. *Ibid.*
8. See, for example, Barbara S. Jacobsen and Janet C. Meininger, "The Designs and Methods of Published Nursing Research, 1956–1983.' *Nursing Res.,* **34**:306–312, Sept/Oct, 1985.

PROBLEMS AND SUGGESTIONS FOR FURTHER STUDY

1. What are the benefits of doing a computerized literature search rather than a manual one? What is the value of a manual search? Describe how a manual search can be efficiently conducted.

2. How can a review of the literature enhance the ability to generalize results?

3. Is all pertinent literature published? What is meant by "fugitive" literature? How does one get access to such material?

4. Make a list of five journals, in fields other than nursing and not included in the list on page 97 that you believe would be useful as a source of literature for nursing research.

5. Apply the "myth of the single decisive study" as discussed by Richard J. Light and David B. Pillemer on page 159 of *Summing Up: The Science of Reviewing Research* (Cambridge, MA, Harvard University Press, 1984) to nursing research.

6. Read Chapter 4 (pp. 63–98), "Finding the Facts," in Jacques Barzun and Henry F. Graff, *The Modern Researcher* (New York, Harcourt, Brace and Jovanovich, Inc., 1977). Develop a study idea in which the data would come from existing sources. What are the advantages to conducting a study from already collected data? What are the disadvantages?

7. Chapter 6 (pp. 73–97) in *Scientific and Technological Communication* by Sidney Paasman (Oxford, Pergamon Press, 1969) discusses "The Secondary Literature." Survey the secondary literature in nursing and name the various kinds of literature that exist (i.e., indexes, abstracts, state-of-the arts review, etc.).

8. Read the following article: Marylou Kiley *et al.,* "Computerized Nursing Information Systems (NIS)," *Nursing Management,* **14**(7):26–35, July 1983. Develop patient descriptors that could be used in a patient classification system related to long-term-care patients.

Suggested Readings

L. DeBakey, *The Scientific Journal: Editorial Policies and Practices.* St. Louis, the C. V. Mosby Co., 1976.
S. DeBakey, and L. DeBakey, "The Abstract: an Abridged Scientific Report." *Int. J. Cardiol.,* **3**:439–445, 1983.
J. L. Binger, and L. M. Jensen, *Lippincott's Guide to Nursing Literature: A Handbook for Students, Writers and Researchers.* Philadelphia, J. B. Lippincott Co., 1980.
K. P. Strauch, and D. J. Brundate, *Guide to Library Resources for Nursing.* New York, Appleton-Century-Crofts, 1980.

8

Formulate the Framework of Theory

OBJECTIVES

- To describe the role of theory in research.
- To show where useful theories are found.
- To explain the use of models in research.
- To clarify the relationship between models and theory.
- To present the various types of models.

Whether stated explicitly or not, theory underlies most research. Without theory a study is isolated and fragmented and cannot contribute to a broader body of knowledge. Theory serves as a reference point and basis for generalization in research.

THEORIES AND MODELS

Role of Theory in Research

The role of theory has been described as:

> ... to summarize existing knowledge, to provide an explanation for observed events and relationships and to predict the occurrence of as yet unobserved events and relationships on the basis of the explanatory principles embodied in the theory.[1]

Theory assists the research process in several ways. First, it can highlight promising research avenues to pursue, thereby performing a function in the process of problem formulation. If the problem selected for research is concerned with the best way of training students for nursing, reference to existing learning theories may suggest the most fruitful approach to developing the problem into a research study.

Second, theories can enrich research by pointing to the way in which the specific findings of research studies relate to a broader and more general body of knowledge. For example, individual studies may show that patients in hospitals request fewer sleeping pills or other depressants on weekends than on weekdays. Although interesting and perhaps attributable to the greater number of visitors on those days who perhaps exert a calming (or exhausting) effect on the patient, such findings do not necessarily offer greater insight into how nursing might be improved unless they are cast into pertinent theories of interpersonal relationships.

And just as theories can enrich research, research can contribute to theory:

> Any research project, considered in its entirety, may clarify theory, reformulate theory, initiate new theory, or deflect theory entirely, as well as verify theory.[2]

To the degree that a research study can be formulated within a framework of theory, the more valuable it is in promoting the advancement of knowledge.

How a Theory Is Developed

Earlier in this discussion a theory was said to involve abstraction or generalization of concrete subject matter or events. To illustrate what is meant by a theory, suppose it was found in a study of the financial status of a group of otherwise similar hospitals that some hospitals showed deficits while others managed to balance their budgets. This finding is a description of concrete events which by themselves may not be especially instructive. However, further investigation may reveal that hospitals that are better off financially are those characterized by a higher degree of community involvement in their operations, such as maintaining a volunteer program and encouraging broad representation of community members on the governing board. Additional studies may confirm this relationship by indicating that community involvement in the affairs of the hospital encourages more enthusiastic participation in fund-raising activities, greater acceptance of higher charges by patients, etc.

The final step then may well be the pronouncement of a theory of the economic success of a hospital that could be worded as follows: The financial health of a hospital is dependent on the intensity of community participation in its internal affairs. This, then, is an example of a theory. It is phrased in the form of a generalization, not in terms of specific events. Its value lies in the ability it affords to control a specific situation by predicting the outcome of certain changes we might make in the situation. Given this theory it is possible to alter the economic well-being of a hospital by influencing the degree of community participation. We can improve its financial health by providing greater community involvement, or we can weaken it by reducing the level of community involvement.

In formulating a research problem it is necessary to conceptualize the problem at a level sufficiently abstract and well defined that findings can be related to those from other studies concerned with the same concepts. Studies in nursing that deal with the same problem and produce similar findings help develop theory. Failure to develop theories is due to the level of abstraction in which the studies are formulated. To illustrate: although a number of studies have examined what nurses do in the care of patients, there has been little effort to integrate their data into a coherent and cohesive body of knowledge, one reason being that many of these studies are based on elementary concepts. There has been no effort to move beyond the specific subject matter into the realm of abstraction and theorizing.

Another limitation to the development of theory from studies in nursing—however tentative these theories might be—is the dividing of the research effort among a large number of different problems. Few studies have dealt with the same topic. The motivation appears to be to do something new each time a piece of research is undertaken. Agencies granting research funds as well as educational institutions offering doctoral programs encourage fragmentation of research by judging the need for the research by its newness. A single study has severe limitations in the development of theory, since it is conducted in a specific setting, uses selected subjects, occurs at a specific time period, and is concerned with a particular, individual problem. What is needed is the development of a systematic body of knowledge based on replicated studies.

Where Are Existing Theories Found?

This question is much simpler to answer for the natural sciences than for the social sciences. While the natural sciences have generated many generally acceptable theories, in the social sciences most theories are tentative and often controversial.

Any textbook in the natural sciences, for example, in the field of physics, contains statements of well-tested theories, laws, and principles, usually identifiable by their titles: Boyle's law of gases, Ohm's law of electricity, quantum theory, the laws of mechanics, the special theory of relativity, the law of gravitation, and so on. Textbooks in the social sciences often catalogue the state of the art in theory development, many of which are continuously being revised. Social science theory includes learning theories, the theory of small groups, psychoanalytic theory, the theory of the business cycles, and so on. Note that the term "law" is rarely applied in the social sciences. The term "theory" is used in a more speculative, transitory sense than is "law," which describes a well established principle. Moreover, a theory is generally broader than a law, the latter being usually confined to a single relationship.

In addition to textbooks, professional journals are a source of current material relating to revisions, modifications, and refutations of existing theory. Whole books are sometimes devoted to a development of a single theory. In the social sciences, for example, we have Veblen's economic theory as contained in his *Theory of the Leisure Class*, Toynbee's theory of history contained in his *Study of History*, and Parsons' all-embracing theory of sociology contained in his *Essays in Sociological Theory*.

Few distinctive theories have been developed in the field of nursing and those that have are still evolving. Some examples of theories in the areas of nursing and patient care were discussed in Chapter 4. Recently, books devoted solely to nursing theories have appeared, which is a good sign.

Models

The use of models in research is related to theories. The term "models" has a recent history. It has appeared in the literature only in the past thirty years, stimulated by developments in the fields of operations research, cybernetics, computer logic, and statistical decision theory. In research, models are symbolic or physical visualizations of a theory, law, or other abstract construct. A model, then, is an analogy of an actual phenomenon expressed in a format that is more readily grasped and understood than the abstract conceptual scheme it is used to describe.

A model is an attempt to free oneself from the restrictions, vagueness, and ambiguities that may arise from the use of language when attempting to verbalize a theory, thereby achieving a clarity and succinctness of expression. Freeing the statement of a theory or some other conceptual scheme from the difficulties inherent in the use of imprecise language not only can achieve greater lucidity and precision of thought, but makes it possible to see additional implications of the theory through its visualization in either a symbolic or physical model. Models based on theories that express relationships among phenomena have a value in making clear the predictive possibilities of a theory. Thus, a schematic model of a patient's needs for nursing care shows that if changes occur in either the patient's self-help ability or in his personal needs, his need for sustenal care will also be affected in a predictable way.[3]

$$N\ Ca\ Sus = f[(SHA-) \times (NP)]$$

Where: $N\ Ca\ Sus$ = need for sustenal care
$(SHA-)$ = reduced state of self-help ability
NP = unsatisfied personal needs
f = indication that the factors are functionally related to each other

Only through a process of abstraction and generalization can the findings of different studies be successfully integrated to form a cohesive body of scientific knowledge. The use of models can help the researcher to apply more of the process of abstraction to the development of a research project as well as to the interpretation of its findings. The process of abstraction focuses the attention of a researcher on the need for precise definition of terms included in the study, on the careful selection of those aspects of the real world that will be incorporated into the study, and on clarifying those phases of the research process concerned with measurement of the phenomenon under study and analysis of the data. In relation to the latter point, the following is particularly relevant:

Models are an abstraction of the properties of the data, and the "fit" of models to the data is dependent upon the quality of the process of abstraction.[4]

Naturally, the use of models in research has limitations. First, although a model can simplify the presentation of a complex idea, it can also oversimplify it. In the natural sciences a brief symbolic formula can completely and accurately describe complex phenomena, as Einstein's $E = mc^2$. In the social sciences not only are the phenomena very difficult to define in a way that would be universally true, but they are usually the product of a multiplicity of causes. One of the problems faced by researchers studying human beings is the necessity of translating complex relationships, concepts, and ideas into simpler representations and, in the process, losing some of the richness and subtlety of the original material. This problem will receive further attention in Chapter 10, in the discussion of measurement of variables.

Bross, in his book *Design for Decision*,[5] points out another danger in the use of models – the attachment of a researcher to a model to the point where he appears to be "riding a hobbyhorse," so to speak. Some research is indeed characterized by the repetitious application of the same

model or theory to a variety of problems. In some applications the model may be completely irrelevant, but is used anyway because the researcher is enamored of it. The application of models should be custom-made to the individual research project and should make a truly creative contribution to the conduct of a study.

A child may become so devoted to the doll that she insists that her doll is a real baby, and some scientists become so devoted to their model (especially if it is a brain child) that they will insist that the model is the real world.[6]

Types of Models

There are many different kinds of models of value to researchers in nursing. These fall under the two main headings of *physical* and *symbolic* and include the following major types of models:

• *Physical Models:* Lifelike physical representations; abstract physical representations; schematic and other diagrams.
• *Symbolic Models:* Mathematical models; statistical models.

A brief description of each model follows:

LIFELIKE PHYSICAL REPRESENTATIONS

Before a new product is fabricated, an exact physical model is usually prepared, often scaled to miniature size. We are familiar with the various models of spaceships and rockets used in the exploration of outer space. Similarly, in hospital construction, a mock-up in miniature of a hospital is usually made of the projected building as well as its equipment and layout. The value of such models is to provide a means for predicting how the finished product will actually work. In the area of patient care, the kinds of questions that can be answered by such physical models are: Can six beds be placed in an intensive care unit in such a way as to provide maximum visibility from all directions? How much walking will a staff nurse have to do to provide care to patients? How can a system of record-keeping be best maintained in the completed hospital?

In addition to answering questions concerning physical layout, facilities, equipment, and supplies, physical models serve other purposes in clarifying problems of nursing and patient care. For example, in research on problems of communications within the hospital, actual models of the work situation might serve to point up places where obstacles to the flow of communications can occur. However, as a tool for facilitating the process of conceptualization and abstraction, a lifelike physical model has limitations. To achieve a higher level of abstraction, abstract physical representations can be employed.

ABSTRACT PHYSICAL REPRESENTATIONS

Like concrete physical models these are also three-dimensional representations of the object. However, they are not lifelike reproductions, but abstractions of the objects they portray. Since models such as these are often used to describe phenomena not directly observable, their abstract character is well justified. The complicated physical model constructed to describe the DNA molecule, consisting of numerous colored balls arranged in an intricate pattern representing the configuration of the atoms, is an abstraction. The actual molecule may not agree with that of the model; no one has ever seen the structure of a molecule.

However, abstract physical models can be used to designate concrete subject matter. Three-dimensional abstract models have been used to portray such tangible phenomena as the components of a patient care system in which three-dimensional symbols rather than exact physical representations were used to designate the components of the system. The inpatient area was represented by one type of symbol, the outpatient area by another symbol, the patient's home by still another abstract symbol, and so forth.

The value of using abstract rather than concrete models is that the former can be employed as a shorthand method of conveying the essential properties of the object it represents. In the model of the patient care system, in which the focus might be on the availability of highly specialized technical care, the inpatient component can be designated by a complicated-appearing symbol rather than a less complicated-appearing symbol for the home component. By comparison, in an exact physical replica of a patient care system, the different elements, such as a hospital facility, would require great skill to construct properly, but would not readily highlight the greater complexity of services rendered by a hospital in contrast to other facilities as would an abstract model. In research this ability of the abstract physical model can underscore certain characteristics of the phenomena under study and reduce a mass of detail into simple, uncluttered symbols. It can also bring clearly to light the essential elements of the problem and the interrelationships among the elements.

SCHEMATIC AND OTHER
DIAGRAMS

These are perhaps the most commonly used devices to assist in visualizing the essential elements in a research study. They are also widely used in work situations. In this category of models are found such devices as organization charts, flow charts, process charts, blueprints, and schematic diagrams.

Like the previously discussed three-dimensional models, two-dimensional diagrams may be either concrete or abstract. Thus, a blueprint containing the layout of a new health center is a two-dimensional representation of the physical structure of the facility. On the other hand, a flow chart showing how a surgical patient moves through a hospital, organized according to the principles of Progressive Patient Care, can be made abstract by using symbols to represent each area of the hospital.

In research studies schematic diagrams are very popular and can be used in various ways. An organization-type chart can be used to show the total research plan. Flow charts, like Gantt charts, can be used to show the sequence of the research tasks. Schematic diagrams can serve as models to portray the theoretical background for the study. Figure. 4.1 on page 63, the scale of self-help ability and nursing care requirements, is an example of such a diagram.

Schematic diagrams are widely used in research because they have numerous virtues. Unlike exact physical models, they can be prepared quickly and are relatively inexpensive. They are also versatile and can take a great many forms, either verbal, symbolic, pictorial, or some combination of these approaches. Their value to a research study can be to clarify concepts and relationships, suggesting fruitful areas for further investigation, and to reveal the links with previous research.

MATHEMATICAL MODELS

A popular model for research that appears to add much to the prestige of a study is the mathematical model. The symbols used in the formulation of a mathematical model do not resemble the actual phenomena they represent; thus it is very abstract. Most mathematical models employ letters of the alphabet, Greek, Roman, or other, to represent the various elements included in the model, while specially devised symbols are used to indicate the mathematical operations (addition, subtraction, multiplication, division, and so on) incorporated by the model.

Mathematical models can be used only where the phenomena represented by the model can be quantified. In the model for optimizing the level of patient care in the hospital system developed by Howland:[7]

$$\text{Patient care} = A_1X_1 + A_2X_2 + A_3X_3 + A_4X_4$$
Where: X_1 = sociological factors
X_2 = psychological factors
X_3 = physiological factors
X_4 = physical factors
A_1, A_2, A_3, A_4 = respective factor weight determined by expert opinion

Mathematical models express a precise formulation of the quantitative relationships among the factors they include. Few phenomena in the social sciences can be formulated in such precise, quantitative terms. However, a mathematical model does not have to be a real representation of the phenomena under study. It can be a theoretical, idealized conception of the phenomena. In the real world most phenomena behave in a probabilistic rather than a deterministic way. We, therefore, have to use such terms as "approximately," "on the average," "in the majority of cases," "it is likely that," "the probability of occurence is," in interpreting the results of the application of mathematical formulations.

The role of mathematical models in nursing research is limited. The use of these models must necessarily be very selective, since the phenomena they deal with must be subject to quantification and manipulation by mathematical processes. Also, these phenomena have to be limited in number because the more phenomena encompassed by the mathematical formulation, the greater the amount and complexity of mathematical manipulation required to solve the equation. With electronic computers this has become a less important consideration.

The value of mathematical models lies in their ability to predict behavior with a high degree of precision. If our mathematical model would state that Y (the quality of patient care) is functionally related to X (the quantity of patient care), then by manipulating the quality of care we can predict the resulting quality of care.

Of course, not all mathematical models are in the form of simple linear, algebraic equations. Other branches of mathematics —such as geometry, set and group theory, and the theory of probability—can also contribute models for research.

STATISTICAL MODELS

One of the most useful types of models for research in nursing is a statistical model. This is a type of mathematical model that states the relative frequency with which certain events will occur. Statistical models are probabilistic and take into account the actual behavior of phenomena in the real world. This behavior is characterized by a considerable amount of variability. Exact relationships can only be approximated by probabilistic equations in which a measure of variability becomes a part of the equation. Thus, the previous example of the relationship between Y and X, where Y is quality of care and X is quantity of care, becomes more realistic when represented as a statistical model.

In most research on human beings the simple equation where one factor is totally and invariably related to another factor does not exist. A more complex equation is needed that expresses the relationship among the factors singled out for study plus a residual term representing other influences not studied, which can be called "chance" influences. To illustrate a statistical model: $Y = b_1X_1 + b_2X_2 + b_3X_3 \ldots b_mX_m + C$ in which $X_1X_2X_3 \ldots X_m$ represents each of the factors we have isolated for study, $b_1b_2b_3 \ldots b_m$ the weights of the factors—i.e., a measure of the extent to which each factor influences Y, the quantity being predicted—and C is measure of the residual influences.

This statistical model is known as the general linear hypothesis. It is one of the most important statistical models in explanatory research. It will be more fully discussed in a later chapter.

SUMMARY

Whether models are physical or symbolic, mathematical or statistical, they can serve a useful purpose in developing a research project. A model can be used to portray a theory or a part of a theory, to clarify concepts, constructs, or definitions, or to develop typologies, classifications, or methods of measurement. Models can reveal relationships among the phenomena being studied and link phenomena to other studies in which the same phenomena have been included. In essence, then, a model, like a theory, can provide a framework for a study. Moreover, models are related to hypotheses, the next topic to be discussed, for as has been said:

> In any research project a model is the set of assumptions, or postulates, not being directly tested. Some efforts may be made to test the model during the research project, but the main objective of the research is to test hypotheses that have been developed from the model. For example, the assumption of the normal curve is frequently part of a statistical model, and this assumption is frequently tested in a preliminary phase of a statistical investigation. The model of one research project may become hypotheses in another project.[8]

REFERENCES

1. Claire Selltiz *et al.*, *Research Methods in Social Relations.* New York, Holt, Rinehart, and Winston, 1962, p. 481.
2. James M. Beshers, "Models and Theory Construction." *Am. Sociol. Rev.*, 22:32, February 1957.
3. Faye G. Abdellah *et al.*, *Patient-Centered Approaches to Nursing.* New York, Macmillan Publishing Co., Inc., 1960, p. 58.
4. Beshers, *op. cit.*, p. 35.
5. Irwin D. J. Bross, *Design for Decision.* New York, Macmillan Publishing Co., Inc., 1953.
6. *Ibid.*, pp. 171–172.
7. Daniel Howland, "A Hospital System Model." *Nursing Res.*, 12:232, fall 1963. For a discussion of cybernetic models in health care see Alan Sheldon, "Adaptive Cybernetic Approaches to Health Care," in Larry I. Shuman, R. Dixon Speas, and John P. Young. *Operations Research in Health Care.* Baltimore, Johns Hopkins Press, 1975.
8. Beshers, *op. cit.*, p. 34.

PROBLEMS AND SUGGESTIONS FOR FURTHER STUDY

1. Can you give an example of a nursing theory? Explain how it meets the definition of a theory given on page 51.
2. A number of theories are presented in Fig. 4–1. Select one of the theories and discuss how it could be useful in a research study. How could it be useful in nursing practice?
3. Differentiate between a theory and a model.

Can a model be a theory? Can all theories be modeled?

4. What is a conceptual framework? Should all research studies have a conceptual framework?

5. Are theories immutable? Can they be modified by research? Do you know of any theories that have been modified? (See, for example, the article by Robert P. Crease and Charles C. Mann, "How the Universe Works." *Atlantic Monthly,* **254**:66–93, August 1984.)

6. Read Chapter 9 (pp. 81–93) in Joanne C. McCloskey and Helen Grace (eds.), *Current Issues in Nursing* (Boston, Blockwell, 1981), by Doris Bloch, "A Conceptualization of Nursing Research and Nursing Science." What is the value of the model on page 86? Discuss the distinction between nursing research and research in nursing.

9

Formulate Hypotheses

WHAT ARE HYPOTHESES?

Hypotheses are statements of the expected relationships among the variables studied. They are formulated prior to data collection and are included as an important part of the research plan or proposal.

Not all research studies are based on hypotheses. The purpose of some research is to obtain new facts about certain phenomena (variables). These studies do not intend to relate the phenomena to each other according to a connecting hypothesis. Such studies are called descriptive studies, whereas in explanatory studies the purpose is to find out why something happens, to search out causes, to discover relationships. For example, the problem to which we might direct a study is: What is the extent of usage of home nursing ser-

vices provided by public health agencies in this country? The variable is "usage of home nursing services." Since we are not interested in studying it in relation to any other variable nor in explaining the extent of usage, this is a descriptive study. It is difficult to conceive what the hypotheses might be for a study like this. The research problem is formulated in terms of a straightforward question requiring a factual answer.

After this study was done, perhaps it showed that a much higher proportion of older people are served in their homes by public health agencies than the proportion of older people among the total population. This finding might well lead to another study, explanatory in purpose, concerned with determining why older people compose such a large share of the home-visiting case load. For this explanatory study, it would be possible to state hypotheses. These would be concerned with the relationship between the variables—age of patients and usage of home nursing services. Whereas the previous study had been concerned with one variable—usage of home nursing services—we have now inserted the variable "age of patients." Based on these two variables, it would be possible to develop the following hypotheses:

- Older patients need more home nursing services than do younger patients.
- Older patients require more nursing time than younger patients.
- The types of nursing services provided in the home are geared to meet the needs of older patients.
- Home nursing care programs are less well publicized to younger persons than to older people.
- Chronically ill patients can be cared for more efficiently in their homes than in the hospital.

These do not, of course, exhaust all the possible hypotheses that could be developed concerning the variables "usage of home nursing services" and "age of patients." The hypothesis selected for study would be the one most closely related to the problem of greatest concern to the researcher. Also, the hypothesis selected for study should meet the same criteria applied in selecting the problem—namely, feasibility, importance, need, interest, and competence of the researcher.

The example of the study of home nursing services illustrates several points concerning hypotheses. First, it shows that a purely descriptive study need not be based on a hypothesis. The absence of hypotheses distinguishes a descriptive study from explanatory research. However, all other steps in the process are applicable to both types of research, that is: formulation of the problem, its framework of theory, and all steps concerned with collection and analysis of data.

Second, the example reveals how a descriptive study can lead to the development of hypotheses that can be tested later

in explanatory studies. Indeed, many descriptive studies are essentially explanatory studies having as their central purpose the generation of other hypotheses for further study. The U.S. Bureau of the Census' *Decennial Census of the Population of the United States* is a descriptive study. It provides a wealth of data for the formulation of problem areas. On the basis of these problems, hypotheses can be developed to guide the undertaking of explanatory studies.

Third, the example illustrates that the same problem can lead to the development of many hypotheses. One of the attributes of a sophisticated researcher is the ability to select the most productive and worthwhile hypotheses to pursue.

In explanatory research, hypotheses serve several purposes. A hypothesis is a tentative explanation of the relationship among the variables studied and is directed toward the solution of the problem. Hypotheses serve as guides to the kinds of data that must be obtained to shed light on the problem. Hypotheses represent statements of the variables to be studied and indicate what is to be measured or enumerated. When defined in as exact terms as possible, hypotheses can suggest how the data concerning the variables will be collected as well as the way in which they will most effectively be analyzed.

EXAMPLES OF HYPOTHESES

The following is a set of twenty-five examples of hypotheses:

1. A degree program produces a more proficient bedside nurse for general hospitals than a diploma program.
2. The hours of nursing care available in general hospitals are related to patient satisfaction with nursing care.
3. Democratic administration of nursing services produces lower turnover among nursing personnel in hospitals.
4. Discharge planning produces better patient care.

5. Professional nurses have more job turnover than female elementary school teachers.
6. Patients in open wards in general hospitals receive more nursing care than do patients in private rooms.
7. Academic performance in high schools is a good predictor of success in a school of professional nursing.
8. The use of diagnosis-related groups lowers quality of nursing care.
9. Disposable surgeons' gloves are better than reusable gloves.
10. Nursing aides can be effectively trained on the job.
11. People who watch television extensively read fewer books.
12. The length of hospitalization of patients with heart disease can be shortened through good nursing care.
13. Better patient care in hospitals can be provided through the use of intensive care units.
14. It is better not to tell a patient that he has a fatal illness.
15. Mental illness is associated with the growth of civilization.
16. The use of tranquilizers is more effective than shock therapy in treating disturbed mental patients.
17. Professional nurses are poorly paid.
18. Obesity causes heart disease.
19. There is a difference between the personalities of surgical nurses and that of medical nurses.
20. It is not necessary to take routine T.P.R.s.
21. Patient's length of stay in a hospital is related to intensity of illness.
22. A public health nurse's case load is increasing.
23. Broken appointments in the outpatient department can be reduced by a good patient education program.
24. Marriage is the main cause of attrition among professional nurses.
25. The school nurse program should be administered by the health department rather than the education department.

Some of the examples have been tested in studies. Others are purely illustrative and, as far as is known, have not been studied. Some are fairly well stated, while others are poorly stated and would need considerable refinement and definition before serving as a basis for a study. All have a high order of concreteness. Some are oversimplified. Hypotheses are often considerably more subtle than these and may be phrased more abstractly. The purpose for presenting these examples is to show the extent to which hypotheses have a common structure. This structure is: *(1) A statement of the relationship between the independent and dependent variables and, (2) the population to which the relationship applies.*

KEY POINT

The variables elucidated in the hypotheses are called *explanatory variables*. The distinction between independent and dependent variables is as follows. The independent variable, also known as the *stimulus, treatment,* or *causal variable,* is the one manipulated (varied) by the researcher. The effects of the manipulation of the independent variable are studied in terms of the dependent variable, also known as the *response* or the *effect variable,* or the *criterion measure.*

Diagrammatically, the relationship between the independent and dependent variables is similiar to the stimulus-response model developed in the field of psychology: A stimulus (*S*) is applied to an organism (*O*) and the response (*R*) in the organism is measured:

$$S \longrightarrow O \longrightarrow R$$

In this ideal model the application of the stimulus is controlled by the investigator. All other stimuli are eliminated. Since the stimulus precedes the response, and since all other stimuli are withheld (controlled), the stimuli can be said to cause the response. This model describes the classical experimental design, which is the fundamental model for studies in which the purpose is to test a hypothesis. The purpose of such studies is to understand the relationship between cause and effect, and these terms can be substituted for stimulus and response. In agricultural studies as well as those in the medical field the terms "treatment" and "effect" are usually applied to the stimulus and response variables.

In the social sciences, few studies can authoritatively demonstrate that one variable is totally responsible for the effects observed in the other variable, because of the complexity of the variables studied, the multiplicity of factors impinging on these variables, and the difficulties in maintaining strict control over the total research process. Often the best that can be achieved is to show an *association* among the variables studied: the variables are related to each other in some predictable way, but not necessarily in terms of cause and effect. For this reason, instead of labeling the variables as cause and effect, it is more appropriate to use the terminology independent and dependent variables.

To assist in the identification of independent and dependent variables in hypotheses, the following designates these variables as well as the applicable population to which they refer, for the odd-numbered hypotheses contained in the previous examples:

Note that many studies are concerned with more than one hypothesis. In the case of multiple hypotheses, the research prob-

INDEPENDENT VARIABLE	APPLICABLE TARGET POPULATION	DEPENDENT VARIABLE
1. Type of educational program	Bedside nurses in general hospitals	Proficiency of nurse
3. Type of administration	Nursing personnel in hospitals	Turnover of nursing personnel
5. Type of profession	Professional nurses and elementary school teachers	Degree of heterosexuality
7. Academic performance in high school	Students in schools of nursing	Success in school of nursing
9. Type of glove	Reusable and disposable surgeons' gloves	Quality of glove
11. Extent of television viewing	People	Extent of readership of books
13. Type of nursing units	Hospitalized patients	Quality of patient care
15. Growth of civilization	People	Prevalence of mental illness
17. Type of profession	Nurses and other professional workers	Level of salary
19. Clinical specialty of nurse	Surgical and medical nurses	Type of personality
21. Intensity of illness	Hospitalized patients	Length of stay in hospital
23. Type of patient education program	Patients in outpatient departments	Frequency of broken appointments
25. Type of organizational control	School health program	Effectiveness of program

lem is usually so broad that it has to be approached through a set of hypotheses. Sometimes multiple hypotheses contain identical variables, but are directed toward different population groups. For example, hypotheses concerning the relationship between the variables "nursing care" and "patient welfare" could be applied to different types of patients: cardiac patients, maternity patients, acutely ill patients, chronically ill patients, and so on. In multiple hypotheses each should make a distinct contribution to the solution of the overall research problem and not merely be a restatement of the same hypothesis.

In addition, hypotheses often include more than one independent or dependent variable. Such hypotheses may be concerned with the simultaneous effects of multiple independent variables on a single dependent variable. To illustrate, hypotheses about the relationship between nursing care and patient welfare can include as independent variables the "proportion of care" provided by professional nurses and the "method of organization" of the nursing staff (team versus primary). An advantage to studies like these that test hypotheses with multiple independent variables is that not only can the effects of each independent variable be tested separately, known as the *main effects,* but the effects of combinations of variables, called *interaction effects,* can also be evaluated.

Similarly, studies may contain hypotheses with a single independent variable and several dependent variables (criterion measures). Thus we may be interested in varying the amount of nursing care provided to patients and measuring the effects on a number of psychological and physiological responses of patients to the differing amounts of care. This type of design was employed in studies conducted at the University of Iowa in which the criterion measures of the patient included skin conditions, mobility, mental attitude, physical independence, length of hospitalization, absence or presence of fever, and usage of sedatives, analgesics, and narcotics.[1]

It is also possible to conceive of hypotheses that would contain multiple independent as well as several dependent variables. The problem here is that it would be more difficult to relate the appropriate responses to the appropriate independent variables than it would be in a simpler design. But techniques are available for coping with hypotheses that contain a multiplicity of variables. The problem is that the variables in such hypotheses need to be even more sharply defined and objectively measured than do those in simpler hypotheses.

Explanatory and Extraneous Variables

In discussing the types of variables included in hypotheses, the distinction has been drawn between independent and dependent variables. These have been called *explanatory variables* and are of primary interest to the researcher. They are often stated in the hypotheses. The explanatory variables are the ones that will be investigated in the study. The independent variable will be manipulated and the effects measured in terms of the dependent variable. The latter is known as the criterion measure and reflects the change in the independent variable. However, these are not the only variables present. Particularly where human beings are the subjects, there are many variables that can enter into the research and affect the findings. The variables not of interest to the researcher are extraneous and need to be controlled so that the hypothesis can be validly tested. Ways of controlling these extraneous variables will be described in Chapter 11.

Because human beings possess so many different variables, the researcher must be aware of the possible impact of extraneous variables in formulating hypotheses. These variables can be classified into two broad categories: organismic and environmental. Organismic variables deal with the many personal characteristics of human beings as individuals—physiological, psychological, demographic, and so on. Environmental variables relate to the many factors in the setting that can impinge on the individual and may include economic, anthropological, sociological, and physical factors. Following is a brief list of some organismic and environmental variables.

- *Organismic:*Age, sex, marital status, education, type of work, personality, height, weight, blood pressure, racial group, nationality, religion, job skill, intelligence, hair color, eye color, political belief, income, level of wellness
- *Environmental:* Climate, family composition, governmental organization, work organization, physical settings (layout, etc.), ideological climate, community setting

Diagrammatically the relationship between independent and dependent variables can be shown as follows:

$$I \longrightarrow O \longrightarrow D$$

Independent	*Organismic*	*Dependent*
Variable	*Variables*	*Variable*

Thus, in hypotheses concerned with the relationship between nursing care and patient welfare a great variety of both organismic and environmental variables can influence the relationship. For example, the organismic variable, age of the patient, can have an important effect on the relationship because older patients may respond differently to nursing care than do younger patients. Similarly, other extraneous variables, such as sex, type of illness, educational level, and so on, can also affect the relationship as can such environmental variables as the physical layout of the nursing unit and its organization.

A major purpose of research design is to control the effects of all extraneous variables so that a valid test can be made of the hypothesis. Ways of controlling these effects are discussed in Chapter 11. One way is to restrict the study population to a certain group, such as patients 65 years of age and over, or patients with hypertension, or patients in intensive care units. Or, instead of eliminating the extraneous organismic or environmental variables they may be brought into the study as additional variables. Thus, the hypothesis could be extended to include the effects of the *type* of nursing care on patient welfare as well as effects of the *amounts* of care provided.

Types of Hypotheses: Causal, Associative

Hypotheses developed from research problems can be concerned with various kinds of relationships. First, they can state *causal relationships:* the independent variable is the causal factor, and the dependent variable is the measure of the effect of the causal factor. Cause and effect have been defined as follows:

> By the cause of some effect we shall understand, therefore, some appropriate factor invariably related to the effect. If A has diphtheria at time t is an effect, we shall understand by its cause a certain change C, such that the following holds. If C takes place, then A will have diphtheria at time t, and if C does not take place, A will not have diphtheria at time t; and this is true for all values of A, C, and t, where A is an individual of a certain type, C an event of a certain type, and t the time.[2]

The testing and proving of causal relationships are desirable goals of scientific research. If we know with certainty the cause, we can predict the effect and thereby have a means of controlling future events. Few studies can establish unequivocal causal relationships. Explanatory variables are too complex and the extraneous variables too numerous.

In the natural sciences, where strict experimental controls can be exerted over the research setting, it may be possible to establish causal relationships. In the social sciences the best we can achieve is to establish a second type of relationship, called an *associative relationship*. Here we know that a change in the dependent variable *is* related to a change in the independent variable, but we cannot with certainty say that the effect on the dependent variable was directly *caused* by the independent variable. This, incidentally, may also be the case in the medical sciences, where, for instance, lung cancer is "associated" with cigarette smoking, the actual cause (s) being not yet discovered. It may be that another, more fundamental variable, not tested in the study—e.g., the genetic make-up of a person that affects both the amount of smoking and the development of lung cancer—is the causal agent. If true, smoking would not be an independent variable but another dependent variable.

Associative relationships are useful for making predictions. To use a rather facetious example, let us assume a study finds that success in nursing school is closely associated with the height of the applicant to the school: all applicants 5 feet 6 inches and under do well, all over 5 feet 6 inches do poorly. To say that level of performance in a school of nursing is related to the height of the students is "silly" since we intuitively know that performance is a function of such variables as aptitude, personality, interest, motivation. If such an association were real, we would have a useful predictive tool in selecting applicants, even though we may have no valid explanation of why students differ in their performances.

Thus, associative relationships, while potentially useful as predictive devices, may be weak as diagnostic tools. The limitations of associative relationships must be recognized to avoid the pitfall of assigning the role of a causal agent to a variable that may itself be affected by the real underlying cause. Moreover, in many associative relationships it may not be possible to specify with assurance which is the dependent and which the independent variable. Sometimes variables are specified as one or the other as a matter of convenience, not because one is really dependent on the other or one is the cause of the other. In fact, in associative relationships the designations of variables can often be interchanged:

> If we wish to compare the frequency of symptom X in patients with diseases A, B, and C, the independent variable is disease, the dependent variable is the symptom (present or absent). If, however, we wish to find the frequency of diseases A, B, and C in patients who come to us with symptom X, the independent variable is the symptom, the dependent variable is disease.[3]

A characteristic of associative relationships is that the variables being considered are related to the same individuals composing the study population. Smoking and lung cancer are variables that are measured in relation to the same individuals. So are heights of individuals and their performance in schools of nursing.

In a third type of predictive relationship, which can be called an *artificial relationship,* the variables may not characterize the same individuals but come from discrete study populations. Thus, data on any two sets of variables may be found to be correlated without having any logical linkage. In relationships like these it is often not possible to say which is the dependent and which the independent variable. However, we know that the variables do behave in a related fashion. For predictive purposes, if we know the value of one variable we can estimate the value of the other. In economics, many relationships like these are used in making forecasts. The behavior of certain economic variables, such as prices of securities, is sometimes linked to certain noneconomic variables, such as birth rates, which, although only remotely connected in logical sense, may be closely related in terms of performance and thus serve as good predictors of each other.

In associative or artificial relationships the incorrect assignment of a cause and effect relationship to variables is termed a *spurious relationship.* A well-known example of a spurious relationship is the study that found a relationship between the number of stork nests contained on the chimneys of different cities and the number of births occurring to residents in the city —the more stork nests, the greater the number of human births. Thus, it can be humorously maintained that human births are *caused* by storks. However, it is obvious that the number of stork nests is a function of size of the human population of a city, and so, of course, is the number of human births. The larger the population the more houses and chimneys and the greater is the likelihood that more stork nests will be found. Both variables, then, number of stork nests and number of human births, are dependent variables, with population the independent variable.

The conditions for establishing true cause and effect relationships are several. First, there must be a consistency, directness, and persistency of the relationship between the dependent and independent variables: "... if C takes place, then A will have diphtheria at time t, and if C does not take place, A will not have diphtheria at time t...." Second, the time interval between the application of the independent variable and the appearance of an effect in the dependent variable should not be too long. If a disease occurs many years after exposure to its supposed cause, it is difficult to establish a causal relationship because of the probable intervention of other independent variables. Thus, smoking as the direct cause of lung cancer is obscured by the fact that most smokers who have developed lung cancer have been smoking for many years prior to the onset of the disease and many other independent factors, such as exposure to air pollution or to radiation, could have also exerted influence on the dependent variable.

Finally, in order to establish a valid causal relationship there must be a logical and plausible connection between dependent and independent variables:

> ... if we stuck postage stamps to the beds of some patients (without knowledge of patients or staff) and found that all those patients recovered, whereas all those without stamps died, we could nevertheless not attribute the recovery to the postage stamps, because the relationship would not be credible, or conceivable, or rationally acceptable.[4]

STATING HYPOTHESES

Hypotheses are stated in a variety of ways. In studies where the hypotheses are to be tested by statistical tests of significance, discussed in Chapter 15, the practice is to employ the concept of the *null hypothesis*. The null hypothesis states that there is no relationship between the variables studied. For example, in studies of the effect of drugs on patients a null hypothesis would state that there is no difference in the recovery rate of patients who receive the drug and those who do not. Our belief may well be that the drug will have a positive effect on patients. But if the data lead us to accept the null hypothesis, we have not established a significant relationship between the dependent and independent variables.

In many studies involving statistical tests of the significance of relationships, alternative as well as null hypotheses are formulated. If the data reject the null hypothesis, one or the other two main alternative hypotheses is accepted. One alternative is that the drug is related to recovery rate in a *positive* way—patients will have a higher recovery rate with the drug. The other alternative is that patients will have a higher recovery rate without the drug. Thus, for each null hypothesis, two main alternative hypotheses can be stated. Actually, many alternative hypotheses are possible since the difference in recovery rates between treated and untreated patients can be formulated in terms of the actual magnitude of difference expected, not just that one group's rate will be higher than the other's.

A psychological advantage of stating a hypothesis in the null or no-relationship format is the sense of scientific objectivity that pervades such a statement. If the hypothesis is stated as, "It is expected that patients who receive the drug will have a more favorable recovery than untreated patients," the impartiality of the researcher in conducting the study can be questioned, since he appears to have a preconceived opinion of the value of the drug. Merely stating the hypothesis in the null form will not ensure objectivity and lack of bias. Various techniques, collectively known as research design, have been developed to reduce bias in research. In fact, it can be argued that a researcher should state the hypothesis in the form of the relationship among the variables that he expects the data to support. Such affirmative statements might instill more reality into the study design and interpretation of the findings.

Sometimes what appears to be a hypothesis may not be a hypothesis at all. Instead it may be a proven fact, at least to the researcher, and the purpose is not really to test it in an objective study, but to demonstrate it—to advertise it to gain acceptance and use. A *demonstration* project is a meritorious activity, but it is not research.

As we move toward the more basic type of study concerned with explaining why something happened, the need for expressing null hypotheses becomes less critical. Studies of the basic phenomena in the social sciences sometimes contain hypotheses stated in the form of the expected outcome of the data: "Prejudice is more widespread where educational level is low." "High morale is a symptom of good interpersonal relationships." "The degree of social integration in a community is affected by the extensiveness of shared purposes and interests among community members."

Assumptions

In addition to the hypotheses actually tested in a study, most studies include assumptions that are not tested. Assumptions can be defined as *statements whose correctness or validity is taken for granted.* Assumptions can be based on several sources. First, they may be so-called "universally accepted truths" or so self-evident that they require no additional testing. Thus, in evaluating the effect of nursing care on patient welfare, we can assume that patients require *some* nursing care without which their lives might be endangered. Therefore, we can design our experimental staffing patterns to be above a certain minimum level of staffing. Second, assumptions can be based on theories accepted as being applicable in the field in which the research is done. A study of patients' physical reactions to nursing care might well contain assumptions based on theories prevalent in the fields of nursing, physiolo-

KEY POINT

gy, medicine, or other related disciplines. Third, assumptions may be based on the findings of previous research, even though such findings are subject to revision. A study of methods of achieving continuity of patient care may use as assumptions findings related to existing practices of coordinating patient care obtained in previous studies.

In formulating research problems and hypotheses based on these problems, assumptions may be stated explicitly in the research plan or, as is true in most research studies, may be implied. Only if an assumption has a significant bearing on the rationale for the study does the researcher need to state it concretely. The careful spelling out of all important assumptions that can significantly affect the course of the study is necessary.

Limitations of the Research

At the time the researcher is considering the assumptions upon which his study is based, he must assess the limitations of the study. While few researchers bother to state assumptions explicitly, it is a mistake not to evaluate the extent to which the study may contain limitations. Knowledge of the limitations is essential to an appropriate interpretation of findings. The limitations of a study are fixed by the study design. They include restrictions on interpretation of findings due to the nature of the hypotheses—particularly the characteristics of the study population, the variables being measured, the extraneous variables not completely controlled, and all other influences that can affect collection and analysis of data.

If the investigator is aware of all possible limitations and restrictions on his research, he can take appropriate precautions to reduce their impact. Thus, if the hypothesis is concerned with an area of study in which many extraneous variables exist, he can design the study in such a way as to keep them under control. One such control is to enlarge the size of the study population to permit statistical analysis of the more important extraneous variables. Moreover, stating this limitation in the research report enables the reader to make a valid interpretation of the data.

From Problem to Hypothesis

Progressing from problem formulation to the establishment of appropriate hypotheses is a process of *definition, delineation, refinement,* and *consolidation.* The process continues throughout the planning stage and ends at the point at which data collection begins. *It cannot be emphasized too strongly that the formulation of hypotheses must be completed before the data are collected.* Too often studies are conducted in which hypotheses are formulated after the data are collected, sometimes being suggested by the findings themselves. Such "ex post facto" hypotheses are legitimate only if they are to serve as the basis for additional research in which new data are to be collected. They cannot be legitimately tested by data from the study from which they arose, because the study design, including definition of variables and selection and development of measuring instruments, was not expressly tailored to the "ex post facto" hypotheses. As a result, hidden biases will distort interpretation of data, if used to "prove" the new hypotheses. Furthermore, in statistical tests of hypotheses it is mandatory that these hypotheses be formulated in advance of data collection to avoid inferring spurious relationships among the variables studied. These errors will be discussed in a later chapter.

To show how a hypothesis may evolve from a broad problem area, the following example is presented. Until the early 1980s one perpetual problem in nursing and patient care was the shortage of nurses. Early research in this area was descriptive, dealing with attempts to measure the magnitude of the shortage through such criteria as vacant positions in institutions employing nursing personnel or by the probing of attitudes of personnel and patients concerning the existence of such shortages. Studies then progressed toward analysis of possible reasons for shortages. Early explanatory studies attempted to describe the things professional nurses do and to evaluate how much of their work load could be done by other personnel—practical nurses, aides, ward clerks, floor managers. Later studies attempted to determine optimum staffing patterns that would maximize the use of scarce nursing time by integrating other types of personnel into the nursing team.

Today's studies have moved beyond those early, somewhat simplistic studies to examination of more complex variables. These variables focus more on patients than on personnel. Prompted by the question of how to alleviate the nursing shortage, other studies have evolved to test hypotheses of the relationship between alternative kinds of nursing practices and patient outcomes. These hypotheses have become more outcome-oriented. Hopefully, these studies will lead to improvement in the quality of patient care.

Although the order of presentation of topics in this book is similar to the order in which they are considered in formulating a research proposal, there is movement back and forth through the steps as the proposal is refined and formalized. However, once data collection begins, all the major elements of the research design must remain stable. Altering any part could invalidate the results.

The elements of research design apply to all types of studies, explanatory, descriptive, experimental, and nonexperimental. The purpose of these elements is to ensure validity of the study and to enhance the efficiency and economy of the research enterprise itself.

The steps in the research process that occur after the problem and hypotheses are formulated, are in some studies the responsibility of a specialist. Specialists in research methodology are concerned with measurement of variables, collection and processing of data, and the statistical analysis of findings. The use of specialists for these tasks depends on the size of the study. Large studies are often administered by a research team of full-time specialists from a variety of subject matter fields and research technology. Small studies are often the responsibility of a single investigator, with consultation from technical experts when required. Whether conducting a large study or small, familiarity with all aspects of the research design is necessary for a proper appreciation of the most effective way of pursuing research.

SUMMARY

Explanatory studies are based on hypotheses that serve to guide the way in which the research will be designed. Hypotheses are statements of relationships between independent and dependent variables in the population to which the relationship is to be inferred. In addition to hypotheses, research plans and proposals should include assumptions made in the research as well as any limitations of the research.

REFERENCES

1. Myrtle K. Aydelotte and Marie E. Tener, "An Investigation of the Relation Between Nursing Activity and Patient Welfare." Iowa City, State University of Iowa, Utilization Project, 1960 (U.S.P.H.S. Grant GN 4786).
2. Morris R. Cohen and Ernest Nagel, *An Introduction to Logic and Scientific Method.* 1982 reprint of 1934 edition, Darby, PA, Darby Books, p. 248.
3. Donald Mainland, *Elementary Medical Statistics.* Philadelphia, W. B. Saunders Co., 1963, p. 17.
4. *Ibid.,* p. 95.

PROBLEMS AND SUGGESTIONS FOR FURTHER STUDY

1. Carefully distinguish the following six terms: problem, theory, postulate, law, model, hypothesis. Show how a problem can be evolved into a hypothesis. How can a hypothesis become a law? Are you familiar with any scientific laws applicable to your field?
2. Discuss the assertion, "Not all research has to be based on hypotheses." What role do hypotheses serve in research? Can an explanatory study be undertaken without a hypothesis?
3. Examine the list of hypotheses on pp. 115–116. Assess these hypotheses in terms of the criteria of feasibility, importance, and need. Select a few of these hypotheses and explain how you would go about testing them in a research study. How would the hypotheses have to be restarted, if at all, to make them researchable?
4. For the even-number hypotheses on pp. 115–116, state the independent and dependent variables and the applicable target population. Which of these hypotheses do you think would lend themselves best to the establishment of causal relationships?
5. In testing a hypothesis, why is it desirable for the researcher to be impartial about whether the data he collects will prove or disprove the hypothesis? Is it possible for a researcher to be completely neutral in his belief concerning the existence or lack of existence of the relationship expressed by the hypothesis?
6. Read the article by M. Johnson, "Some Aspects of the Relation Between Theory and Research in Nursing," in *Journal of Advanced Nursing,* 8:21–28, 1983. On page 24 the author discusses inductive and deductive methods in nursing research. Is the role of hypotheses different in each of these methods?

CHAPTER

10

Define and Quantify Variables

OBJECTIVES

- To explain how variables are defined.
- To describe how variables are quantified.
- To present various physiological, psychological, and sociological instruments for measuring variables.

- To provide guidance on how to select a measure for a study.
- To explain how measures of variables are evaluated.
- To describe efforts to measure quality of care.

The success of a research study depends on how well the various steps in the research process have been formulated. These steps are like links in a chain. If one is defective the entire chain may fail. Often, the weakest link is determining how to define and measure the variables in the study. The purpose of this chapter is to discuss ways of defining and measuring the variables being studied, to describe criteria for evaluating this process of definition and measurement, and to give examples of some measures of variables useful in patient care studies.

HOW TO DEFINE VARIABLES

In descriptive research no distinction is made between dependent and independent

variables. When quantitative data are to be collected on variables in descriptive studies, the research plan should contain a skeleton outline of the statistical tabulations, called dummy tables, made from the data. Their preparation before the study will assist in sharpening the definitions of the variables as well as demonstrating how they are to be measured.

Explanatory research is concerned with testing a hypothesis about a relationship between an independent variable and a dependent variable. In explanatory research the independent variable is manipulated by the researcher. The effects produced by these manipulations among a group of study subjects are evaluated by measurement of the response in the dependent variable. In addition to these variables, explanatory research includes variables not of specific interest to the researcher but present in the research situation and that can influence the relationship among the explanatory variables. These are called extraneous variables and are of two major types: organismic variables, defined as the characteristics of individual research subjects themselves, and environmental variables, defined as the characteristics of forces external to the subjects.

While it is generally necessary to identify only the major extraneous variables, it is essential that all explanatory variables be operationally defined. An operational definition is a series of words that clearly describe acts or operations that can be performed or observed and, therefore, verified by other individuals. If our hypothesis is that the quality of nursing care (independent variable) is related to patient welfare (dependent variable), we must define each variable operationally. Quality of nursing care must be defined as certain actions on the part of the nursing staff that can be consistently observed and evaluated by independent observers. Patient welfare must be defined in terms of some objective indicator of a patient's response to the care received.

KEY POINT

Direct and Indirect Definition of Variables

In defining variables in research we need not always use literal constructs. It may be more advantageous to define variables indirectly. A literal definition of patient welfare might be the degree to which the patient is well—that is, free from illness. However, a literal measure of this variable is not available. Therefore, we might use a more indirect definition as the basis for measurement. Thus, patient welfare might be defined as the extent to which a patient requests a tranquilizing, sleep-inducing, or pain-relieving drug. While not a direct measure of patient welfare if defined as the degree of freedom from illness, it may be a correlated variable, so that low usage of such drugs is consistently associated with freedom from illness, and vice versa.

Indirect measures of variables are widely used in psychological measurement. The variable "personality" can be assessed in terms of literal evidence such as the way in which the subject responds to such questions as, "Do you like to be with other people?" "Do you like members of the other sex?" "Would you rather be a politician or a hermit?" "Do you like to watch fires?" Personality can also be assessed in terms of nondirective measures such as the thematic apperception test, where the respondent describes what he sees in a series of pictures, or in terms of even more nondirective measures, as the Rorschach test in which the subject describes what he sees in inkblots.

The variable "creativity" has been given considerable attention in the search for people with scientific talent. Literal measures of this variable assess a person's capability to produce something original. Originality can be measured, for example, by asking the respondent to provide titles to a synopsis of a movie plot, or to create new things from such disparate items as a nail and a stick, or a piece of string and a stone. Somewhat more nondirective is the type of measure of creativity based on respondent's reaction to such questions as, "What would happen if there were no longer any nighttime?" "What would happen if people lost their ability to speak?" "What would happen if money became valueless as a medium of exchange?"

DEFINING THE INDEPENDENT VARIABLE

The independent variable describes the characteristic by which the alternative groups we are studying are distinguished. Usually the independent variable is divided into a few discrete groups distinguished from each other in meaningful ways. In the hypothesis linking smoking to lung cancer, the independent variable may be divided into two categories, smoker or nonsmoker, with a smoker defined as someone who smokes at least one cigarette a day. For greater refinement more than two categories can be established—nonsmoker, light smoker, moderate smoker, and heavy smoker. Definition of these categories might be nonsmoker: no cigarettes smoked; light smoker: less than fifteen cigarettes smoked a day; moderate smoker: fifteen to thirty cigarettes a day; heavy smoker: more than thirty cigarettes a day.

In the hypothesis relating type of nursing education program to proficiency as a graduate nurse, the independent variable might consist of the categories: diploma program, associate degree program, and baccalaureate degree program. For the hypothesis testing the relationship between nursing care and patient welfare, the independent variable could be various arrangements of the nursing team: 25 percent professional nurses, 25 percent practical nurses, 50 percent nursing aides; or 50 percent professionals, 25 percent practical nurses, and 25 percent nursing aides. In some studies the independent variable might be numerous finely graded classes of the variable, such as different dosage levels of a drug, different amounts of caloric intake of food, or varying amounts of exposure time to a medical treatment, an education program, or some other stimulus.

KEY POINT There are three important objectives in defining the independent variables. First, the various subdivisions or categories of the variable should be sharply and clearly distinguished from each other. Moreover, they should be mutually exclusive. This means that a subject can be placed in only one category with no overlapping. If our independent variable is the amount of cholesterol intake in the subject's diet, and if the variable has three categories—high, medium, and low—it should be possible to classify a subject in only one of the categories.

Second, the distinction between the categories should be meaningfully directed toward the research problem. If we are interested in measuring the effect on patient recovery of various types of physical facilities in hospitals, such as intensive care units versus conventional units, the alternative versions of the independent variable being tested—types of patient care facilities—should be defined so as to truly and completely represent the different facilities. The definition cannot refer to only one aspect of the variable, such as the ready availability of certain supplies and equipment, or to some other variable altogether, such as nurse staffing pattern.

Third, the definition of the independent variable must remain constant throughout the period in which the subjects are exposed to it, as well as during the analysis of data. If we were to shift definitions, so that some subjects are exposed to one definition and other subjects to another, we would be introducing a new variable. To illustrate, if we want to test the effect of a certain dosage level of a drug on the responses of patients, and if after a series of trials we find no response among the patients, we may be tempted to increase the dosage level. If we do, we establish a new alternative of the independent variable. Unless we treat it as such, we cannot make the proper interpretation of our data.

More subtly, in a partially controlled experimental study of the effect of a new method of ordering and delivering drugs on the incidence of medication errors, some physicians and nurses may continue to order and deliver drugs as before. In such a situation an alternative version of the independent variable is now present in the study. If the investigator were unaware of this situation, the relationship found between the independent and the dependent variables would be spurious.

DEFINING THE DEPENDENT VARIABLE

While the independent variable is applied to the study subjects as a group, with all members of a group receiving the same alternative, the response in the dependent variable is measured for each subject separately. While our concern with the independent variable is primarily one of definition, with the dependent variable we must consider the dual problem of definition and measurement.

To illustrate this point we can begin by stating that the fundamental design for explanatory research is one in which differences in the independent variable—usually just a few fixed groups (values)—are assessed in terms of differences in the dependent variable—often numerous values. In testing the effect of an appetite-depressing drug on weight reduction, we give one group of subjects the drug and the other group a placebo. After a period of time we measure the body weight of *each* subject in the alternative groups and compare the weight change in the two groups. The independent variable in this example posses just two values—administering the weight-reduction drug and withholding the drug. On the other hand, the dependent variable, defined as change in body weight, possesses many values and is measured in terms of a highly refined, multivalued scientific scale, in this case, body weight.

In some studies the dependent variable may have as few groups as the independent variable. In the study discussed in the last chapter in which the effects of a health education program on the polio immunization rates were evaluated, the independent variable had two categories—exposed to the educational material and not exposed to the material—and so did the dependent variable—vaccinated, not vaccinated. The main difference between the two variables is that while both had to be carefully defined—What is a health education program? What do we mean by vaccinated?—it was the latter variable that was "measured," the measurement consisting of counting the number of people in each category of the vaccination scale.

The remainder of this chapter will deal with the dependent variable, the definition and measurement of which are crucial to explanatory research.

QUANTIFICATION OF VARIABLES

Definition of the variables provides a framework for determining how they will be measured. Measurement depends on the gradations, levels, or degrees of difference of the variable. In the process of measurement we are determining into which of these graded categories the phenomenon we are observing belongs. These categories may be qualitative—as, for example, the statement that the patient feels warm. Here the variable is body temperature, and gradations of our measuring device, called a scale, may simply be below normal, normal, warm, hot. Or the measuring device may have a quantitative scale and be graded into finely distinguished numerical values, ranging from 94.0°F. to 109.9°F, a total of 160 different points, not merely 4, as in the qualitative scale.

Both types of scales provide a means of obtaining numerical values for the observations made of the variable. In a qualitative scale we observe the subject, and on the basis of the definition of the variable we place him into one of its categories. We observe the next subject and place him into the applicable category, and so on. If we applied the qualitative temperature scale to a group of 100 subjects, we could accumulate data like these:

TEMPERATURE	NUMBER OF PATIENTS
Below normal	5
Normal	70
Warm	20
Hot	5

Through a process of counting, we have derived some interesting quantitative (numerical) data which serve as a measurement of the condition of our subjects. As a summary we can say that 70 percent of our subjects have normal temperatures.

Qualitative scales of measurement are sometimes called *enumeration scales*. The numerical data they yield are called *frequency data*. They show the frequency with which the subjects studied possess each of the discrete categories of the scale.

Variables such as body temperature are measured by a thermometer, a scale in quantitative form, ranging from 94.0°F. to

109.9°F. Such quantitative scales are sometimes called *measurement scales* because of the wide and continuous range of values to which a subject can be assigned and because the properties of the scales are such that we can assess the meaning of the intervals along the scale. With the qualitative temperature scale we cannot objectively evaluate differences in temperature. In comparing a subject classified in the "hot" category with one in the "warm" group, we know one is hotter than the other, but the term "hotter" is subjective. But we can say that a subject with a temperature of 104°F. is 5° hotter than one with 99°F. This 5° difference has important significance in evaluating the health status of the two patients.

The quantitative data yielded by the measurement scale for body temperature would be recorded as follows:

TEMPERATURE IN FAHRENHEIT	NUMBER OF PATIENTS
98.1	1
98.2	3
98.3	0
98.4	4
98.5	5
98.6	12
98.7	9
98.8	8
98.9	4
99.0	6
99.1	4
99.2	3
99.3	5
etc.	

These data, for convenience in analysis, can be grouped as follows:

TEMPERATURE	NUMBER OF PATIENTS
Under 98.6	13
98.6–99.6	61
99.7–100.9	19
101 and over	7

Whether the scale is verbal or numerical, it can yield numerical data of value. The verbal scale yields a qualitative classification value for each subject and provides a count of the total number of subjects possessing each of the qualitative values. The numerical scale provides a quantitative measurement value for each subject and can also provide a count of the total number of subjects possessing each quantitative value.

Use of Nonquantitative Data in Research

Not all research requires data to be numerical. Certain types of descriptive research, such as case studies, contain verbal descriptions of the study subjects called anecdotal data. Anthropological research is largely of this type, and so is psychologically oriented research employing the psychoanalytic approach.

Most studies use both quantified and nonquantified data. Narrative descriptive statements are included in the analysis of the data not only to add interest to the report, but to make the interpretation of the data more meaningful.

One of the most frequent uses of narrative data is the quotation of verbatim statements by individual subjects. An example of such a quotation, from a study of nurses' attitudes toward the people they work with, illustrates the usefulness of quotations in clarifying the meaning of variables and other concepts employed in the study.

Another recurrent theme in these early talks with nurses was deep concern about "the move away from the bedside." But there was by no means complete agreement about what this meant or what should be done about it. Some were worried because nurses did not have, or would not take, enough time for individual and intimate contact with patients. One typical head nurse, assailed with increasing paper work and administrative duties, was waiting for the proverbial day when the utilization of ward clerks or floor managers would free her to devote more time to her patients and her nursing staff. One supervisor, taking another tack, blamed the training of present day graduates for their "carelessness about details" and "their lack of devotion"; she felt that "something fine had gone out of nursing."[1]

Sometimes anecdotal data are used as a substitute for quantitative data. This is done to avoid overwhelming the reader with excessive amounts of numerical data or to guide the reader's attention to the main interpretative points the writer wishes to make. A typical statement of this kind is:

> In those services for which there are few incidents reported, the medication load is relatively light and most of the medicines are given by graduate nurses and doctors. The close correspondence between the proportion of medicines given by student nurses and the proportion of incidents they reported suggests that the job classification may not be as important a variable as the medication load or other factors associated with a particular service.[2]

Where verbal presentation is employed the numerical data are often also included. Nonquantified data do not replace quantified data but serve to elaborate them. It is rare that nonquantified data can provide the total data for a study.

Nonquantified data are subjective. The data on the body temperatures of the 100 research subjects can be described as follows: "A few subjects had below normal temperatures, the majority had normal temperatures, some were warm, and a small group had temperatures that could be described as hot." The shortcoming of this statement is that terms "a few," "some," "a small group," and "the majority" mean different things to different people. Such terminology lacks the precision of numerical data. Nonquantitative data should be used selectively. They are most useful in enriching the analysis of the research findings and in providing insights into the meaning of the phenomena being observed:

KEY POINT

> The inspection of nonquantified data may be particularly helpful if it is done periodically throughout a study rather than postponed to the end of the statistical analysis.

Frequently, a single incident noted by a perceptive observer contains the clue to an understanding of a phenomenon. If the social scientist becomes aware of this implication at a moment when he can still add to his material or exploit further the data he has already collected, he may considerably enrich the quality of his conclusions.[3]

The Importance of Quantification in Research

The use of quantification in research enables us not only to state, in our example, that a subject's temperature is warmer or colder than normal, but how much different from normal. Being able to state the extent of difference provides a sensitive description of the variables. As Cohen and Nagel[4] have remarked:

> Both in daily life and in the sciences, however, it is often essential to replace propositions simply affirming or denying qualitative differences by propositions indicating in a more precise way the degree of such differences. It is essential to do so in the interest of discovering comprehensive principles in terms of which the subject matter can be conceived as systematically related. Thus we may believe that there is more unemployment this year than last, or that winters during our childhood were more severe than those during the past few years. But it may be important to know how much more unemployment there is, or how much less severe the winters have become; for if we can state the differences in terms of degrees of differences, we not only guard ourselves against the errors of hasty, untutored impressions, but also lay the foundation for an adequately grounded control of the indicated changes.

Quantification provides the following benefits:

1. It enhances the preciseness and objectivity of the data. Evaluative statements like "after treatment the patient's temperature became warmer" or "most patients were discharged after a short stay in the hospital" are imprecise. But statements like "after treatment the patient's temperature rose from 99°F. to 101°F" and "90 percent of the patients were discharged from the hospital in seven days or fewer are exact

and have universal meaning. Indeed, numbers are a universal language. It is possible to understand the statistical data in a research report written in a foreign language even when the text is incomprehensible.

2. Quantification performs the function of shorthand in the collection, tabulation, and analysis of data. How useless it would be if the observations made in a study, in which the dependent measure was body weight, were in a qualitative rather than quantitative form. How would we record such observations, and how would we analyze the data if we did not use numbers?

3. Highly developed statistical techniques are available for analyzing numerical data. Such techniques permit us to obtain the maximum amount of information from the data. Quantification provides for efficiency and economy in research.

4. When data are in numerical form, a researcher can compare his results with those of other studies. Quantification provides a means of linking the data from different studies.

5. When data are in quantitative form, the investigator has greater control over the research than if nonquantitative data are used. Certain checks which depend on mathematical models requiring numerical data such as the normal curve of error can be performed to test the reliability of the data.

6. When a relationship is found among variables that can be expressed in quantitative form, a high degree of control over the behavior of the dependent variable is available. Through such a relationship we know that when we change the independent variable a certain quantitative amount we will also change the value of the dependent variable by a certain predictable amount.

SCALING TECHNIQUES

The idea of the scale underlying the variable has been introduced in the example of the qualitative and quantitative evaluation of patients' temperatures. In the qualitative scale a set of verbal categories are established, each distinguished from the other in terms of meaningful characteristics. For the variable "temperature" we developed four categories: below normal, normal, warm, and hot. Each class should be described in such a way as to permit the user of this scale, the observer, to unequivocally place a subject into one of the alternative classes. This could be accomplished by the observer's touching of the subject's brow or by some other means that would provide the observer with sufficient information to make a suitable rating.

The quantitative scale for determining a patient's body temperature consists of an instrument whose scale is calibrated in finely divided numerical gradations. When the instrument is applied to the subject, it provides a numerical reading of the temperature.

There are several differences between the two types of scales:

1. In the qualitative scale the assignment of the subject to the appropriate category depends on the observer's ability to interpret the characteristics distinguishing one class of the scale from another. For many qualitative scales such characteristics may be subjective in that appropriate distinctions depend on the observer's senses—touch, in the case of temperature—or other judgmental and interpretative factors not easily standardized and varying from observer to observer in unpredictable ways. In the quantitative scale, a so-called scientific measuring instrument is used and objectivity is enhanced through the elimination of the observer's personal judgment. But even a quantitative measure is not free of observer bias. The instrument still is read by the observer, and in this reading process, as many studies have shown, subjective elements associated with the ability, attitudes, and personality of the observer may create bias.

2. A qualitative scale usually has only a few discrete categories, while a quantitative scale has many gradations. Theoretically these gradations are infinite, since numbers can be expressed not only in whole units

but in fractions of whole numbers. If our thermometer were refined enough we might be able to read a subject's temperature as 98.66754°F. in contrast to another subject's temperature of 98.66755°F. For all practical purposes these temperatures are identical, but this illustration indicates the potential power of the quantitative scale in making very refined distinctions.

Many qualitative scales consist of just two categories: male-female, dead-alive, sick-healthy, nurse-nonnurse, inpatient-outpatient, but there are qualitative scales that contain hundreds or even a thousand categories. Studies of the functions of professional nurses have developed a classification of over 400 distinct activities. The *International Classification of Diseases* lists thousands of diseases.

3. A major advantage of a quantitative scale is that it provides a means for determining not only that one subject is different from another in terms of the variable, but *how much* different. A subject who weighs 180 pounds is 30 pounds heavier than one who weighs 150 pounds. Additionally, we can say that the first subject is 20 percent heavier. A qualitative body weight scale consisting simply of the categories underweight, normal, and overweight cannot provide discriminating information.

4. The major advantage of a qualitative scale is its descriptive value. To the consumer of research findings it is more meaningful to state that "40 percent of the patients went from overweight to normal after being subjected to a weight reduction program" than to report that "the average reduction in body weight for the patients in the program was 22.5 pounds." Sometimes, in reporting the results of research, data originally collected by use of a quantitative scale are transformed into a qualitative scale. Data collected by use of a thermometer may be reported as "70 percent of the patients had normal temperatures after treatment, while 30 percent of the patients had elevated temperatures." Thus two qualitative classes, normal and elevated, have replaced a wide range of numerical values.

TYPES OF SCALES

We have used the terms "qualitative" and "quantitative" to distinguish the two major types of measurement scales. With a qualitative scale we can "measure" by determining how many subjects possess each discrete scale category. With a quantitative scale we can measure the numerical extent to which each subject possesses the variable. These scales represent different phases in the development of a measuring instrument. We may in the early stages of development employ a crude, qualitatively differentiated scale to distinguish between the objects we are classifying. In early nursing care, whether a patient had fever or not was determined by touching the patient and making a subjective evaluation. With the perfection of scientific instrumentation a numerical scale became available in the form of a thermometer, which when applied to a body cavity gives a quantitative measurement.

For many variables of today for which only qualitative scales are available, a numerical scale may be developed in the future. The variable "sex" is usually differentiated in terms of two classes—male and female. However, it may someday be possible to develop a quantitative measure of the degree of maleness or femaleness based on measurement of a biological or physiological characteristic. The variable hair color is usually scaled in terms of four qualitative categories: black, brown, blond, red. Since color can be measured quantitatively in terms of the wavelength of the light it emits, it is possible to scale hair color (or eye or skin color) numerically.

Similarly we have shown that quantitative scales are often transformed into qualitative scales. This is done to clarify the meaning of the data as well as to put them into a more useful form. Every numerical scale can be recast in the form of a verbal one, although the reverse procedure requires appropriate measuring instruments.

There are four types of scales. Two are qualitative and two are quantitative.

Qualitative Scales

Nominal Scale

This is the most basic and widely used scale. As its name implies, a nominal scale is a scale in name only. It consists of discrete, mutually exclusive categories of a variable, each possessing a distinctive attribute, but there is no necessary relationship between the categories. In applying such a scale, an individual is assigned to the appropriate category according to its definition. Among the many variables found in studies in nursing that are nominal scales are: occupational field, race, marital status, religion, nationality, type of illness, and cause of death. Nominal scales can have just two categories or many. An example of the former is the variable "sex": male-female. An example of the latter is "type of illness."

Quantitative data are generated with nominal scales by counting the number of subjects in each category of the scale. Such data, called frequency or enumeration data, are usually summarized in terms of the percentage of subjects in each category: the number of subjects in each category is divided by the total number of subjects and the resulting number (the quotient) is multiplied by 100.

Sometimes numbers are assigned to represent the different categories. For the variable "marital status," the number 1 might be assigned to married, 2 to single, 3 for widowed, and 4 for divorced or separated. The assignment of these numbers is known as *coding*. It is a form of shorthand that expedites tabulation of the data and has no other quantitative meaning.

It is possible to relate data on variables possessing nominal scales by a statistical technique known as *attribute correlation*. Suppose we are able to classify a group of patients composing a case load of a visiting nurse association according to their marital status and whether they are receiving service because of cardiovascular illness or some other illness. It would be possible to determine if there were a relationship between the two variables (associative, of course, not causal) by a procedure known as cross-tabulating the data:

MARITAL STATUS	ILLNESS CATEGORY		
	CARDIO-VASCULAR	OTHER	TOTAL
Single	5	95	100
Married	50	100	150
Total	55	195	250

The data indicate that for the 250 patients in the study there was indeed a high relationship between the two variables—most patients with cardiovascular illness are married. Such a relationship does not mean that a married person is more likely to acquire a cardiovascular illness than is a single person. The true interpretation might well be that another variable, age, which has not been controlled in the data analysis, is the underlying causal factor, being directly related both to marital status (the older a person, the more apt he is to be married) and to illness (the older a person, the more apt he is to have a cardiovascular illness).

As criterion measures, nominal scales leave much to be desired. Many describe invariant properties of people, such as race, sex, nationality and cannot be used as criterion measures of whether a change in the dependent variable is indicative of, for example, improvement or lack of improvement among the subjects. A nominal scale is essentially a sorting device for grouping the subjects into different categories which, evaluatively, may have no connection with each other.

Ordinal Scale

A more highly developed form of qualitative scale is one that grades the different categories in the scale in an order. This grading or ranking may be according to some underlying sequence of intensity, as in most to least intense; or quantity, as in highest amount to lowest; distance, nearest to furthest; strength, strongest to weakest; emo-tion, happiest to saddest; preference, love to hate; and so on.

Ordinal scales are utilized in a manner similiar to nominal scales. Definitions of each scale category are provided, and the observer places the subject into that category which the subject most closely fits. Ordinal scales can be used as self-rating instruments in which the subject places himself in the category he feels is most appropriate. An example is the rating scale given to patients to evaluate nursing services: "How did you like the nursing care you received: Excellent, very good, average, poor?"

Most ordinal scales have only a few categories, mostly three or five, a middle, neutral point and one or two classes on the upper and lower ends. Few scales of this type have more than ten groups, since it is difficult to make qualitative distinctions beyond that number.

Quantification of data collected with ordinal scales is similar to that used in nominal scales. Counts are made of the number of subjects in each category and are converted to percentages to show the relative frequency of occurrence of each scale value. The most typical scale value, an average called the *mode*, is the one in which more of the subjects are placed than in any other. Also, numbers may be assigned to each scale value to show the rank order of the values (excellent—1, very good—2, average—3, poor—4). Through such a ranking procedure it is possible to analyze the relationships between several variables that are ordinally scaled by using a statistical procedure known as *correlation of ranked data*. Suppose we obtained a rating from a group of ten patients, each in different hospitals, of satisfaction with nursing care and placed these on an ordinal scale having four categories ranked from 1 to 4. At the same time suppose a group of expert judges rated the adequacy of the nursing services provided to the patients, also in terms of a four-point scale. The data we gather might appear as follows (1 = best, 4 = worst):

PATIENT NO.	RATING OF ADEQUACY- OF CARE	RATING OF SATISFACTION WITH CARE
1	2	3
2	1	1
3	2	2
4	1	2
5	4	3
6	4	4
7	1	1
8	2	3
9	3	3
10	1	2

By inspection it can be seen that there is quite a high relationship (correlation) between the two ratings. For five patients, both ratings are identical. For the others the ratings are never more than one category apart. Statistical techniques are available for measuring the magnitude of correlation between the two variables.

A limitation of the ordinal scale is that there is no way of evaluating the interval between one scale category and another. We do not know in the example just given whether the difference between 1 and 2, excellent and very good, is the same as the distance between 2 and 3, very good and average. Nor can we say that the interval between 1 and 3 has twice the value as the interval between 1 and 2, or 2 and 3.

But even with this limitation, ordinal scales can serve useful purposes as criterion measures because they do provide a means of evaluating the effects of manipulating an independent variable. A scale like the one just mentioned of adequacy of nursing care can be used to evaluate different types of staffing patterns, physical facilities, nursing care provided, or some other kind of independent variable. However, in such uses another shortcoming of an ordinal scale often becomes apparent. This is a lack of sensitivity in a scale that consists of only a limited number of categories. With only four or five, or even seven, scale points it is difficult to detect fine differences produced by the independent variable. Only more sensitive measuring instruments can detect such subtle effects.

ORDINAL SCALES IN SOCIAL SCIENCE RESEARCH

Numerous ordinal scales have been developed in the field of social psychology. Thurstone, Likert, Guttman, and others have developed scales for measuring such variables as morale, prejudice, and political orientation. Brief descriptions of the more widely used of these scaling methods follow.

Graphic Rating Scales In this method the variable is qualitatively scaled along a continuum from one extreme to the other. The rater, who may be the study subject himself, an expert judge, or other type of observer, places a check mark at the point on the scale which most closely represents his evaluation of the degree to which the object being rated possesses the variable studied. An example of such a scale for evaluating adequacy of nursing care is Figure 10–1.

Although equally spaced, the true intervals between the five scale points have not actually been determined. Therefore, the scale is ordinal. One of the disadvantages of such a scale is the tendency of the rater to avoid the extreme categories, which results in a pile-up in the central classes and reduces the sensitivity of the measuring instrument. One way of avoiding this bias is to omit the central category. This forces the rater to take a position in one direction or the other.

In order to increase sensitivity, some rating scales permit the rater to indicate the evaluation by placing a mark between the categories. The rating might then be scored as a fractional estimate of the distance between the two categories: 2.8, 3.4, 4.1, and so on. The fallacy in such a procedure is that it assumes that the intervals between the scale points are equal, or that they have some quantitative significance. If this assumption were correct, this type of scale would be quantitative rather than qualitative. However, such scales are indeed qualitative and the only meaning that can be assigned to the numbers on the scale—1, 2, 3, 4, 5—is a positional one. They provide an indication of the rank order of the scale categories. That is to say, they show the ordinal relationship of the categories to each other rather than the quantitative degree to which the object being rated possesses the variable.

Thurstone-Type Scale In this scale, an attempt is made to establish the quantitative distance between the categories included in the scale. Instead of having a rater make a direct rating on the scale, as in the graphic type of scale, a battery of statements—as many as 20 to 25—is presented to the rater who checks those statements which most closely represent his position. Since each statement has a previously established scale value which is not shown on the checklist, it is possible to obtain a numerical rating for the individual rater by computing the average scale value for the statements checked.

The scale values for the statements

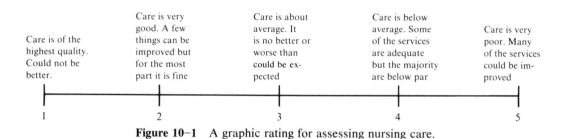

Figure 10–1 A graphic rating for assessing nursing care.

included in such a checklist are determined through a method known as "equal-appearing intervals." First, the variable is clearly defined. Then the scale developer collects as many statements as possible representing different evaluative positions along the continuum underlying the variable. If the variable were "adequacy of patient care," defined as patient's feelings toward the care he receives, a few examples of typical statements might be:

1. My nurse is very friendly and pays a lot of attention to me.
2. I feel that I am not told enough about my care.
3. I cannot wait until I am able to go home. This institution is very poorly run.
4. Everybody seems so rushed around here, I often feel that I am imposing on the staff when I request a needed service.
5. The food they serve here is as good as that in some of the best restaurants I have eaten in.
6. I cannot sleep very well; there is too much noise and the light shines in from the hallway.

The procedure for selecting and scaling the items for the final checklist is to have a number of expert judges sort all the statements, which could number a hundred or more, into eleven piles. The piles are considered to be equally spaced in value and represent different scale points along the continuum. For the variable "adequacy of patient care," the first pile would be for the statements representing highest adequacy of care, the second pile for the next highest, and so on down to the eleventh pile, which would contain statements representing the lowest adequacy of care. The sixth, or middle, pile is the center point representing care that is neither adequate or inadequate. For each of the sortings by the judges a statement is assigned a value from, say, 1 to 11, depending upon which pile it is placed into. After all sortings have been completed, the average value is computed for each statement. A final selection of statements is made to compose a checklist consisting of about fifteen to twenty items

whose average values spread over the scale from one extreme to the other. Statements are selected that have been consistently rated and are clear and unambiguous in meaning. When completed by a respondent the checklist yields a numerical score arrived at by summing up the values of the checked items.

Unlike the numbers on a graphic rating scale, which only show the rank order position of the categories, a Likert-type scale produces a numerical score that supposedly expresses the degree to which the variable is possessed by the object rated. For this reason it is considered superior to an ordinal scale, as it is reputed to be a quantitative scale whose values can be analyzed by refined statistical techniques. However, many authorities in the field of scaling techniques have questioned whether the method of equal-appearing intervals does in fact produce a numerical scale in which the intervals between the scale points have a valid numerical meaning. The main criticism concerns the assumption that the distance between the eleven piles can be quantitatively assessed:

> Even though judges consider the eleven piles as being equal distances apart, this does not mean that the processes inferred from the statements actually change linearly with these perceived equal distances. This places on the unsophisticated judge the responsibility for interpreting not only the relative amount of unfavorableness implied by agreement with certain statements but also the increments of unfavorableness. In other words, he must do, without any knowledge of the problems involved, what the experts have found impossible.[5]

Other limitations of the scale include the extent to which competent judges can be selected to make the sortings of the items, as well as the ability of the scale developer to make an initial selection of items that are meaningful in terms of the variable being scaled. For these reasons, the Thurstone-type scale may be considered as an ordinal scale, although one in which more finely graded categories can be developed than in the graphic rating method.

Likert-Type Scale In this scale the variable is also evaluated by a series of statements which when responded to by study subjects can provide a criterion measure of the variable. The Likert scale, unlike the Thurstone, is not based on the notion of equal-appearing intervals but rather is an ordinal scale. The form of the scale is such that the subject is given a battery of statements which can vary in number according to the type of variable being measured. He

responds to each statement in terms of a scale expressing favorableness or lack of favorableness toward the statement or aggreement or disagreement with it. The scale might consist of three or five or even a larger number of categories. An overall scale value is obtained for the rater by summing up the values of the responses to each of the items. An example of a statement from a Likert-type scale for the variable "adequacy of patient care" might be:

The nursing personnel employed by this hospital are trying to do the very best job they can in providing good care to patients:

STRONGLY DISAGREE	DISAGREE	NEITHER AGREE OR DISAGREE	AGREE	STRONGLY AGREE
1	2	3	4	5

The method for developing a Likert-type scale is, first, to define carefully the variable to be scaled. Then, many statements are collected concerning the variable. The statements are worded so that a rater can express his evaluation in terms of categories representing agreement—disagreement or favorableness—unfavorableness. The statements are given to a representative group of subjects, who are asked to rate each statement according to the applicable scale category. Each statement is scored in terms of a rating that ranges from 1 to 5 (or 1 to 3, depending on the number of scale categories) with the numerical values assigned in a consistent order to represent the degree of favorableness or unfavorableness toward the statement. A score is computed for each respondent. Responses to each statement are then analyzed to select for the final checklist those items which correlate most highly with the score, as well as those that consistently discriminate between raters whose scores are high (very favorable) or low (very unfavorable). The illustrative item just presented would be considered a good item for inclusion in the final checklist if a rater who marked category 5 for the item—strongly agree—obtained a score

showing a high degree of favorableness toward the adequacy of patient care. Conversely, one who strongly disagreed with the statement should obtain a score indicating a very unfavorable attitude toward adequacy of care.

The Likert-type scale has several advantages over the Thurstone scale. Among these is the greater simplicity of construction of the scale. A group of expert judges is not required since the scale is developed among study subjects representative of the target population. Moreover, the content of the statements included in the Likert scale does not have to be as carefully selected as in the Thurstone method, where it is necessary for the validity of the sorting process to include only statements with comparable subject matter.

In the nursing field several Likert-type scales have been developed for research purposes. In an attempt to measure the variable "job satisfaction among nursing personnel," Wright developed a checklist of 215 items concerning job conditions in hospitals.[6] The rating scale for each of the items consisted of four values: agree, disagree, neither agree nor disagree, and don't know. Examples of the items contained on the checklist were:

- I like my assignment as well as any other for which I am fitted in the hospital.
- There is a lot of confusion around here as to what each kind of personnel is supposed to do.
- Our patients get adequate emotional support as well as physical care.
- Staff nurses spend too much time doing work that could be handled by clerical personnel.
- The teamwork and cooperation among the various departments are good.

Another type of Likert scale was developed in a study of nursing student's perception of patients' needs for nursing care.[7] A four-category scale was used to determine the extent of agreement between patients and students as to the importance of certain aspects of patient care. The scale categories were: very important, important, less important, not important. Among the items were:

- To have nurses who are friendly.
- To have the nurse come promptly when I call.
- To be able to sleep.
- To understand why I am getting my medicines.
- To know that a nurse will come when I need her.

In a study of patient and personnel satisfaction with nursing care provided, a variation of the Likert-type scale was used.[8] Instead of having the rater respond to the statements in terms of a scale of favorableness, importance, or agreement, the scale categories represented frequency of occurence of the items: this happened today; this happened some other day; this did not happen. Among the items included on the patient checklist were:

- Nurse did not seem interested in me.
- Got waked too early for temperature taking.
- Not propped up, making it hard to enjoy my meal.
- My nurse was especially nice to me.
- Air in room was poor.
- My nurse is always in a hurry.

In an example of the use of an ordinal scale to measure a physiological phenomenon, Hasselmeyer[9] employed the following graded scale to describe different stages of the variable "sleep behavior" as applied to premature infants:

- Asleep.
- Eyelids slit.
- Undecided
- Awake

Guttman-Type Scale This scale is of the variety known as cumulative scales. It consists of a set of statements to which the rater indicates agreement or disagreement. But unlike the Likert or Thurstone scales, the statements are related to each other in a graded fashion so that a positive response by a rater to item 2 is also accompanied by a positive response to item 1. Also, a positive response to the fifth item in the graded series would indicate a positive response to the preceding four items. A main purpose of Guttman's technique, called scalogram analysis, is to test whether the items form a unidimensional scale.

Unidimensionality of a scale means that the variable being studied is considered to exist in a single plane if it can be scaled cumulatively. The scale for assessing adequacy of patient care would be considered unidimensional if a series of statements concerning this variable could be graded in such a way that a score of three favorable responses in a series of ten graded statements would invariably—or in most applications of the scale—indicate a favorable response to the first three items and negative responses to the succeeding seven items. Similarly, a score of seven would indicate a favorable response to the first seven items in the series. As other investigators have pointed out, however, it is highly unlikely that the variable "patient care" would meet the test of unidimensionality.[10]

However, by selecting one aspect of patient care, for instance, the friendliness of the nursing staff, it may be possible to establish a graded series of statements that have a cumulative property. An example of a series of four statements pertaining to the friendliness of the nursing staff in which the patient might respond in terms of agreement of disagreement might be:

- The staff usually says "Good morning" to me.

- I know the names of most of the nurses.
- The nurses seem interested in me even though they have a lot of work to do.
- My nurses spend a lot of time talking to me and cheering me up.

The cumulative property of these items is such that agreement on any item should also mean agreement with all preceding items. If not, the items cannot be considered to have formed a scale in the scalogram sense.

Q-Sort This technique was originally developed as a device to explore the personality of individuals, not as a scaling method.[11] However, it has become widely used in research as a device to derive an ordinal scale for measuring certain kinds of variables. The procedure for conducting a Q-sort resembles that of the development of a Thurstone scale. The rater is given a set of statements, often numbering 100 or more, related to the variable being scaled. He is instructed to sort the statements into a given number of piles, usually seven, nine, or eleven, in terms of some graded scale. If the statements are concerned with adequacy of patient care, the scale categories might represent degrees of adequacy ranging from very adequate to very inadequate, and each pile would represent a different category.

One difference between the Thurstone method and the Q-sort is that the sorting process for the Q-sort is often employed to determine the rater's own attitudes toward the object being rated whereas the Thurstone sort is aimed at obtaining an expert judge's rating of the degree to which the *content* of the statement itself reflects favorableness or unfavorableness toward the object being rated.

A second difference between the two sorting methods is that in the Thurstone approach only the number of piles into which the statements are to be sorted is specified. The number of statements that can be placed in each pile is not specified, so that, theoretically, the sorter could put them all into one pile. In the Q-sort approach the number of statements to be placed in each pile is specified, and the sorter can put no more or less in each pile. The number to be placed in each pile in the Q-sort generally follows "the normal curve" in that few statements can be placed in the extreme piles, with the numbers increasing as the center pile is approached. Thus in a sort of fifty statements into five categories, the number of statements placed into each pile would be:

Pile:	1	2	3	4	5
Number of Statements:	4	12	18	12	4

One advantage of stipulating the number to be placed in each pile is that it forces the rater to distribute the items over all scale values. In the case of the graphic rating scale, there is often a tendency for a rater, when he uses an ordinal scale to choose the center or least controversial or extreme position on the scale. To counteract such a tendency, "forced choice" methods have been developed, such as the Q-sort technique.

Another forced choice method is Thurstone's method of *paired comparisons*. In this approach every item is evaluated in terms of every other item according to the scale criterion. The results of these comparisons form a graded scale. Suppose we want to determine which components of patient care are least adequate, and which most adequate. For simplicity, since each additional item to be compared greatly expands the number of comparisons, assume we select five components for study:

A. Efficiency of admitting procedure
B. Friendliness of the nursing staff
C. Quality of the food
D. Cheerfulness of the room
E. Opportunity to rest

We pair each item with every other item and instruct the rater to check the one item of the pair that was more adequate. The following paired comparisons would be possible: AB, AC, AD, AE, BC, BD, BE, CD, CE, DE. In mathematical terms the number of different combinations of five items taken two at a time would be:

$$\frac{5 \times 4 \times 3 \times 2 \times 1}{(2 \times 1)\ (3 \times 2 \times 1)} = 10$$

Assume a rater responded as follows by underlining the member of the pair he felt to be more adequate: A<u>B</u>, <u>A</u>C, A<u>D</u>, A<u>E</u>, <u>B</u>C, <u>B</u>D, <u>B</u>E, C<u>D</u>, C<u>E</u>, <u>D</u>E. The items would then fall into the following rank order in terms of adequacy of service.

1. Friendliness of the nursing staff
2. Cheerfulness of the room
3. Opportunity to rest
4. Efficiency of admitting procedure
5. Quality of the food

Quantitative Scales

INTERVAL AND RATIO SCALES

KEY POINT

True quantitative scales are those that assign a numerical value to an object to the degree that it possesses the variable being measured. Quantitative scales are often called *measurement* scales because they provide a numerical value for the variable they are measuring. On the other hand, qualitative scales are called *classification* scales because they are a means of placing the objects to which the scale is applied into discrete classes in terms of qualitative criteria.

Although qualitative scales do use numbers to distinguish one class from another, they do not have a real quantitative meaning. In nominal scales the numbers may be a shorthand way of designating the different categories, called *coding*. In ordinal scales, the numbers designating the different classes show the rank order of the categories in the scale so that in a scale representing adequacy of nursing care, a value of 1 could indicate more adequacy than a value of 2, a value 2 more adequacy than 3, and so on, although we have no way of assessing how much more.

If we can measure the distance between the scale points—that is, if we can actually say how much more a value of 1 is, say,

than a value of 5—then we have a true numerical scale. A thermometer will tell us not only that Mr. Jones's temperature is above normal (an ordinal ranking), but it will also tell us that it is three degrees (or intervals) higher than normal if the thermometer reads 101.6°F. In a five-point ordinal scale of adequacy of nursing care, ranging from 1 as the most adequate rating to 5 as the least adequate, with 3 as the middle, it would not be meaningful to say that Mr. Jones's evaluation of adequacy of care, which he checked as 1, is two intervals above the middle. We have no way of interpreting this distance except in terms of the qualitative distinctions established for the five categories on the scale.

If the quantitative value of the intervals between the scale points on an ordinal scale can be determined, and that is the aim of the Thurstone "equal-appearing intervals" method, then we have upgraded it to a numerical scale, called an *interval* scale. A major advantage of the interval scale over an ordinal scale is its greater sensitivity. An ordinal scale consists of a limited number of discrete scale points which cannot be subdivided further, since the distance between the points is unknown. On an interval scale the distance between the points is equal, so we can break the intervals into finer subdivisions which will provide us with more refined distinctions among the objects we are measuring.

KEY POINT

Quantitative scales possess two properties. One, common to all quantitative scales, is that the intervals between the scale points can be measured. The other, not present in all quantitative scales, is that the scale contains a zero point—a point at which the variable being measured can be said to be totally absent. A quantitative scale without a zero point is called an *interval* scale. One with a zero point is called a *ratio* scale. A ratio scale is so named because having a scale point of absolute zero—the total absense of the variable—it is possible to determine not only *how much* greater one measurement is from another, but also *how many times* greater it is.

The scale for the variable "time" is a ratio scale, since it has a zero point. If we measure how long it takes for nursing aide A to make a patient's empty bed, we might find that it took three minutes. Nursing aide B took two minutes for the same task. It took aide A one minute longer to make the bed than aide B. We can also say that aide A took one and a half times as long to make the bed as did aide B (the ratio 3/2).

The scale for the variable "body temperature" is an interval scale, since it does not have a zero point, but usually begins at about 94°F. If we measure patient A's temperature, we might find it to be 100.5°F. Patient B's temperature might be 99.5°F. We can say that patient A's temperature is one degree higher than patient B's. However, we cannot say that A's temperature is 1.010 warmer than that of B (The ratio 100.5°/99.5°), since in the absence of a true zero point such a ratio is meaningless. Moreover, bear in mind that the numbers assigned to the body temperature scale are purely a matter of convention. There are other types of numerical scales for measuring temperature.

On the centigrade scale, patient A's temperature would be 38.05°C. and B's would be 37.50°C., a difference of 0.55 degree. Superifically, this would seem that the difference between the two patients' temperatures is less than that found when the Fahrenheit scale was used, where the difference was a whole degree. Yet in terms of a ratio comparison of the temperatures, A's temperature seems to be 1.015° "warmer" than B's (the ratio 38.05°/37.50°) as compared to only 1.101° "warmer" on the Fahrenheit scale.

In ratio scales, even when different types of numerical scales are used for measuring the variable, the ratio of two values on the same scale is identical with the ratio of the corresponding values on the other type of scale. For the variable "weight," either the avoirdupois or the metric scale can be used, both being a true ratio scale. On the avoirdupois scale two pounds is twice as heavy as one pound. The corresponding values on the metric scale would be 908 grams (2 pounds) and 454 grams (1 pound) also a ratio of 2 to 1.

In interval scales the ratio of two *differences* in scale values (not the values themselves) on one type of scale is identical with the ratio of two *differences* in the corresponding scale values on the other type of scale used to measure the same variable. To illustrate: a rise in temperature on the Fahrenheit scale from 99.5° to 101.5° is numerically twice as much as a rise from 99.5° to 100.5°, the ratio of the *differences* being 2/1. A rise in temperature on the centigrade scale corresponding to a rise from 99.5° to 101.5° is 37.5° to 38.6°, a difference of 1.1°. The rise corresponding to 99.5° to 100.5° on the Fahrenheit scale is 37.50° to 38.05° on the centigrade scale, a difference of 0.55°. Thus, on the centigrade scale the ratio of the differences is also 2/1 (1.1/0.55.). In interval scales, then, it is possible to speak of ratios of *differences* in scale values even though the ratios of the actual scale values themselves are not meaningful.

Actually, it is possible to construct a temperature scale with a true zero point. *Absolute zero* temperature is at $-273.1°C.$ and $-459.6°F$. It is possible to transform these scales so that on the centigrade scale, for example, instead of having the zero point at the temperature where water freezes (or ice melts), it could be at absolute zero, defined as the total absence of heat—when all molecular action ceases. Such a scale would be a true ratio scale.

Most quantitative scales are of the ratio type. Often called scientific scales, many have been developed in the "hard" scientific fields of physics and chemistry. A distinguishing characteristic is that they are generally highly sophisticated, and some times highly complicated, mechanical apparatus. Most ordinal and nominal scales, by contrast, are "paper and pencil" types of questionnaires, tests, or scales.

In the area of patient care, many scientific scales are available for making quantitative measurements. Table 10–1 lists

TABLE 10–1.

Examples of Some Quantitative Measuring Instruments Used in Patient Care, the Variables They Measure, and Their Uses

NAME OF INSTRUMENT	VARIABLE MEASURED (INDICATORS) PHYSICAL*	USES
Arteriography	Identifies site of arterial damage	Useful for patients with transient ischemic attacks to determine surgical accessibility and treatment
Audiometer	Hearing	Tests the power of hearing
Balance	Weight	Increased weight due to edema often associated with congestive heart failure
Biophotometer	Dark adaptation of eye	Indication of vitamin A deficiency
Calorimeter	Metabolism: rate of basal metabolism expressed in calories per hour per square meter of body surface in a subject at absolute rest, 14–18 hours after eating	Diagnosis of diseases of the thyroid gland
Cardiac catheterization	Intracardiac pressure	To secure blood samples
Cardiograph	Heart movements: measures the force and form of the heart's movements	Detection of cardiovascular heart diseases
Cardiotachometer	Heart beats: counts the number of heart beats over long periods of time	Useful in detecting arrhythmias that occur periodically
Clock	Time: beats of pulse per minute	Indicator of state of vital function of the heart
Computed tomographic (CT) scanner	X-ray of head and body using CT scanner	Used in field of diagnostic radiology for early detection of tumors in head and body
Electroencephalography (EEG)	Measures electrical activity of the brain that may be caused by structural or biochemical lesions	Useful in distinguishing between cerebral and brain stem lesions
Electrometrogram	Uterine contractions: records uterine contractions	Measurement of progress of labor
Electromyography	Electric potential of muscle: use of needle electrodes into the muscle to determine if muscle is contracting	Detection and location of motor unit lesions; recording electrical activity evoked in a muscle by stimulation of its nerve, as following a laminectomy or in a paralytic patient
Erythrometer	Color scale for measuring degrees of redness	Useful in diagnosis of erythromelalgia, a disease affecting chiefly extremities of the body marked by bilateral vasodilation
Goniometer	Angles	Measurement of the degree to which a patient can raise or lower a limb, as following a mastectomy or laminectomy

* Physical indicators are measurable signs and symptoms and can be used as nonintrusive evaluative tools.

TABLE 10-1 (continued)

NAME OF INSTRUMENT	VARIABLE MEASURED (INDICATORS) PHYSICAL*	USES
Kinesimeter	Movements: quantitative measurement of movements	Useful in exploring the surface of the body to test cutaneous sensibility
Kinesthesiometer	Muscular sensibility	Study of muscular sensibility as in Hasselmeyer's study of premature infants
Kinomometer	Motion in fingers and wrist	Useful in measuring progress being made by the patient following cerebral vascular accidents
Mecometer	Length of fetus or an infant	Accurate measure of human who cannot stand
Optometer	Measurement of the power and range of vision	Used in diagnosis of eye diseases
Oxyhemoglobinometer	Oxygen content of the blood	Various forms of anemias
Ruler	Distance: holding ruler between the eyes and the printed page	To test binocular and stereoscopic vision
Sphygmomanometer	Blood pressure: the force of the pressure exerted within the arterial vessels during each of the phases of cardiac action—contraction and relaxation—(normal—120/80)	A marked increase or decrease in the differential is an indication of disturbed physiological homeostasis as in the hypertensive cardiac patient or shock
Spirometer	Respiratory volumes	Separates total gas content of the lung into tidal volume, inspiratory reserve volume, expiratory reserve volume and residual volume. Used to assess pulmonary function in patients with pulmonary disease.
Telethermometer	Body functions	Records body functions as temperature, pulse, respirations, blood pressure
Thermometer	Temperature (Normal 98.6°F. or 37°C. on a clinical thermometer)	To measure the balance of heat maintained between that which is produced and that which is lost from the body. Disturbance in homeostasis is a measurable deviation in body temperature above or below the established norm
Vital capacity	Air in lungs: the number of cubic inches of air a person can forcibly expire after a full inspiration	Ability of the blood to absorb oxygen from the lungs and carbon dioxide from the tissue

TABLE 10–2.

Examples of Some Measuring Instruments Developed in the Social Sciences Used in Patient Care and Measurement of Human Behavior, the Variables They Measure, and Their Uses

NAME OF INSTRUMENT	VARIABLE MEASURED (PSYCHOLOGICAL INDICATORS)	USES
MEASUREMENT OF HUMAN BEHAVIOR		
Williams and Leavitt (1947) sociometric index	Leadership performance	Identification of leaders in ward groups
Zeleny scale (1940)	Social status: measurement of satisfaction and morale	Assessment of environmental settings
Patient satisfaction (1953)	Adequacy of nursing care	Assessment of patients' needs
Patient classification (1957)	Degree of illness	Grouping of patients in areas where they can receive nursing care best suited to their needs
Simon (1957) sociometric scale	Mental attitude of patient	Assessment of mental attitude as one criterion of patient welfare
Wooden (1962)	Patient independence	Degree of independence used as a basis for carrying out a program of family-centered care
Dumas (1963) stress scale	Stress prior to and after surgery	Use of nursing care as a way of reducing postoperative vomiting
Meltzer-Pinneo-Ferrigan (1964)	Degree of cardiac damage following coronary: assessment of both physical and psychological factors that might contribute to cardiac damage	Useful in predicting arrhythmias associated with coronary occlusion
Aptitude tests	Aptitude and ability	To predict success in nursing
Stanford-Binet's test	Mental age of subject; evaluation of overall intellectual level	Mental capacity of children and youth
Wechsler test		
Projective techniques Rorschach test	Human behavior: (a) measurement of personal and spontaneous impulses; (b) signs of insecurity and anxiety; (c) response to promptings from within or without	Provides clues to maladjustment, balance, and control of personality structure
Murray thematic apperception test (T.A.T.)	Deep-lying roots of personality	Gives some understanding of human motivations and inner needs
Self-inventories	Traits, likes and dislikes, attitudes, emotional tendencies	Helps to determine the meaning with which individuals respond to a situation
Self-rating scales	Traits and behavior patterns easily overlooked	Encourages self-analysis and improvement

some common types of instruments and briefly describes their uses. Table 10–2 shows some of the scales developed in the social sciences that have been found useful in nursing research, many of which are essentially qualitative.

A major advantage of quantitative scales, in addition to their objectivity and sensitiv-

TABLE 10-2 (continued)

NAME INSTRUMENT	VARIABLE MEASURED (PSYCHOLOGICAL INDICATORS)	USES
MEASUREMENT OF HUMAN BEHAVIOR		
Standardized tests Multiple-choice Completion Alternative-response Simple recall Matching analogies	Comprehension; facts and skills	Used in nursing curriculums to measure program content
Minnesota multiphasic personality inventory (M.M.P.I)	Personality	Helpful in measuring tendencies toward different kinds of psychiatric difficulty
Stimulation program (Brown and Hepler, 1976)	Provision of sensory and perceptual stimluli experienced by normal full-term new borns	Stimulation used in the care of the critically ill newborn, particularly the premature to provide contact of infant and mother

ity, is their versatility. One quantitative scale can serve many research needs. A weight scale for measuring body weight not only is a clinical diagnostic tool, but can serve as criterion measure for a variety of studies, each directed toward quite dissimilar research problems. For example, it has been used in psychological research to test the effects of psychotherapy on weight reduction and in research on space travel to measure the effects of simulated conditions of weightlessness. A weight scale has also been used as a criterion measure to evaluate the influence of nursing care on premature infants.

Patient outcome indicators (physical, psychological, social) can be most useful in descriptive, experimental, and analytical explanatory studies. Indicators can link appropriate background theory with empirical research methods, facilitating the development of an appropriate research design within a selected frame of reference.*

Generally, ordinal and nominal scales do

not have this versatility. They are frequently developed for a single study and are not used again. In using scales developed in other studies great care must be taken to see if they have applicability beyond their original purpose.

Developing a Quantitative Scale from a Nominal Scale

As an illustration of the effort to quantitatively scale a variable of interest to nursing research we can examine the development of a scale to measure patient's needs for nursing services. The most rudimentary method for classifying such needs is diagnostic categorization according to the patient's illness. Classification by diagnosis can be very detailed; the total list of diseases contained in the *International Classification of Diseases* is over ten thousand. Diagnostic classification can also be in broader classes such as the diagnosis related groups, which combines these into 470 categories. It can be more aggregated as in the typical service categories of a public health agency: cardiovascular illness, cancer, communicable diseases, mental illness, etc. Or it can be in still

*University of Alberta School of Nursing, *Development and Use of Indicators in Nursing Research*. Proceedings of the 1975 National Conference on Nursing Research. G. N. Zilm, S. M. Stinson, M. E. Steed, and P. Overton, (eds.). Edmonton, University of Alberta School of Nursing, 1975

broader classes, as in the typical grouping of patients in a hospital: medical, surgical, obstetrical, pediatric.

These classifications are clearly nominal scales. There is no underlying continuum that connects the different categories. Although they are related in that each represents a distinctive type of illness—a departure from health—the scale provides no quantitative assessment of the extent of this departure nor does it provide any indication of the amount of nursing services required by patients in the different categories.

Taking the variable "nursing needs" it is possible to construct a scale in which the underlying continuum would be a graded scale representing intensity of needs. Many such scales have been developed. In one, developed at Johns Hopkins Hospital, patients' requirements for nursing service can be assessed according to a scale that possesses three categories: intensive care, intermediate care, self-care. This is an ordinal scale which provides a more analytical evaluation of the needs of patients than does the nominal scale of classification by diagnosis or service category. To illustrate, suppose we select two hospitals, each with 100 patients. By the conventional classification of patients we might find the following distribution:

SERVICE CATEGORY	NUMBER OF PATIENTS	
	HOSPITAL A	HOSPITAL B
TOTAL	100	100
Medical	30	40
Surgical	40	30
Obstetric	20	15
Pediatric	10	15

Examination of these data reveals little understanding of the nursing needs of the patients in the two hospitals. We might conjecture that hospital A's patients have more needs because it has a larger number of surgical patients. But, this is offset by a smaller number of pediatric patients. Nothing definitive can be said about nursing needs until a scale that measures these

needs is applied to the patients. Such a scale might reveal the following data:

NURSING NEEDS CATEGORY	NUMBER OF PATIENTS	
	HOSPITAL A	HOSPITAL B
TOTAL	100	100
Intensive care	10	25
Intermediate care	70	50
Self-care	20	25

These data show a picture of patients' nursing needs somewhat different from that conjectured by analysis of the data yielded by the nominal scale. Hospital B has in fact a larger share of patients with more intensive nursing needs than does hospital A. The use of the ordinal scale has provided more meaningful data about the variable being investigated than did the nominal scale.

The next stage in the development of a scale to assess patients' nursing needs would be to advance from an ordinal to a quantitative type scale. By detailed study of groups of representative patients it is possible to determine the average amounts of nursing care required by patients in each of the three categories. On the basis of these data, a crude quantitative scale can be established that provides values for the intervals between the three classes. The following scale (Figure 10–2) shows the quantitative relationships among the classes:

This means an intermediate care patient requires twice as much nursing care as does a self-care patient. An intensive care patient has five times the requirements of the self-care patient. These values provide a method for quantitatively assessing the needs of patients which could yield useful data for research as well as for administrative purposes.

The highest stage in the development of a scale to measure the nursing care needs of patients would be to develop a truly comprehensive quantitative measure of a patient's total care needs. Such a measure might well be part of a larger concept of the

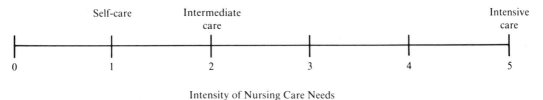

Figure 10-2   A quantitative scale for assessing intensity of nursing care needs.

measurement of a person's level of wellness. Although it is difficult to conceive of such a scale as possessing unidimensionality, since we can speak of wellness in terms of physical, psychological, or sociological factors, it may be possible to develop an abstract measure that would synthesize these various factors.

The importance of a wellness scale to nursing is that it would be concerned with a person's total health status. Present patient classification methods are directed primarily toward the needs of a patient who has some morbid condition in need of correction. A wellness scale would be valuable not only as a criterion measure for many different kinds of studies concerned with assessing the impact on patient welfare of different methods, procedures, or programs, but also as a tool for planning and evaluating patient care.

There is, indeed, a long way to go in applying exact quantitative measurement to the study of human beings. As Cochran[12] has remarked:

In the study of human beings many of the problems of measurement are formidable. Not only have we to measure fairly concrete attributes like the state of disease in the individual (which the doctors will assure us is not easy to measure well) but we need to classify and if possible to measure many things that are hard enough to define in the first place, like motives, morale, intentions, feelings of stress. This means a vast undertaking that has had to start from the ground with crude homemade tools. Thus far, for want of anything better in sight, we have obtained our raw data mainly from what the individual tells us. And the recording instrument has usually been another individual.

HOW TO SELECT A CRITERION MEASURE FOR A STUDY

The type of criterion measure or measures used in an explanatory study is influenced by the research problem and the hypotheses developed to explore the problem. The hypothesis is a statement of the explanatory variables with which the research will be concerned. After defining the variables as concretely and operationally as possible, the researcher must decide how the dependent variable will be measured— whether to use a direct or an indirect measure. This decision will be influenced by the ease with which the variable can be directly measured and the extent to which a subtler measure might yield more meaningful data. In many instances indirect measurement of a variable may be simpler to accomplish than direct measurement of the phenomenon.

But indirect measurement may be more efficient than direct measurement. For example, it is rather simple to measure the density of liquids on the basis of the law that expresses density as a constant function of the ratio between the weight and the volume of the particular liquid, but it would be tedious and less precise by direct procedures. By a direct procedure we might, for example, use a standard set of solid bodies, which we would place in the various liquids. We would agree to call one liquid more dense than another if we could find a solid body which would float in one but not in the other. Following this procedure systematically for all liquids, we would assign the numbers 1, 2, 3, 4, 5, etc., to designate the position of the liquids in the density scale. Clearly, the direct procedure is more cumbersome and less precise than the indirect procedure.[13]

In some studies the researcher has available a variety of criterion measures of the dependent variable. If the variable can be measured in terms of physiological response, many scientific instruments can yield highly refined numerical measurements.

If the variable is a psychological or sociological phenomenon, there are many satisfactory tests and scales that can be used. Such variables as personality, motivation, perception, creativity, abilities of all types, intellectual and mechanical aptitudes, as well as a great variety of social attitudes such as prejudice, authoritarianism, and morale, can be measured in terms of ordinal scales by standardized paper and pencil tests. For many important variables, useful nominal scales already exist. A variable such as "type of illness" has been developed into a highly refined nominal scale.

In retrospective studies the researcher must accept the measures of variables developed by others, since he is using data originally designed for another purpose. With such data care must be taken that they do actually meet the needs of the research in which they are used. If our criterion measure in a retrospective study is rate of patients' recovery from their illnesses and we obtain our data from hospital charts, we may find gaps in these records. Moreover, the definitions used may differ from our own. Such deficiencies can seriously weaken the measurement process and can damage the total research effort.

Many researchers must develop their own measures of the explanatory variables—namely, the dependent variables. In the case of highly complex variables, measurement can be difficult, requiring the assistance of experts. There are specialists in the field of measurement, and a researcher should not hesitate to enlist their services when necessary. Most researchers, however, follow a "do-it-yourself" course in developing criterion measures. For many variables this task does not present too much difficulty. For others,

it can represent a formidable effort, perhaps the single most time-consuming and difficult step in the entire research process.

Review of the literature can often be helpful in the development of a criterion measure. A researcher can sometimes find a measure that he can use either directly or with some adaptation. If it is necessary to develop his own measure, useful ideas can sometimes be suggested by the literature.

Knowledge of existing instrumentation that can be used for research measurement is available from textbooks, manuals, encyclopedias, and similar types of reference works. A good textbook on physiology will contain descriptions of the more common types of measuring apparatus in this field. In the social sciences several specialized journals deal with problems of measurement. These include *Psychometrika, Sociometry, Mathematical Biosciences*, and the *Journal of Mathematical Psychology*. Occasionally, the literature in the statistical field includes material on measurement. Information pertinent to patient care research is most likely to appear in such statistical journals as *Biometrics* and *Biometrika*.

CRITERIA FOR EVALUATING SUFFICIENCY AND EFFICIENCY OF MEASURES OF VARIABLES

Whether the method for measuring the variables in a study has been designed by others or developed by the researcher, the measures used must meet certain tests to be considered acceptable. Four of the most important criteria for evaluating the adequacy of measures are validity, reliability, sensitivity, and meaningfulness.

Validity

The criterion of validity is the most important of the four tests. If a measure is not valid, it does not really matter that it meets other tests. The concept of validity, also called relevance, simply means: does the measure actually measure what it is suppose to? If a measuring instrument is supposed to measure patient satisfaction with nursing care, does it really measure satisfaction as it has been operationally defined, or is it measuring some other variable, or nothing? As a check on whether a variable such as patient satisfaction is operationally defined, the following questions can be raised. What is satisfaction? Does it have substance and meaning so that it manifests itself in terms of observable, tangible behavior? Such behavior might be, for dissatisfied patients—vocal complaints including a firm resolve never to return to the hospital; for satisfied patients—unsolicited compliments.

A succinct and humorous illustration of what is meant by validity follows.

> We hear of a museum in a certain Eastern city that was proud of its amazing attendance record. Recently a little stone building was erected nearby. Next year attendance at the museum mysteriously fell off by 100,000. What was the little stone building? A comfort station.[14]

Understandably the museum was using the number of persons entering the museum as a measure of interest in its exhibits. This measure was invalid because what attracted many people to the museum as it turned out was another purpose.

The object of measurement is to determine the true value of the variable for the individual being measured. If we measure satisfaction with patient care and find differences among the patients included, we hope that these differences reflect true differences in the level of satisfaction of the patients. However, we must recognize that there are certain sources of variation in measures that do not reflect true differences in the variable. In the discussion of research design, we have mentioned two—the extraneous organismic and environmental variables. To illustrate, patient care studies have shown that age is related to how a patient responds to the scale of satisfaction with adequacy of nursing care —older people generally react favorably to

their nursing care regardless of its actual quality. Thus in an explanatory study of adequacy of patient care, it is possible that more older patients would be assigned to one group than to others. If we were unaware of the relationship between age and satisfaction and examined only the average satisfaction scores for the groups as a whole, we may conclude that the group with more older patients was receiving more adequate care, when, in fact, by other criteria it was not. Errors due to the intrusion of these variables can be largely controlled by such techniques as randomization, balancing, and pairing, which distribute them so that they offset each other. Unfortunately, some effects of extraneous organismic and environmental variables are always present in a study no matter how well controlled.

In addition to the variation in measurement attributable to extraneous variables there are errors arising from the measuring process itself that can also affect the validity of the findings. These arise from defects in the measuring instrument—a weight scale that goes out of order occasionally, an achievement test that contains ambiguous items misinterpreted by respondents—or from errors made by the observer who reads the instrument or the rater who scores a test. Such inconsistencies in the measurement process, known as unreliability, also harm the validity of the measure.

Therefore, validity can be influenced by errors arising from the subjects themselves, from outside influences on the subjects, and from inconsistencies in the measuring process. An otherwise quite valid measure can have its relevance destroyed by these sources of error. However, even if all these sources of error were controlled, we would still have no guarantee that our measure was valid.

Validity must be assessed on its own merits. Assume we used a measure such as blood pressure as a criterion of the variable "patient well-being" in an experimental study of alternative types of nurse staffing

KEY POINT

patterns. Further, assume we kept all possible sources of error under control—we randomized our experimental subjects to the alternative groups, the environment of the patients was kept identical, and expert observers used the best available apparatus. The results could still be invalid because blood pressure may not be a relevant measure of patient well-being. That is to say, variations in blood pressure measurements may not truly reflect variations in the well-being of subjects. When an indirect measure is used as a criterion measure of a dependent variable, special care must be taken to see that it is relevant.

For many variables it is possible to make an empirical check of the validity of the measure by testing the accuracy of predictions based on the measure. In this procedure we correlate the results obtained by the measure with an outside criterion. An example of the empirical validity of a measure is contained in a study of job satisfaction of nursing personnel in which an ordinal scale was developed based on a battery of 215 items representing different aspects of the work situation.[15] A group of representative nursing personnel responded to the items and were ranked according to high and low job satisfaction. Job turnover was the validity criterion, since it was assumed that personnel with low satisfaction would leave the organization at a higher rate than those with high satisfaction. This relationship was found in studies of other occupations. Some correlation was found between turnover behavior and job satisfaction, but it was not high enough to validate satisfactorily the job satisfaction scale in terms of the variable "turnover behavior." Possibly an outside validation criterion other than turnover would have been better predicted by the satisfaction measure.

Most desirably, validation of a measure should be done empirically by correlating it with an independent behavioral criterion—a criterion that describes a meaningful, objective, observable action. If we are measuring the variable "proficiency as a nurse" by a pencil and paper instrument we should be able to validate it in terms of the behavior of the nurse in actual practice. For many measures, particularly those dealing with somewhat vague sociological or psychological concepts, this type of validation cannot be done too easily, if at all. Look at the previously mentioned variable, satisfaction with nursing care. What practical behavioral criterion can we use to make predictions from the measure?

As a substitute for empirical validation of such variables we can use the technique of validation by independent expert judges. The judges observe the patients who ranked low on the measure of satisfaction with nursing care and, using a set of objective criteria, decide whether they are different in some meaningful way from those who ranked high. This procedure is more subjective than correlating the measure with a behavioral criterion, but if the only other alternative is no formal validation of the measure at all, it should be given consideration.

Up to this point we have described the concept of validity primarily in terms of the *predictive* power of the measure: the ability of the measure to predict some outcome or event that is hypothesized to be related to the fundamental concept. Thus, the measure "nurse satisfaction" should be able to distinguish between high turnover and low turnover. A nurse with a high satisfaction score would be less likely to quit her job than one with a low score.

Predictive validity is a desirable way of assessing the validity of measures from either the physical or social sciences. In the social sciences other ways of assessing validity also have been developed. These are especially applicable to measures that are composed of a battery of items such as Likert scales. They are called *face, content,* and *construct* validity. *Face* validity is essentially a common-sense evaluation of a measure. If a measure "feels right," if it agrees with the investigator's concept of what the measure is supposed to describe, it has face or pragmatic validity. *Content* validity, closely related to face validity, assesses the comprehensiveness and representativeness of the content of the measure. *Construct* validity refers to whether the measure is consistent with the purpose to which the measure is addressed and the theoretical framework on which the measurement is based.

Construct validity is difficult to assess empirically. In one approach to construct validity, a measure is said to have construct validity if it discriminates among groups in a logical and expected way. For example, a measure of intensity of nursing needs of patients in acute care hospitals would possess construct validity if patients with different measures had varying lengths of stay: those with greater needs would remain in the hospital longer than those with lesser needs. It is clear that construct validity is similar to predictive validity except that in the latter there does not have to be a theoretical connection between the measure and the predictor variable.

Reliability

This criterion is also known as the reproducibility or the repeatability of a measure and concerns the consistency or precision of the measure. A measure is reliable only if it is consistently reproducible.

The concept of reliability can be best understood when it is considered that variation in measurement can arise from two main sources, assuming control of all extraneous organismic and environmental variables. If we measure a patient's temperature at two different times we may note a rise in the reading. This could be due to two factors: a real rise in temperature due to physiological change, or a false rise due to either a mistake by the observer or a failure of the instrument. A false reading due to either observer or instrument error would mean a lack of reliability of the measuring process. If both errors occur frequently during a study, the measure is unreliable. In this example, temperature may well be a

valid measure—that is, it relevantly describes the variable under study—but it may not be reliable.

Stated the other way, if measurement of an object is made over a period of time, and if the variable being measured has undergone no real change, the measure is reliable if the observer reports no change. Or if in repeated measurements a real change occurs, reliable measurements must reflect this change.

Perhaps the most likely source of error that renders a measure unreliable is that due to the observer. Mechanical instruments, especially those of high quality, are generally stable. Some can be calibrated and adjusted to account for deterioration. Many electronic instruments have controls to adjust for the aging of components, changes in temperature, variations in the electric supply, and so on. Scientific instruments such as thermometers, weight scales, and clocks can be checked for accuracy and consistency either by comparing instrument readings against another known to be exact, or by subjecting the instruments to analysis by test equipment especially made for assessing reliability.*

Reliability of physiological and sociological instruments can be checked by such techniques as the split-half or odd-even method, in which the score on half of the items in an instrument is compared with the score on the other half. Since the items are distributed randomly, it can be assumed that the scores on the two halves are identical. To the degree that they are not is an indication of the unreliability of the measure.

Still another way of checking the reliability of tests and scales is the test-retest method. For variables whose measures for a given individual should remain stable over time, such as intelligence, personality, interest, and basic attitudes, repeated measurement should yield approximately the

* The National Bureau of Standards, Office of Technical Information, Gaithersburg, Maryland, will test an instrument for its reliability and when possible standardize it (there is a charge for this service).

same scores. To the extent that the values are different the reliability of the measuring instrument is questionable.

Observer error in reading scientific instruments can be checked by having independent observers read the same instrument simultaneously and comparing the readings. Interrater reliability is measured by the extent to which the readings of the observers agree. Unlike the method of repeated measurements over time which tests reliability in terms of the stability of the instrument, comparison of simultaneous measurements eliminates the possibility of differences in the measure related to the passage of time. In a study of the reliability of blood pressure readings by nurses, Wilcox[16] employed a double stethoscope having one head and two sets of earpieces. Two observers, using a single, accuracy-checked sphygmomanometer, could make simultaneous readings of the same patients' blood pressure. Three pairs of nurses read the blood pressure of the same patient over a brief period of time. The findings revealed considerable variation (lack of reliability) in blood pressure readings of the same patients, both systolic and diastolic, among the observers.

Observer error in other methods of data collection, such as an observer making narrative recordings of what she sees, can be similarly checked for reliability through a comparison of recordings made simultaneously of the same events by independent observers. To illustrate, a check of the reliability of a patient classification instrument consisted of having two observers, the head nurse and her assistant, both having an equal amount of information about the patient, make simultaneous independent ratings of the same patient's needs for nursing care. The two ratings were compared, and a high level of agreement was found, particularly on those items reflecting physical care needs of patients.

Simultaneous measurement can also be made of the same phenomenon using different instruments, which would check the consistency or equivalence of the different measuring instruments.

Errors in measurement will not disturb the validity of the measurements made of large groups of study subjects if the errors are randomly distributed, since they would tend to offset each other. Only when they are consistently skewed in one direction can they bias the findings of a study. However, when measurements are needed for individual cases, as in diagnosis of a patients' illness, unreliability cannot be tolerated, since wrong measurements may negatively affect the course of treatment.

Reliability of measurements can be controlled if the sources of error are known. The following summarizes the main causes of unreliability in measurements:

1. Defects in measuring instruments —usually mechanical in the case of physical instruments; wording and other structural defects in the case of pencil and paper instruments.
2. Lack of adequate training and/or experience of the observer in reading the instrument or in scoring or interpreting the results of a pencil and paper test.
3. Psychological biases on the part of the observer affecting the reading of the measure.
4. Errors arising from the person being measured—as, for example, misinterpreting instructions on a test and responding incorrectly.

It is important to note that even if an instrument is reliable there is no guarantee that it will produce a valid measure of the variable. For example, half a dozen experts independently reading the same electrocardiograph measurements could arrive at the same interpretation, but their interpretation would be quite irrelevant if the apparatus were defective and produced normal readings for patients who actually had abnormal heart conditions, and vice versa. On the other hand, unreliable measurements seriously harm the relevance of findings based on a measure that is a valid one.

Sensitivity

This test refers to the ability of the measure to detect fine differences among the subjects. One limitation of many ordinal

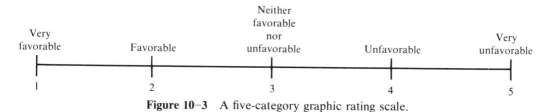

Figure 10–3 A five-category graphic rating scale.

and nominal scales is crudeness. Having only a few global categories, these scales cannot really distinguish significant differences in the dependent variable, thus masking what may be important effects of the independent variable. If we use, for example, a scale consisting of only two categories—improved, not improved—to measure the effects on patients of some nursing procedure, we will be lumping together in the improved category patients whose conditions vary widely, some showing considerably more improvement than others. However, dividing such a scale into many categories may not really increase the sensitivity, since some of the categories may represent distinctions too fine for the measure to detect properly. Thus, if the improved class were subdivided into "much improvement, moderate improvement, little improvement," we would have to be sure that the specifications for each value were sufficiently clear and distinct to ensure that the use of the scale would have a high degree of reliability. Moreover, we would also have to be certain that these more refined categories would have practical significance. That is, they should add substantively to our knowledge of the independent variable.

With psychological and sociological phenomena there is often the temptation to expand an ordinal scale by treating it as an interval scale. The intervals between the scale points are subdivided into smaller and smaller segments, and the scale is then treated as a numerical one. Assume that a five-category graphic rating scale consisting of the following classes was developed to measure attitudes of the respondents toward phenomenon (see Figure 10–3):

To introduce greater sensitivity the researcher might subdivide each of the four intervals into five equal parts and instruct the respondent to check the scale at the point that represents his feelings most closely. The researcher might then treat these data as being truly quantitative and expose them to the full battery of statistical methods. With such "refinement" the number of values on the scale has been increased four times (see Figure 10–4):

That this type of refinement is unreal becomes obvious when it is considered that the numbers on this scale have no quantitative meaning, per se. They are purely positional values, and indicate the rank order of the subject's response. We can say that a respondent with a value of 1 has greater positive feelings toward the phenomenon than one with a value of 4, but we cannot say how much greater his feelings are.

The addition of the refined subdivisions has not increased the sensitivity of the measurements, since most users of the scale would not be able to make these dis-

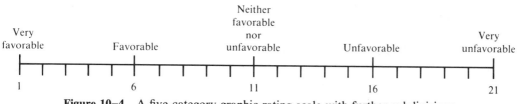

Figure 10–4 A five-category graphic rating scale with further subdivisions.

tinctions validly. In fact, confused by such a large number of choices, they might be inclined to make erroneous ratings. Refinement in such a case actually reduces the reliability of an instrument.

True numerical scales have a high degree of sensitivity. Theoretically such scales can be infinitely subdivided. A thermometer with gradations for each tenth of a degree can be scaled in terms of one-hundredth of a degree, if such sensitivity were required. However, for readability a much bigger scale would be needed than the one commonly used. The instruments then might become impractical. Also, enlargement of a numerical scale may result in unneeded refinement. In most studies it makes little difference if a patient's temperature is read at 98.60°F. or 98.61°F. Refinement of a scale, even where mathematically justifiable, must be tempered by the practical significance of the small differences in values obtained by such refinement.

Meaningfulness

KEY POINT   The concept of meaningfulness of a measure can also be called the pragmatic test of the measure as a whole. Does the measure have practical, real-life meaning and application? If an instrument is used to measure patient satisfaction and it is found that by varying the independent variable—for instance, hours of nursing care available—the scores on the patient satisfaction instruments are increased, does this mean that the patients are better off when increased care is provided? What is meant by "better off"? Do they have higher recovery rates? Do they live longer? Do they become more productive? Are they able to enjoy life more? The researcher must be able to translate the criterion of satisfaction and the measurement scale into something tangible and meaningful.

Meaningfulness of a measure is related to the three tests of validity, reliability, and sensitivity. If a measure of a variable is not valid, it certainly cannot be meaningful. If the measure is not reliable, it cannot yield meaningful results, and if it is insensitive, it loses its meaningfulness.

The quest for a meaningful criterion measure is perhaps the most difficult and most important aspect of the design of nursing research. Unless the criterion measure used in a study meets the test of relevance and practicality, the findings are ineffective and sterile.

It is difficult to find relevant and practical criterion measures in nursing research. How much simpler a task the medical researchers often have in this regard. Salk demonstrated the effectiveness of his polio vaccine by showing an impressive reduction in the incidence of this disease among children who were vaccinated. His criterion was not only relevant, it was practical and meaningful in a most important way —in a life and death way.

The social sciences have been accused of attempting to measure meaningful variables by scales that reduce them to meaningless and artificial constructs. Krutch[17] attacks the attempt to measure a variable such as "happiness" as follows:

> Misguided attempts to deal quantitatively with so complex a thing as happiness are the enemies of literature and perhaps of happiness itself because they encourage us to assume both that one kind of happiness is the same as another and that they are equally valuable. In fact nothing is more important, prudentially or morally, than the realization that whether or not the pursuit of happiness is a legitimate chief aim depends upon which of the many happinesses one chooses and upon the means used to pursue it. Taken seriously, statistical studies are all too likely to teach us only how to become dismally "adjusted." Is it safe to take seriously a study in which you put in the same category everyone who says that he frequently feels "on top of the world," even though feeling on top of the world may mean anything from the friskiness of a puppy to the joy celebrated in the Ninth Symphony?

Direct meaningful measurement of variables such as "happiness" or "patient care" may not be possible because, for one thing, they are not undimensional. Instead they consist of numerous subvariables each having its own distinct underlying continuum. Moreover, like the difficulties encountered in attempting to measure directly the density of water, such complex variables may be measured more meaningfully through indirect methods. It was found that the variable "job morale" was assessed more adequately, not by constructing the scale from items whose content referred to the specifics of the actual work situation, but rather from items oriented to the total life situation of the worker.

THE ROLE OF CRITERION MEASURES IN RESEARCH IN NURSING

KEY POINT Measurement of patient care in terms of valid and reliable criterion measures is crucial to research in nursing. Because of the multi-dimensional nature of patient care, it is difficult though not impossible to measure this variable. Measurement of patient care can be approached by evaluating the adequacy of the facilities in which patient care is provided, the effectiveness of the administrative and organizational structure of the agency providing patient care, the professional qualifications and competency of personnel providing care, and the effect on the comsumers of care—the patients.

Patient care in hospitals is appraised by four techniques.[18] The first is the examination of the prerequisites for adequate care, such as the minimum and optimum levels of facilities, equipment, professional training and distribution of personnel, and the organizational structure of the institution.

Second is the evaluation of performance, particularly of tasks related to patient care. Here such observable quantitative measures can be used as the time nursing personnel spend on activities with patients, the utilization rates for specific procedures, length of patient stay, use of chest x-rays, laboratory and other diagnostic procedures, autopsy rates, pathological reports on surgical specimens, and correlations between preoperative and postoperative diagnosis.

The development of rating scales to measure levels of adequacy of patient care is the third way of measuring the quality of care. Scales must be developed which provide appropriate yardsticks to estimate qualitative levels of care. Most desirably such scales should be quantitative.

The fourth way of measuring quality is direct measurement of the patient by clinical evaluation. This can become highly subjective and less relevant than the three previous methods, but in many respects it is the most ideal measure, since it focuses on the product of patient care.

Criterion Measures of Patient Care

Criterion measures of nursing practice must derive from the dependent variables that indicate the effects of practice upon patient care.

The criterion measures of patient care may be categorized into four main groups.

Group I. Criterion measures of patient care related to preventive care needs.[19] These measures are observable in all patients. The patient's ability:
- A. To maintain good hygiene and physical comfort
- B. To achieve optimal activity, exercise, rest, and sleep
- C. To prevent accident, injury, or other trauma and prevent the spread of infection
- D. To maintain good body mechanics and prevent and correct deformities

Group II. Criteria of patient care related to sustenal and restorative care needs. This group of criterion measures of patient care relates to normal and disturbed physiological body processes that are vital to sustaining life. The patient's ability:
- A. To facilitate the maintenance of a supply of oxygen to all body cells
- B. To facilitate the maintenance of nutrition to all body cells
- C. To facilitate the maintenance of elimination
- D. To facilitate the maintenance of fluid and electrolyte balance
- E. To recognize the physiological re-

sponses of the body to disease conditions—pathological, physiological, and compensatory

F. To facilitate the maintenance of regulatory mechanisms and functions

G. To facilitate the maintenance of sensory function

Group III. This group of criterion measures of patient care involves those related to rehabilitative needs, particularly those involving emotional and interpersonal difficulties.

A. To identify and accept positive and negative expressions, feelings, and reactions

B. To identify and accept the interrelatedness of emotions and organic illness

C. To facilitate the maintenance of effective verbal and nonverbal communication

D. To promote the development of productive interpersonal relationships

E. To facilitate progress toward achievement of personal spiritual goals

F. To create and/or maintain a therapeutic environment

G. To facilitate awareness of self as an individual with varying physical, emotional, and developmental needs

H. To accept the optimum possible goals in light of limitations, physical and emotional

Group IV. This group covers those criteria of patient care related to sociological and community problems affecting patient care. The patient's ability:

A. To use community resources as an aid in resolving problems arising from illness

B. To understand the role of social problems as influencing factors in the cause of illness

Measurable Components of Patient Care

At present, the components of patient care easiest to measure fall into Group II—those observations that report disturbed physiological and body processes, including vital signs such as T.P.R., blood pressure, EKG, and oxygen content in the blood.

Difficulties in Identifying Criterion Measures

Nurses themselves cannot agree upon measurable criteria of effective nursing care. A scientific body of knowledge that is uniquely nursing has yet to be identified to provide a theoretical basis against which nursing practice can be measured. Unlike the use of criterion measures in a controlled environment, in nursing the measures must be employed in the framework of the patient's complex environment. Because there are so many extraneous variables both organismic and environmental. It is difficult to keep them under control.

The difficulties in identifying criterion measures in nursing have directed much of the research in nursing into areas that are more easily researchable. To illustrate, the study of the nurse—what she does, how much time she spends on patient care—provides empirical knowledge. This knowledge has value in that it helps to discover problem areas that need in-depth study. Ultimately, how the nurse functions must be measured against the effects (criterion measures) of nursing practice upon the patient's care.

Studies of the role of the nurse give direction to the nursing profession. These studies are important but will have little impact on the improvement of patient care if there are no adequate criterion measures of the effects of changed practice upon the patient care. We may think that we have improved nursing care, but we may not really know. We may be meeting the hospital's, the physician's, and the nurse's needs, but not the patient's!

Donabedian in the paper, "Some Basic Issues in Evaluating the Quality of Health Care," presented at the ANA, National Invitational Conference, "Issues in Evaluative Research," 1975, stated that there is not enough knowledge at present to base any program of quality assessment assurance exclusively on any one structure, process, or outcome. All three must be used simultaneously. The system also must be designed to show the relationship among the three. Desirable outcome criteria related to health care are controversial and some are not economically feasible.

Progress Made in the Measurement of the Quality of Nursing

Research in nursing can produce new knowledge, better methods of caring for people, and sounder rationales for tested nursing practices. Nurses may undertake studies that throw light on patient problems or reveal characteristics of the community setting of health problems. Research is an important means of improving quality nursing practice.

The first significant early attempt to measure quality nursing care was made by Reiter and Kakosh in 1950.[20] They identified twelve components of nursing care to define some standards for appraising observed nursing care. These components are:

1. Control of environment
2. Mental adjustment
3. Condition of skin and mucous membranes
4. Elimination
5. Posture, position, and exercise
6. Rest and sleep
7. Nutrition
8. Observation of signs and symptoms
9. Administration of laboratory tests
10. Administration of medicines
11. Administration of treatments
12. Teaching health

Each component was defined in operational terms and an observational guide was developed to record these observations.

Next, six qualitative categories were developed and defined to form criterion measures that could be quantitatively scaled:

• *Dangerous:* The patient's health or welfare is endangered by the nursing care he received.
• *Safe:* No harm comes to the patient for having had nursing care; patient's life and values protected.
• *Adequate:* To the extent possible, the patient's standards and customary way of living are kept as normal as possible; that he recov-

ers to the greatest extent his former state of health at his own rate of recovery.
• *Optimum:* The patient's integrity is respected and he is helped to improve his state of health and is better able to care for himself.
• *Maximum:* The design of patient care is based on the best known scientific advances to date.
• *Ideal:* Patient care is examined and evaluated for the purpose of improvement through controlled research in nursing.

Quality nursing practice is based on scientific findings that emerge from a study of nursing practice itself. Quality nursing practice has been defined as follows:

> For the patient it means that the best present nursing practice is not good enough and for the nurse it means incorporating research in nursing into the practice of nursing. The components of such care not only include the conscious and continuous search for the reasons underlying the nursing care but also the creation of new ways of care.[21]

Recent Attempts to Measure Quality

Several other direct attempts have been made to measure quality nursing practice. A long-range study was initiated in 1955 by Aydelotte and Tener[22] at Iowa in which measures of the skin condition, mental attitude, and mobility were developed. Simon[23] continued the work by studying activity patterns of hospitalized medical and urological patients with the aim of deriving patient activity indices that might be used as measures of patient welfare. Sampling was carried out by nurse observers who used a special code to record what each patient was doing at the moment he was observed. Twenty-eight different indices were computed for each patient, each representing the proportion of time the patient spent in a given category of activity. These indices were correlated with other patient welfare measures and were found to be significant.

A four-year study of nursing care of the hospitalized patient with a diagnosis of myocardial infarction was undertaken by Nite and Willis[24] at Community Studies, Inc., Kansas City. A nurse and a social scientist participated in giving direct care to patients and were able to identify some of "measuring rods" that could be used in evaluating a special type of care given to these patients. The conceptualization underlying this research is that nursing practice can be therapeutic when directed toward correctly identified problems of specific patients, and which when administered to the patient will give evidence of resolution of these problems.

The researchers were able to identify specific criteria of improvement to measure the progress of the cardiac patient. They were: the patient will gradually show less apprehension toward pain as he is given an understanding of the physiological process causing pain; the patient permits the nurse to perform necessary activities for him; the patient will tend to sleep during the day after major activities and during the entire night without medication.

Meltzer and associates[25] at Presbyterian Hospital in Philadelphia sought to answer this question: Can the modification of nursing practices result in the reduction in the death rate of cardiac patients? In the study attention was directed at lowering the fatality rate of coronary patients developing arrhythmias during the first seventy-two hour period of hospitalization. Intensive nursing care and observation by utilizing special monitoring systems to identify subtle changes in the patient's status might make it possible to take action during the precatastrophic period. Specific steps were then outlined for the nurse to follow once the catastrophe had occurred. Because of this study, lives have been saved owing to the professional nurse's ability to recognize signs early and to begin countershock therapy within *a few seconds* of the detection of the arrhythmia. The researchers also developed tools to assess the patient's condition on admission and during hospitalization in order to predict patient behavior prior to the occurrence of the catastrophe.

Attempts to measure quality nursing by the nurse's performance have had only limited use in measuring the effect of nursing care upon patient recovery. A small but sig-

nificant study conducted by Dumas and Leonard,[26] showed that clinical experiments in nursing practice are feasible and can be used to measure quality nursing. The aim of this research was to observe the effect of an experimental nursing process on the incidence of vomiting during recovery from anesthesia.

One experiment included the study of a sample of patients scheduled for surgery. Patients assigned to the experimental group were given nursing care by research nurses who used the experimental nursing process directed toward helping the patient obtain a suitable psychological state for surgery. Specific steps in this process are: (1) the nurse observes the patient's behavior and explores with him whether or not he is experiencing distress; (2) the nurse further attempts to find out what is causing the distress, if any, and what is needed to relieve it; (3) an appropriate course of action is undertaken to relieve the stress; and (4) the nurse follows through on her action(s) to see if the distress was relieved. This experimental nursing process was proved to be successful in reducing postoperative vomiting.

An important theoretical basis for this study is that emotional reactions of surgical patients to their illness and treatment have important consequences for their postoperative course. The study has demonstrated further that the relief of emotional distress is a part of the nurse's professional role.

A major problem in measuring quality nursing is the lack of instrumentation to measure it directly. Smith[27] at the University of Florida proposed that we measure nursing practice more indirectly than directly. Measurement of the nursing care of a "patient as a whole" may not be possible. Measurement of quality nursing may be made on the basis of the "scientific rightness" of our assessment of the patient's nursing problems and our management of them. It is proposed that "... we need a system—an organized framework wherein we can see plainly and definitely what is to be done and what we must do to accomplish it." It is proposed that the nursing problems that professional nurses are called upon to assess and manage daily could form the basis for evaluating quality nursing care. Quality nursing might be measured indirectly by examining the system or organization that deals with nursing problems. For example, the degree to which communications are systematized could be one of the most important criterion measures used in assessing quality nursing practice.

Hegyvary and Haussmann[28,29] developed a methodology for monitoring the quality of nursing care that focuses on the nursing process and the actual delivery of nursing care. Begun in 1972, this research resulted in a project designed to develop an improved methodology for monitoring the quality of care by:

- Synthesizing and incorporating methodologies available.
- Establishing a conceptual framework for nursing care, one that could accomodate both existing and new criteria.
- Designing an observation and scoring methodology using a set of criteria to maximize measurement efficiency.
- Testing the methodology and refining criteria.

The basis of the quality monitoring methodology is a master list of 220 criteria applicable to medical, surgical, and pediatric nursing units. Not all are used with each patient.

The researchers pilot-tested the research in two hospitals for applicability, comprehensiveness, and reliability of criteria. Intensive testing and analysis demonstrated the instrument to be reliable and valid. Trained nurse observers can achieve reliability in interpretation of evaluation criteria. The quality-monitoring methodology developed proved to be an important tool for nursing management in controlling nursing performance at the unit level. It was found that it is not enough to assess patient outcomes. Nursing management must know and understand both process

and outcomes to be able to make decisions regarding quality of care.

This research also identified important problems in developing criteria: establishing and maintaining validity and reliability in quality monitoring; observers general ability and willingness to interview patients; nurses' loyalty to hospital policies; poor quality of records; and writing criteria for specific populations.

The American Nurses' Association (ANA) has a long history in the involvement in efforts of quality assurance. A major effort beginning in 1974 resulted in a milestone document, *Guidelines for Review of Nursing Care at the Local Level.*[30] The guidelines had been developed as one part of the contract between ANA and the Department of Health, Education and Welfare (DHEW). The manual is intended to help registered nurses develop a system for evaluating the quality of nursing care.

Examples of guidelines suggested in developing outcome criteria are:

- Screening criteria is a crucial factor (outcome or process) that, if not met, may indicate a significant deficiency in nursing care. Screening criteria are used to survey a large number of cases to determine acceptable levels of patient outcomes.
- The outcome stated in the criterion must be possible to achieve.
- Each criterion should be a statement of one specific outcome representing its optimal achievement.
- In establishing criteria, select the most critical time for the measurement of the identified outcome for a particular population.
- A criterion must be appraisable and phrased in positive terms.
- Criteria are not static and change as values and scientific knowledge change.

STEPS IN WRITING OUTCOME CRITERIA

- Choose a category.
- Identify the target population.
- Select the appropriate population variables.
- Select criteria subsets.

- Generate outcome criteria.
- Establish critical time of measurement.
- Establish the standard.
- Establish any exceptions to the criteria and standards.
- Document the sources for the criteria.
- Select screening criteria.

The development of outcome criteria in nursing is particularly significant as nurses become more involved in peer review mechanisms such as Professional Standards Review Organization (PSROs) enacted by Congress in 1972 under P.L. 92–603. PSROs are modeled after the fundamental concept of peer review, which holds that health professionals rather than third party payors are the most appropriate individuals to evaluate the quality of services they deliver and that Medicare reviews should be done at the local level.

In 1974, Lang[31] developed a Model for Quality Assurance, which was later adapted for use by ANA/DHEW. The components of the model are:

- Clarification of values.
- Establishment of outcome, process and structure standards, and criteria of nursing care.
- Assessment of the degree of discrepancy between the standards and criteria and the current level of nursing practice.
- Selection and implementation of an alternative for changing nursing practice.
- Improvement of nursing practice.

The Lang model provides a mechanism into which one may feed specific data and accommodate a variety of practice situations.

The development of patient assessment approaches and related outcome criteria for long-term care patients started more than 25 years ago and culminated in the work of Densen, Jones, Flagle, Katz and Danehy[32] of which a dictionary of common definitions and a single database were significant parts.

In 1974, DHEW launched a nationwide Long Term Care Facility Improvement Campaign.[33,34] A significant finding was that in order to improve the quality of care in nursing homes one must first assess the patient's/resident's needs for care, then develop a plan of care with specific goals, and, finally, determine through outcome criteria if the goals have been met. DHEW has now developed, tested, and modified a systematic process for assessing health care known as Patient Appraisal and Care Evaluation (PACE). PACE can provide a single data source which is consistent and a current source of patient/resident data including demographic descriptors, impairments, functional status, services provided, etc. Specifically, PACE provides accessible and measurable data on appropriateness of care as well as outcome criteria for use by such groups as PSROs, JCAH, PRO's, Federal, state, and regional surveyors. The PACE system needs to be adapted for use in hospitals and in noninstitutional care settings such as home care, day care centers, hospices.

SUMMARY

Variables are fundamental to nursing research. They are essential to all forms of research, but particularly to research in which hypotheses are posed. R. A. Fisher has said that research and statistics are basically directed toward the study of variation.

Variables have to be carefully defined and quantified. Measurement of variables takes many forms. Some variables can be measured precisely with scientific instruments. For many psychosocial variables, a variety of "pencil-and-paper instruments" have been developed in which the variables are quantified through scales. Scales vary in refinement from the quantitative nominal scale to the precise quantitation of the ratio scale.

Various criteria have been developed for evaluating measures of variables. These include validity, reliability, sensitivity, and meaningfulness.

Valid and reliable criteria measures are

essential in explanatory and evaluation research. The measurement of the quality of nursing practice is one of the most important and challenging areas in nursing research. This identification of criterion measures of nursing practice poses many problems because of its complexity. Multiple studies will have to be undertaken before definitive measures of quality nursing can be identified. Measurement of quality care will have to be both direct and indirect before a complete assessment of the effect(s) of nursing practice upon patient welfare can be made.

REFERENCES

1. Genevieve R. Meyer, *Tenderness and Technique: Nursing Values in Transition.* Los Angeles, Institute of Industrial Relations, University of California, 1960, p. 13.
2. Miriam A. Safren and Alphonse Chapanis, "A Critical Incident Study of Hospital Medication Errors." *Hospitals, J.A.H.A.,* **34:**62, 64, May 1, 1960.
3. Claire Selltiz *et al., Research Methods in Social Relations.* New York, Holt, Rinehart and Winston, 1962, p. 435.
4. Morris R. Cohen and Ernest Nagel. *An Introduction to Logic and Scientific Method.* 1982 Reprint of 1934 Edition. Darby, PA, Darby Books, p. 263.
5. Helen Peak, "Problems of Objective Observation," Chapter 6 in Leon Festinger and Daniel Katz (eds), *Research Methods in the Behavioral Sciences.* New York, The Dryden Press, 1953, p. 256.
6. Stuart Wright, "Turnover and Job Satisfaction," *Hospitals, J.A.H.A.,* **31:**47–52, October 1, 1957.
7. Rena E. Boyle, *A Study of Student Nurse Perception of Patient Attitudes.* U.S. Public Health Service Publication No. 769. Washington, DC, Government Printing Office, 1960.
8. Faye G. Abdellah and Eugene Levine, "Developing a Measure of Patient and Personnel Satisfaction with Nursing Care." *Nursing Res.,* **5:**100–108, Frebruary 1957.
9. Eileen G. Hasselmeyer, *Behavior Patterns of Premature Infants.* U.S. Public Health Service Publication No. 840. Washington, DC, Government Printing Office, 1961.
10. Macolm W. Klein *et al.,* "Problems of Measuring Patient Care in the Out-patient Department." *J. Health Human Behavior,* **2:**138–144, 1961.

11. W. Stephenson, *The Study of Behavior, Q-technique and Its Methodology.* Chicago, University of Chicago Press, 1953.
12. William G. Cochran, "Research Techniques in the Study of Human Beings." *Millbank Memorial Fund Quarterly,* **33:**125, April 1955.
13. Selltiz *et al., op. cit.,* pp. 196–197.
14. W. Allen Wallis and Harry V. Roberts, *Statistics: A New Approach.* New York, The Free Press of Glencoe, 1956, p. 133.
15. Wright, *op. cit.*
16. Jane Wilcox, "Observer Factors in the Measurement of Blood Pressure." *Nursing Res.,* **10:**4–17, winter 1961.
17. Joseph Wood Krutch, "Through Happiness with Slide Rule and Calipers." *The Saturday Review,* **XLVI:**14, November 2, 1963.
18. Mindel C. Sheps, "Approaches to the Quality of Hospital Care." *Publ. Health Rep.,* **70:**877–886, September 1955.
19. Faye G. Abdellah *et al., Patient-Centered Approaches to Nursing.* New York, Macmillan Publishing Co., Inc., 1960.
20. Frances Reiter and Marguerite E. Kakosh. *Quality of Nursing Care,* A Report of a Field Study to Establish Criteria 1950–1954 (P.H.S. Grant #RG 2734). Institute of Research and Studies in Nursing Education, Division of Nursing Education, Teachers College, Columbia University, 1963.
21. *Ibid.*
22. Myrtle K. Aydelotte and Marie E. Tener, "An Investigation of the Relation Between Nursing Activity and Patient Welfare." Iowa City, State University of Iowa, Utilization Project, 1960.
23. J. Richard Simon, "Patient Activity as a Measure of Patient Welfare." State University of Iowa, October 1962 (P.H.S. Grant, GN 7610, unpublished).
24. Gladys Nite and Frank Willis, *The Coronary Patient: Hospital Care and Rehabilitation.* New York, Macmillan Publishing Co., Inc., 1964.
25. Lawrence E. Meltzer, Rose Pinneo, and J. R. Kitchell, *Intensive Coronary Care.* A Manual for Nurses. Philadelphia, The Charles Press, 1970.
26. Rhetaugh G. Dumas and Robert C. Leonard, "The Effect of Nursing on the Incidence of Postoperative Vomiting." *Nursing Res.,***12:**12–15, winter 1963.
27. Dorothy M. Smith, "Myth and Method in Nursing Practice," *Am. J. Nursing,* **64:**68–72, February 1964.
28. Sue Thomas Hegyvary and R. K. Dieter Haussmann. "Monitoring Nursing Care Quality." *J. Nursing Administration,* **69:**9:3–9. November 1976.
29. R. K. Dieter Haussmann, Sue T. Hegyvary, and John F. Newman, *Monitoring Quality of Nursing Care.* Part II, Assessment and Study of Correlates.

Bethesda, Md., DHEW Pub. No (HRA) 76-77, July 1976.

30. American Nurses' Association, *Guidelines for Review of Nursing Care at the Local Level,* Rockville. MD DHEW Contract HSA 105-74-207, September 1976.

31. Norma Lang, "A Model for Quality Assurance in Nursing." Unpublished doctoral dissertation, Marquette University, Milwaukee, WI., May 1974.

32. Ellen W. Jones, *Patient Classification for Long-Term Care: User's Manual.* Rockville, MD, DHEW Pub. No. HRA 74-3107, December 1973.

33. DHEW, *Long-Term Care Facility Improvement Study.* Rockville, MD, DHEW Pub. No. (OS) 76-50021, July 1975.

34. Faye G. Abdellah, "Patient Assessment. Its Potential and Use." *Am. Health Care Assoc. J.* 1(3):69-80, November 1975.

PROBLEMS AND SUGGESTIONS FOR FURTHER STUDY

1. Describe five variables that could serve as either dependent or independent variables in patient care research. What kinds of dependent variables could never conceivably serve as independent variables?

2. Study the 25 hypotheses listed on pages 115–116. Describe how you would go about quantitatively measuring the dependent variables stated in these hypotheses. Do measuring instruments already exist to measure these variables, or will fresh ones have to be developed?

3. Review some periodicals containing reports of research in nursing and patient care (like *Nursing Research*) to obtain some examples of the use of nonquantified data in a study. What are some of the limitations in using nonquantified data in research? What are the benefits to be gained by the use of such data?

4. Describe five types of nominal scales commonly used in nursing and patient care. Can you conceive of a way in which these scales can be converted into quantitative scales? How meaningful would such quantitative lowing variables.

5. Develop a graphic rating scale for the following variables
   a. Quality of performance of a nursing aide
   b. Cooperativeness of a patient
   c. Ability of the patient to verbalize his feelings
   d. The sleep behavior of an adult patient
   e. Degree of mobility of a patient
   f. The severity of a surgical operation

6. What are the essential differences between the graphic rating scale, the Thurstone-type scale, the Likert-type scale, and the Guttman scale? How would you rank these scales in the order of their usefulness to research in nursing and patient care?

7. The Q-sort technique has been occasionally used in research in nursing. Referring to the journal *Nursing Research,* locate a report of a study in which the Q-sort method has been used (several have been reported). Write a summary and critique of the use of the method in the reported study.

8. Perform the following experiment. Take the temperatures (orally) of a group of patients, say, a dozen or so. Have a few nurses independently read the same patient's thermometer and record the readings. In comparing the readings for the same patients, do you find any variation? Next, take the same patient's temperature with two thermometers simultaneously. Do this for a number of patients. Do the readings always agree exactly?

9. Make the following scale conversions:
   a. 200°F. to the centigrade scale
   b. 25 pounds avoirdupois to the metric scale
   c. 34 centimeters to linear measure
   d. 44°C. to the Fahrenheit scale
   e. 8 quarts (liquid) to the metric scale
   f. 100 yards to the metric scale

10. Analyze the criterion measures used in the following studies:
   a. Anayis K. Derdiarian and Alan B. Forsythe, "An Instrument for Theory and Research Development Using the Behavioral Systems Model for Nursing: The Cancer Patient." *Nursing Res.,* 32:260–266, October 1983.
   b. Florence C. Austin, Ellen Donnelly Davis, and Judith Rubenstein Steward, "Characteristics of Psychiatric Patients Who Utilize Public Health Nursing Services." *Am. J. Pub. Health,* 54:226–238, February 1964.
   c. Edith M. Lentz and Robert G. Michaels, "Comparisons Between Medical and Surgical Nurses." *Nursing Res.,* 8:192–197, fall 1959.
   d. Leonard I. Pearlin and Morris Rosen-

berg, "Nurse-Patient Social Distance and the Structural Context of a Mental Hospital." *Am. Sociol. Rev.,* 27:56–65, February 1962.

e. Kathryn M. Lillesand and Sarah Korff, "Nursing Process Evaluation: A Quality Assurance Tool." *Nursing Admin. Q.,* 7:9–14, spring 1983.

f. Marie E. Meyers, "The Effect of Types of Communication on Patients' Reactions to Stress." *Nursing Res.,* 13:126–131, spring 1964.

g. Robert A. Hoekelman, Harriet J. Kitzman, and Anne W. Zimmer, "Pediatric Nurse Practitioners and Well Baby Care in a Small Rural Community," in *ANA Clinical Sessions,* 1972, pp. 103–113. New York, Appleton-Century-Crofts, 1973.

h. Geraldine V. Padilla and Marcia M. Grant, "Quality of Life as A Cancer Nursing Outcome Variable." *Advances in Nursing Science* 8:45–60, October, 1985.

11. Read the article by Faye E. Spring and Herman Turk, "A Therapeutic Behavior Scale" (*Nursing Res.,* 11:214–218, fall 1962). How do the authors employ the scalogram analysis in this study? How was reliability of the scale assessed? Do you think the scale developed could have applicability in other studies? A more recent application of scalogram analysis is presented in the article by Richard N. Nonickoff and others, "Limitations of Provider Interventions in Hypertension Quality Assurance." *Am. J. Pub. Health,* 75:43–46, January 1985. Comment on this study.

12. In her article "Evaluation of Nursing Care—Could It Make a Difference?" *Int. J. Nursing Stud.,* 19:53—60, 1982, Rebecca Bergman discusses the variable "nursing care." Could these definitions be used in nursing research?

13. Read the article by Linda Farrand and others, "A Study of Construct Validity: Simulations as a Measure of Nurse Practitioners' Problem-Solving Skills." *Nursing Res.* 31:37–42, January/February, 1982. Explain how construct validity was measured in the study. How does construct validity differ from "predictive" validity? Which, if any, is a more important measure of validity?

14. Read the article by Alex Barr and others, "A Review of the Various Methods of Measuring the Dependency of Patients on Nursing Staff." *Int. J. Nursing Stud.,* 10:195–208, August 1973. What are some of the measurement problems in developing an index of patients' dependency on nursing staff?

15. Read the article by Fabienne Fortin and Suzanne Kérouac, "Validation of Questionnaires on Physical Function." *Nursing Res.,* 26:128–135, March-April 1977. Is the CICCHETTI statistic a good method of testing reliability?

16. Clearly distinguish between a direct measure of a variable and an indirect measure. Are some measures more indirect than others? Describe some direct and indirect measures of patient care that could serve as criterion measures in research.

17. The article by Philip E. Clark and Mary Jo Clark, "Therapeutic Touch: Is There a Scientific Basis for the Practice?" *Nursing Res.,* 33:37–41, January/February 1984, is an excellent example of a literature review. What are some of the dependent variables the authors found in the review? Do these suggest further research?

CHAPTER
11

Determine the Research Design

OBJECTIVES

- To describe the essentials of experimental design.
- To clarify the various types of experimental designs.
- To explain how to conduct an experiment.
- To describe the various kinds of nonexperimental designs.
- To describe how to conduct nonexperimental research.
- To show how to choose between an experimental and nonexperimental research design.

Research design is concerned with the overall framework for conducting the study. Although the design of a study begins when a topic for research is selected, the detailed work of determining the study format takes place after the problem has been formulated and the hypotheses, if any, have been stated.

KEY POINT The essential question that research design is concerned with is how the study subjects will be brought into the research and how they will be employed within the research setting to yield the required data.

Basically, there are two types of research design, the experimental and the nonexperimental. The main difference between the two is that in experimental research all major elements of design are largely under the control of the researcher. These include research setting, explanatory variables, study subjects—particularly assignment of these subjects to different study groups—and method for collecting data from study subjects. In nonexperimental research, sometimes called surveys, the researcher does not have as stringent control over the various elements of design.

EXPERIMENTAL RESEARCH

Experimental research is conducted for the purposes of diagnosis and explanation. Although numerous examples of experimental research can be cited from the physical sciences where the purpose of the experiment is descriptive—for example, a microscopic analysis of the characteristics of chromosomes—the most used application of the experimental technique is to explain: what happens to A when B occurs. Experimental research finds its greatest application today in evaluating products, programs, techniques, or methods or procedure. In these evaluations, called comparative experiments, the effects produced by the independent variable are compared in terms of some criterion measure to find out which produces the most desirable effect.

The experimental approach to testing is ideally one in which all factors except the one being tested are strictly controlled so that only the tested factor will exert an effect on the study subjects. Experimental research should be able to accurately relate the effect to its appropriate cause with an economy of effort.

The field of comparative experiments —where the purpose is to test some procedure, or program—is young. Early comparative experiments were conducted in agriculture where the effects on crop yield of different levels of such variables as chemical fertilization, depth of plowing, and moisture were studied. The study of experimental design as a systematic method for carrying out comparative experiments dates back to the 1930's with the publication of Sir Ronald A. Fisher's famous treatise, *The Design of Experiments.*[1] Most of the major books on the subject have been published since the 1950's: Cochran and Cox, Kempthorne, and Federer—writing about the design of agricultural experiments; Edwards—psychology; Chapin—sociology; Chew—industry; and Finney—biology and medicine.[2-8]

Not only is the experimental approach a powerful tool for testing alternative ways of doing things, but it is the only valid approach to establishing and understanding causal connections between phenomena. It has made important contributions to the advancement of knowledge in modern science.

Cause and Effect

The previous chapter defined cause and effect; that is, the *cause* of a certain *effect* was some appropriate factor invariably related to the effect. The experimental method was developed to uncover causal connections between phenomena. John Stuart Mill's five rules or canons of experimental research, contained in Book III of his *System of Logic.*[9] described how to study relationships. Two of the fundamental rules of Mill's method of experimental inquiry are his *method of agreement* and *method of difference*. Mill describes these rules as follows:

> The simplest and most obvious modes of singling out from among the circumstances which precede or follow a phenomenon, those with which it is really connected by an invariable law are two in number. One is, by comparing together different instances in which the phenomenon occurs. The other is by comparing instances in which the phenomenon does occur, with instances in other respects similar in which it does not. These two methods may be respectively denominated, the Method of Agreement, and the Method of Difference.[10]

METHOD OF AGREEMENT

The method of agreement states that if the circumstances leading to the occurrence of a given event, B, have, during every occurrence of the event, only one factor in common, A, then A is probably the cause of B. This is a useful principle, particularly in the development of hypotheses. However, it has certain limitations. First, the event, B, must have constant meaning during each occurrence. Second, the circumstances leading to the occurrence of B must be confined to a single, isolated factor, A. This method is not useful to deal with such complicated problems as cancer, in which the causes are suspected to be multiple, although it is effectively utilized in the narrowly defined experiments that add small bits of information to the larger puzzle of cancer.

METHOD OF DIFFERENCE

The method of difference states that if two or more sets of circumstances are different in respect to only one factor, A, and if a given event, B, occurs only when A is present, then A is probably the cause of B. For example, if two groups of patients are provided with identical kinds of nursing care in identical settings, except that in one group the team method of assignment is used and in the other the functional method is employed (one nurse responsible for all medication, another for all patient teaching, and so on), and if patients in the team assignment group appear to get well faster than those in the other group, we might say that we have demonstrated the truth of the hypothesis that the higher recovery rate is caused by the team method of assignment. The shortcoming of this approach is that there is no way to be sure that the circumstances—nursing care, environment, and, most important, patients—are different with respect to only one variable, type of organization for providing care. Perhaps in some subtle, difficult to perceive way the patients in the two groups really are different, and this characteristic is actually the cause of the difference in recovery rates. Or, perhaps it is not the method of patient care organization per se that influences recovery rates but some sociopsychological factor intrinsic to the form of organization employed.

Such pitfalls as these in the application of the method of difference have given rise to the principles of statistical design of experiments. An essential aspect of these principles is the technique of randomization, discussed later in the chapter. Through randomization the groups under study can, theoretically at least, be equated in all factors. Except for chance differences attributable to randomization itself and measurable by statistical methods, the only difference between the groups should be the independent variable being manipulated.

Joint Method of Agreement and Difference

A third canon of experimental research, called the joint method of agreement and difference, combines the two methods in an attempt to make a more valid assessment of cause and effect. In the joint approach, the method of agreement is applied first to discover the one characteristic, A, common to all occurences of the phenomenon, B. Then the method of difference is applied to determine that B does not occur when A is absent. If we first show that the team method of assignment is the one characteristic common to all instances in which high recovery rates are found, and that the team plan is never employed where low recovery rates occur, we can say that the team plan is the cause of higher recovery rates. However, we are again faced with the problem of standardization of the groups for all factors except the independent variable—type of nursing care organization. Randomization is a way of achieving this.

Concomitant Variation

A fourth rule of experimental research is that of concomitant variation. As formulated by Mill, the canon states: whenever two phenomena vary together in a consistent and persistent manner, either the variations represent a direct causal connection between the two phenomena, or else both are being affected by some other common causal factor.

Note that this rule merely broadens the ideas contained in the previous canons. However, here the phenomena (the independent and dependent variables) are variables that differ in degree and can assume a wide range of values, whereas the previous canons were concerned with independent variables that differed in kind—team plan versus functional assignment—or were of the all-or-nothing variety—smoke, do not smoke.

Three main types of relationships can be found among dependent and independent variables—causal relationships, where the dependent variable is causally related to the independent variable; associative relationships, where both variables are causally related to a third independent variable; and artificial relationships, where the variables are statistically related to each other, but may not be causally connected to the same independent variable. The rule of concomitant variation, while useful for explanatory research, has limitations as a method for causal discovery.

As Cohen and Nagel[11] have stated:

Even very high correlations, especially in the social sciences, do not necessarily signify an invariable connection. For the phenomena between which such correlations can be established may be in fact unrelated in any way which would warrant our believing them to be invariably connected. A little statistical skill and patience make it possible to find any number of high correlations between otherwise unrelated factors. We do not discover causal connections by first surveying all possible correlations between different variables. On the contrary, we suspect an invariable connection, and then use correlations as corroborative evidence.

METHOD OF RESIDUES

Mill's fifth canon of experimental research is called the method of residues. This method makes use of previously established causal relationships. Its object is to discover causes by a process of elimination. The method of residues states: when the factors that are known to cause a part of some phenomenon are isolated, the remaining part of the phenomenon is the effect of the residual factors. The eliminative approach is especially useful in research on human beings where the effects observed are frequently due to many causes and not a single factor. Thus, lung cancer may be related to other factors as well as inhalation of cigarette smoke because some persons who die of lung cancer do not smoke cigarettes. Conversely, many cigarette smokers do not develop lung cancer. Similarly, it is not possible to demonstrate that there is a complete and invariant relationship between nursing care and patient welfare because many factors in the patient care situation in addition to nursing care impinge on patient welfare, not least of which are the organismic variables found in the patients themselves.

Mill's five canons have been most useful in providing a logical basis for conducting explanatory research—that type of research which has as its purpose the discovery of causal connections among variables studied. Research design is the means by which such research is conducted most efficiently and validly. The most valid way of finding causal connections among variables is by the kind of research design known as an experiment.

Experimental Design

In the classic design of an explanatory experiment the researcher establishes two groups from the study population. The groups are standardized for all possible extraneous variables, by a deliberate matching procedure or by random assignment to one of the two groups, or by a combination method. One of the groups, the experimental group, is then exposed to the independent variable—treatment, method, procedure, or other factor. The other group, the control, contrast, or comparative group, does not receive the independent variable. Or the experiment may consist of applying different levels of the independent variable to the groups (e.g., different dosages of a drug). At a certain point in time the effects of the independent variable on the two groups are compared in terms of a criterion measure (dependent variable). Differences in the values of the criterion measure for the two groups are compared with an estimate of the differences attributable to the randomized extraneous variables in order to assess the significance of the effects produced by the independent (casual) variable. To the degree that these effects are significantly greater than would be expected by chance alone, and to the degree that all relevant extraneous variables have been accounted for, the greater is the confidence that a causal connection has been established between independent and dependent variables.

Modern experimental design, building on Mill's canons, has added the features of randomization to standardize the groups studied and statistical assessment of differences produced among the groups through application of probability theory. Modern experimental design incorporates the following canons of Mill:

1. The method of difference is used in setting up two study groups, experimental and comparison group, identical in all important respects, except the independent variable to be manipulated. According to this canon, any response in the dependent variable must be attributed to the independent variable. Moreover, by standardizing the characteristics of the experimental and the comparison group, starting with a clean slate, so to speak, it can be demonstrated clearly that the application of the independent variable preceded the response measured by the criterion variable.

2. The rule of concomitant variation is the basic statistical model for experimental research. In its fundamental form this model is the general linear hypothesis which states:

where Y = dependent variable
and X = independent variable
then $Y = f(X)$

and any change in Y is associated with a change in X.

3. By different experiments concerned with the same explanatory variables the method of agreement can be shown to apply in drawing causal inferences from data. If it is found in repeated trials that similar effects are produced by a common factor, this common factor can be designated the causal agent.

4. Repeated proofs of the same hypothesis in identical experiments (replications) uphold the relationship among the variables as invariant.

5. By a series of experiments, each testing different independent variables as possible causes of the phenomenon, we apply the method of residues. Each experiment eliminates independent variables having no relationship to the dependent variable. In cases of multiple causality—a number of factors causing an effect—we can see the extent to which each partially causative

variable contributes to the explanation of the dependent variable.

Experimental research is a highly controlled, forward-looking study conducted in a specially created setting in which the researcher manipulates the independent variable and controls any extraneous variables that could affect the dependent variable. By contrast, in a nonexperimental explanatory study the independent variable is not manipulated. It is accepted as it occurs naturally in the study population. Often, a nonexperimental explanatory study looks backward in that the researcher first observes the effects in the dependent variable and then traces back to the possible independent variable(s) that could have caused them. In a nonexperimental study the independent variable has often been applied before the study began whereas in an experimental study application of the independent variable always precedes measurement of the dependent variable. An experiment is prospective.

Application of independent variable	→	Study population	→	Measurement of dependent variable

A nonexperimental explanatory study is retrospective.

Measurement of dependent variable	→	Study population	→	Observation of independent variable

ADVANTAGES AND DISADVANTAGES OF THE EXPERIMENTAL DESIGN

Advantages of experimental design over the nonexperimental approach are:

1. Where the purpose of the research is explanation, causal relationships may be established among the variables by experimentation, especially in studies involving physical objects, where the variables are more easily controlled than in human studies.
2. In descriptive studies, the controlled environment in which the study is conducted

can yield a greater degree of purity in observation.

3. Conditions not found in a natural setting can be created in an experimental setting where the independent variable is manipulated by the investigator.

4. In the experimental approach we can often create conditions in a short period of time that may take years to occur naturally. In genetic studies we can breed strains of animals in a fraction of the time that it would take nature.

5. The experimental approach to research, when conducted in a laboratory, experimental unit, or other specialized research setting, is removed from the pressures and problems of the real-life situation and the researcher can pursue his study in a more leisurely, careful, and concentrated way.

However, the experimental design has its own disadvantages. Some are so severe that this design may be automatically ruled out in certain types of studies. In brief, the main disadvantages are:

1. Although theoretically the experimental approach can yield insight into the causes of certain phenomena, in research involving human beings the phenomena are usually so complex and derive from such a plurality of causes that the simple experimental model, $Y = f(X)$, does not apply. What may be required is a more complicated multivariate nonlinear model, which may only with great difficulty be amenable to the experimental approach.

2. For many important human variables—for example, patient welfare or level of wellness—there are no valid criterion measures available at present. The use of the refined, experimental approach in studies involving such variables is a mismatch of study design and measuring instrument. In many studies the independent variables may be so crude or gross—for example, the variable "nursing care"—that a mismatch between degree of refinement of design and measurement of explanatory variables would be like shooting flies with an elephant gun. When variables are crude and ill-defined, it is better to use the more flexible nonexperimental approach.

3. For certain research problems, because of danger to the health and well-being of the study population, it is improper to conduct experiments on humans. Certain drugs or treatments are so dangerous that we use animals for our study population, realizing that it may not be possible to make valid generalizations from animal to human. Or the independent variable may be psychologically harmful to study subjects and would create difficulties in securing and maintaining their cooperation, for example, studies of sensory deprivation.

4. In some research it may not be possible to create experimentally the conditions to be studied. To attempt to study the effects on patient well-being of a global independent variable such as the organizational and physical structure of a hospital would be totally impractical.

5. Experiments are often impractical where the effect of the independent variable may require a lengthy period of time before it emerges as a response in the criterion measure. This situation exists for many of the variables in nursing. One of the main drawbacks to conducting experiments on the effects of nursing care on acutely ill hospitalized patients is that the patients are discharged from the hospital in such a short period of time that there is little opportunity for the effects we are studying to occur. Only by a difficult and costly procedure of following up discharged patients in their homes is it possible to observe experimental results.

6. Another limitation of the experimental design is the difficulty in obtaining cooperation of study subjects. Participation in an experiment usually imposes more of a burden on subjects than other types of studies. Therefore, in experiments with human subjects it is best to keep the study population as small as possible and consistent with the requirements for obtaining sufficient and meaningful data. With small-sized populations assigned to the different study groups it becomes especially important that members of groups be kept intact. Dropouts, and possible contamination of one

group by members of another, can destroy the validity of an experiment. The administrative problems in securing and maintaining cooperation of study subjects are formidable and sometimes discourage the selection of this design as the method for a study.

7. Because the population for experiments involving human beings is often kept small, there is a question as to how representative the findings of such studies can be. If the target population is diverse, if the explanatory variables are complex, if the extraneous variables are numerous, and if these extraneous variables can exert spurious influences on our dependent variable when uncontrolled, there is some question as to whether a small number of study subjects can provide findings meaningful for a larger population even if they have been carefully selected and kept intact during the study.

The use of experimental design is ruled out in many research problems because the number of subjects required to provide meaningful data would be impractically large. In order to be approached experimentally, many research problems have to be delimited to permit the use of small study groups. Such narrowing down, of course, restricts the importance of the findings so that the studies become nothing more than sterile exercises.

8. Artificiality is an issue in the application of the experimental method to patient care research. To what extent can findings be generalized from an unnatural setting in which the variables tested are artifacts, created and manipulated by the researcher among subjects who may not represent the population at large? These limitations are especially restrictive where the aim of the research is a practical application of the findings. Many experiments conducted in the social sciences suffer from artificiality because, first, they often use a specially selected population, such as students or patients in hospitals who are not representative of any larger target population. It is difficult to say to what extent data collected in experiments like these can be generalized at all. Second, the setting in which such experiments are sometimes conducted—a classroom, a laboratory, or some specially devised experimental unit—may not have any resemblance to reality, making it difficult to apply the findings to real life. Third, the independent variable being manipulated, for instance, the size and composition of the nursing team, may be so artificial as to make application to an actual nursing situation impossible.

The limitations inherent in the experimental approach are greatest where the experimental subjects are human beings. Since most conceivable patient care studies involve humans, the use of the experimental method in such research is limited. However, this method serves as the ideal model for all types of studies where the aim is to discover causal relationships among variables. Indeed, some aspects of the experimental method can be incorporated into the nonexperimental design to improve the quality of data collected.

ADVANTAGES AND DISADVANTAGES OF THE NONEXPERIMENTAL DESIGN

The distinguishing feature between experimental and nonexperimental explanatory research is that in the latter the investigator does not manipulate the independent variable. That is to say, its application to study subjects is not under his direct control. In fact, in many retrospective studies the application of the independent variable occurred before the study was initiated. Nevertheless, the nonexperimental approach to research does have certain advantages:

1. Generally, nonexperimental studies are less expensive to conduct. In surveys the subjects are not brought together in a specially designed study unit, but remain in natural settings. Often mailed question-

naires are used to gather data, or data may be obtained from existing sources. Per unit cost of collecting data is much lower than in an experiment.

2. A survey can usually be completed in a much shorter time than can an experiment. A retrospective study of the variables associated with deaths from certain diseases can be done in a relatively short time, usually less than a year. A prospective study in this area may extend over many years and will not be complete until all study subjects have died.

3. The problem of obtaining the cooperation of study subjects is generally less formidable in nonexperimental research than in an experimental study. Frequently, all that is required from the subject in a survey is information, which may take only a short time. On the other hand, an experimental subject not only may have to devote a considerable amount of time to participation in the research, but may also be exposed to unusual, unpleasant, or burdensome conditions.

4. The nonexperimental approach is the method of choice where there is a large time lag between application of the independent variable and appearance of a response in the dependent variable. It is easier to keep track of subjects when they are able to function in normal setting rather than in the highly controlled environment demanded by the experimental approach.

5. Nonexperimental studies involving human beings possess more realism—in terms of variables studied and setting for the research—than an experiment. Thus generalizations of nonexperimental research findings beyond the boundaries of the research setting are more widespread.

6. In general, findings of nonexperimental studies are more representative of a larger target population than are findings from experimental studies. In some experiments the subjects may be brought into the study merely as a matter of convenience. Because it usually is less expensive and less burdensome to collect data in a nonex-

perimental study, more subjects can be included, increasing the representativeness of the research. Moreover, it is usually possible to obtain wider geographical representation of subjects through the nonexperimental approach by the use of mailed questionnaires and other means of data collection that cannot be employed in a highly controlled experiment.

There are drawbacks to the use of the nonexperimental approach in research, the most serious of which are:

1. The nonexperimental method cannot establish causal relationships with the same degree of confidence as can the experimental method. The main attribute of the experimental method is the higher degree of control over extraneous variables. Often the best that can be achieved in a nonexperimental study is the establishment of associative relationships. These, of course, are useful for predictive purposes but weak for diagnosis and explanation. Even with the experimental approach it is not always possible to establish cause-and-effect relationships. The extraneous variables can be so numerous and so potent in their effects on the explanatory variables that they cannot be entirely eliminated by experimental procedures such as randomization. However, the danger that exists in nonexperimental research to a much greater extent than in experimental studies is the erroneous ascribing of a causal relationship among variables that may only be artificially or spuriously related.

2. It is obvious that the experimental approach, particularly the retrospective or cross-sectional, cannot be applied to test out a newly developed product, program, or procedure. A nonexperimental study has its greatest usefulness where the variable being studied is already established. The purpose of the experimental approach—the prospective study—is to describe and evaluate an event or phenomenon.

3. The nonexperimental approach is not useful in the development of new theories, ideas, or principles. Experimentally we can

create the conditions necessary for an investigation of a theoretical construct. Nonexperimentally, we must take them as they exist. Natural conditions may not be very efficient raw materials for a theoretically oriented investigation.

4. Among some researchers, only a study based on the experimental method is considered true research. Nonexperimental studies are often entitled "surveys" to distinguish them from so-called "real" research, and acceptance of survey findings may be less enthusiastic, more qualified, than findings of experimental studies. This attitude toward nonexperimental research often makes it harder to obtain funding for such studies. Moreover, there may be reluctance to accept the findings of such studies as being truly scientific.

Comparison of Experimental and Nonexperimental Design

As a summary of the main features of the two methods the following illustration shows how the same problem can be approached by the different types of design.

Suppose someone were interested in finding out whether a graduate of a degree program in nursing is more proficient as a bedside nurse in a general hospital than a graduate of a diploma program. Whether this study were to be conducted experimentally or nonexperimentally, certain common elements in the design of both types of studies must be considered. First, the total population to which the study findings apply must be specified. Second, the method for selecting subjects has to be determined. Third, the alternative versions of the independent variable to be tested—the degree curriculum and the diploma curriculum—must be defined. Fourth, the criterion measure to be used to evaluate the effects of the two types of programs on proficiency as a bedside nurse is developed. Finally, the statistical method to analyze results is selected.

If the study were conducted experimentally, a group of high school graduates would be selected, randomly assigned to an experimentally developed and administered diploma or degree program. They would be followed after they had graduated from their program and been employed as graduate nurses in hospitals. Then, their proficiency as nurses would be measured to see whether there was a difference in proficiency between the graduates of the two types of programs.

If the study were conducted nonexperimentally, a random sample of graduate nurses in hospitals would be selected, their proficiency as bedside nurses would be measured, a determination made of whether they had attended a degree program or a diploma program, and a statistical analysis performed to test the difference in proficiency scores. The study, if carried out experimentally, may take a minimum of five years and require much money and effort. If carried out nonexperimentally, it could possibly be done in about a year with considerably less expense. However, the experimental approach would provide data that would permit the drawing of inferences about the effect of type of curriculum, which would more likely be free from the impact of such uncontrolled variables as innate ability of the study subjects, their values, goals, and ideals, quality of teaching in the two types of programs, and other extraneous organismic and environmental variables.[12]

The main difference between the two types of design illustrated by this example is, first, the experimental approach allows greater control over the character of the independent variable—the type of educational program. In the experimental design such relevant variables as content of curriculum, physical facilities, quality of instruction, could conceivably be standardized and controlled. In the nonexperimental approach, these environmental factors are not manipulated by the researcher but accepted as they exist. The only control the researcher can exert over these environmental variables is by an "ex post facto" approach of sorting the data according to the variables after they have been collected, assuming such "cross-tabulation" could be done retrospectively.

For example, if quality of instruction were considered a potentially significant extraneous variable that could affect the proficiency scores, perhaps even overriding the effect of type of program, pertinent data could be collected to control it. Thus, each study subject, in addition to supplying data on the type of program in which she trained, would be asked to rate the quality of instruction received. If this kind of subjective rating were not deemed valid, then the experimental might be the better approach.

The value of "ex post facto" data on important extraneous variables can be demonstrated by the following fictitious data. Suppose in the nonexperimental study of the comparison of nursing proficiency of graduates of diploma and degree programs the following average proficiency scores were obtained for samples of 1,000 graduates from each program (assume a range of scores of 0 to 100 percent, where 100 percent represents excellent proficiency and 0 poor proficiency):

TYPE OF PROGRAM FROM WHICH GRADUATED	PROFICIENCY SCORES (%)
Average, both types of programs	75
Degree	90
Diploma	60

These data make it appear that the degree graduate was more proficient than a graduate of a diploma program, and we may infer that a degree program prepares a better nurse than does a diploma program. But the difference in scores may not be causally related to type of program at all but to some other variable, such as quality of instruction. This variable could be the major influence on proficiency regardless of type of program. If we were able to obtain ratings of the quality of faculty and introduce this variable into the tabulation we might find the following relationship:

PROFICIENCY SCORES BY QUALITY OF INSTRUCTION (%)			
TYPE OF PROGRAM FROM WHICH GRADUATED	AVERAGE, BOTH TYPES OF INSTRUCTION	HIGHER QUALITY INSTRUCTION	LESSER QUALITY INSTRUCTION
Average, both types of programs	75	95	57
Degree	90	95	55
Diploma	60	97	58

When quality of instruction is accounted for, diploma graduates score at least as well as degree graduates in both categories of instruction—higher and lesser quality. Thus, a different interpretation can be drawn from these data than when only the variable "type of program" is considered. This interpretation is: the graduate of a diploma program is at least as proficient as a degree graduate when their schools are standardized for quality of instruction.

The following question may be raised concerning the data just presented: How can the average proficiency scores for the two types of instruction *combined* show a greater proficiency for the degree program graduate when the diploma graduate scores higher in proficiency than degree graduate in *each* category of quality of instruction? The answer becomes evident when the number of study subjects in each category is tabulated:

TYPE OF PROGRAM FROM WHICH GRADUATED	NUMBER OF NURSES BY QUALITY OF INSTRUCTION		
	TOTAL, BOTH TYPES OF INSTRUCTION	HIGHER-QUALITY INSTRUCTION	LESSER-QUALITY INSTRUCTION
Total, both types of programs	2,000	950	1,050
Degree	1,000	850	150
Diploma	1,000	100	900

We see from the number of nurses in each category that there are as many nurses who graduate from degree programs with higher-quality instruction as there are graduates from diploma programs with lesser quality instruction. Thus the average proficiency scores, when quality of instruction is not considered, is weighted by these highly skewed distributions.

From these data we see that quality of instuction is related to type of nursing program. Degree programs are characterized by higher-quality instruction, diploma programs by lesser quality. It may well be that the "cause" of high or low proficiency scores is not type of program, per se, but quality of instruction. To raise the level of proficiency of graduates, it is not necessary to eliminate the diploma program, but to raise the level of quality of instruction. This example indicates that the independent variable, "type of nursing program" is much too broad. It must be redefined to take account of the significant elements that really distinguish a diploma and a degree program.

A second difference between the experimental and nonexperimental research design is the greater control over organismic variables in the experimental approach through random assignment of the subjects to different groups. The purpose of random assignment is to standardize the composition of the different groups for all relevant organismic variables. If the groups are not standardized, it may well be an uncontrolled organismic variable that would influence the dependent variable rather than the independent one, as in the case of the environmental variable, quality of instruction.

In nonexperimental research there is no standardization of groups by random assignment of subjects; the groups have been formed by self-selection.

The nonexperimental study to evaluate the proficiency of diploma and degree graduates commences at the point where the subjects have already graduated and are practicing as graduate nurses. They themselves had selected their educational program.

The difference in proficiency scores may be due to a variable that is highly correlated with type of nursing program selected. This variable could be the intelligence level of the student which is correlated with the student's selection of an educational program: high-I.Q. students choose a degree program, lower-I.Q. students select a diploma program. Moreover, high-I.Q. nurses may score better on the proficiency scale than do low-I.Q. nurses, irrespective of the type of educational program they attended. Consequently, it is intelligence that determines proficiency, not type of program.

There are several methods by which the comparison groups can be equated in a nonexperimental design, according to the relevant organismic and environmental variables, to avoid inferring spurious relationships. One way is to broaden the analysis of data by treating all important extraneous variables as additional independent variables. This means that data would be gathered on all these variables and cross-tabulated with the criterion measure. Analysis of all significant organismic and environmental variables could lead to a standardization of the study groups similar to that achieved through random assignment.

A third difference between experimental

and nonexperimental research designs is that an experimental study is generally easier to reproduce. Reproducibility is necessary to experimentation. It permits other researchers to repeat the original work in order to verify it. Such verification is important in the establishment of a scientific body of knowledge, since the results of a single experiment cannot be considered conclusive.

An experiment is easier to reproduce —or, in statistical terminology, to replicate —because the elements are controlled and standardized. The protocol for the experiment—the detailed design or the study—is the plan for repeated testing. In nonexperimental studies, where there is less control over the research elements, exact replication of the design by other investigators is difficult to attain. For example, because the independent variable is not manipulated, it is difficult to achieve uniformity of definition of the alternative study groups from one study to the next. In the study of the relationship between type of educational program and proficiency of the graduate nurse, it is impossible to assure that the alternative groupings for the "type of program" variable—degree and diploma—remain the same from study to study even if the replicated study were to be conducted in the same schools. Because of this lack of control over the independent variable, significant changes could have been made in the programs offered by the schools from one study to the next that could make them noncomparable.

KEY POINT Basically, then, the main virtue of the experimental approach lies in the degree of control over various elements in the study —setting, subjects, and variables. The particular advantage lies in the researcher's ability to control the extraneous variables —variables not of interest, but which if uncontrolled could exert a significant and perhaps misleading influence on the dependent variable.

Variables in Explanatory Studies

The variables present in every explanatory study fall into two major categories: (1) the explanatory variables, those among which the researcher is seeking a relationship, and (2) the extraneous variables in which the researcher is not interested and is attempting to control with an appropriate research design. (See Figure 11–1.)

I. **Controlled Extraneous Variable(s)**

    A. By random assignment of study subjects to different comparison groups representing alternative versions, levels, gradations, or types of independent variable.

    B. By random assignment of study subjects to comparison groups with matching of subjects on relevant organismic variables.

    C. By random assignment of study subjects with application of the covariance technique to the analysis of data.

    D. By limiting the target population to subjects with certain specific characteristics, reducing the number of different organismic variables present among subjects, and providing greater homogeneity.

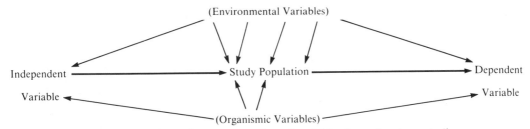

Figure 11–1 Schematic representation of variables in explanatory studies.

E. By limiting study settings to a small number of homogeneous units.

F. By ex post facto standardization of study groups through elaboration of data by a cross-tabulation with additional variables—essentially a process of introducing additional independent variables and relating them to the criterion variable.

II. Uncontrolled extraneous variable(s)

The variables that are confounded, that is, mixed with and confused with the explanatory variables and can result in spurious relationships among these variables.

TYPES OF EXPERIMENTAL DESIGN

In its simplest form the objective of an experiment is: (1) to vary the independent variable among study subjects while holding other relevant organismic and environmental variables constant, and (2) to measure the effect of this variation on the dependent variable. The major design problem lies in the phrase, "holding other relevant organismic and environmental variables constant." Numerous experimental designs have been developed to accomplish this as well as provide efficient ways of analyzing the data after they are collected in (Table 11–1). A brief explanation of each follows.

One-Group Design

The weakest of all the experimental designs is the one in which a stimulus is applied to a study population and the response measured in the dependent variable. To illustrate, we may institute a program of

TABLE 11–1.
Types of Experimental Design

TYPE OF DESIGN	STRUCTURE OF DESIGN		FORM OF DATA ANALYSIS
1. One-group	I D*		Evaluate magnitude of D
2. One-group, before-after	D I D		Compare change from D to D
3. Two-group	Study group Comparison group.	I D_1 D_2	Compare difference between D_1 and D_2
4. Two-group, before after	Study group: Comparison group:	D_1 I D_1 D_2 D_2	Compare difference between change D_1 to D_1 and change D_2 to D_2
DESIGNS WITH RANDOM ASSIGNMENT TO ALTERNATIVE GROUPS			
5. Two group with control group	Experimental group: Control group:	I D_1 D_2	Compare difference between D_1 and D_2
6. Multiple comparison groups, single independent variable	Experimental group 1: I_1 D_1 Experimental group 2: I_2 D_2 Experimental group 3: I_3 D_3 etc.		Compare difference between D_1 D_2, D_3, etc.
7. Multiple comparison groups, multiple independent variables	Exp. group 1: I_1 I_1' I_1'' D_1 Exp. group 2: I_2 I_2' I_2'' D_2 Exp. group 3: I_3 I_3' I_3'' D_3 etc.		Compare difference between D_1 D_2, D_3, etc., in terms of main effects of each of the independent variables as well as the interaction among the variables

*I = Application of independent variable to the group of study subjects; D = Measurement of the dependent variable before application of the independent variable; D = Measurement of the dependent variable after application of the independent variable

Note: Subscripts (e.g., D_1, D_2) signify the different study groups.

self-medications for hospitalized patients as part of the study. Patients are given a supply of the prescribed medications, excluding those where an error would have serious consequences, and allowed to take them according to the required dosage and time schedule. The criterion measure to evaluate this procedure would be the frequency with which patients correctly follow their medication regimen. If we find a high level of cooperation among patients and low rate of medication errors, we can regard the new system as a success. If medication errors are high, we would evaluate the system as a failure.

In this example the one-group type of design might be workable because there is an implicit standard of comparison by which to evaluate the effect of the change in the medication procedure. This standard states: the system is workable if it operates with perfect or nearly perfect accuracy.

However, consider a different type of study. Suppose we want to measure the effect of a new drug on the rate of a patient's recovery. If we gave a group of patients the new drug and then observed the percentage of patients who recovered, we would not be able to attribute this result to the drug because we have no knowledge of what would have happened to the patients if they had not been given the drug. Assuming that the illness was not one that was invariably fatal, most patients would recover even without the drug. In order to evaluate the impact of the drug we must have a standard of comparison that would tell us the patients' recovery rate without the drug.

Another example of the one-group design is an attempt to influence people to obtain polio immunization by distributing a pamphlet aimed at achieving this purpose and afterward measuring the level of immunization in the community. The problem in evaluation here is that if the level is low we would probably be correct in saying that the educational campaign was a failure. But if the level is high, we cannot automatically attribute this to our independent variable because we do not have any assessment of the change in the immunization level that

resulted as a direct consequence of the health education program. The level may have been high initially.

A final example concerns the reorganization of the nursing unit to include ward secretaries and then measuring the "effect" in terms of the proportion of time the professional staff spends in providing direct nursing care to patients as opposed to indirect activities such as charting. If we found that the staff spent a fairly high proportion of time on direct care to patients after the introduction of the ward secretary we still would not be able to attribute this effect to this independent variable because: (a) we do not have a basis for comparison to show what proportion of time would be spent on direct care in the absence of ward secretaries (it may be higher because with more pressure on her time the nurse might make better use of it), and (b) even if a standard of comparison did exist to show an improvement in expenditure of time on direct care, it would be difficult to attribute this to the independent variable—the use of ward secretaries—because we have not controlled any of the possible extraneous variables that could also influence our dependent variable—time spent on direct nursing care. These extraneous variables might be any of a whole host of uncontrolled organismic variables, such as the educational level of the staff, their personality, their perceptions of their jobs.

Because the subjects selected have insight into how to schedule their time, they devote to patient care most of the time that has been freed from clerical work by the provision of ward secretaries. However, such insight may not be typical of nurses in general, in which case we may well be incorrect if we infer that the use of ward secretaries would typically permit nurses to spend more time on patient care.

Another type of extraneous variable that can confuse findings of studies like this one can be labeled the sociopsychological reaction that human beings often exhibit to change, which may be stronger than the reaction to the independent variable. Doing something for a patient that seems to indicate that you are interested and want to be helpful can produce a positive reaction independently of the substantive nature of what you are doing. A back-rub may well have a more important psychological than physical impact. Therefore, in bringing together a group of people in a specialized research setting, we may create a group feeling among the subjects and generate interactions among them that can cause them to respond in unexpected ways to the independent variable.

Reaction to novelty introduced by a study was first observed in the classic experiments at the Hawthorne plant of the Western Electric Company in Chicago, during the late 1920s and early 1930s, and has become known as the "Hawthorne effect."[13] In this study the investigators wanted to measure the effect of such independent variables as physical environment on the subjects' productivity. Contrary to expectations, no direct relationship was found between physical working conditions and the amount of goods produced. However, the study pointed out a methodological principle of great value to the development of research design. As described by French,[14] the principle is as follows:

KEY POINT

> From a methodological point of view, the most interesting finding was what we might call the "Hawthorne effect." In order to manipulate more precisely the physical factors affecting production, the experimenters had set up a special experimental room for a small group of girls who were wiring relays. This wiring room was separated from the rest of the factory, and the girls working in it received special attention from both outside experimenters and the management of the plant. Careful studies of this wiring group showed marked increases in production which were related only to the special social position and social treatment they received. Thus, it was the "artificial" social aspects of the experimental conditions set up for measurement which produced the increases in group productivity.

In the one-group type of design the "Hawthorne effect" is especially trouble-some because there is no way of either controlling this effect or measuring its impact on subjects. For this reason alone it should be ruled out as a design for most studies. Moreover, except where standards are already established from other studies or similar authoritative sources, it does not provide its own basis of comparison for assessing any changes produced by the independent variable. Finally, we cannot be sure that the changes produced in the study would hold true beyond our study subjects, because we have no control over or even assessment of the effect of important organismic variables related to the specific characteristics of the study subjects.

In brief, the one-group design is not a research design at all. It is nothing more than the trial and error approach. Like trial and error, it is inefficient and subject to spuriousness.

One-Group, Before-After Design

This design makes a modest improvement over the simple one-group design. Here a measurement is made of the dependent variable before the independent variable is applied. The independent variable is then applied. After an appropriate time, the dependent variable is measured again. The main distinction between this design and the previous one is that an initial measurement is made the basis for comparing the final measurement. In the analysis of data the difference between the first and last measurements represents the effect of the independent variable.

To illustrate this design, suppose we were interested in the same research problem mentioned previously, that of measuring the effect on the population of a community of an educational campaign to convince people to obtain immunization against polio. Our criterion measure is the percentage of the total population immunized against polio. Our dependent variable is the distribution by mail to every home in the community of an attractive pamphlet describing the value of polio immunization and urging everyone to obtain it. We measure the rate of immunization prior to the distribution of the pamphlet by sending a mailed questionnaire to all residents of the community asking if they have been immunized. We repeat this questionnaire six months after the pamphlet has been distributed. If we find that the rate of immunization has increased significantly, can we attribute this to the educational campaign?

Actually this design is not much better than the previous one. We do have a standard of comparison—the "before" measure—but we have certain biases. Because this design is weak, we cannot draw causal inferences with assurance. There are at least four kinds of extraneous variables that could have influenced the change in rate of immunization in a positive way. First, the residents may have been exposed to other stimuli during the study period, for instance, a television program about the suffering that a family undergoes when a member contracts polio. Without the influence of this program, the immunization rate may not have shown a significant change.

A second type of extraneous variable could be the passage of time during which forces related to aging and maturation of the subjects exert influences on the dependent variable. These can override or mask the effect of the independent variable. A disposition to obtain immunization may have had its origin before the study began and would contribute to an increase in the rate, although totally unrelated to the independent variable. For example, the birth of a baby may reinforce a long-standing intention to obtain immunization independently of the educational material. In "before and after" research on patients this kind of extraneous variable is especially important to control. In studying the effect of nursing care on patients in which we observe the patients over a long period of time, changes in the patient that are purely a function of the passage of time must be sorted out and controlled so that they are not confused with the effects of the nursing

care that we expect to measure. We know that over time patients with various types of illnesses undergo changes in their physiological and psychological states associated with the maturation of the illness process and not necessarily with the care they receive.

A third type of extraneous variable that can confuse the findings of "before and after" studies is exposure to the measuring process itself. In the study described, the subjects are asked in a questionnaire about their immunization status prior to being exposed to the educational campaign. Asking people whether they are immunized or not may serve as a stimulus to those who would otherwise not seek immunization. Thus, the success of the distribution of the educational pamphlet can be exaggerated, since part of increase in the immunization level may be due to the questionnaire. Another aspect of this type of spuriousness is the use of the same psychological test to obtain before and after measurements. Initial exposure to the test may make the subject "test-wise." As a result the final responses may be more closely related to this factor than to the independent variable. Even physiological measurement can affect behaviour. As described by Campbell:[15]

> In general, any measurement procedure which makes the subject self-conscious or aware of the fact of the experiment can be suspected of being a reactive measurement. Whenever the measurement process is not a part of the normal environment it is probably reactive. Whenever measurement exercises the process under study, it is almost certainly reactive. Measurement of a person's height is relatively nonreactive. However, measurement of weight, introduced into an experimental design involving adult American women, would turn out to be reactive in that the process of measuring would stimulate weight reduction.

A fourth source of bias can result from the Hawthorne effect, which the design makes no attempt to either control or measure. The values of the before and after measurements may well reflect the sociopsychological reaction to the change introduced by the application of the independent variable and not to the variable itself.

Two-Group Design

This design improves upon the two previous ones. Unlike design "one," there is a comparison group against which change in the study group can be evaluated, and unlike design "two," this comparison group is an external one. In the polio example, we can select two communities for study of the effect of an educational pamphlet on the level of immunization and distribute the pamphlet to the residents of one community and not to the other. After an appropriate time we measure the rates of immunization in both. If, in comparing these rates, we find a difference, can we attribute it to the educational program?

We cannot. First, we do not know the previous levels of immunization in the two communities. The level may well have been higher in the community in which the pamphlet was not distributed. Therefore, the effect of our educational campaign may be masked unless we can, on an ex post facto basis, standardize our two communities in terms of initial level of immunization. Even if we can retrospectively standardize the two groups, we are still faced with the problem of the differential effect of our independent variable among groups with different immunization patterns to begin with. Assume that before we distribute the pamphlet, the community receiving it has a higher rate of immunization than the community not receiving it. It would undoubtedly be more difficult to raise the immunization level by the distribution of the pamphlet, because the few who are not immunized may include individuals who would resist any appeal. Conversely, with a low immunization level in the community receiving the educational material, substantial improvement might occur because there is potentially greater room for improvement.

Furthermore, there are a number of other extraneous variables that could affect the dependent variable in addition to the independent variable. Thus, if the city in which we distributed the pamphlet had a more highly educated population than the other, we may have achieved greater success than with a less educated population. It is known that the appeal of a health education program is greatest among those whose educational level is, in general, high.

Moreover, this design is also affected by the biases of the Hawthorne effect. We cannot be sure that any effects produced in the study group—even having available to us the criterion measurement for the comparison group—were related to extraneous sociopsychological variables rather than to the educational program. Finally, there is the bias that could arise from the uncontrolled occurrence of an event (the television drama is shown in only one of the cities) that could influence the dependent variable in ways unknown to the researchers.

The one advantage this design has over the previous one—the one-group, before-after—is that it eliminates the possible bias attributable to exposure to the measuring process itself. As an experimental design it is very weak and is rarely used in prospective studies.

However, this design is widely used for retrospective nonexperimental studies. In such a study two groups may be found to differ in terms of a particular variable and, by Mill's method of difference, may also differ in terms of another variable. If there appears to be a logical connection between these two variables, one may be designated as the independent and the other as the dependent variable. If we observe a high rate of attrition in one school of nursing and a low rate in another, and upon further investigation find that the school with the high dropout rate has poor physical facilities while the other school does not, we may then infer that quality of physical facilities is related to drop-out rates in schools of nursing. The shortcoming of the approach is that for the "method of difference" to apply we must be sure that the schools are more or less identical in terms of all relevant variables except that of physical facilities.

Two-Group, Before-After Design

This design attempts to correct the weakness of the previous one—that of making comparisons among study groups not standardized according to extraneous variables. Here the lack of initial standardization is compensated for in some part by the data analysis in which we compare the changes in both groups from the time before the independent variable was applied to the changes after it was applied. In the analysis, differences in the before and after measures for each group are calculated. The changes in each group are compared to see if the change in the study group is larger than that in the comparison group.

If it is, it can be attributed to the independent variable. If the difference in the before and after rate of immunization is larger for the group that received the educational material than for the comparison group, we are better able to attribute this effect to the educational program than in the case of the previous designs.

Many of the faults of the three previous designs are corrected by controlling most of the extraneous variables that could influence our dependent variable. In the immunization study the immunization levels of both groups would be tested initially so that effects of extraneous variables—such as the measuring process, the passage of time, etc.—are equal in both groups. If these extraneous variables were to exert an influence on the level of immunization, this influence could be estimated by the difference in the before and after immunization rates for the comparison group. Assume we had collected the following data:

	TOTAL POPULATION	NUMBER FOUND TO BE IMMUNIZED INITIALLY	NUMBER FOUND TO BE IMMUNIZED AFTER EDUCATIONAL CAMPAIGN
Study group	1,000	400	700
Comparison group	1,000	600	700

If we had used design "one" (one group only), we would know only that after the educational campaign 70% of our study group had been immunized; but without a comparative measure we have no way to evaluate this statistic. If we had used design "two" (one-group before-after), we could have compared the 70 percent final rate with the 40 percent initial rate and could perhaps have attributed this significant rise in immunization level solely to the program of health education, which may have not been a valid inference. In design "three" (two-group), we could have compared only the final measures, 70 percent for both groups, and undoubtedly would have concluded that the educational campaign had no effect.

But if we had used design "four" (two-

group, before-after), we may be able to come closer to the truth. In this design we can estimate the increase in immunization level attributable to extraneous factors as: the increase in the immunization rate in the comparison group. We can then estimate the increase attributable to the explanatory variable as: the increase in immunization level of the study group *after* subtracting the increase attributable to extraneous factors. Thus, in the comparison group there were 400 persons who were *not* immunized at the time of the first measurement. At the final measurement, 100 of these had been immunized. Therefore, the percentage of the 400 who had been immunized during the study was 25 percent: $(100 \div 400) \times 100$. This percentage can be considered an estimate of the effect of the extraneous variables. Applying it to the number in the study group who were initially not immunized—600—we can say that 25 percent or 150, were influenced to seek immunization during the study period as a result of the uncontrolled factors, and the remaining 150 of the 300 immunized during the study period were influenced by the educational campaign. Our conclusion using this design would be that the campaign was *more* effective than in the two-group after-only design where all we knew was that both groups had the same level of immunization at the final measurement, but that it was *less* effective than in the one-group before and after design where the 300 immunizations that occurred during the study period were all attributed to the educational campaign.

KEY POINT The two-group, before-after design is perhaps the most widely used design in partially controlled experiments in the social sciences, particularly those conducted in natural settings. It is unquestionably superior to the first three designs, but does have a serious shortcoming. It assumes that both groups have been standardized for all important extraneous variables. For this design to yield valid data any extraneous factor that significantly affects one group should also affect the other. If the composition of the groups is not comparable, study results cannot be valid. The simple fact is that if the two groups are not as alike as possible (standardized), there can be no basis for comparison.

Finally, the Hawthorne effect is not eliminated by this design and could be particulary troublesome in patient care studies. For example, if our independent variable were a nursing procedure, we have no way to measure how much of a change in our dependent variable is related to the procedure itself and how much to the Hawthorne effect, even if we used design "three". If the Hawthorne effect cannot be kept from influencing the study group, we must also expose the comparison group to it so that its influence is measured with other extra-

neous variables in the before-after evaluation.

In partially controlled experiments and in nonexperimental studies there is great difficulty in standardizing the groups being compared for all the relevant organismic and environmental variables that can influence the results. These difficulties have given rise to the development of what are considered to be "true" or fully controlled experimental designs, in which maximum control over all extraneous variables is achieved. The key element is *random assignment* of study subjects to alternative groups. Through such assignment, equalization is achieved for extraneous organismic variables, although it is not always perfect. A measure of the effects of randomized extraneous variables, known as experimental error, can be computed. To control the influences of environmental variables, the study setting is kept as identical as possible for the different groups, and external events are prevented from affecting the groups differentially. Certain techniques are employed to keep the Hawthorne effect from biasing the study.

Ideally, then, the good experimental design creates conditions for both the study and comparison groups, called the experimental and control groups, in which the two groups are identical in every respect, except in terms of the independent variable. Any difference that occurs in the values of the dependent variable for the two groups can then be attributed to the independent variable.

Experimental Designs with Random Assignment

Two-Group with Control Group

This is the classical experimental design and the basic model for the more complex types of controlled experimental designs. In this design the target population is first delineated. A random sample of subjects is selected from the target population, and these are further subdivided into the experimental and control groups by random assignment. (Methods for selecting a random sample from the target population will be described in Chapter 12, and methods of random assignment of the sample will be discussed in this chapter.) Random assignment means that neither investigator nor study subjects shall determine whether a subject is assigned to the experimental or the control group. This randomization procedure standardizes the composition of the two groups in the same way that tossing a coin yields, over the long run, the same number of heads and tails.

The independent variable in the fully controlled experiment may be of the all-or-nothing variety in which the "all" alternative (an educational campaign, a nursing procedure, a drug) is applied to the experimental group while the control group receives nothing. In other fully controlled experiments the independent variable may be graded so that, for example, the experimental group receives one dosage level of a drug whereas the control group receives a different level. In still other studies the independent variable may involve different versions of some phenomenon such as different types of teaching methods: the experimental group would be exposed to a teaching machine whereas the control group would be taught by conventional methods. More complex designs consist of more than two groups, as in experimenting with a variety of nursing staffing patterns (the team, functional assignment, case method, primary nursing). Still further complicated designs involve the simultaneous testing of a number of different independent variables. Instead of the terms "experimental and control groups," a more general terminology such as "contrast groups" or "comparison groups" is used, since in many experiments each group receives some positive value of the independent variable.

Randomization The purpose of randomization is to standardize the composition of the groups under study so that they are identical with respect to all pertinent organismic variables and differ only in terms of the explanatory independent variable. Any differences found among the groups in the values of the criterion measure are then ascribed to the influence of the independent variable. Randomization requires allocation of subjects to different groups according to the laws of chance, which, in its simplest aspect, is drawing names out of a hat and placing the first name in the control, the next in the experimental, and so on, alternately. In our immunization study if we had 2,000 subjects, half in the experimental group to receive the educational campaign and half in the control group not to receive it, by random assignment to the two groups we should allocate about the same number who have already been immunized to each group, as many highly educated people to each group, the same number of older people, and so on.

Randomization attempts to control bias from extraneous organismic variables that could influence comparisons among the groups by making the groups similar in composition. However, it will not completely eliminate these influences, particularly if the size of our group is small. **KEY POINT**

Random assignment is important because through randomization we can compute the "experimental error," which is a measure of the effect of the extraneous variables. One example is found in design "four", where the effect of the extraneous variables was estimated by the change in the before and after measure for the group from which the educational campaign was withheld.

How can one be sure that the differences measured between the experimental and control groups are actually caused by the (controlled) independent variable? This is done by dividing these differences by the amount of experimental error, using the "t-test," a statistical procedure. The resulting figure is the extent to which observed dif-

$$\begin{pmatrix} \text{Level of significance} \\ \text{of difference ob-} \\ \text{served (probability} \\ \text{that observed differ-} \\ \text{ence could have} \\ \text{arisen by chance)} \end{pmatrix} = \frac{\begin{pmatrix} \text{Value of measure of} \\ \text{dependent variable for} \\ \text{experimental group} \end{pmatrix} \text{ minus } \begin{pmatrix} \text{Value of measure} \\ \text{of dependent variable} \\ \text{for control group} \end{pmatrix}}{\text{Value of measure of experimental error}}$$

ferences can be attributed to the independent variable.

A third benefit of random assignment is that it can be used in more complex, highly sophisticated types of designs in which efficient and sensitive tests of significance can be applied to the data. In these designs, a test known as the "analysis of variance," in which more than two alternatives of the independent variable are tested simultaneously or where the experiment involves more than one independent variable, can be used to provide information concerning not only the effects on the dependent variable of each independent variable (main effects), but also the effects of combinations of these variables (interactions). For our immunization study we could simultaneously test numerous independent variables—the pamphlet, the educational level of the study subjects, age of subjects, and so on. Through the analysis of variance we could test the effects of each variable separately as well as the combined effects of several variables (e.g., does exposure to the pamphlet among poorly educated subjects have less effect on immunization level than exposure among highly educated subjects?)

As would be expected, the practical application of randomization is not without limitations. Foremost is a drawback common to all highly controlled studies—the difficulty of actually putting and keeping people in the alternative groups.

In the study of the impact of health education on the level of polio immunization, how practical would it be to assign subjects to one group or another and still keep them uncontaminated by outside influences, such as one group interacting with the other? Randomization works best with inanimate objects or with animals in the laboratory setting. In partially controlled settings, where a classroom, a patient's unit, or a physician's office is used for the experiment, it may be possible to randomly assign the subjects to the alternative groups of the independent variable, but very difficult to control the environmental variables. Thus, if two subjects are side by side and one is in the control group and the other in the experimental, they will interact with each other, and this interaction may significantly influence the values of the criterion measure.

A second limitation of random assignment is that while it can promote standardization of characteristics of members of the various groups, it cannot *guarantee* it. It is possible, but not likely, that random assignment will do a poor job in standardizing the composition of the groups on relevant organismic variables. After all, the probability of shuffling a deck of fifty two playing cards (randomizing them) and dealing a perfect bridge hand to each player (thirteen cards of the same suit to each player) is highly remote, but is as equally likely as dealing out any other specific distribution of cards stipulated in advance by the dealer. In other words, sometimes by randomization we may not achieve the effect we desire—that of shuffling subjects so that the composition of the groups is closely similar.

Several techniques have been developed to provide added assurance that alternative groups will be standardized for all relevant characteristics beyond that of randomization. They are: *pairing, balancing,* and *covariance,* sometimes embraced under the general heading of "matching."

Pairing The most commonly used method of standardizing the experimental and control groups is to determine the extraneous variables for which subjects in the two groups are to be matched and to assure that these variables are equally represented among subjects in the groups by a method that combines purposive assignment with randomization, that is, pairing. Pairing is described by Cochran[16] as follows:

Matching of the experimental and control samples with respect to the covariables can be accomplished in a number of ways. Conceptually, the simplest is the method of pairing. Each member of the experimental samples is taken in turn, and a partner is sought from the control population which has the same values as the experimental member (within defined limits) for each of the covariables. One way of doing this is to perform a multiple classification of the control population by the variables. We then examine the first member of the experimental sample, pick the cell which contains all control members having the desired set of covariables, and choose as the partner one control member at random for this cell. This procedure is repeated for each member of the experimental sample.

If an occasional cell is found to be empty, it is usually preferable to choose the control partner from a neighborhood cell, rather than to omit the experimental member. If numerous cells are found to be empty, this is a danger signal. Either the limits of variation allowed in the covariables are too narrow or the control population is not satisfactory.

The analysis of the results is very simple. The difference (experimental-control) is computed for each pair, and any t-tests are applied directly to this series of differences.

An ideal type of pairing that has been used in a few psychological studies is the so-called co-twin control, in which one twin is assigned to the experimental group and the other to the control group.

The method of pairing subjects in establishing experimental and control groups was employed by Hasselmeyer[17] in her experimental study of the effect of the diaper roll on the behavior (crying, sleeping, eating, etc.) of premature infants. In this study the variables selected for matching the infants were birth weight (four groups), sex (two groups), and race (two groups). A total of sixteen cells were established ($4 \times 2 \times 2$). For each cell there was an even distribution of experimental and con-

trol subjects. The placement of a specific infant into either the experimental and control group was determined by chance, providing the randomization necessary to justify computation of experimental error and application of statistical tests of significance of differences between the experimental and control groups.

There are several drawbacks to the use of the matched pair design. One is the subjectivity introduced by the researcher in the selection of the variables upon which the pairing will be based. The variables selected should be those organismic variables most likely to affect the dependent variable and confuse the results if proper standardization of the experimental and control groups is not done. Using unimportant variables in pairing will not contribute to the control of extraneous influences on the data and will only add an unnecessary burden to the research design. In patient care studies typical matching variables for patients include diagnosis, age, sex, education level, and severity of illness.

Pairing also complicates the study design and can slow down its progress, particularly where the size of the groups is large and where there are a number of matching variables, each having numerous subdivisions. Pairing then becomes tedious and difficult. When the experiment extends over a long period of time, there is danger of loss of some of the subjects, which will spoil the balanced pattern of the pairs.

With all of its drawbacks, pairing is helpful in matching the composition of the experimental and control groups on important organismic variables. It can be particularly helpful and usually easy to administer in patient care studies where, if uncontrolled, some of the organismic variables can have a significant impact on the behavior of the dependent variable.

Balancing The purpose of balancing is similar to that of pairing. The difference between the two methods is that matching by balancing is accomplished in terms of the groups as a whole rather than of the individuals composing the groups, as in matching by pairing. If age is one of the balancing variables, the assignment of members to the two groups is arranged so that the average age of the group is identical. If sex is another matching variable, the percentage of males or females assigned to the alternative groups is the same. Assignment of a subject to either group is still accomplished through randomization. However, unlike unrestricted random assignment there is a deliberate attempt to match the groups as a whole in terms of those extraneous organismic variables of sufficient importance to be specially controlled.

Balancing is generally easier to do than pairing and provides about the same amount of precision in standardizing the two groups. However, in testing the statistical significance of differences in the values of criterion measures for experimental and control groups a more complicated type of analysis has to be used.[18]

Covariance The analysis of covariance is another procedure applied to data to take account of important extraneous variables (called in statistical terminology, covariables). Unlike the two previous methods, where matching of the groups is done by assigning individuals to study groups on the basis of certain covariable characteristics *before* the independent variable has been applied, covariance analysis is a procedure for adjusting data to standardize groups *after* the independent variable has been applied to the subjects and measurements made of the dependent variables.

Actually the analysis of covariance combines the two statistical techniques of regression analysis and analysis of variance. The computations involved in the analysis of covariance are rather complicated, especially if the number of covariables is large. However, as a device for ex post facto matching of groups it can be extremely useful, particularly when it is not feasible to match the groups during the assignment process by either pairing or balancing. Sometimes the covariable used in the analysis is an initial measure made of the dependent variable. In essence then,

covariance analysis becomes a type of "before and after" design with the "before" measures used to adjust the "after" data. If we were studying the effects of a drug on weight reduction, and our experimental group consisted of subjects given the drug and the control group of subjects not given the drug, we would make weight measurements of subjects before application of the independent variable. These measurements would be used in the covariance analysis to adjust data obtained on the "after" measurement of the subjects.

Other Matching Methods Another method of standardizing study groups is not a formal method at all but a restriction of the study population to subjects with homogeneous characteristics. If we wish to evaluate the effects of a referral system on reducing the rate of patients' readmissions to hospital, we may restrict the study population to patients in a particular age group, with a particular diagnosis, and in a certain income group, to eliminate the effects of these variables and ensure that experimental and control groups are closely matched. Naturally, restriction of the study population means that the target population has also been narrowed, thereby limiting any generalizations made from the data collected.

Still another method of matching groups, widely used in nonexperimental research although applicable to experimental studies as well, is the cross-tabulation of data in terms of relevant organismic and environmental variables. Like the covariance technique this is an ex post facto approach, although the variables should be selected before data collection. Stipulation in advance is necessary to ensure that data pertaining to these variables will be collected and available for analysis when that stage of the research is reached. In the study of the effect of an educational campaign on immunization levels, not only can the data be tabulated to show the immunization levels *after* exposure to the educational campaign according to whether the individual was or was not exposed, but they can also be analyzed in terms of age of the subjects, educational level, income, sex, and other organismic variables deemed important in influencing immunization behavior.

It is through randomization that the "two-group with control group" design standardizes the study groups according to extraneous organismic variables and prevents them from exerting a spurious influence on the relationship between independent and dependent variables. In fully controlled experimental research, extraneous environmental influences are controlled by standardizing the study setting for both experimental and control groups. All external disturbances are eliminated or at least standardized for both groups.

There still remains the problem of the Hawthorne effect—the sociopsychological reaction of the subjects to the study situation itself. Coupled with this is the need to control biases originating in the collection of data, known as observer bias. In experimental studies of the effects of drugs on patients, called clinical trials, these problems have been largely resolved by the development of two techniques for controlling psychological biases, known as the "placebo" and the "double-blind".

Placebo   The term placebo, (Latin, "I will please") is used in clinical trials of drugs to describe an inert capsule, tablet, or injection that is made to look exactly like the experimental drug. While subjects in the experimental group receive the experimental drug, the placebo is given to subjects in the control group to assure a similar psychological response in both sets of subjects. Any difference in the values obtained on the criterion measure for the experimental and control groups should be above and beyond the psychological reaction to the study situation itself. The difference should provide a real measure of the true physiological effect, if any, of the drug.

In studies not concerned with testing drugs, it is possible to develop a "dummy" treatment to be applied to the control group to induce psychological reactions similar to those of subjects in the experimental treatment group. This reaction would provide a measure of the Hawthorne effect. For example, in a study testing a new nursing procedure on a group of patients, the amount of professional nursing time that would normally be spent with patients would be increased for patients in the experimental group. Therefore, instead of withholding the procedure from the control group, added nursing time should also be provided to control subjects to equalize the attention both groups receive. In other words, for every exposure to the independent variable given experimental subjects, an equivalent "dummy" exposure should be provided to the control group. In this way we can be more certain that the difference we measure between the two groups is more purely related to the independent variable and is not contaminated by extraneous social or psychological factors.

Double-Blind   The placebo is employed to provide a further control that the experimental and control groups are identical in every way except in terms of the independent variable. Whereas randomization attempts to equalize the groups at the start of the study by controlling bias that could arise from organismic variables, the placebo equalizes them by controlling any psychological biases arising from the subject's reaction to receiving the medication, apart from any therapeutic benefits. A further control on the psychological biases that could arise during the course of an experiment is the double-blind technique. Through its use, neither the research workers in contact with the study subjects nor the subjects themselves are aware of who is in the experimental group and who is assigned to the control group.

In the double-blind approach the randomization of subjects to the alternative groups is done by someone who has no contact with the study subjects. In drug trials using placebos, neither subject nor investigator should know who is receiving the experimental drug or the placebo. Concealing the placement of a patient in experi-

KEY POINT

mental or control group is intended to eliminate the bias that could occur where, for example, an otherwise well-meaning nurse might interfere with the course of the study by giving a patient in the control group the drug being tested rather than the placebo because she felt that to deprive him of the drug would cause undue suffering. Similarly, if a patient knows which group he is in, he may react in a way that could bias measurements of the dependent variable. He might be fearful or upset if he knew he was in the control group and thought he was being deprived of a potentially beneficial drug. Or, conversely, aware of being in the experimental group he might be concerned as to whether he was being exposed to a potentially harmful drug.

In studies other than drug trials or similar types of independent variables where a placebo can be developed, it is not possible to use the double-blind approach. For example, in measuring patient responses to a nursing procedure it is not possible to conceive of a "dummy" alternative that could be applied to the control group. Also, in studies testing alternative versions of some variable—say, different methods of obtaining information from patients (structured interviewing compared with nondirective interviewing)—the double-blind approach is inappropriate because each group receives a "treatment" of some kind.

Placebos and the double-blind technique have their best use in experiments in which a treatment, drug, or stimulus of some kind is being tested. However, in all types of studies the researcher must guard against possible psychological or physiological biases, arising during the study from either subjects or investigators, that could distort the relationship among the explanatory variables. It must be constantly borne in mind that the paramount objective is the attainment of ideal experimental conditions in which the comparison groups are identical in every respect except the independent variable. Practically, this ideal is rarely achieved outside of strictly controlled laboratory studies or theoretical exercises.

In studies of human beings, because of the vast number of extraneous variables present, we can only hope to approximate this ideal. We must be alert during the entire course of human experiments to possible biases. If we cannot eliminate them, at least we should be aware of the limitations and effects they impose on the quality of our data. With such awareness we can make a more valid and meaningful interpretation of the data.

MULTIPLE COMPARISON GROUPS, SINGLE INDEPENDENT VARIABLE

In many studies, the independent variable can be grouped into more than two categories. Some variables can be scaled according to a quantified continuum in which many gradations are possible. One independent variable for a patient care study might be hours of nursing care available to patients. Another is the dosage level of a drug. Still others might be size of nursing unit (number of patients) or hospital, school, or community.

Other types of independent variables with multiple categories are those scaled according to a qualitative characteristic. The variable "patient observation method" may consist of such categories as direct observation by the professional nurse, indirect observation by the professional nurse through the use of television, or monitoring by electronic devices. The variable "educational program for training in nursing" may consist of four groupings: practical nurse training, associate degree preparation, diploma education, and college education.

From the standpoint of research design the major advantage of the multiple comparison group design is that it provides more information than does the two-group design. The two-group design, particularly the experimental-control group, all-or-nothing variety, is relevant only where there are no meaningful alternatives to the one being tested in the experimental group, or as in drug studies, where it is not certain that the drug being tested will have any beneficial effect, regardless of the dosage level. The latter, the two-group, all-or-nothing design, can serve as a prescreening trial study. If, in such a trial, the drug or other dichotomized variable being tested appears to have promising therapeutic benefits, further study will test finer gradations of the variable to determine the optimum therapeutic level.

When the independent variable can be scaled according to quantitative (numerical) gradations, the analysis of the relationship among independent and dependent variables can be expressed as a mathematical equation. This equation, once improved and perfected, should make apparent the value of the independent variable that will produce the optimum value of the dependent variable. Nonexperimental research studies concerned with the relationship among independent and dependent variables that can be scaled quantitatively, are sometimes called correlational studies, and are useful in many fields of research. In experimental research, since the elaboration of the study to include additional groupings of the independent variable increases the number of subjects required, and since the cost of increasing the number of subjects is considerably higher than in nonexperimental studies, such correlational studies are less frequently undertaken.

However, the one-group before-after design is frequently elaborated to vary the independent variable according to graded levels in order to determine which level produces the best effect. Thus, the dosage level of a drug will be gradually increased until optimum patient response is noted. The danger in the use of this design, in addition to all the limitations of the before-after design, is the cumulative effect on the patient of repeated applications. Since each treatment is not really independent of previous treatments, it may not be possible to ascribe any specific effect observed to a particular level of treatment.

A drawback, then, to the use of multiple comparison groups is the need to expand the study to include additional study subjects, which, of course, adds to the expense. Moreover, with additional comparison groups the problem of standardizing the composition of the various groups so that everything is a least theoretically held constant, except the independent variable, is compounded. However, through the use of the technique of statistical analysis of experimental data known as analysis of variance, the multiple comparison groups design can yield more information per unit cost of conducting the experiment than the simpler, two-group design. As such it is a more efficient design.

Latin-Square Design An experimental design involving multiple comparisons, developed to make efficient use of subjects, is the so-called latin-square design. In this design the number of times each alternative of the independent variable is replicated is equal to the number of comparison groups. If we were studying the effect of four different patterns of nursing care (team plan, functional assignment, etc.) on patient satisfaction, each pattern would be replicated four times among different study groups to provide sixteen measures of our dependent variable. The assignment of study groups to each of the replications would be by randomization.

The latin-square design originated in the agricultural field, where it offered a means not only of efficiently analyzing study results, but also of randomly assigning the plots of land to the alternative versions of the independent variable. For example, if four kinds of fertilizer were to be tested, each containing different proportions of nitrogen, phosphorus, and potash (5-10-5, 10-6-4, 10-10-10, 20-10-5), the experimental field would be divided into four equal parts north to south (rows), and four equal parts east to west (columns), making a total of sixteen equal-sized plots. Each of the four types of fertilizer would be randomly assigned to four plots, a crop planted on all plots, and the yields measured and compared to see which produced the greatest output. The latin-square method of assignment of the four kinds of fertilizer to each plot would ensure that each kind would appear only once in each of the four

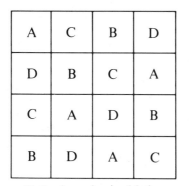

Figure 11-2 A randomized latin-square.

rows and once in each of the four columns and thus fertility variations in both directions are randomized. If each type of fertilizer were labeled A, B, C, D, the method of assignment to the plots would be a latin-square. (see Figure 11-2):

Now instead of this randomized latin-square pattern of assignment, suppose it were decided to systematically assign the different types of fertilizers to the plots. R. A. Fisher told the anecdote, somewhat altered for simplicity, of the experimenter who thought the systematic type of allocation of treatment to the experimental subjects would be better than the random method, so instead of using a randomized latin-square he assigned the different fertilizers along the diagonal of the field. He felt he would thereby achieve better representation of the fertilizers among the different parts of the field (see Figure 11-3).

He fertilized, planted, and watched the crops grow. He measured the yields, com-

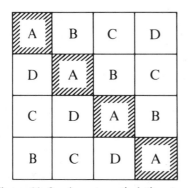

Figure 11-3 A systematic latin-square.

pared the results, and discovered that the plots treated with type A fertilizer had a much greater crop yield per plot than those fertilized with any other type. Fertilizer A was then marketed and extravagant claims made for its effectiveness in producing rich yields of wheat.

Some time later, complaints were received by the fertilizer company that fertilizer A was not living up to claims made for it. The experimenter went back to his experimental plots to recheck the design. To his horror he discovered, on closer examination of the geography and soil conditions of the sixteen plots, an underground stream that ran in a perfect diagonal straight through the four plots he had selected for fertilization with Type A. Thus, his dependent variable—crop yield—was at least as much affected by this uncontrolled independent variable, moisture content of the soil, as by the independent variable he actually controlled—chemical fertilization. Had he used the latin-square design, which would have randomly allocated the plots to alternative groups, he most likely would have eliminated the effect of this extraneous factor.

MULTIPLE COMPARISON GROUPS, MULTIPLE INDEPENDENT VARIABLES

Perhaps the most efficient of all is this design, which tests simultaneous effects of several independent variables. Such a design may also involve multiple alternatives for each independent variable. These designs, known as *factorial designs*, were originally used in research on nonhuman subjects in the fields of agriculture, botany, and genetics, and although potentially useful in studies of human beings, they still have their widest use in the physical and biological sciences.

In an agricultural experiment using the factorial design, our dependent variable might be the yield of a crop; our subjects, plots of land; our independent variables (factors), depth of plowing, amount of fertilizer used, and amount of irrigation of the plots. Assignment of the plots to each of the numerous combinations of variables would be on a random basis. Each of the many possible combinations of factors would be represented by at least one of the plots.

The number of possible combinations in a factorial experiment is equal to the product of the number of alternative groupings of each independent variable. If the depth of plowing factor had two alternative groupings, the amount of fertilizer three groupings, and the amount of irrigation four groupings, the number of different comparisons (combinations of factors) would be $2 \times 3 \times 4 = 24$.

Applied to nursing research, a possible factorial design might be a study of the effects on quality of care (assume a valid quantitative measure of this dependent variable existed) of such factors as size of hospital (small, medium, large), layout of the unit (large open ward, a ward of all semiprivate units, a private ward), and amount of nursing care (high, medium, low). In this experiment, known as a 3^3 factorial, the number of combinations that can be formed from the different factors is $3 \times 3 \times 3 = 27$. To conduct this experiment as a fully controlled one, patients would be randomly assigned to one of twenty seven groups upon admission to the hospital. Each group would consist of a different combination of factors. Assuming that we want twenty patients in each of the twenty seven comparison groups, the allocation of the patients would be as in Table 11-2. Note that the number of patients exposed to each of the three variables as a whole, as well as to the alternative versions of each variable, is the same, or, in experimental design terminology, perfectly balanced. This type of design is part of a family of experimental designs, such as the latin-square, called balanced designs. They are designs in which subjects are matched according to exposure to different combinations of independent variables. One of its major virtues can be seen from Table 11-2. Each of the three main variables consists of 180 subjects: 180 patients in each of the three different amounts of nursing care groups, 180 patients in each type of nursing unit, and 180 in each size hospital. For each combination of two variables, there are sixty subjects: sixty patients in private units of small hospitals, sixty in private units of medium-sized hospitals, sixty in private units of large hospitals, and so on for a total

TABLE 11-2
Number of Patients Assigned to Each Combination of the Independent Variable

HOSPITAL SIZE AND TYPE OF NURSING UNIT	AMOUNT OF NURSING CARE			
	LOW	MEDIUM	HIGH	TOTAL
Small hospital				
Private unit	20	20	20	60
Semiprivate	20	20	20	60
Ward	20	20	20	60
Medium hospital				
Private unit	20	20	20	60
Semiprivate	20	20	20	60
Ward	20	20	20	60
Large hospital				
Private unit	20	20	20	60
Semiprivate	20	20	20	60
Ward	20	20	20	60
Total	180	180	180	540

of 9 groups. For each combination of three variables, there are twenty patients in each of the twenty seven combinations: twenty in private units of small hospitals with low care, etc.

If, instead of a factorial design we had designed the study to test the effect of only one independent variable, say, amount of nursing care, on our dependent variable, quality of care, we may well have needed sixty subjects in each of the three comparison groups to produce valid findings. With this design, we would have only been able to make three comparisons—among the three levels of amounts of nursing. Through the factorial design with just *three* times the number of subjects, we can make *nine* times the number of comparisons. Moreover with the factorial design, not only can we compare the effects of each of the three main variables themselves, known as the main effects, to see which, if any, exerts the greatest influence on our dependent variable, but we also have important information on the interactions between these variables. As Edwards[19] says:

> This in turn means that the outcomes of the experiment provide a sounder basis for generalizing about the effectiveness of the experimental variables, since they are tested not only in isolation, but in conjunction with the effects of other variables.

The factorial design is an efficient form of experimental design, perhaps the most efficient developed to date. By using the analysis of variance to analyze the data, the amount of information yielded by the study as well as the precision of the data analysis is maximized. In the sample cited we would learn not only whether providing more hours of nursing care produces higher quality of patient care, but whether hours of care in conjunction with (interaction with) size of nursing unit and size of hospital affect quality.

Consideration of the effects of several variables simultaneously is a more sophisticated approach to explaining why some-thing happens than is the approach to understanding causation by examining only one variable at a time. This is particularly true in research concerned with human beings, where there usually is no single explanation for an event.

However, one drawback exists in the application of factorial designs to human subjects. A balanced design, such as the factorial design, is a symmetrical design and requires the assignment of the same number of subjects to the alternative groups. If, as so often happens in research on humans, a subject drops out of the study, the quality of the data is threatened. Even with techniques available to estimate missing values for lost cases, attrition of subjects remains a serious problem not only in factorial designs, but in all the experimental designs. And, as Mainland[20] points out, statistical analysis of data obtained by experimental designs in which multiple comparisons are made—the analysis of variance methodology—is most efficient and (some say) only applicable where the dependent variable is a quantitative variable having a finely graded numerical scale and not a qualitative variable with broad, crudely defined classes.

HOW TO CONDUCT AN EXPERIMENT

The previous discussion has provided a rapid overview of the various types of experimental designs, beginning with the weak type of partially controlled designs without random assignment of study subjects to alternative groups, moving through the fully controlled designs with random assignment, and ending with the highly sophisticated factorial design, in which the effects of several independent variables are studied simultaneously. Understanding of the experimental approach can be acquired only through further study of the subject by reading the specialized literature in the field, as well as obtaining personal experience in conducting experiments. The material presented here can be considered only as an introduction to the subject. While these designs provide the structure of an experiment, determination of the design to use in an actual study is only one of twelve important steps in the experimental process. The major steps in conducting an experiment are chronologically and substantively nearly identical with the twelve steps in the research process outlined earlier. The following is a brief review of these steps with special emphasis on the experimental approach.

1. *Formulate the experimental problem:* A clear, precise statement of the problem is especially urgent in experimental research where large expenditures of time, effort, and money are often required to collect data. Determine the purpose of the study —is it to acquire knowledge or to test a product, program, or procedure? Question the *need* for the experiment, its *feasibility,* the *importance* of the problem as to requiring an experimental approach, the degree to which findings can be *generalized,* the *interest* of the investigator in the subject matter, and his *competence* to pursue the experiment.

2. *Review the literature:* In some areas little experimental work has been done. In others, the literature is vast. Much can be gained from learning about another investigator's firsthand experiences in approaching a problem experimentally.

3. *Formulate the framework of theory:* A research study will have greater meaning and importance if it can be placed within a theoretical framework. Even a practical study on a specific subject such as evaluating an alternative procedure or method can usually be placed within a broader conceptual base. Linking study to theory can contribute to the accumulation of a comprehensive body of scientific knowledge.

4. *Formulate hypotheses:* Most studies are explanatory, seeking insight into the causation of observed phenomena. For such experiments the formulation of clearly stated hypotheses is essential. The hypoth-

esis should contain a statement of the expected relationship among the variables as well as the population whom such relationship concerns.

5. *Define variables:* In studies comparing the effects of an independent variable or variables on a dependent variable, the alternative groups of the independent variable must be clearly differentiated. The criterion measure by which the alternative groups will be evaluated must be meaningful and consistent. All variables must be defined in terms of performable acts and in such an objective way that they can be consistently and accurately observed by independent observers.

6. *Determine how variables will be quantified:* The analysis of results of experiments employ highly sophisticated statistical techniques that require the data to be in a quantitative form. Moreover, the use of perhaps the most refined statistical tool for analyzing experimental data—the analysis of variance—requires that the dependent variable have a numerical scale of measurement, most desirably with a finely graded continuous scale—as for example, temperature, weight, blood pressure, time, etc.

7. *Select the research design:* A fully controlled, explanatory study requires the establishment of comparison groups representing the alternatives of the independent variable, the assignment of experimental subjects to alternative groups on a strictly random basis, and keeping of the conditions constant during the entire experiment so that the only differences are in the independent variable. Greater efficiency in experimental design can be achieved by testing the effects of several independent variables simultaneously. Among the more complex designs are the latin-square and the factorial. The main objective in an experiment is to control the effects of any extraneous variables, organismic or environmental, that could bias the relationship among the explanatory variables. Lack of randomization can lead to a mismatching of the characteristics of the alternative groups with

possible biasing of results by extraneous organismic variables. Lack of control over the uniformity of study conditions can invite the spurious influence of extraneous environmental variables.

8. *Delineate the target population:* For a study to have value beyond its own subjects and setting, the subjects must be drawn from a larger population, called a "target population." This selection must be made in such a way as to insure that the experimental subjects are representative of the members of the target population. The greater the extent to which the findings of a study can be generalized, the greater is the contribution to scientific knowledge.

9. *Select and develop the method for collecting the data:* Numerous methods are available for collecting data from experimental subjects. In many studies the data are obtained directly from subjects through use of human observers. In data collection, as well as in the process of exposing the subjects to experimental conditions, the sociopsychological biases—the Hawthorne effect—that can result when human beings are placed in novel situations or are treated in a special way must be controlled. The use of such techniques as the *control group* to whom the experimental treatment is not given and the *placebo* or *dummy treatment* given to the subjects of this group are examples of these controls. The *double-blind* technique, to completely disguise which subject receives the experimental treatment and which the dummy treatment, can also help control psychological bias in many types of studies such as drug trials, or those in which the independent variable consists of the all-or-nothing variety.

10. *Formulate the method of analyzing the data:* In comparative experiments using random assignment of subjects to alternative groups, the statistical analysis of data is well-defined and fully described in numerous textbooks on statistical methodology. In comparing the values of criterion measures for two groups, a test known as the "t test" evaluates the difference found

in the measures in relation to an estimate of the effect of the randomized extraneous variables, called experimental error. In making multiple comparisons the analysis of variance is used in which the evaluation of the effects of the various experimental alternatives is accomplished by means of an "F test."

11. *Interpret the results of the experiment.:* The statistical tests of the results of an experiment—such as the t test, and F test—give a measure of the statistical significance of the findings—i.e., the extent to which the differences found among the alternative groups exceed that which can be attributed to chance. The practical or substantive meaning of data can be extracted only through the interpretative skills, sophistication, and the subject matter expertise the investigator brings to the data. Interpretation of results must be tempered by due recognition of the limitations of the study.

12. *Communicate the results of the experiment:* A single study cannot provide the final word on any conceivable research problem. The findings of one study are limited by the fact that it is generally based on a small group of subjects and conducted in a specific place at a specific time. Publication of the method and findings of a study can stimulate replication of the study by others as well as providing a link with the body of scientific knowledge.

Some Practical Problems in Conducting an Experiment

Not all decisions that need to be made in conducting an experiment are technical, theoretical, or statistical. An investigator is continually faced with a variety of practical problems. The solutions to these problems often depend on the individual's accumulated practical experience and wisdom as well as his intuitive grasp of the implications of the decisions. Some of the more important of these problems require discussion.

1. *Choice of experimental setting:* Ideally, the most desirable setting for an experiment is one especially developed for that purpose, such as a laboratory or some other type of experimental unit where it is generally easier to exert control over extraneous influences. In animal or other types of studies, such specialized facilities are highly desirable, but in experiments with humans they may have limitations. One drawback is the problem of obtaining the cooperation of people placed in an unnatural environment. A related, and perhaps more important limitation is the difficulty of controlling the psychological biases that can result from a novel setting. The Hawthorne effect was first identified in the atmosphere of an artificial experimental situation. Finally, the artificiality of the specially constructed experimental setting puts restraints on the extent to which findings can be generalized. Nursing care provided in an experimentally devised setting may have little relevance to care provided in a real hospital.

Of course, the content of many experiments does require specially devised settings. The independent variable may necessitate radical alterations of the normal setting. A study of the use of television in monitoring patients would require significant changes in the usual facilities of the hospital. Also, the extensive use in a study of a complicated mechanical instrument to measure the dependent variable—for example, a cardiotachometer—certainly represents an "unnatural" environmental factor.

The main concern in the choice of an experimental setting is the degree to which possible disturbing influences of extraneous variables can be controlled. Fortunately, a high degree of control can be exerted in many settings that could be used for research in nursing and patient care. In hospitals, facilities such as operating rooms, intensive care units, recovery units, and nurseries can serve as highly controlled settings for studies involving patients. Other types of highly controlled natural settings of possible use in experimental research in nursing include classrooms, outpatient clinics, and employee health units.

The problem in controlling the influences of extraneous variables introduced by the study setting varies directly in magnitude with the time lag between application of the independent variable and observation of the effect in the dependent variable. If the time lag is short, as in an experiment concerning alternative ways of assisting a patient with eating as evaluated in terms of both nurse and patient acceptance, extraneous environmental influences have little opportunity to bias the experiment. In such studies natural settings can be used without fear of loss of control over the experiment. If the time lag is long, however, extraneous influences have more opportunity to affect the experiment. If we attempt to test, in the patient's home, the effect of teaching family members how to provide certain elementary nursing services, there may be a lag of weeks or even months before the effect (skill at providing such services) can be observed. During this time many outside variables could influence this dependent variable and might well confound the effect of the independent variable. Of course, the longer the time between stimulus and response, the more difficult and impractical it is to conduct a fully controlled experiment. There are definite limits as to how long a "captive audience" can be expected to remain cooperative.

2. *How many subjects shall an explanatory experiment include?* The number of subjects (replications) to be included in an experiment is not a simple, cut-and-dried determination. Other things being equal, the larger the size of the study population (the sample of the target population), the more precise will be the findings of the experiment. But size of sample must be balanced against the practical problems involved in obtaining cooperation of subjects and in keeping them in the study during the experiment. Attrition from an experi-

ment can seriously damage the data and suggests that keeping the sample size small enough to be manageable, but large enough to provide definitive findings is a practical requirement.

Discussion of methods for determining the appropriate number of experimental subjects is contained in Chapter 12. Briefly, the size of the sample depends on six factors:

a. A primary consideration in determining size of sample required is the degree of precision desired. This precision, which in testing hypotheses is called the level of statistical significance, is a measure of the confidence that can be placed in the fact that any difference in the values of the criterion measure found among the comparison groups is truly related to the independent variable and not to extraneous factors. Generally, greater precision in study results requires a larger number of subjects.

b. The uniformity of members of the target population in relation to significant organismic variables influences the number of subjects needed. If there are large differences in important extraneous variables such as age, health status, education, and so on, a larger sample would be required to assure representation of the target population than if there were greater uniformity among members.

c. With greater control over possible confounding environmental variables, a smaller sample can be used to achieve the same level of accuracy than when more environmental variables are uncontrolled. Obviously, a perfectly controlled experiment is more efficient than one less perfectly controlled, since it yields just as precise findings with fewer subjects.

d. Sample size is influenced by the amount of difference (among comparison groups) perceived as having real and substantive significance. If a large difference is established as being truly significant, a larger sample size is required

to prove statistical significance than if the researcher accepts a small difference as truly significant. While a large sample is more likely to demonstrate the statistical significance of experimental findings, the essential meaning of these differences also needs to be understood.

e. The sensitivity of the measuring instrument used to evaluate the effects of the independent variable can also influence the sample size. With a crude instrument having only a few gradations it may be necessary to use a larger sample to detect statistically and practically significant differences among the comparison groups than if a more sensitive instrument were used. Whether sensitive or crude, the measuring instrument must yield valid and reliable data to assure the veracity of the experiment.

f. With greater numbers of independent variables and more alternative groups for each variable, the number of experimental subjects required grows larger. But, factorial experiments involving the simultaneous testing of several independent variables are much more efficient than designs with single independent variables, because the amount of information gained substantially exceeds the increase in sample size.

3. *How are the experimental subjects randomly assigned to each of the comparison groups?* Through randomization, neither the experimenter nor the experimental subject deliberately determines to which of the groups the subject shall be assigned. Many procedures are available for achieving a truly random allocation of experimental subjects such as tossing a coin, drawing names by lot, and shuffling cards. Probably the best method of randomization is a table of random numbers. This table is simple to use. Suppose in a study of different methods of infant feeding we wanted to divide forty nursery infants into two groups, A and B, each receiving a different method of feeding. We would write the names of each infant (or its number) on

a separate index card, shuffle all the cards carefully, open the book containing random numbers to any page (at random), select a two-place digit from anywhere in the table (at random), and write the digit down on the first card. We would then copy consecutive two-place digits on succeeding index cards by moving in any order in the table of random numbers—up or down, right or left. After we had assigned a random number to each card, we would arrange them in order of magnitude of the random numbers (from 00 to 99). The twenty lowest numbers would be assigned to group A, and the twenty highest numbers to group B. By what appears to be rather involved but actually is a simple procedure we have assigned the infants to each group in a completely random fashion. Random allocation increases the likelihood that the two groups of infants were equalized in terms of extraneous variables as well as enabling the computation of a measure of the influences of such randomized variables.

4. *How long shall the experimental subjects be exposed to the independent variable?* The answer to this question depends on the nature of the independent variable. For some variables that elicit a quick response, short exposure may be sufficient. For others, where reactions are slower to develop, a longer period of exposure would be required. Suppose we are experimenting with the best way (i.e., the cheapest, the most efficient, providing the highest quality of care) to organize a hospital. Our independent variable may consist of two alternatives: the progressive patient care type of organization and the conventional hospital organization. Such an experiment may require a period of study over a number of years before any differences between the two systems can be detected in the criterion measures. Such a lengthy period is required because the influences exerted by such complicated independent variables are subtle and indirect. Also, it will often take long periods of time for the subjects to settle down within the experi-

mental situation and begin to respond normally to the independent variable itself rather than to the novelty of the situation.

5. *How long a time lag shall there be between exposure to the independent variable and measurement of its effect on the dependent variable?* The answer depends on the nature of the explanatory variables. Generally, a strong independent variable will produce a quicker effect than a weaker one. Similarly, a sensitive dependent variable should detect the effects of the independent variable in a shorter time than a less sensitive one. There is danger in too great a lag between exposure of subjects to the independent variable and measurement of response in the dependent variable. Problems of attrition of subjects are magnified, as well as the greater likelihood that intervening extraneous variables will affect the study.

6. *Can an experiment include several dependent variables as criterion measures?* Many experiments include numerous dependent variables to measure the effect of the independent variable. For example, a study of methods of organizing a hospital (progressive patient care versus conventional organization) can have as criterion measures: an evaluation of the hospital's financial status, a measure of personnel satisfaction, an audit of the quality of patient care, and a comparison of patient mortality. Hasselmeyer[21] in her study of the effect of the use of a diaper roll on the behavior of premature infants used five criterion measures: time required to regain initial birth weight, sleep behavior, crying behavior, bodily movements, and eating ability. Where multiple criterion measures are employed each should make a distinctive and substantial contribution to the understanding of the independent variable. One variable should not duplicate another. When studies contain multiple dependent variables they are usually analyzed separately in terms of their relationship to the independent variable. However, techniques are available in an area of statistical methodology known as *multivariate analysis,* in

which these criterion measures are analyzed as simultaneous responses and each weighed against the other.

7. *How can the experimental groups be kept intact during the whole course of the experiment?* There are no hard and fast rules for maintaining the cooperation of the study subjects throughout the course of the study. Some subjects may drop out because of circumstances beyond anyone's control. In patient care studies we must continually be aware that some subjects may leave the study for any number of reasons. In out-of-hospital studies, people move, change jobs, or otherwise alter their status, which removes them from the study. One approach to the dropout problem is to try to motivate the subjects and to see that they fully understand its aims, methods, and importance.

The Use of the Experimental Approach in Studies of Patient Care

With increasing frequency the experimental method is being applied to problems in nursing and patient care. In general it can be said that research employing the experimental approach has been limited to narrowly defined problems conducted in settings where experimental controls could be feasibly applied: team method of assignment on a hospital ward, use of a diaper roll as support for premature infants, closed-circuit television as a method of teaching nursing students, and so on. Such narrowing of the research problem is required by the nature of the experimental method.

Close analysis of the studies that have employed the experimental method will frequently reveal lack of full control over the experimental situation. At best, most experiments in nursing and patient care can be classified as partially controlled experiments. In few studies has the random assignment of the subjects to the alternative groups been attempted. Most experimental studies in nursing have been conducted in natural settings where control over extraneous environmental variables has been difficult to achieve. Moreover, for most of the independent variables included in nursing studies it is difficult to control sociopsychological biases. The double-blind method of assignment and the placebo treatment are difficult to apply in such studies.

The problem of applying rigorous controls in experiments involving human beings can be illustrated by examining a study to test the comparative pain-relieving effects of five popular aspirin-containing analgesic preparations.[22] The five drugs included two containing aspirin alone, one with aspirin and additional ingredients to avoid a gastrointestinal upset, and two containing aspirin and other pain-relieving ingredients. As a control on psychological biases, a sixth group was given a placebo. The double-blind method was used.

The study contained three phases. In phase 1, the analgesic potency and rapidity of onset of relief from pain was measured in a group of postpartum patients. In phase 2, the gastrointestinal side effects were assessed in a group of elderly patients. In phase 3, a group of nine arthritic patients were studied for the effect of the drug on pain relief and gastrointestinal disturbance.

In none of the phases were the subjects selected at random. Consequently, it is not possible to make *statistical* generalizations of the results beyond the study population. However, in all phases of the study the drugs were randomly assigned to the patients. In phase 1, medications were randomly and "blindly" administered to patients on request. Patients were interviewed prior to administration and seven times after the drug was administered, beginning fifteen minutes after the drug was given and ending four hours later. Patients were asked to rate their pain as absent, slight, moderate, severe, or very severe. A quantitative score was applied to these ratings indicating a change from one level of severity to the next. One of the criterion measures used was the percentage of patients reporting complete pain relief at selected intervals. The data for the one- and three-hour intervals are as follows:

DRUG	PERCENT OF PATIENTS REPORTING COMPLETE PAIN RELIEF AFTER:	
	I HOUR	3 HOURS
Buffered aspirin	71	67
Combination of ingredients I	67	73
Plain aspirin I	59	60
Plain aspirin II	52	59
Combination of ingredients II	49	67
Placebo	24	40

Statistical analysis of these data (the well-known "chi-square test") revealed that for one- and three-hour intervals there was no significant difference among the five drugs in the percentage of patients reporting complete relief. However, the percentage was significantly greater for all drugs than for the placebo.

In phase 2, a 6 by 6 latin-square design was employed in which sixty patients were randomly divided into six groups of ten patients each. Concurrently each group was given a different drug for five days until all groups had received all five drugs and the placebo. One hour after a drug was given, the patient was interviewed to find out whether he had experienced a gastrointestinal disturbance. The following occurrences were reported:

DRUG	NUMBER OF DOSES GIVEN	PERCENTAGE OF ALL DOSES GIVEN IN WHICH GI UPSET REPORTED
Buffered aspirin	812	0.6
Placebo	833	0.8
Plain aspirin I	818	1.1
Plain aspirin II	829	1.1
Combination of ingredients I	799	2.9
Combination of ingredients II	760	4.5

The researchers found that the incidence of upset stomach was significantly higher for the combination of ingredients than for the three other drugs and the placebo. No statistical significance was found among the rates of upset stomach for these three drugs and the placebo. In phase 3, a group of nine arthritic patients who had been receiving regular doses of aspirin three times a day over a long period were given the five drugs in random order and interviewed afterward in relation to pain relief and gastrointestinal upset. No differences were found in the patients' reactions to the drugs.

Here, then, is a clear example of the use of the experimental method in pursuing a research problem among human beings directly concerned with patient care. That the problem is of sufficient importance to warrant an elaborate experiment is easy to demonstrate. The use of aspirin is more widespread than the use of any other drug. As the authors remark, "Analgesic compounds have assumed a leading position among the proprietary drugs that are most widely and most stridently advertised."

In the conduct of the experiment, every possible control was employed, including random assignment to alternative groups, placebo, and double-blind. Control over extraneous environmental factors was attained by the very short lag between administration of the independent variable (the different pain-relieving drugs) and measurement of the dependent variable (pain and gastrointestinal upset).

We have in this research the elements of an experiment involving human beings where a very high degree of control can be achieved, perhaps higher than can be attained in most conceivable patient care studies. Yet with all its controls it still possesses weakness in design that make it not completely free of the influences of extraneous variables. The lesson learned from this study is that it is extremely difficult, if not impossible, to conduct a fully controlled experiment among human beings.

Some of the weaknesses of this experiment are:

1. There is no target population to which the findings can be statistically generalized. The study subjects—hospitalized patients—are unquestionably different from the typical aspirin user: an out-of-hospital, ambulatory, otherwise healthy individual. However, this does not preclude the experimenters from generalizing the data beyond the experimental setting if they are convinced by their knowledge and experience that their findings would apply to other people, in other places, and at other times.

2. In phase 1, randomization was used without any further attempt at matching the groups. We have no assurance, then, that the influences of extraneous organismic variables were equally distributed among the groups. However, in phases 2 and 3, the use of balanced designs essentially matches the groups, since each subject in each group receives each of the drugs being compared.

3. The criterion measures used, the patients' own evaluations of the occurrence of pain and gastrointestinal upset, are subjective measures. Because of their subjectivity, their validity and reliability can be questioned. However, it can be argued that these variables represent subjective phenomena and that self-reporting is the only realistic and meaningful type of measurement.

4. Although the double-blind approach was employed in the experiment, there is some question as to whether the identity of the drugs could be completely disguised. Physically, the drugs tested do differ in appearance, and although this difference may be slight, it could introduce psychological bias.

5. Some question can be raised as to cumulative effect of the application of the independent variable. In phase 2, for example, the drugs were given three times a day for five days. Repetitive dosage may build up an effect differing from that of a one-time or at least short-term use, the most common type of use. Therefore, the findings of the experiment may not be directly relevant to the research problem that precipitated it—that of the widespread use of analgesic compounds.

6. In all phases of the study, repetitive measurements were made of the dependent variable. In repetitive measurements there always exists the danger that the measuring process itself will introduce psychological bias. Although, of course, the use of the placebo serves as a control and a measure of the influence of such bias, the unnaturalness of the experimental situation is thereby increased.

NONEXPERIMENTAL DESIGNS

Nonexperimental designs are probably the most widely used type of designs in research involving human beings. Descriptive studies, where the aim is to generate new facts, are largely nonexperimental. Nonexperimental design is especially suited to such studies, since description implies natural observation of the characteristics of the research subjects without deliberate manipulation of the variables or control over the research setting. If we are interested in determining descriptive facts about the nursing needs of home care patients, we will attempt to observe and record these needs in their actual settings.

Nonexperimental explanatory research, also called analytical surveys, have the same objectives as explanatory experiments: to discover causal patterns or relationships. Nonexperimental research can rarely establish causal relationships. Because of the lack of control over all extraneous variables that can confound the relationship between the explanatory variables, the best generally achieved is the establishment of associative relationships. Such studies can be useful in making predictions as well as in suggesting controlled experiments that may ultimately lead to causal explanations.

The model for nonexperimental explanatory research is the controlled experiment. The essential difference between the two types of designs is the absence of deliberate randomization of the study subjects to the alternative groups. While in the experimental design the experimenter manipulates the independent variable through assignment of subjects to the various alternative groups, the manipulation of the independent variable in the nonexperimental design is done by bringing subjects into the study who already possess that quality of the independent variable. In other words, in the nonexperimental approach to explanatory research the subjects already have been exposed to the independent variable by forces other than deliberate assignment to the alternative groups through a random process.

In nonexperimental explanatory research there are several methods available for achieving the equalization of groups that in experimental research is accomplished by random assignment and the matching techniques of pairing, balancing, and covariance. In one method the comparison groups are selected so that as many as possible of the important extraneous variables are alike, much as in the matching methods. Assume we want to nonexperimentally study differences in the rate of readmission to a hospital between patients discharged from a hospital with a home care program and those discharged from a hospital without such a program. We select the alternative hospitals so that, except for the home care program, they are similar in all important extraneous variables, such as amount and type of nursing care available, educational level, economic status, diagnoses of patients, and characteristics of the patients' home environment.

Another way of enhancing comparability of groups is to restrict the target population to homogeneous subjects. A nonex-

perimental study of the effect of different patterns of outpatient department care on the general health status of patients could limit the patients to those in certain age, economic, education, and diagnostic groups. Such restrictions of the target population limit the scope of generalization of the findings.

Basically there are two kinds of nonexperimental designs: cross-sectional and longitudinal. In addition, a longitudinal design may be either retrospective or prospective.

Cross-sectional Design

A cross-sectional survey can be thought of as analogous to the taking of a snapshot of some situation and analyzing it. We "stop" the action at a point in time and examine it. Most descriptive surveys are of this type. When a nurse renews her license to practice she supplies data concerning her age, employment status, and field of practice. These data are compiled to provide a composite picture of the characteristics of the registered nurse at a point in time. Similarly, the American Hospital Association routinely collects data from a panel of short-term general hospitals concerning the utilization of the hospitals as of a certain time period. Every few years the United States Public Health Service samples the characteristics of registered nurses in the United States.

The cross-sectional design can also be used in explanatory surveys. In a study of the relationship of the amount and type of nursing care available in hospitals, a sample of hospitals was selected that included hospitals with different staffing patterns (the independent variable).[23] Evaluation of the adequacy of nursing services provided at that time was obtained from patients and personnel in each hospital (the dependent variable). The two variables were analyzed to see whether there was a relationship.

It can be clearly seen that in the cross-sectional design the researcher has not randomly assigned the subjects to the various alternatives. In the study just cited, patients and personnel were not allocated at random to the different staffing patterns. Although theoretically a sort of random process is in operation in that the distribution of the patients to the different hospitals can be considered a function of chance factors, we cannot be sure that all conditions are more or less equivalent for the different groups.

Restrospective Design

One of the most popular types of nonexperimental designs, particularly in explanatory studies, is retrospective. The dependent variable is observed first and then traced back and related to relevant independent variables that are hypothesized as being associated with the dependent variable. For example, in a study of birth injuries reported on the birth certificate, it was noted that the incidence of injuries appeared to be higher in some hospitals than in others. In checking these statistics, it was found that hospitals with lower rates of birth injuries had better designed and equipped delivery rooms than those with higher rates.

Another important retrospective study was the one that brought to light the association between smoking and lung cancer. The impetus was a startling increase in deaths from lung cancer among men. Case histories were developed on the lifelong smoking habits of men with lung cancer and of those who had died by interviews with relatives. As a "control group," life histories were compiled on men who had died from other causes. A comparison of the two groups showed a much higher percentage of cigarette smoking among those who died from lung cancer than among those who died from other causes. Recent reports show a large increase in the incidence of lung cancer among women, which coincides with a huge increase in the number of women who have begun smoking since World War II. The number of deaths from this disease in women is expected to continue to rise in future years because the number of women smoking increased steadily until 1982, when a slight decrease was noted. In fact, the recent so-called "epidemic" of cancer was actually due almost entirely to a big jump in lung cancer in women.

Retrospective studies are popular because they are relatively inexpensive and easier to administer than other types. Basically, a retrospective explanatory study is the reverse of the experimental design. In experimental explanatory studies, exposure to the independent variable precedes observation of the dependent variable. In the retrospective method the dependent variable is observed first, and then the independent variable that may have caused the behavior of the dependent variable is sought.

Retrospective explanatory studies are essentially longitudinal in that the relationship between the dependent and independent variables extends over time. For such variables as smoking and lung cancer, a lengthy period of time has elapsed. A limitation of this approach is the lack of control over the research setting, subjects, and variables. Consequently there are difficulties in establishing relationships among the variables that are free of spuriousness. Moreover, retrospective studies often make extensive use of data originally collected for a purpose other than that of the researcher's, such as data contained in birth and health records, health histories, patient records, and personnel records. Or, they may use data that are heavily dependent upon the respondent's ability to accurately recall some past event. Such data are not as valid and reliable as that controlled in prospective studies. The advantage of retrospective designs is the relative ease and inexpensiveness of collecting data. As hypotheses-generating, exploratory-type studies, retrospective studies can be most valuable.

Prospective Design

Prospective explanatory surveys, also called longitudinal studies, are similar to experiments in that the study begins with alternative groups of subjects followed over a period of time and compared in terms of some criterion measure. We may, for example, follow over a period of time two groups of premature infants after discharge from the hospital, one group from a formally organized premature nursery, and the other from a regular nursery, to see whether differences occur in their physical development. Or we may follow two groups of high school students, one school in which future nurse clubs are organized and the other where no such clubs exist, to determine whether there are differences in the proportion of subjects in each group choosing nursing as a career.

The major difference between the prospective nonexperimental and experimental designs is the absence in the former of random assignment to comparison groups. Also in the survey there is no control at all over the many variables to which the subjects are exposed during the study period.

Prospective nonexperimental studies are popular in following a group of subjects over a long period of time to observe what happens to them. Studies that focus on the same group of subjects over time are also known as *cohort* studies. The term "cohort" refers to a set of subjects who are grouped according to certain characteristics and observed longitudinally. In explanatory studies these characteristics would be the independent variables. Thus, we can select a group of graduates from a degree program in nursing and another from a diploma program and observe them at regular intervals over a long period of time to see how many remain in nursing and how many leave. Of those remaining in nursing we can find out how many become supervisors and administrators and how many remain as staff nurses and, of those leaving, how many are housewives and how many take jobs in other fields. The experience of the subjects over time can be related to their cohort characteristic, which in this example is the type of nursing program.

Cohort studies are widely used in the field of demography where the mortality or morbidity experience of a group of individuals may be observed over a long period of time. In one type of cohort study "life tables" are produced which statistically quantify the experience of the cohort groups. Thus, we can take a group of individuals who have a disease such as cancer, follow them over a period of time, and record the number of deaths that occur at different time intervals: one year after onset, two years, three years, etc.

Cohort studies such as the ones described are essentially a series of cross-sectional studies involving the same subjects repeated over a period of time. Subjects from a given group are tested at regular intervals and measurements of the same phenomena made. The cohort-type study, particularly where only one group is involved, is similar to the "before-after" type of experimental design in which control over possible confounding organismic variables is achieved by restricting the study to the same subjects.

Mixed Designs

In research practice, mixed types of design are sometimes employed. We may begin our study as an experiment and then employ a prospective, cohort-type nonexperimental study. For example, the experimental phase may consist of randomly assigning one group of hospitalized cardiac patients to a comprehensive program of patient teaching while another group would receive no formal teaching. After discharge, patients in both groups (the cohorts) would be followed to determine whether there is any difference in their mortality experience. Due to the many intervening variables that could exert an influence on the mortality rates, however, it would be difficult to demonstrate a causal relationship among the variables.

Another common type of mixed design is one that incorporates a cross-sectional approach and an experiment. Through this approach certain relevant clues may be obtained in a cross-sectional survey concerning the variables of interest to the researcher, and these may be incorporated into an experimental study. Also, a retrospective study often precedes a prospective one, the former serving as an exploratory phase to generate hypotheses and to suggest fruitful avenues of approach in the forward-looking study.

Historical Research in Nursing

Historical research in nursing is a neglected area and yet it should be one of highest priority for the researcher.

> Research into present day problems without adequate search into the past to examine the course of events which produced the present problems, or to bring to light past investigations of the same or similar problems by nurses or others, results in research which only scratches the present surface and may even duplicate previous work.[24]

Historical research is sometimes referred to as documentary research and is recognized as an appropriate method of inquiry. Such research goes beyond the collection of facts and dates and considers the relationship of facts and incidents to current and past issues and events. "A major contribution of historical inquiry is in the development of a broader, more complete perspective to enhance our understanding of the present and our approach to the future."[25] It is different from the scientific method only in that historiographers are concerned with "the conscious or thought-side of human existence."

The historical method has similarities to the methodology of the natural sciences in that both must deal with discovery, verification, categorization, and interpretation of facts and events.

Criteria of Historical Research

Historical research must pass the same rigorous tests of validity and reliability as other forms of research. The historiographer seeks to establish truth, ascertain facts and form the basis of conclusions and generalizations. Christy[26] points out that historiographers have evolved two separate processes for the critical examination of data. The first is external criticism which establishes the validity of documents such as manuscripts, letters, and books, and internal criticism which determines the reliability of the information contained within the document.

All important is that the historiographer compare documents with the originals and whenever possible use primary sources. This is the best way to establish fact. If available, two independent primary sources that corroborate should be used. If only one primary source can be found and there is no contrary evidence, the evidence can be considered probable.

Fitzpatrick[27] identifies the following key criteria used in evaluating historical research:

1. Nature, adequacy, and completeness of sources. The historiographer uses a systematic approach in collecting and verifying data. Primary sources are used and are not limited to one. Further, varied sources are used—documentary materials (letters, minutes, proceedings) as well as published materials.
2. Completeness with which the identified subject is treated. Are the important components addressed? Are varied and key questions asked? Are limitations stated? Are explanations of why different approaches were or were not used provided?
3. Recognition of bias in selection of hypotheses. Is the researcher directed to certain data and issues without consideration of alternatives? Is information provided that leads to preconceived judgements? Does the researcher recognize the complex nature of the area being researched?
4. Contextualism. Historiographers must have concern for context and time that make events unique.
5. Interconnectedness. The historiographer is concerned with the relationship of parts to the whole; the weaving together of disparate parts to form a coherent explanation that communicates meaning.
6. Organization.
7. Clarity.

8. Logical sequence.
9. Originality of interpretation.

Selected Examples of Historical Research in Nursing

The National Organization for Public Health Nursing, 1912–1952: Development of a Practice Field by M. Louise Fitzpatrick.[28]

This superb example of historical research makes a significant contribution to the all too few efforts of historians in the field of nursing. The author provides a fully documented and scholarly report of the origin, development, and activities of the National Organization for Public Health Nursing from 1912 to 1952. Particularly important is the author's unique approach to describing public health nursing as it was reflected in the interests and activities of the National Organization for Public Health Nursing. A span of forty years is covered in which the work of NOPHN contributed to the advancement of public health nursing and the educational preparation of public health nurses.

A Cornerstone for Nursing Education by Teresa E. Christy.[29]

Historical research contributes a valuable perspective to the analysis of current activities by providing a sense of continuity over time through the analysis of persons, movements, events, and concepts. Through the process of reconstructing events of the past and the analysis of why events occurred as they did, the historian has the capacity to assist professional groups in measuring, evaluating, and predicting social change.[30]

This was the sentiment expressed by Eleanor Lambertsen in describing the Christy historical research:

"The author provides a history of the Division of Nursing Education of Teachers College, Columbia University, and places the main events in juxtaposition with parallel events at the beginning of the twentieth century. The historical presentation is not limited to the history of one institution but particularly important is the thorough documentation of the broad movement toward better, more uniform education for nurses. The international influence of M. Adelaide Nutting and Isabel M. Stewart is clearly portrayed."

Mary Adelaide Nutting: Pioneer of Modern Nursing by Helen E. Marshall.[31]

This is a biographical study in which the author attempted to trace the development of nursing as a profession by reporting the achievements of one of its great leaders, Mary Adelaide Nutting. The author had access to Miss Nutting's papers preserved by Isabel Stewart and Mary Roberts. Miss Virginia Dunbar collated the correspondence between Miss Stewart and Miss Nutting and indexed the Nutting family papers. What resulted in Dr. Marshall's biography of Miss Nutting is a very personable account of a leader in the nursing profession.

Watch-Fires on the Mountains: The Life and Writings of Ethel Johns by Margaret M. Street.[32]

The biography of a pioneer nurse of the Canadian west whose leadership helped to shape American nursing. Of particular importance is the historiographer's approach to relating events of the first half of the twentieth century to nursing affairs at the local, national, and international levels.

From Nightingale to Eagle: An Army Nurse's History by Edith A. Aynes.[33]

An example of the experiences of an army nurse before, during, and after World War II. She portrays her personal experiences and documents these with significant events of the times, thus producing a historical document with a personal assessment and point of view.

The Lamp and the Caduceus. The Story of the Army School of Nursing by Marlette Conde.[34]

A well-documented account of the history of the Army School of Nursing. Several notable leaders who were graduates of this program have had great influence on American nursing. The author had access to a number of primary documents such as army and alumnae records.

A School of Nursing Comes of Age: A History of the Frances Payne Bolton School of Nursing, Case Western Reserve University by Margene O. Faddis.[35]

An excellent example of how the history of a professional school can become an important part of the history of a profession. The development of the Frances Payne Bolton School of Nursing clearly reflects the evolution of nursing toward a true profession. Primary sources were used from the university archives, the archives of university hospitals and alumnae records.

Historical Research Tools and Resources

MANUSCRIPTS AND ORAL HISTORIES

The historiographer has available both the tape-recorded interview and the historical record although these research tools are not without problems.

Manuscripts continue to be the main resources for the historiographer. These may include letters, drafts, a variety of historical records exclusive of archives and other documents.[36] Oral tape-recorded interviews have come to be an accepted historical record and research tool and now fall within the range of primary research materials. Oral histories may serve as single historical documents or one aspect of the total research effort.

The historiographer using the oral history "attempts to capture the recollections and interpretations of those participants in the development of contemporary medicine who are judged to be knowledgeable about the subject under study."[37] Thus the oral history can provide information related to a specific subject or an autobiographical memoir. The oral history has one major limitation in that it lacks the footnote or citation considered basic to scholarship. Interpretations by other historians are limited, and additional verification of the facts and opinions on tape may be needed. Thus, related historical documents to verify the facts in the oral history become extremely important. Historiographers using the oral

history as a research tool should preserve primary records for possible future research. Such histories can also extend the usefulness of manuscripts.

Oral history materials to be used by researchers must be cataloged and administered by qualified personnel in historical libraries. The historian will find *The American Archivists, The Journal of the Society of American Archivists,* helpful in that it publishes an annual bibliography covering subjects related to archives and manuscripts. Also helpful is *Library Trends.*[38]

A unified manuscript-oral history approach has merit for the historiographer in that a single and combined catalog of related subjects would be available.

Significant progress has been made at the National Library of Medicine (medicine is used here in the generic sense as it refers to all health literature) in developing and handling archival material. Sizable manuscript collections housed at the National Library of Medicine have cataloged together manuscripts and oral histories.

The Nursing Archives at the National Library of Medicine.

At a historic meeting on April 6, 1973, the Executive Director and the president of the National League for Nursing (NLN), Deputy Chief of the History of Medicine Division, Dr. Peter D. Olch, and Chief Nurse Officer of the USPHS met to discuss the establishment of a nursing archives at the National Library of Medicine. It was agreed that the NLN would transfer the material in their archives to the National Library of Medicine. This material, which included early records of the NLN, the American Society of Superintendents of Training Schools, and the National Organization for Public Health Nursing, was received on December 12, 1973. At the meeting, participants also agreed that the NLN would make an effort to identify the location, content, and accessibility of manuscript items important to the history of nursing in the United States. In those instances where materials could not be adequately processed and preserved at the parent institution, the representative of the National Library of Medicine would discuss with a designated NLN committee the advisability of transferring the material to the National Library of Medicine.

Recognizing the importance of the preservation of manuscript materials documenting the history of the American nursing profession, the repository at the National Library of Medicine has welcomed the receipt of the NLN collection and hopes their action will stimulate other individuals and nursing organizations to seriously consider the preservation of their personal papers and records in this or other repositories where they can be organized and made available for scholarly research.

A catalog entry of the NLN collection appears in the 1976 volume of the *National Union Catalogue of Manuscript Collections,* which originates in the Descriptive Cataloging Division of the Library of Congress.

Reference inquiries pertaining to NLN material in the library will be answered, but MEDLINE has no information about manuscript collections within the library.

Steps are being taken by the Public Health Service to encourage faculties at Teachers College, Columbia University, Wayne State University, Boston University, and other universities to have a historian or archivist develop registers for special collections, which could then be made available at the National Library of Medicine for cross-reference. Historians would then have a total picture of what is available at the National Library of Medicine as well as at the on-site location of private collections.

At the present time historical documents of the Federal Nursing Services cannot be accepted at the National Library of Medicine due to a regulation published in the *Code of Federal Regulations,* Title 41, Public Contracts and Property Management, Chapter 101 (Revised July 1, 1974), which requires records of the Federal Nursing Services to be filed with the Federal Archives. After full exploration, it was found that 85 to 90 percent of records submitted to the National Archives are destroyed and a separate nursing collection is not maintained. For this reason, other avenues are being explored that will permit the Federal Nursing Services to submit their historical documents so that they can be added to the nursing collection at the National Library of Medicine. At present the National Library of Medicine can only accept private collections such as the National League for Nursing (NLN) historical documents. The preservation of importat historical nursing documents is critical and every use should be made of the superb resources at the National Library of Medicine located in Bethesda, Maryland.

HOW TO CONDUCT NONEXPERIMENTAL RESEARCH

The twelve steps in the research process discussed in detail in chapter 5 provide the sequence of activity involved in developing a nonexperimental as well as an experimental study. We begin with formulation of the problem and end with reporting the findings. While the steps involved in developing all types of research studies are identical, the emphasis on certain of the steps differs somewhat for the various designs. The major differences are as follows:

1. In nonexperimental research more effort is usually devoted to the statement of the problem than in experimental. Many nonexperimental studies come to grips with thornier, more broadly conceived problems than do experiments. Hypotheses in such studies are often less specific and may not lend themselves to simple statistical tests.

2. In nonexperimental studies the variables are usually less clear-cut, the relationships among them more complex, and the need to consider the impact of extrane-

ous variables more pressing than in experimental studies.

3. In an experimental study much more concern is focused on the specific design, particularly the randomization procedure, the form of statistical analysis of data, in fact, the total mechanics of administering the study, than is devoted to similar matters in the nonexperimental approach.

4. More time is spent in nonexperimental studies analyzing data through statistical tables and in interpreting them above and beyond their statistical significance.

5. In a nonexperimental study more concern is usually devoted to the method of random selection of study subjects from the target population. An experimental study is more concerned with the random assignment of the subjects to the alternative groups.

6. Collection of data is often different for the two approaches—the experimental approach usually involves direct collection of data through observation, interview, or use of mechanical instruments. The nonexperimental approach is more likely to employ indirect methods such as the mailed questionnaire.

7. The types of criterion variables are frequently different in the two approaches. The experimental method employs more refined tools of measurement, often using scientific instrumentation. The nonexperimental is more apt to employ more crudely measured variables.

HOW TO CHOOSE BETWEEN AN EXPERIMENTAL AND NONEXPERIMENTAL DESIGN

One type of research design can often serve as a substitute for another type. The actual choice of design for a study depends on the evaluation of numerous factors, such as:

1. *Nature of the research problem:* Some research problems do not lend themselves to the experimental approach because they cannot be set up outside of an uncontrolled natural setting. Similarly, other problems may not be capable of study nonexperimentally because the ingredients of the research may not exist in nature and may have to be experimentally constructed.

2. *Amount of resources available to do the research:* Generally speaking, it is more expensive in money, manpower, and materials to conduct an experimental than a nonexperimental study on the same problem.

3. *Amount of time available to do the research:* An experimental study will generally take longer for completion than will a nonexperimental study concerned with the same problem. Many retrospective or cross-sectional studies can be completed in several months. In an experimental study this length of time may be needed just to plan the study.

4. *Possible danger to health or safety of people:* Some research cannot be pursued experimentally because of potentially harmful effects to the subjects. Nonexperimental studies are far less likely to have such negative consequences on the study population.

5. *The exploratory nature of the study:* In the field where little research has been done previously and where it may be presumptuous to launch a full-blown, highly structured experiment, a nonexperimental study can be useful in exploring the field, clarifying concepts, developing hunches, and formulating the problem and the hypotheses.

6. *The degree of refinement of the measurement of the variables:* The success of an experiment is heavily dependent on the ability to clearly and operationally define the various alternatives of the independent variable as well as on the availability of valid, reliable, sensitive, and meaningful measurements.

7. *The extent to which we can enlist the cooperation of our study subjects:* Generally, it is easier to obtain cooperation from study subjects in a nonexperimental study. Fewer demands are likely to be made of

subjects in a nonexperimental study. This factor must be given serious attention in the choice of a design, since the validity of an experimental study will be severely damaged by high attrition of subjects.

8. *The degree to which we hope to explain causality:* The major attribute of the experimental method is the greater likelihood that we will be able to discover causal relationships. If the explanation of the cause of some effect is the aim of our research, the more closely we can model our design after the experimental method, the greater is the assurance we will have of achieving it.

SUMMARY

The aim of the experimental method is to control the influences of all extraneous variables that could bias the data in the study. In experiments involving human beings, total control of all extraneous variables is seldom achieved. Nevertheless, it

is the goal to which the task of designing a valid experiment is dedicated. The means for controlling the major sources of bias in explanatory experiments are shown in Figure 11–4. In this diagram of an "ideal" experimental design involving two comparison groups, one of which receives the treatment and the other a placebo or dummy treatment, the four major ways in which the design controls the influences of extraneous variables are as follows:

1. The experimental subjects are drawn at random from the target population in order to insure representativeness of subjects as well as to be able to quantitatively estimate the extent to which the subjects are an adequate sample of the total population.

2. The subjects are randomly assigned to the alternative groups to ensure equalization of the characteristics of the subjects composing the groups. By the techniques of pairing, balancing, and covariance analysis, additional control over the matching of the composition of the groups can be achieved.

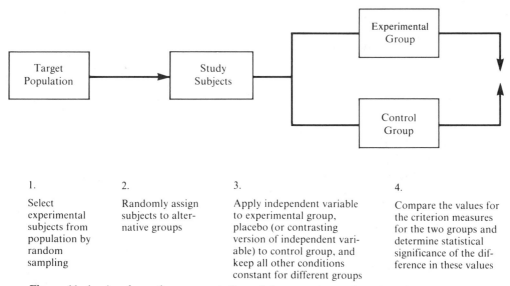

Figure 11–4 A schematic representation of the experimental method for explanatory research (showing four stages of experimental control). (*Courtesy* Greenburg, B. G. "The Philosophy and Methods of Research." In Harriet H. Werley (ed.): *Report on Nursing Research Conference.* Walter Reed Army Institute of Research, Washington, D.C., 1961.)

3. After the administration of the treatment, all environmental variables are also controlled, so that the only difference between the alternative groups is the effect of the independent variable. By the use of a dummy treatment (placebo) and the double-blind technique, sociopsychological biases (Hawthorne effect) can be controlled.

4. Differences found in the criterion measures for the alternative groups are compared to differences attributable to extraneous (chance) factors and are computed by taking into account the number of subjects in the study group (sample size) and their variability in relation to the criterion measure. The resulting index is a measure of the degree to which the differences exceed that which can occur due to chance alone and in the statistical significance of the differences found.

Even with all these safeguards against bias, there is always the possibility that our experiment may produce results that can be erroneously interpreted, a problem to be discussed later. Moreover, a critical area of control not included in the ideal design mentioned is that concerning the definition and measurement of the explanatory variables. No matter how well the experiment is otherwise controlled, weaknesses in measurement will seriously damage its validity. Therefore, all conclusions based on a single experiment, particularly among such variable subjects as human beings, are considered as tentative until confirmed by replicated experiments.

Nonexperimental research generally lacks some of the important controls found in experimental research. It is, therefore, weaker in control of extraneous variables. Although nonexperimental explanatory studies may employ random sampling of subjects from the target population, the researcher does not randomly assign the subjects to the alternative groups being studied. In other words, he does not deliberately manipulate the independent variable except through bringing into the study subjects already assigned to the alternative groups or by an ex post facto sorting of subjects into alternative groups through statistical manipulation of the data (cross-tabulation). An important value of nonexperimental research is the broader scope that such studies can have, since it is less costly to use large samples of subjects than in experimental research. Therefore, more independent variables can be studied, with perhaps a greater depth of analysis possible than in an experimental approach to the same problem. Moreover, the artificiality of the experimental situation is eliminated, providing findings that have more relevant application to the real world. Nevertheless, the experimental approach to research remains as the ideal model for establishing trustworthy scientific knowledge.

REFERENCES

1. R. A. Fisher, and G. T. Prance, *The Design of Experiments*. Darien, CT, Hafner, 1974.
2. W. G. Cochran, and Gertrude M. Cox, *Experimental Designs* (2nd ed.). New York, John Wiley and Sons, 1957.
3. Oscar Kempthorne, *The Design and Analysis of Experiments*. New York, Robert E. Krieger Publishing Co., Inc., 1973.
4. W. T. Federer, *Experimental Design: Theory and Application*. New York, Macmillan Publishing Co., Inc., 1955.
5. A. L. Edwards, *Experimental Design in Psychological Research* (4th ed.). New York, Holt, Rinehart and Co., 1973.
6. F. S. Chapin, *Experimental Design in Sociological Research*. Westport, CT, Greenwood Press, 1974.
7. Victor Chew, *Experimental Designs in Industry*. New York, John Wiley and Sons, 1958.
8. D. J. Finney, *Experimental Design and Its Statistical Basis*. Chicago. University of Chicago Press, 1955.
9. John Stuart Mill, *A System of Logic*. New York, Harper and Brothers, 1873.
10. *Ibid.*, p. 222.
11. Morris R. Cohen and Ernest Nagel, *An Introduction to Logic and Scientific Method*. 1982 Reprint of 1934 Edition. Darby, PA, Darby Books, p. 263.
12. Adapted from Eugene Levine, "Experimental Design in Nursing Research." *Nursing Res.,* **9:**203–212, fall 1960.
13. Elton Mayo, *The Human Problems of an Industrial Civilization*. New York, Macmillan Publishing Co., Inc., 1933.
14. John R. P. French, Jr., "Experiments in Field Settings," in *Research Methods in the Behavioral*

Sciences, Leon Festinger and David Katz (eds.). New York, The Dryden Press, 1953, Chapter III, p. 101.

15. Donald T. Campbell, "Factors Relevant to the Validity of Experiments in Social Settings." *Psychol. Bull.,* **54:**297–312, 1957.

16. William G. Cochran, "Matching in Analytical Studies," *Am. J. Pub. Health,* **43:**684–691, June 1953.

17. Eileen G. Hasselmeyer, *Behavior Patterns of Premature Infants.* U.S. Public Health Service Publication No. 840. Washington, DC, Government Printing Office, 1961.

18. Bernard G. Greenberg, "The Use of Analysis of Covariance and Balancing in Analytical Surveys." *Am. J. Pub. Health,* **43:**692–699, June 1953.

19. A. L. Edwards, *op. cit.,* p. 233.

20. Donald Mainland, *Elementary Medical Statistics.* Philadelphia, W. B. Saunders Co., 1963, p. 17.

21. Eileen G. Hasselmeyer, *op. cit.*

22. Thomas J. DeKornfeld, Louis Lasagna, and Todd M. Frazier, "A Comparative Study of Five Proprietary Analgesic Compounds." *J.A.M.A.,* **182:**1315–1318, December 29, 1962.

23. Faye G. Abdellah and Eugene Levine, *Effect of Nurse Staffing on Satisfactions with Nursing Care.* Hospital Monograph Series No. 4. Chicago, American Hospital Association, 1958.

24. Mildred E. Newton, "The Case for Historical Research." *Nursing Res.,* **14:**1:20, winter 1965.

25. Lucille E. Notter (editorial), "The Case for Historical Research in Nursing." *Nursing Res.,* **21:**6:483, November-December 1972.

26. Teresa E. Christy, "The Methodology of Historical Research: A Brief Introduction." *Nursing Res.,* **24**(3):189–192, May-June 1975.

27. M. Louise Fitzpatrick, Critique of Philip and Beatrice Kalisch's paper: "Congress Copes with the Nurse Shortage, 1941–1971: Dynamics of Congressional Education Policy Formulation." Ninth Nursing Research Conference, Kansas City, Missouri, American Nurse's Association, 1973.

28. M. Louise Fitzpatrick, *The National Organization for Public Health Nursing, 1912–1952: Development of a Practice Field.* New York, National League for Nursing, 1975.

29. Teresa E. Christy, *A Cornerstone for Nursing Education.* New York, Teachers College Press, Teachers College, Columbia University, 1969.

30. *Ibid.,* p. vii.

31. Helen E. Marshall, *Mary Adelaide Nutting: Pioneer of Modern Nursing.* Baltimore, The Johns Hopkins University Press, 1972.

32. Margaret M. Street, *Watch-Fires on the Mountains: The Life and Writings of Ethel Johns.* Toronto, University of Toronto Press, 1973.

33. Edith A. Aynes, *From Nightingale to Eagle: An Army Nurse's History.* Englewood Cliffs, N.J, Prentice-Hall, Inc., 1973.

34. Marlette Conde, *The Lamp and the Caduceus: The Story of the Army School of Nursing.* Washington, DC, Army School of Nursing Alumnae Association, 1975.

35. Margene O. Faddis, *A School of Nursing Comes of Age: A History of the Frances Payne Bolton School of Nursing, Case Western Reserve University.* Cleveland, The Alumni Association of the Frances Payne Bolton School of Nursing, 1973.

36. T. R. Schellenberg, *The Management of Modern Archives.* Chicago, The University of Chicago Press, 1965.

37. Peter D. Olch, "Oral History and the Medical Librarian." *Bull. Med. Library Assoc.* **57:**1–4, January 1969.

38. Robert L. Brubaker, "Manuscript Collections." *Library Trends.* **13:**226–256, October 1964.

PROBLEMS AND SUGGESTIONS FOR FURTHER STUDY

1. Discuss the following statement by Camilleri ("Theory, Probability and Induction in Social Research," *American Sociological Review.* **27:**173, April 1962): "A fundamental criticism of Mill's methods of experimental inquiry is that to use them to discover the causes of a phenomenon or to prove that a particular factor is the cause of a phenomenon requires the *a priori* assumption that all the possible causes are known and examinable."

2. Select five hypotheses from pages 115–116. Briefly outline how research would be conducted to test these hypotheses experimentally and nonexperimentally. What are some of the practical problems in pursuing this research experimentally? Would it be possible to establish causal relationships for the variables stated in the hypothesis if the research were conducted nonexperimentally?

3. What kinds of studies can be done experimentally that cannot be done nonexperimentally? Conversely, what kinds, if any, can be done nonexperimentally that cannot be done experimentally?

4. Is it possible in research on human beings to conduct a completely controlled experiment? How would a researcher know that he had controlled all possible extraneous variables?

5. A dictionary definition of "chance" is "something that befalls as the result of unknown or unconsidered forces." Does the term "forces" in this definition mean the same as "extraneous variables" as used in

research design? Look up the definition of the term "random" and discuss its relationship to "chance."

6. Explain the following mathematical terms:
   a. Linear equation
   b. Function
   c. Nonlinear equation
   d. Slope of a line
   e. Parameter
   f. Coefficient
   g. Exponent
   h. Stochastic process
   i. Nonparametic
   j. Algorithm
   k. Subjective probability

7. How does random assignment differ from random sampling? How are these procedures alike? Why is the use of a table of random sampling numbers a better way of randomizing than a lottery-type drawing of names?

8. Read the book *Explanation in Social Science* by Robert Brown (Chicago, Aldine Publishing Co., 1963, 198 pp.). How many different methods of explanation about social phenomena does the author present? Comment on the following statement by the author, "Most work in the social sciences, like most work in history and in the natural sciences, is not directly concerned with the furnishing of explanation. It may well be true, as is so often said, that the tasks of any empirical science are to explain, predict, and to apply. But in any such field these tasks are embedded in a workload that may be referred to as identification, classification, description, and measuring and reporting as well." (p. 47.)

9. The following references report on studies that have at least some aspects of an experimental design. Read them and determine which of the designs summarized in Table 11-1 were employed in each of the studies:
   a. Eugene C. Nelson *et al.,* "Medical Self-Care Education for Elders: A Controlled Trial to Evaluate Impact." *Am. J. Pub. Health,* **74:**1357–1362, December 1984.
   b. Mildred Struve and Eugene Levine, "Disposable and Reusable Surgeon's Gloves." *Nursing Res.,* **10:** 79–86, spring 1961.
   c. Katherine Wiley, "Effects of a Self-Directed Learning Project and Preference for Structure on Self-Directed

Learning Readiness," *Nursing Res.,* **32:**181–185, May/June 1983.
   d. Theresa K. Cheyovich, Charles E. Lewis, and Susan R. Gortner. *The Nurse Practitioner in an Adult Outpatient Clinic.* DHEW Publication No. (HRA) 76-20, Washington, D.C, U.S. Government Printing Office, 1976.
   e. M. R. Kinney, "Effects of Preoperative Teaching Upon Patients with Differing Modes of Response to Threatening Stimuli," *Int. J. Nurse. Stud.,* **14:**49–59, 1977.
   f. Loretta T. Zderad, "A Study of the Effectiveness of a Cooperative Group Method in Teaching Basic Psychiatric Nursing." *Nursing Res.,* **2:**126–137, February 1954.
   g. Mark Mulder and Al Stemerding, "Threat, Attraction to Group, and Need for Strong Leadership." *Human Relations,* **16:**317–334, November 1963.
   h. Sally O'Neil, "The Application and Methodological Implications of Behavior Modification in Nursing Research," in *Communication Nursing Research: The Many Sources of Nursing Knowledge.* Boulder Co, 1972, pp. 177–191.

10. Why is it important to equalize the composition of the comparison groups in an experiment? Discuss the various methods for achieving such equalization in an experiment. Is it ever possible to obtain perfect equalization of the groups? Discuss methods for equalizing the groups in an explanatory survey and in this connection read Chapter 7 of Hyman's *Survey Design and Analysis* (Glencoe, IL, The Free Press, 1955, pp. 295–329), "The Introduction of Additional Variables and the Elaboration of the Analysis."

11. In experimental studies of patient care, what are some of the sources of sociopsychological biases? What are the methods by which they can be controlled? Is it really possible to eliminate completely the "Hawthorne effect" from the usual kinds of patient care studies that are conceived?

12. Comment on the following statement by R. A. Fisher in his *The Design of Experiments* (Darien, CT, Hafner, 1974), "Experimental observations are only experience, carefully planned in advance, and designed to form a secure basis of new knowledge. That is, they

are systematically related to the body of knowledge acquired, and the results are deliberately observed and put on record accurately."

13. What are the advantages and disadvantages of introducing more explanatory variables into an experimental study? What are some guidelines that a researcher can use in determining the most pertinent explanatory variables for his study? Why is a "factorial design" considered to be an efficient experimental design?

14. Read the following article: Ada Sue Henshaw, Rose M. Gerber, Jan R. Atwood, and Janice R. Allen, "The Use of Predictive Modeling to Test Nursing Practice Outcomes," *Nursing Res.*, 32:35–42, January/February 1983. What do the authors mean by describing their study as *quasi-experimental, partially* double-blind? What were the limitations of this study?

15. A factorial experiment in which each factor is tested at two levels is called a 2^n factorial experiment. If the number of different factors is 3, there would be 2^3 different combinations possible or 8 ($2^3 = 2 \times 2 \times 2$). If the factors are tested at three levels it would be called a 3^n experiment. How many different combinations would be possible in an experiment that consisted of six factors: two of which have two levels, two have three levels, and two consist of four levels? Does the term "interaction" mean the same as "combination" as used here? (Note: see a book such as Cochran and Cox, *Experimental Designs* [New York, John Wiley and Sons, 1957, Chapter V, "Factorial Experiments"] for a discussion of interaction in factorial designs.)

16. Obtain a copy of a table of random numbers, such as in appendix B of Phillips and Thompson *Statistics for Nurses* (New York, Macmillan Publishing Co., Inc., 1967). Using the table, create a hypothetical experiment in which 100 subjects are randomly allocated into four comparison groups.

17. Discuss the statement that a cohort study is "actually a series of cross-sectional surveys repeated over a period of time for the same study population." Give five examples of well-known cross-sectional surveys that are conducted in the health field. By definition are all experimental studies prospectively longitudinal? Are they also cohort studies?

18. Critique the study conducted by Lenn, Gurel and Lenn, "Patient Outcome as a Measure of Quality of Nursing Home Care" (*Am. J. Pub. Health,* 67:337–344, April 1977). What techniques were used to control extraneous variables? What extraneous variables would affect patient outcome?

19. Read Chapter 3 of Philip J. Runkel and Joseph E. McGrath, *Research on Human Behavior: A Systematic Guide to Method* (New York, Holt Rinehart, and Winston, Inc., 1972, pp. 35–80.). Discuss some of the practical advice the authors give in relation to planning a study.

20. Read Theodore X Barber's *Pitfalls in Human Research: Ten Pivotal Points* (New York, Pergamon Press, Inc., 1976). Which of the pitfalls are most serious? Which of the pitfalls can be controlled by careful research design?

21. What are some of the difficulties in long-term longitudinal research? What are some of the advantages of this type of research? In this regard read Lucille Knopf's *RN's One and Five Years After Graduation* (New York, National League for Nursing, 1975). What was the attrition rate among study participants? Was this a high rate as compared to other longitudinal studies?

22. What is a clinical trial? Is it a type of experimental research? Refer to the book *Fundamentals of Clinical Trials* by Lawrence M. Freidman, Curt D. Furberg, and David L. DeMets (Littleton, MA, John Wright, 1984). Do you agree with the authors that a clinical trial is the most definitive tool for evaluation of the applicability of clinical research?

23. Read the article by Karen Buhler-Wilkerson, "Public Health Nursing: In Sickness or in Health" (*Am. J. Pub. Health* 75:1155–1161, October, 1985). Comment on whether this is an example of what has been described in this chapter as historical research.

12

Define the Study Population and Sample

OBJECTIVES

- To explain how to define a target population for a research project.
- To describe the process of sampling.
- To define a random sample.
- To present the various kinds of random samples.
- To describe nonrandom samples.
- To delineate the advantages of sampling.

This chapter will be concerned with three related topics: first, the selection of study subjects from the target population; second, the means by which data are obtained from the study subjects; and third, the ways in which data are processed and organized.

Decisions made concerning how the data will be gathered and processed are closely related to the other elements of the research process. In a highly controlled experimental type of research design, collection of data would most likely involve direct contact with the study subjects. On the other hand, in a nonexperimental design, indirect means of collecting data such as a mailed questionnaire can be used.

If the variables can be quantitatively measured, scientific measuring instruments requiring direct observation of the study subjects are needed. Data on qualitative variables can often be gathered by indirect methods such as self-administered tests or scales. Moreover, the ease with which the measurements can be made will influence the number of study subjects. If measurements are difficult and time-consuming to make, the number of subjects may need to be restricted.

Each method of selecting subjects and collecting data on the variables being measured has advantages and limitations. The method for a study should be tailor-made for the research problem.

SELECTION OF THE STUDY SUBJECTS

The subjects included in the study can be human beings, animals, plants, cells, or inanimate objects such as equipment, buildings, chemicals, plots of land, or even nonmaterial subjects such as words, constructs, processes, or procedures. The subject of a study is the person or thing from whom data are collected. In some studies the whole subject is the concern of the measurement—for example, determination of the level of wellness of a person. In others only a part of the subject is measured, such as dental cavities among children. The definition of the variable being studied—in the first example, level of wellness, and in the second, condition of teeth—describes that aspect of the subject examined.

Definition of the Target Population

The first step in selecting subjects is to define the *target population*. The target population consists of the total membership of a defined set of subjects (people, animals, plants, etc.) from whom the study subjects are selected and to whom the data will be generalized. The target population must be defined with respect to the nature of the individual subjects as well as its geographical and temporal scope. We may speak of the population of professional nurses in the United States who were licensed to practice in 1986, or we may define the target population as all hospitals in the state of New York accepted for listing by the American Hospital Association in 1986.

Each individual nurse or each individual hospital composing the target population is potentially a study subject. The individual members of the target population are called the *sampling units*. A study usually focuses on the measurement of particular variables relevant to the sampling units, for example, the nurse staffing (variable) of general hospitals. Thus, a population consists of all the measurements that could theoretically be made of the variables under study. In this example the population would be hospitals, called the *primary sampling units*, not the measurements of staffing in the hospitals. Similarly, if we are studying the effect of different brands of toothpaste on prevention of dental caries, the target population would be defined as individual people, not

as measurements of teeth, and the primary sampling units would be whole people.

Theoretically, the same individual can be a member of many different target populations at the same time, depending on how the scope of the population is defined as well as the types of variables being measured. For example, the nurse licensed to practice in 1986 could be a sampling unit in various geographically defined target populations of registered nurses. These populations could encompass the entire world, or be limited to the country, state, or city. The same nurse could also be a sampling unit in target populations defined according to different characteristics, as, for example, populations of working mothers, people who voted in the last election, alumnae of a certain school of nursing, residents of urban areas, or nurses who work in the field of public health.

One should make a distinction between the *target population* and the *sampled population*. The target population is considered to be the entire population to whom the findings of the study are applicable, while the sampled population is considered to be the aggregate of all the identifiable sampling units from whom the subjects were drawn. In many studies the two populations are identical. However, if we select our subjects from all nurses registered in the state of New York and make generalizations from the data for all nurses in the United States, the latter would be considered the target population and the former the sampled population.

In the following discussion the term target population is used interchangeably with the sampled population—as the population for whom the data can be statistically generalized. The concept of the "hypothetical universe" to be discussed shortly will be used to designate a broader population that exists beyond the sampled population.

A target population, as used here, is a finite population, its boundaries fixed and described by time, geography, and the characteristics of the individual members composing it, as well as the nature of the variables being studied. The importance of precisely defining this population arises from the fact that in most research studies the aim is to generalize to some larger population the findings obtained from the study subjects. If we are testing the effect of increased nursing hours to psychiatric patients in one hospital, we would undoubtedly be interested in applying the data from our subjects to psychiatric patients in other hospitals. Only through a widespread application of the findings will the time, effort, and money expended be worthwhile. It is indeed a rare study that does not look toward generalization of its findings beyond the immediate study setting. *Generalization of findings is considered an essential characteristic of meaningful research.*

The boundaries of statistical generalization of research findings are fixed by the limits of the population from which the sample was drawn. In many studies, a population is not defined in advance. Instead a group of subjects is studied, for example, all the freshman students in a particular school of nursing. In these studies implicit generalizations of findings to a larger population are often made through the style in which the data are interpreted. The use of the present rather than the past tense in reporting the findings of such studies creates a sense of generality: "Students whose initial exposure to the nursing situation in a hospital is a traumatic one are more apt to withdraw from school before the end of the first year than those whose exposure is pleasant."

Even where a target population has been defined in advance and the study subjects carefully chosen from the population so as to be representative of it, generalizations often extend beyond the population limits, particularly those limits imposed by time. Research findings are frequently extended into the future, and in so doing the fact is often overlooked that a study has been conducted during a specific period in the past. Because most situations are not static, the same findings may not be true for an indefinite time.

Generalizations are frequently made from findings obtained in experimental research even though the study was conducted in a limited way, as when subjects are brought into the experiment because of convenience—e.g., patients who happen to be in the hospital at the time. On the other hand, in nonexperimental studies the subjects are more likely to be representative of some larger population and are frequently selected through scientific means. Sweeping generalizations of the findings of experiments are considered warranted because of the strict controls exerted over the extraneous variables. Such generalizations are possible when the subjects are inanimate and the variables are precisely and relevantly quantified. When the subjects are human beings and when the measuring instruments are not precise, the caution offered by McGinnis[1] should be borne in mind:

> There is no such thing as a completely general relationship which is independent of population, time, and space. The extent to which a relationship is constant among different populations is an empirical question which can be resolved only by examining different populations at different times in different places.

Studies in which findings are generalized beyond the boundaries of target populations, whether the target population is specified in advance or not, are being generalized to a *hypothetical universe*. The idea of a hypothetical universe has been postulated to enable a researcher to extend the findings beyond the finite target population and provide them with more general applicability. As described by Hagood and Price:[2]

> This superuniverse must be a universe from which our finite universe can be considered a random sample. It has been defined as an unlimited or infinite universe of all the possible finite universes that could have been produced at the instant of observation under the conditions obtaining. It is therefore only an imagined possibility and whether or not one wishes to utilize the concept is still at the discretion of the individual research worker.

It can be argued that the idea of a hypothetical universe is vague and somewhat contrived. General principles can be established only by replications of studies in which findings are confirmed or reinforced from one study to the next. If repeated tests of the same hypothesis produce the same findings, the formulation of a general relationship has been strengthened. Multiclinic trials of drugs is an example of repeated studies that broaden the scope of generalizations. Before the Salk and Sabin vaccines were released for general usage, their effectiveness in reducing the incidence of polio was tested and retested in many clinical trials.

The importance of carefully defining the target population in advance of a study is illustrated by the famous *Literary Digest* poll undertaken to predict the presidential election in 1936. The *Literary Digest* was a popular magazine during the 1930's, but went out of business soon after erroneously predicting that Landon would defeat Roosevelt. The error in the survey arose from the way in which the sampling units were selected. Telephone directories and other specialized lists were used to obtain a listing of the names and addresses of persons to whom straw ballots were mailed. The target population for the poll was supposed to be all voters in the United States, but the sampling frame actually was restricted to owners of telephones, thereby overrepresenting persons with high income.

The reason for the erroneous prediction was that income level was related to voting behavior in the 1936 election. In general, lower-income people voted for Roosevelt, higher-income people for Landon. The distorted result was inevitable given the sampling method.

SAMPLING

After the target population for a study has been carefully defined, the subjects are selected. If the target population is small, all the sampling units may be used as subjects. If we are studying types of patients who receive home nursing care from public health agencies in the United States, and if the total number of primary sampling units (agencies) in this population is around 1,000, we may decide to include all of them in the study, particularly if our measurements can be made simply and quickly. If the number of sampling units is very large and the data difficult to obtain, the number selected for study will be fewer than the total number composing the target population.

The process of selecting a fraction of the sampling units of a target population for inclusion in a study is known as *sampling*. The set of sampling units chosen for the study is called the *sample*. Studies that include the entire target population are sometimes known as 100 percent samples. Summary measures—such as percentages, means, medians, percentiles, and standard deviations—that are computed from measurements obtained from a sample of the total population are called *statistics*. Summary measures based on all the sampling units in the target population are known as *parameters*. Statistics, therefore, are estimates of population parameters.

One objective of sampling is to obtain a sample of subjects that will be representative of the total population in terms of important organismic variables. If our target population consists of patients receiving home nursing care, and if 40 percent of the patients are males and 60 percent are females, if 30 percent are 65 years of age or over and 70 percent under 65 years of age, and if sex and age are considered to be important organismic variables in relation to the hypothesis, our sample would be representative if the characteristics of the sampling units selected approximated these percentages. *A sample should be a replica in miniature of the total population.* The extent to which our sample findings are different from what they would be if we had studied all the sampling units is known as *sampling error*.

History of Sampling

The process of selecting a sample of the total members of a population is an ancient one. Thousands of years ago, Greek scientist philosophers made valid generalizations of the behavior of celestial bodies by observing a portion of the visible stars. Sampling of human populations began in England prior to the 1700s when estimates were made from small samples of the number of people composing the total population of cities. In the 1800s, stimulated by Bentham and his philosophy of utilitarianism, health surveys were undertaken based on samples of the total population.[3]

The application of the mathematical theory of probability to sampling began in the twentieth century, although probability theory was well established 200 years ago. A. L. Bowley, considered the father of scientific sampling, undertook a sampling study of the economic classes in England in 1912.[4] In 1927, L. H. C. Tippett[5] produced his table of random sampling numbers, which facilitated the selection of probability samples. In the 1930s many descriptive surveys were done in the fields of health, welfare, and social relations which used probability sampling. And in the 1950s and early 1960s, partly based on the extensive work on sampling done by the U.S. Bureau of the Census, several major texts were produced in the field,[6-8] one specifically directed to the sampling of hospitals.[9] Today the theory and practice of sampling are of major importance in the work of statisticians. Indeed, many applications of sampling in research require the specialized attention of sampling experts, since the quality of a sample vitally affects the validity of the research findings.

Advantages of Sampling

The benefits of sampling, particularly where the target population is very large or difficult to reach, are many. Briefly, they can be summarized as follows:

1. We must sample in studies where complete measurements of all members of the target population is not possible. If we intend to test the effects of a drug in the treatment of patients with cancer, we could not practically include every patient who has cancer as study subjects, even if we had large amounts of time, money, and personnel, because the total number of sampling units is too large and too dispersed.

2. It is usually cheaper and quicker to measure a sample of study subjects than all the members of a target population. Sampling reduces the cost and time of research.

3. The gain in accuracy from inclusion of all members of a population is often not worth the time and expense. Sometimes sample data can be almost as precise as data obtained from the total population. For example, it has been found in the decennial census of population that a sampling produces almost as precise data for some of the variables as does the complete enumeration.

4. In some studies the process of measurement can introduce spurious influences into the research. The Hawthorne effect is the reaction of the subjects to the study process itself and can obscure or bias the effects of the independent variable. By keeping the number of subjects as small as our need for precision will permit, we can more easily control the Hawthorne effect as well as other psychological biases that can be introduced during the measuring process.

5. The number of subjects should be kept as small as is feasibly possible when the independent variable could have unpleasant side effects on the study subjects. Trials of experimental drugs, especially when not all of the effects of the drug on the patient can be assessed in advance, are based on samples. Potentially dangerous phases of the study are restricted to animal subjects and computer simulation.

6. In studies involving nonhuman subjects, the measuring process sometimes destroys the sampling units. In such studies economics would dictate a limitation of sample size. For example, in the evaluation of alternative products—e.g., X-ray equipment produced by different manufacturers—we might have to break down the equipment to obtain certain measurements.

To keep the cost of such tests from getting out of hand, the number of sampling units must be kept to a minimum.

Scientific Sampling

The aim of sampling is to obtain a group of study subjects that is a replica in miniature of the target population. The method of probability sampling has been developed to provide a measure of how good a replica of the population the sample is. Probability sampling, also called random sampling, is a method whereby each sampling unit in the target population has a known—greater than zero—probability of being selected in the sample. Moreover, in drawing a probability sample, neither sampler nor sampling unit has any deliberate influence over the inclusion of a specific sampling unit. In other words, the process of drawing a probability sample is a random one. This process is analogous to that of random assignment of study subjects to the various alternative groups of an experiment. Random sampling can be achieved in the same manner as random assignment. We can put the names or numbers of each sampling unit on slips of paper, put the slips in a bowl, and then draw a number of slips at random which will compose the sample. More scientifically, we could assign numbers to each sampling unit and then select the sample members by choosing the numbers from a table of random numbers.

Instead of drawing a probability sample we might deliberately select the sampling units according to certain criteria that we as subject-matter experts in the field know to be important. Thus, if the sampling units in a study of nurse staffing patterns consist of hospitals, we might stipulate which hospitals are to be included because we are familiar with their characteristics and feel that the hospitals chosen are typical of hospitals in general.

Probability samples have two advantages over deliberately selected, nonrandom samples:

1. Statistical techinques can be applied to evaluate the precision of summary measures based on randomly selected samples. We can compute the *sampling error* of these statistics, which tells us how good an estimate they are of the parameter values. In nonrandom samples we have no adequate way of estimating sampling error.

2. By random selection of sampling units we can help to avoid the possible unconscious selection of a biased sample. An example of a biased sample that was drawn nonrandomly is the Kinsey study on sexual behavior in females. The subjects were invited through advertisements to enter the study voluntarily. Here randomness was missing. By volunteering, the subjects controlled who was to be included in the study. Unless adequate procedures for controlling the parameters of such studies are devised, their applicability to broader segments of the population is at best questionable.

Random selection of the sampling units does not guarantee that the sample will be representative or typical of the target population. It may well be possible to select a more typical sample by nonrandom selection, but these gains in representativeness must be weighed against the inability to evaluate statistically the precision of summary measures obtained from nonrandom samples.

Types of Probability Samples

There are numerous methods by which a probability sample may be drawn. The ones most applicable to research in nursing and patient care will be briefly discussed.

SIMPLE RANDOM SAMPLES

This is the most fundamental type of sampling design. In this design each sampling unit has an equal probability of being selected as the first member of the sample; after the first member is selected each of the remaining units in the population has an equal chance of being the second member of the sample, etc. If the target population consists of a total of 100 units, each sampling unit has a 1 percent probability (chance) of being chosen as the first member in a sample of size 1, a 10 percent chance in a sample of size 10, and so on. Most important, in a simple random sample each possible combination of the various sampling units has an equal chance of being chosen. In a sample of 10 units drawn from 100, each possible combination of 10 (and there are millions of them) is as equally likely to be selected.

Selection of a simple random sample includes the following steps: (1) we define the target population; (2) we establish a complete listing, sometimes called a frame, of all the sampling units in the population. Such a listing might be in the form of a roster or a deck of index cards containing the names and addresses of all the people, hospitals, schools, or public health agencies composing the target population; and (3) we decide how many sampling units to include. Determination of sample size is a rather technical matter often best handled by a professional statistician, whose determination takes into consideration the following factors:

1. *The amount of precision required in the statistics (summary measures) that are computed.* Precision means how accurate we want to be in estimating the values of the parameters of the target population. The amount of precision needed in a study depends upon the nature of the research problem. If the findings of the study can affect the health of people, we want a high degree of precision. If we can tolerate rough approximations of the values of the parameters, a smaller sample might suffice.

The basic formula for computing the sampling error of a sample estimate of a population parameter is as follows:

$$\text{Sampling error} = \frac{\text{Variability of values of measurements among sampling units}}{\sqrt{\text{Size of sample}}}$$

This formula is applicable to estimates obtained from simple random samples. For other types of sample designs an elaboration of this formula is required. As can be seen, precision depends on the ratio of the variability of the measurements among the individual sampling units to the square root of the number of sampling units. Precision can, therefore, be increased either by reducing the variability among the sampling units, accomplished by changing the method of selection from simple random sampling to other methods, or by increasing the size of the sample. Because of the "square root" operation, however, doubling the sample size (with variability of the measurements held constant) will only increase the precision by the square root of two, ($\sqrt{2}$, or 1.4), not by two. Quadrupling the sample will double the precision.

2. *The variability of the measurements among the sampling units.* The greater the variability among the measurements, the larger the sample needed to attain a desired level of precision among sampling units. If the measurements had varied little among the sampling units, it is obvious that a smaller number of units would be required to make a precise estimate of the population parameter than if variability were high. Suppose we were interested in estimating the average number of hours of nursing care per patient per day in a target population of five hospitals. If there were little variability among the sampling units, the data might look as follows:

HOSPITAL	AVERAGE HOURS PER PATIENT PER DAY
1	4.6
2	4.1
3	4.5
4	4.9
5	4.8
Average	4.6

If we chose any one of these hospitals as our sample, we would have a fairly precise estimate of the average hours per patient in all hospitals—4.6—since none of the hospitals deviates by more than one-half hour from this average. However, if the individual values varied as widely as in the following target population, a sample of only one hospital could differ from the average as much as two hours.

HOSPITAL	AVERAGE HOURS PER PATIENT PER DAY
1	4.6
2	1.8
3	3.7
4	5.9
5	4.3
Average	4.1

3. *Sensitivity of the measuring instruments.* Other things being equal, the more sensitive the instruments used to measure variables, the smaller the sample required to detect significant differences among subjects. Let us assume that our study involved the testing of the relationship between alternative methods of training nursing aides, and our criterion measure was a rating scale of the proficiency of the aide. We would need a larger sample to detect significant differences among the subjects if the scale consisted of only two broad qualitative categories than if it were a highly refined quantitative scale that could validly and reliably detect small but significant differences in proficiency.

4. *Amount of detailed descriptive data required.* In experimental studies the end product might simply be a test of statistical significance of the differences among the values of summary measures for the alternative groups. In nonexperimental studies, where the time and expense involved per sampling unit in collecting the data usually are less, we are often interested in obtaining detailed descriptive data relevant to the research problem, even when the purpose of the study is primarily one of explanation. Such descriptive data might refer to important organismic variables concerning study subjects—age, marital status, educational level, occupation, and so on. We may wish to cross-tabulate these variables against the dependent variable—that is, to simultaneously tabulate the summary measures by the organismic variables as well as the explanatory variables. To the extent that we desire detailed, meaningful cross-tabulations of the data, the size of the sample will have to be enlarged in order to provide sufficient data for the additional cells of the table. Assume we are interested in assessing the relationship between the size of a public health agency (the independent variable with four size groups according to case load) and the cost per visit to patients in home nursing care programs (dependent variable); the table showing this relationship would need only four cells—one for each of the four size groups. If we were interested in seeing the effect of the control of the agency (official, nonofficial, combination) on this relationship, we would need a larger sample, since the table showing this relationship would now have twelve cells:

CASE LOAD OF AGENCY	CONTROL OF AGENCY		
	OFFICIAL	NONOFFICIAL	COMBINATION
Fewer than 50 patients			
50–99 patients			
100–199			
More than 200 patients			

Another reason for enlarging the sample size is to be able to detect rarely occurring events. For example, the effectiveness of the vaccines to combat polio was measured in terms of the reduction in the in- cidence of paralytic polio. Since this type of polio rarely occurs, even among unvaccinated populations—only a few cases are reported each year—it was necessary to include a very large number of individuals in order to detect any significant reduction in this rare event after vaccination.

5. *Number of sample units in the target population.* When the target population is small, a smaller number of sampling units can provide more precise statistics than if the target population is very large—assuming, of course, relatively equivalent variability among the sampling units of the different-sized populations. Data from a sample of 100 would very precisely measure the parameters of a target population consisting of 100 units—there would be no sampling error. This same-sized sample would produce less precise data if the target population consisted of 1,000 units, and even less precise data if it contained 100,000 units.

6. *Practical limitations.* Size of sample is often restricted by such practical limitations as time and money. Such criteria as precision of sample estimates and detail desired in results must be balanced against availability of resources. The aim of sample design is to secure an efficient sample, one that produces the most information at the lowest possible cost per sampling unit.

SELECTING A SIMPLE RANDOM SAMPLE

When size of sample has been determined, the next step is to select the sampling units from the target population. The previously described table of random numbers provides the best selection procedure. If we choose a sample of 100 patients' records from files containing 50,000 records, each having a five-digit identification number, we would open the table of random numbers to any page and copy 100 five-digit numbers, beginning at any place in the table, and continuing up and down the columns or across the rows of figures until we obtained 100 numbers. The patient records bearing these numbers would compose our sample.

The simple random sample has perhaps more applicability in research in nursing and patient care than other types of sampling, particularly in studies involving the selection of a sample of patients, person-nel, students, or records from within an institution or a limited geographic area. In such studies the target population consists of a relatively small, fairly homogeneous number of sampling units, so that the simple random sample is an adequate method. For large, heterogeneous target populations, other sampling methods are generally more efficient. Even in the more elaborate sample designs, which involve grouping the sampling units in terms of certain criteria before selection of the units, simple random sampling is often employed.

Systematic Sampling

When the sampling units are arranged in some order, such as names on a list or geographical location, it is sometimes simpler to select the sample in a systematic way: every tenth name on the list, patients in the odd-numbered rooms, every fifth house on a block, every tenth baby born in the hospital. The random element in such a sampling method is provided by the random start. That is, if a list contains 1,000 names and we need 100 for our sample, we would select every tenth name, but we would start by selecting the first name by chance and then take every tenth name after that. Thus, if the first randomly selected name were the seventh on the list, the next sample subject would be the seventeenth name, the next would be the twenty-seventh, and so on.

A variation of the systematic sampling technique is the work sampling method recommended by the U.S. Public Health Service's Division of Nursing.[10] In this method, after a random start, the activities of nursing personnel are observed every fifteen minutes and classified in terms of variables such as the area of activity (patient care, housekeeping, maintenance of environment) and skill level of activity (head nurse, staff nurse, aide, clerk, and so on). This systematic sampling of activities is in contrast to the simple random sampling advocated by work sampling theorists in other fields.[11] Tests of the two sampling approaches show that both provide approximately the same precision.

Systematic sampling has two limitations. One is that the sampling error formula for such samples is difficult to derive. This hinders the computation of the sampling error of any statistics computed from such samples. Another is the danger that the order in which the sampling units are arranged on a list, or their geographical arrangement, or, as in the case of work sampling, their time ordering, would be systematically related to some extraneous variable, which if unknown to the researcher may result in the selection of a biased sample. In other words, the use of a systematic sample assumes that the order in which the units are arranged is essentially random in relation to the variables being studied. But this assumption may not always be correct. We might find that the patients in the odd-numbered rooms had certain special characteristics. Perhaps the rooms, because of peculiarities of construction of the hospital, are higher-priced, and the patients in them in higher income brackets. Consequently our sample, like the *Literary Digest* poll, would be over-weighted with wealthier people. Or in the systematic time sampling there may be a cyclical pattern of activities in the work of the nurses we observe: certain activities begin every hour. If our observation schedule coincides with these cycles, it gives us a distorted picture of the range of activities. In systematic sampling, then, we must be sure that there is randomness in the arrangement of the sampling units in the population. This can be done by taking a number of random starts, not just one.

Stratified Random Sample

In this type of sample the target population is subdivided into homogenous subpopulations. Then a simple random sample, or a systematic sample, or some other type is selected from each subpopulation. If we select for study 200 patients from a target population of 5,000, we might first subdivide the 5,000 sampling units in terms of certain important organismic variables— say, the age and sex of the patients. If we establish four groups for age and two for sex there would be eight cells, called *strata*. From each stratum we would take a certain proportion of sampling units for a total of 100. The proportion of sampling units selected from each stratum for the sample is identical with the proportion of sampling units in each stratum in the population. This is illustrated in Table 12–1.

TABLE 12–1.
A Stratified Sample (Proportions in percent are in parentheses)

AGE	POPULATION			SAMPLE		
		SEX			SEX	
	TOTAL	MALE	FEMALE	TOTAL	MALE	FEMALE
Total	50,000 (100)	20,000 (40)	30,000 (60)	200 (100)	80 (40)	120 (60)
Under 21	5,000 (10)	4,000 (8)	1,000 (2)	20 (10)	16 (8)	4 (2)
21–44	15,000 (30)	3,000 (6)	12,000 (24)	60 (30)	12 (6)	48 (24)
45–64	10,000 (20)	5,000 (10)	5,000 (10)	40 (20)	20 (10)	20 (10)
65 and over	20,000 (40)	8,000 (16)	12,000 (24)	80 (40)	32 (16)	48 (24)

For the same-sized sample, stratification generally increases the precision of summary measures above that of simple random sampling by making the various strata as homogenous as possible. Such homogeneity tends to reduce the value of the numerator in the formula used to compute the sampling error—the variation of the individual measurements among the sampling units—for each stratum. This results in a reduction of the sampling error for all strata combined.

Essentially, stratification is a process of sampling from subdivisions of the target population. The most common procedure is to select the number of sampling units from each stratum proportionately, as in Table 12–1, since this simplifies the computations. However, this is not a necessary feature of this type of sample design. A disproportionate number of sampling units could be selected from each stratum. For example, a stratum consisting of only a few sampling units may represent an important group regardless of its small numbers. Thus, when all nonfederal, short-term hospitals in the United States are stratified by size, one would find only about twelve hospitals with more than 1,000 beds. Such a stratum may be sampled in its entirety, even though it represents only a tiny fraction of all sampling units—five hospitals compose less than 1 percent of all general hospitals in the United States. Disproportionate sampling requires the adjustment of any summary measures computed from such samples by weighting each stratum according to its relative contribution to the value of the summary measure for all strata combined.

A technical procedure known as *optimum allocation* can be used to determine the best possible allocation of the sampling units into strata. This procedure determines the most efficient size sample for each stratum, balancing precision against cost per sampling unit.

For many sampling situations in nursing and patient care research, a simple random sample will suffice. The next most frequently used design is stratified random sampling with proportionate allocation. Disproportionate allocation is the least frequently used. The gain in precision may not always be worth the additional complexities in selecting the sample and in determining the sampling error of estimates obtained by the latter design. Its use is generally limited to those research situations where a significant enhancement of the precision of estimates can be obtained.

Cluster Sampling

In large-scale descriptive studies involving target populations with geographically dispersed sampling units, it is often necessary to use *cluster sampling*. Suppose, the research problem requires that we obtain certain measurements on hospitalized psychiatric patients by visiting each sample hospital. Our basic sampling unit is the patient. But since we do not have a list of such patients, we must select our sample in terms of some other identifiable sampling unit, such as the hospital in which they are located. Moreover, since the more than 500 psychiatric hospitals in the United States are geographically well distributed, it will be costly and time-consuming to select the sample of patients from a list even if one were available, because we will probably find our sample patients widely scattered. Our procedure is to randomly select sample hospitals (our clusters of patients). Then we either include all patients in the selected hospitals as subjects or we subsample by randomly selecting a portion of the patients in each hospital. This sample design involving more than one stage of sampling is called a multistage sample. In this case the hospital or other entity serving as the unit selected first is called the primary sampling unit. The patients are the secondary or second-stage sampling units.

Multistage sampling can have numerous stages. The primary sampling unit may be a hospital, the second stage a random sampling of various nursing units in each hospital, and the third stage a sampling of patients on whom the actual measurements are made.

Multistage sampling is applicable where the target population can be grouped according to a formal or informal organizational or structural entity. In cluster sampling, the cluster, or primary sampling unit, may represent a hospital, as in the previous example, or school, state, city, neighborhood, block, house, association, family, agency, work team, and so on. An advantage of this type of sampling is that it is usually possible to obtain a larger amount of data at a lower cost than with other methods. In the example of the psychiatric patients, it is obvious that it would be cheaper to collect data from 100 patients all located in one hospital than from one patient in each of 100 hospitals.

Cluster sampling is often the only kind of sample design that can feasibly be employed in many research situations. If no lists are available to identify the basic sampling units in a target population—as in a study of part-time nurses working in public health agencies—we can only reach the individual members of the target population through the group to which they belong. Cluster sampling is an especially good approach to find data that cannot be obtained in any other way. In epidemiological studies cluster sampling can be most helpful. If we wish to determine the prevalence of certain diseases among people in a community, we select the sample so that the primary sampling unit is a block of streets in the community, the second stage of sampling would be a house on a block, and the third and final stage a resident of a house. The U.S. Public Health Service has frequently used such designs in studies of the prevalence of illnesses among the population of the United States.[12,13]

There are several disadvantages to cluster sampling. One is that for the same-sized sample it will usually yield less precise data than other sample designs such as stratified random sampling. Another is the greater complexity in determining the sampling error of estimates based on cluster sampling. Such error formulas must take account of the fact that the individual sampling units being measured were not selected independently. Therefore, they may not be independent of each other in relation to relevant environmental variables that could influence the variables being measured. In the sample of patients in psychiatric hospitals, all patients in a particular hospital have been exposed to a similar set of environmental variables. These variables may well be different from those to which patients in other hospitals have been exposed. Thus, if we measure two patients from the same hospital to determine the kind of nursing they receive, the measurements are correlated, because both patients would probably receive similar care. If we measure two patients independently and randomly selected from different hospitals, the measurements are not correlated. The latter sample is more apt to be "representative" of the total target population than is the cluster sample.

The effect of clustering must be taken into account in determining the precision of summary measures computed from cluster samples. As Kish[14] points out, the formula for a simple random sample is used to compute sampling error in many studies when in fact the sample was based on a cluster design. The wrong formula results in an incorrect determination of the sampling error.

The researcher generally finds it economical and convenient to use for his sampling units existing clusters (blocks, cities, counties, work groups, school classes, etc.). These clusters usually exist as ecological, perhaps geographical units, and sometimes as "psychological groups" as well. The individuals in these units tend to resemble each other—there is usually some homogeneity of characteristics, of attitudes, of behavior—but homogeneity is generally not complete. It may be due to common selective factors, or to joint exposure to the same effects, or to mutual influence (interaction), or to some combination of these three causes. Because of this homogeneity, the use of these clusters for sampling units has definite consequences: it destroys the independence of the characteristics of the sample elements. The correspondence with the "well-mixed urn," inherent in the assumption of independence, is neglected; and formulas that depend on that assumption fail to apply.

Cluster sampling has not been widely used in nursing and patient care research because most studies have involved geographically limited target populations, and lists identifying sampling units have been readily available. An example of a cluster sample was in a study of the relationship between hours of nursing care available and satisfaction of patients and personnel with care provided.[15] Here the primary sampling unit was a hospital, and a total of sixty were randomly selected for inclusion. The sampling was actually done at one stage only, as all patients and personnel in the hospitals selected were included. In another study of hospitals conducted by the Bureau of Hospital Administration at the University of Michigan, described in the monograph *Probability Sampling of Hospitals and Patients,*[16] the technique of *controlled selection* was used to select a sample of hospitals in Michigan. The hospitals served as clusters for a study of the characteristics of a sample of patients discharged from the hospitals.

Mixed Sampling Designs

Combinations of the major types of sampling techniques can be used to maximize economy and efficiency in data collection. Thus, stratification and clustering can be combined into a single design. In a study of nursing students, we might first stratify all the schools of professional nursing by size of student body and type of program. Then we would select a sample of schools from each strata as the primary sampling units, a sample of students from each school being selected as the second-stage sample.

Sequential Sampling

In sample designs discussed thus far, the number of sampling units to be included in the study is fixed in advance of data collection. Such designs are sometimes called "fixed sample plans." In sequential design the sampling units are taken into the study sequentially, and the number included is not fixed in advance. That is, we start with a sample of one and measure it. Then we select another sampling unit, measure it, combine it with the first, and obtain a summary measure for the two. Then we select another unit, measure it, and so on. The sampling stops when the summary measure for the cumulated sampling units reveals that we are within the sampling error range established prior to the sampling. The process of deciding when to terminate the sampling is known as the "stopping rules."

Sequential sampling has proved useful in testing hypotheses. It has been used to experimentally test the effects of drugs on patients.[17,18] In these studies it has been found that sampling always terminates at a level below the number of sampling units that would have been included in a fixed-sample-size design. Sequential sampling is, therefore, an economical sampling method.

However, it does have limitations. Such a design should not be used in testing hypotheses where there is a large time lag between application of the independent variable and measurement of the effects produced in the dependent variable. Because the decision to either terminate or continue sampling depends on the sequential measurement of each sampling unit, the progress of the study would grind to a halt if it took months for an effect on the subjects to appear.

Another limitation is the narrow focus of studies based on sequential sampling. A sequential sample is geared to providing information on a specific and limited set of variables—the variables formulated in the hypothesis. Many studies of patient care are more broadly conceived than a specific test of a hypothesis concerned with "what happens to dependent variable Y when we make a certain change in independent variable X?" The small-sized sample generally required by the sequential approach to test such narrow hypotheses would be inadequate to investigate the multivariable, complex research problems so frequently encountered in patient care. Even though a fixed-sample-size design may overshoot the number of sampling units actually needed, it will yield more information concerning the variables being measured and is, therefore, not a wasteful design.

Types of Nonprobability Samples

Many studies are conducted with subjects who have not been chosen by truly random sampling methods. This does not mean that such studies are bad or that their data are inaccurate. The main limitation of the use of data obtained through such samples is the difficulty of generalizing them to a larger target population. Basically, nonprobability samples are not samples at all but are complete populations from which no *statistical* generalizations to larger populations can be made.

There are various kinds of nonprobability samples. All are popular because they are usually cheaper and more convenient than probability samples. In some types of nonprobability samples a target population is specified in advance of sample selection, but the sampling units are not selected randomly. In other types the target population is defined ex post facto—that is, after the data have been collected and analyzed and the characteristics of the sampling units have been fully investigated. In still others a certain element of randomness may be present in the selection of the sampling units in that the selection is not done purposively but by chance or accident. A few of the more common types of nonprobability samples are described below.

Purposive Samples

Many samples are of the kind where the researcher deliberately selects the sampling units to be included in the study because he feels that they are representative of the target population. Such handpicked samples, also known as *judgment samples,* are widely used in research in nursing and pa-

tient care. If we are interested in studying the differences between a "good" school of nursing and a "bad" school or a "well-run" health agency and an "inefficient" one, we might rely on the judgment of knowledgeable people to select the actual institutions. Also, if we are conducting a study involving patients we might select Mr. X, Mr. Y, Mr. Z, and so on, because we are sure they have typical or average characteristics that would make them representative subjects. In other studies we might select the most typical day to observe the patients in hospital, or to test students, or to interview personnel.

The danger in the use of such purposive samples is that there is no way of measuring the precision of the estimates. Also, unconscious bias may exert an influence, so that we choose Mr. X, not because he is the typical patient, but because he is cooperative and we are sure he will be a good subject.

Convenience Samples

Another common type of nonprobability samples is the kind where we select for study the patients who happen to be in the hospital at a certain time, or patients who will be receiving home nursing care on the day when the agency has a large staff making home visits, or students who happen to be receiving their field experience in psychiatric nursing, or the first fifty visitors who come to the hospital that afternoon, and so on. It is true that there is an element of randomness in the entry of such subjects into the study; the subject has not been purposively selected as in the earlier sample. But a convenience sample is not a true random sample, because the subjects have not been selected from a larger population in which all members had some stated chance —greater than zero—of being selected.

Quota Samples

This, too, is essentially a convenience sample, but it has controls to prevent overloading the sample with subjects having certain characteristics, e.g., a sample of patients with too many males or too many younger patients. The controls are established by determining the distribution of the members of the target population according to certain significant variables. The distributions serve as limits or quotas for the number of subjects with these characteristics to be taken into the study. By using the data in Table 12–1, the selection of a quota sample of 200 patients from a population of 50,000 can be established in terms of the age and sex of the patients. The quota would be sixteen males under twenty one years of age, four females under twenty one, twelve males between twenty one and forty four, forty eight females between twenty one and forty four, and so on. The appropriate number of patients with these characteristics would then be selected as they conveniently could be found, rather than through random selection. This design resembles stratified sampling with the omission of randomization.

In another type of quota sample, used frequently in market research, the quotas are not established in accordance with the proportionate distribution in a target population. Instead the data collector interviews a group of subjects well-distributed according to sex, marital status, income level, and so on. The interviewer selects cases by seeing that they are dispersed more or less evenly among the different strata.

Quota samples do have an element of chance or accident in the selection of a particular subject for inclusion in the study, but we cannot be sure that bias has not entered into the selection process. In quota sampling the tendency to choose the most convenient or the most cooperative subject can result in a distorted sample.

VOLUNTEERS

Samples composed of volunteers are the reverse of judgment samples. In judgment samples, the sampler hand-picks the sampling units. In voluntary samples, the individuals do the selecting by deciding whether they will enter the study or not. Many studies require volunteers. The National Institutes of Health in Bethesda, Maryland, maintains a continuing "normal volunteer" program for the large number of studies conducted "on campus." Studies in which questionnaires are mailed to a random sample of a target population and where only a fraction respond are a voluntary, not a random sample. The danger in the use of volunteers as sampling units is that they may not be representative of the target population in terms of the variables being measured, making it difficult to draw unbiased generalizations from sample to target population.

Random sampling, if strictly adhered to, is a disciplined and quite difficult approach to the selection of study subjects from a target population. Once an individual has been selected for inclusion by the method of random sampling, he must enter the study regardless of lack of cooperativeness or inconvenience in collecting the data. If a household is selected for interviewing we would have to keep calling until we found someone at home regardless of the expense. In actual practice, however, many studies using random sampling allow for a certain amount of nonresponse or provide for a substitute sampling unit for an uncooperative individual. Nevertheless, random sampling is a more time-consuming and more expensive method of selecting subjects from a target population than is nonprobability sampling. However, it can yield more valid data than other sampling methods.

SUMMARY

Research applies to a specific population, which must be carefully defined. Since it is usually not feasible to include the entire population in a study, a sample is selected to serve as research subjects. A sample should be drawn *randomly* from the population, otherwise it will not be possible to assess, through statistical techniques, the precision of the sample or to draw valid inferences from the sample to the population. There are numerous ways of drawing random samples, which are also known as probability or scientific samples. The sampling method chosen depends on the nature of the population, including the ability to identify and locate the individuals who compose the population.

REFERENCES

1. Robert McGinnis, "Randomization and Inference in Sociological Research." *Am. Social. Rev.,* **23:**412, August 1958.

2. Margaret J. Hagood and Daniel O. Price, *Statistics for Sociologists,* rev. ed. New York, Henry Holt and Co., 1952, Chap. 16.

3. Sidney and Beatrice Webb, *Methods of Social Study.* New York, Cambridge University Press, 1975 ed.

4. Frederick F. Stephan, "History of the Uses of Modern Sampling Procedures." *J. Am. Statistical A.,* **43:**12–39, March 1948.

5. L. H. C. Tippett, *Random Sampling Numbers.* Cambridge, Cambridge University Press, 1927.

6. M. H. Hansen, W. H. Hurwitz, and W. G. Madow, *Sample Survey Methods and Theory,* Vol. 1. New York, John Wiley and Sons, Inc., 1953.

7. W. E. Deming, *Some Theory of Sampling.* Mineola, N.Y. Dover, 1984.

8. W. G. Cochran, *Sampling Techniques.* New York, John Wiley and Sons, Inc., 1977.

9. Irene Hess, Donald C. Riedel, and Thomas B. Fitzpatrick, *Probability Sampling of Hospitals and Patients.* Bureau of Hospital Administration, Research Series No. 1. Ann Arbor, University of Michigan, 1975.

10. Faye G. Abdellah and Eugene Levine, "Work Sampling Applied to the Study of Nursing Personnel." *Nursing Res.,* **3:**11–16, June 1954.

11. C. L. Brisley, "How You Can Put Work Sampling to Work." *Factory Management Maintenance,* **110:**84–89, July 1952.

12. Theodore D. Woolsey, *Sampling Methods for a Small Household Survey.* U.S. Public Health Service Monograph No. 40. Washington, D.C., Government Printing Office, 1956.

13. Staff of the U.S. National Health Survey and Bureau of Census, *The Statistical Design of the Health Household-Interview Survey.* U.S. Public Health Service Publication, No. 584-A2. Washington, D. C., Government Printing Office, 1958.

14. Leslie Kish, "Confidence Intervals for Clustered Samples." Am. Sociol. Rev., **22:**154, April 1957.

15. Faye G. Abdellah and Eugene Levine, *Effect of Nurse Staffing on Satisfactions with Nursing Care.* Hospital Monograph Series No. 4. Chicago, American Hospital Association, 1958.

16. Hess *et al., op. cit.*

17. Peter Armitage, *Sequential Medical Trials.* New York, John Wiley and Sons, Inc., 1975.

18. E. J. Anscombe, "Sequential Medical Trials." *J. Am. Statistical A.,* **58:**365–383, June 1963.

19. Faye G. Abdellah and Eugene Levine, *Appraising the Clinical Resources in Small Hospitals.* U.S. Public Health Service Monograph No. 24. Washington, D. C., Government Printing Office, 1954.

20. Eugene Levine, "Turnover Among Nursing Personnel in General Hospitals." *Hospitals, J.A.H.A.,* **31:**50–53, 138, 140, September 1, 1957.

21. Marion J. Wright, *Improvement of Patient Care.* New York, G. P. Putnam's Sons, 1954.

22. Monroe Lerner and Odin W. Anderson, *Health Progress in the United States.* Chicago, University of Chicago Press, 1963.

23. Deming, *op. cit.*

24. Gladys L. Palmer, "Factors in Variability of Response in Enumerative Studies." *J. Am. Statistical A.,* **38:**148–152, 1943.

25. Deming, *op. cit.,* p. 24.

26. Christopher Rand, "Center of a New World." *The New Yorker Magazine,* April 1964, pp. 58, 60.

27. Charles D. Flagle, "How to Allocate Progressive Patient Care Beds," Chapter 6, in Lewis E. Weeks and John H. Griffith (eds.), *Progressive Patient Care: An Anthology.* Ann Arbor, University of Michigan, 1964, pp. 47–57.

PROBLEMS AND SUGGESTIONS FOR FURTHER STUDY

1. Define the target populations for the hypotheses listed on pages 115–116. For which of these target populations would listings of the sample units be readily available? Discuss the pros and cons of defining the target population as broadly or as narrowly as possible.

2. Read the article by Morris J. Slonim, "Sampling in a Nutshell" *(J. Am. Statistical A.,* **52:**143–161, June 1957). Discuss the following statements by the author, "In addition, many who insist that the only accurate way is to make a complete count, overlook the fact that often there are many sources of error in the basic data and that a 100 percent count can be highly erroneous, as well as nearly impossible to achieve." (See pp. 146–147 in Slonim article.)

3. It has been said in this chapter that the same

person is simultaneously the member of many different conceivable target populations that could be defined for a study. Can you list at least five different target populations of which you are a member that could be the populations for a study (e.g., a target population of voters, a particular occupational group, the alumni of a school, etc.)? Is it possible for one individual to participate in more than one study at the same time?

4. Suppose we wanted to experimentally test the effects of a nursing procedure on patients who are hospitalized with a certain type of illness, say, a chronic disease. If we selected our patients from only one hospital would we be able to generalize our findings to other hospitals? If we included two hospitals would we be in a better position to generalize findings? What about a dozen or two dozen hospitals?

5. In agricultural experiments a plot of land is subdivided into smaller plots, each representing a different sampling unit. Is it possible to take a human being and treat him similarly? Could we, for example, in testing out various sunburn preventatives apply a different preventative to various part of a person's body, expose him to the sun, and determine which does the best job in preventing sunburn? Would each part of the body represent a different sampling unit? What are the limitations of such a design?

6. Discuss the sampling designs employed in the following studies. Which of the studies employed probability sampling? How would you classify the nonprobability samples?

   a. Dorothy E. Reese and Stanley Siegel, "Educational Preparation of Nurses Employed in Non-Federal Hospitals." *Hosp. Mgmt.*, **89:**108–112, April 1960.

   b. James K. Spencer, "Nurses' Cigarette Smoking in England and Wales." *Int. J. Nursing Stud.* **21:**69–79, 1984.

   c. Sharon Ringholtz and Miriam Morris, "A Test of Some Assumptions About Rooming-In." *Nursing Res.*, **10:**196–199, fall 1961.

   d. Janice E. Mickey, "Findings of Study of Extra-Hospital Nursing Needs." *Am. J. Pub. Health,* **53:**1047–1057, July 1963.

   e. Janet Rosenaur, Dennyse Stanford, Walter Morgan, and Barbara Curtin, "Describing Behaviors of Primary Care Practitioners." *Am. J. Pub. Health,* **74:**10–13, January 1984.

f. John S. Hathaway *et al.,* "The Role of the Nurse in a University Health Service." *Nursing Outlook,* **10:**533–537, August 1962.

g. Margaret L. Schell and Peter J. Korstad, "Working Sampling Study Shows Division of Labor Time." *Hospitals, J.A.H.A.,* **38:**99–102, January 16, 1964.

h. Irene S. Palmer, "Surgical Intervention and Social Class." *Nursing Sci.,* **2:**15–37, February 1964.

i. Louis E. Davis, George M. Parks, and Samuel R. Wickel, Jr., "A Sampling Technique for Estimating Linen Supply." *Hospitals, J.A.H.A.,* **37:**118, 120, 122, 123, 141, March 16, 1963.

j. Christine Webb and Jennifer Wilson-Barnett, "Self Concept, Social Support and Hysterectomy." *Int. J. Nursing Stud.,* **20:**97–107, 1983.

k. Ada Sue Hinshaw and Jan R. Atwood, "A Patient Satisfaction Instrument: Precision by Replication." *Nursing Res.,* **31:**170–175, 191, May/June 1982.

7. On pages 10 and 11 of their *Probability Sampling of Hospitals and Patients* (Bureau of Hospital Administration, Research Series No. 1, Ann Arbor, University of Michigan, 1975), the authors (Hess, Riedel, Fitzpatrick) describe a method of selecting a simple random sample of patients admitted to a hospital during a period of a year. Since some patients may be admitted more than once to the same hospital during the course of a year, what technique do the authors propose to obtain a sample of different persons?

8. How would you classify the following types of samples that are selected for a study? Discuss their adequacy as sample designs.

   a. After a random start, select every fifth patient who visits the outpatient department during the week.

   b. Select all the home visits made by the public health nurses to patients whose last names begin with an odd letter (i.e., A, C, E, G, I . . . etc.).

   c. Select all patients admitted to the hospital on Tuesdays and Thursdays during a three-month period.

   d. Select at random six diploma nursing schools out of thirty five located in a state. For the study population choose at random the first-year class in two of the schools, the second-year class from two of the remaining four schools, and the third-year class from the remaining two schools.

e. Obtain a copy of the classified telephone directory (yellow pages) for a dozen large cities. Select every twentieth name listed under "Nurses."

f. Obtain the latest copy of *State Approved Schools of Practical Nursing* (published by the National League for Nursing, 10 Columbus Circle, New York). Number the schools consecutively, beginning with 1. Choose twenty five schools for a sample by selecting the numbers from a table of random numbers.

g. Choose a sample of medication orders by putting a copy of all medication orders written during a month into a box, mixing up the slips (as in a lottery), and selecting 100 slips at random.

9. Why does the design of a sample have to consider the other phases of the research process—e.g., definition and measurement of variables, types of data-collecting methods used, methods for analyzing the data? What are some of the pitfalls in designing a sample for a study without considering other phases of the research process?

10. Read the article by Abdellah and Levine in *Nursing Research* (3:11–16, June 1954), "Work Sampling Applied to the Study of Nursing Personnel." How would you go about designing a study to demonstrate that systematic work sampling is as reliable as random work sampling? What is the basic sampling unit in a work sampling study?

11. Define the following:
   a. Random start
   b. Confidence level
   c. Level of significance
   d. Self-coding
   e. Pencil-and-paper instrument
   f. Parameter
   g. Response error
   h. Standard error

12. Read the article, "On the Use of Sampling in the Field of Public Health" (*AM. J. Pub. Health,* **44**:719–740, June 1954). What are some of the guidelines offered in the article as to when to enlist expert assistance in the design of a sampling plan? Discuss the disadvantages of sampling that are presented in the article, and indicate at least three situations in which sampling is inappropriate or will offer no advantages over study of the whole target population.

13. In the article by Betty Alexy, "Goal Setting and Health Risk Reduction" (*Nursing Res.,* **34**:283–288, September/October 1985), a *convenience sample* is described. Why, do you think, was this type of sample used? Could a random sample have been used in this study? Would it have been a better sample?

13

Collect the Data

OBJECTIVES

- To describe the various methods of collecting data in research.
- To explain how to select a data collection method.
- To delineate criteria for evaluating data collection methods.

- To show how to enhance data collection precision.
- To clarify various types of errors.
- To show how to compute sampling error.

METHODS OF COLLECTING DATA

The ways by which data on the variables being studied can be collected are outlined as follows:

    I. Use of existing data
   II. Use of the observer to collect the data
      A. Nonparticipant observer: use of quantitative scales
      B. Nonparticipant observer: use of qualitative scales
      C. Participant observer
      D. Interviewing
  III. Self-recording collection of data
      A. Factual questionnaires
      B. Psychological and sociological pencil and paper instruments
      C. Mechanical instruments
  IV. Combined methods

Existing Data

Existing or secondary data play a role in all types of research. In nonexperimental studies, existing data may provide all of the needed data. In experimental studies, existing data may provide a background for the new data and assist in the analysis and interpretation of the findings.

Existing data can be found in two forms, raw and tabulated. In its raw form there are basic documents such as patients' records, personnel folders, birth, death, and other vital records, licensure forms, applications of various kinds, and financial records. Such records are originally designed as administrative documents, not as research instruments, but it is often possible to prepare valid and reliable statistical tabulations from them. From existing patients' hospital records, it is possible, for example to tabulate the number of discharged hospital patients who are in each of the major diagnostic categories. The data can then be used to assess the variety of clinical experiences the hospital could provide to nursing students.[1] In another study, personnel folders of all the members of the nursing department can be used to provide an analysis of the stability of the work force.[2] Another study can use the Kardex to obtain data on the work load of the nursing department.[3]

Data already tabulated can be used either as supplementary data or as the major source of data in a study. Data produced by governmental organizations such as the Bureau of the Census, the Public Health Service, and the Bureau of Labor Statistics can serve many purposes in addition to those for which they were primarily designed. Such a report as that by Lerner and Anderson[4] largely consists of an analysis of data from agencies such as these.

In the field of nursing and patient care there are a variety of useful source documents that can provide data for a study. These include the Public Health Service's *Health Manpower Sourcebook* and *Health United States* series, the American Hospital Association's Annual Directory Issues, and the American Nurses' Association's *Facts About Nursing.*

A major limitation to the use of existing data is that the definitions of the variables for which data are available may not correspond to the definitions of the study in which they are to be used. That is, they may lack content validity. If we were to use as a criterion measure of the effectiveness of a public health program a tabulation from existing records of the number of deaths from different diseases, we may not have a valid measure, since the death rate may not be a function of how well a program is executed, particularly on a short-run basis.

A second drawback to the use of existing data is the difficulty in evaluating its quality. Tabulated data, particularly if published, look authoritative. However, published data may sometimes have limitations. They may be incomplete or contain errors of one kind or another, or have some other deficiency that may destroy their usefulness as research data. Such deficiencies may not be known to the potential user unless the user is sophisticated in a statistical and subject content sense. It is advisable to be cautious in the use of secondary data and to maintain at all times a skeptical attitude regarding their quality.

Use of an Observer to Collect the Data

In many studies the requirements are such that data collection must be tailor-made. Data available from existing sources are either nonapplicable, or not sufficiently reliable, or not complete enough. Thus, new data, called primary data, must be collected. One of the most widely used methods of collecting new data is through the use of an observer. The several means by which an observer obtains the required data are described below.

NONPARTICIPANT OBSERVER: USE OF QUANTITATIVE SCALES

In Chapter 11 discussion of the measurement process mentioned various types of quantitative scales that could be used to measure variables. These scales are usually incorporated into mechanical instruments such as weight scales, thermometers, or clocks to provide a precise and sensitive source of data. The observer using mechanical instruments records the data by applying the instruments to the subjects and taking readings. If the observer is well trained, a high degree of precision can be achieved since subjective judgment is kept to a minimum.

NONPARTICIPANT OBSERVER: USE OF QUALITATIVE SCALES

The use of an observer to obtain data on qualitatively scaled variables permits the observer to exert more judgment than in the use of quantitative scales. As a nonparticipant in the events being observed, the observer stands outside the phenomena being measured and as objectively as possible records the required data. The recording may be in the form of a direct scaling of the observed event. For example, the observer could rate the performance of nursing personnel on a graphic rating scale with categories ranging from "high proficiency" to "low proficiency." Instead of a direct scaling, the recording could be a narrative description of what transpires, or entries on a checklist, or a questionnaire type of form—material that will later be classified in terms of a nominal or ordinal scale.

Many examples of this method of observation can be cited from research in nursing and patient care. In the assessment of the activities of nursing personnel by work sampling, the observer either makes a narrative recording or directly classifies the activities into a nominal scale. In another approach to the study of the work of nurses, a watch is used to quantitatively measure how long different types of activities take as well as to classify the activity.

The use of an observer to gather data on qualitative variables requires a high level of control to insure the reliability of the observations, because the observer must use considerable judgment in making decisions about the categorization of the observed phenomena. Nurses do make very precise observers, because they have been trained to assess the behavior of patients, but there is often a substantial difference between the kinds of observations made in patient care and those required in research. Research observations are often concerned, not with signs and symptoms of patients, but with subtle and intangible phenomena that are detected through the use of unstructured data-collecting instruments. A high level of skill is required on the part of the observer to insure the relevance and precision of such observations.

The usefulness of data collected by an observer on qualitative variables will depend not only on how well trained the observer is, but on the clarity, meaningfulness, and sensitivity of the scale used to measure the variables, the definitions of the categories included in the scale, and the format of the instrument used to gather the data. In making unstructured observations, the observer has maximum freedom to record what is observed, since the instrument used to collect the data is a blank piece of paper. Here the burden of classifying and scaling the data is upon the editor of the data, who must be provided with definitive guidelines. In more highly structured observations, the observer must fit the observations into predetermined categories. This relieves the editor of much of the burden of classifying and scaling, but requires the observer to have a thorough understanding of the scale.

PARTICIPANT OBSERVER

One limitation to the use of the nonparticipant observer is the possibility of introducing psychological bias by the presence of the observer—the Hawthorne effect. In observing people at work, for example, those being observed may work harder, or at least may behave differently from normal. One way of eliminating observer bias is to disguise the observer by having her blend into the situation. Maximum blending is obtained when the observer participates in the situation being observed.

The use of the participant observer is very popular in sociological research. The term "sociometry" has been applied to measurement of the social interactions among a group of people. A participant observer may be a member of the group, collecting the required data while taking part in the activity, for instance, assessing the attractions and repulsions among the group's members by plotting their interactions on a device called a sociogram. This device has been used to analyze leadership wielded at meetings and conferences by recording who talks to whom, who initiates topics, and so on.

Nonsociological evaluations can also be the subject of participant observation. In evaluating the service provided in a hospital the observer can be disguised as a patient, rating not only the services received but all activities that come within her purview. A question can be raised as to the ethics of such a procedure, since it can be called "spying."

It appears that for much of the research in nursing and patient care, the participant observer technique has value if a dual observer (another outside partner) is involved to corroborate the participant observer's observations. A major principle of nonparticipant observation is for the observer never to intrude into the situation being observed. This may be difficult to do for a nurse observer who sees something being done that is regarded as harmful to a patient.

INTERVIEWING

In interviewing, the observer gathers data by questioning the subjects to elicit data on the variables being studied. The format of the interviews can vary from the highly structured kind where the interviewer actually reads the questions to the subject and records the answers, to the highly unstructured interview where only a general framework is provided for the content of the questions and the interviewer is given much leeway in framing the actual questions and the extent of coverage of the material. The unstructured interview permits greater probing into the responses of the subjects to verify meaning and to obtain data of depth and breadth. However, the highly structured interview usually allows the interviewer to probe in order to clarify and broaden responses. One advantage of the structured interview is the greater ease with which the data can be processed. Another is that the observer need not be highly skilled in interviewing. To obtain valid and reliable data in an unstructured interview, the interviewer must be well trained.

Direct Collection of the Data

In direct collection of data an observer is not used and the study subjects themselves supply the material needed. This can be in the form of a rating on a qualitative scale, a reading on a quantitative scale, a narrative description, or responses to a checklist, test, or questionnaire.

By eliminating the observer three important benefits are achieved. First, the cost of collecting the data can be reduced. In studies where large amounts of observation are required, such costs can be quite high. The savings obtained by elimination of the observer can be used to increase the *size* of the sample.

Second, elimination of the observer removes a source of possible bias from the study—observer error, although this may well be offset by the introduction of a new source of bias—response error. Without an observer trained to interpret the meaning of the information being sought, the respondent can frequently misinterpret the items on the instrument thereby reducing the precision of the data.

Third, with self-recording techniques it is possible to guarantee the study subject that his responses will be kept anonymous. When a study deals with sensitive or highly personal data this may be an important advantage.

A major disadvantage of the self-recording method of data collection, as compared to the use of an observer, is the lesser depth of response that can be obtained. This can be a particularly serious disadvantage if the research problem is a thorny one and the variables studied are highly complex. An observer asking questions in an interview can probe the meaning of a response. This cannot be done easily when the subject is responding to questions on a standardized form.

Also, there are many variables of importance to research in nursing and patient care that can be studied only through the use of an observer. For example, in studying the flow of an ongoing process or activity, such as the provision of nursing care, we would usually employ an observer to record the observations. Such substitutes as recording by a motion picture or television camera would be much more costly if done on a large scale. Moreover, such instruments do not entirely eliminate the observer, but only make the process of observation an indirect one.

KEY POINT Three of the ways in which data can be collected directly from the study subjects without the need for an observer are by the use of factual questionnaires, psychological and sociological tests and scales, and mechanical instruments.

Direct Collection Without an Observer

FACTUAL QUESTIONNAIRES

Perhaps the single most widely used instrument for data collection, particularly in nonexperimental studies, is the factual questionnaire. This often consists of a battery of questions aimed at eliciting data on demographic variables such as age, marital status, occupation, educational level, size of family, or on economic variables such as possessions owned, salary earned, expenditures made, as well as on variables concerned with behavioral characteristics such as kinds of books read, hobbies pursued, hours of work performed, television programs watched, jobs held. Included also are variables that describe preferences—Who is your best friend? What food do you like best? Who is your favorite political can-

didate? Factual questionnaires also deal with specific events—When were you last ill? Where did you purchase your car? How many times did you visit a dentist last year? How long did you spend on different activities on your job last week?

Responses to many kinds of factual questions are readily amenable to validation. If a study subject claims to be twenty nine years of age, an independent check is available—the respondent's birth certificate. If the respondent's favorite television program is listed as the evening news, corroboration may be possible by checking with family members, friends, or fellow workers.

Although a low response error is expected in factual questionnaires, such is not always the case.[5] A major source of error in responses to factual questions, particularly questions relating to past events, is faulty memory. Bell and Palmer reported a study[6] in which the identical factual questions were presented to the same respondents one week to ten days apart. There was an amazing lack of agreement in the responses to some of the variables.

VARIABLE	PERCENT OF AGREEMENT IN RESPONSE
Race	99.9
Marital status	98.2
Number of persons in household	85.3
Occupation	78.1
Age	68.5
School grade completed	55.8
Length of service in present job	40.0

For many factual questions, standardized wordings are available that can be used from one study to the next. One of the virtues of standardized items is that the comparability of data from different studies is insured.

Factual questionnaires can serve as useful criterion measures for a study. Since they contain questions related to concrete, observable behavior, it is possible to use such questions to measure the effects of the independent variable. If, for example, the independent variable represents different kinds of treatment given to patients while they are hospitalized, a factual questionnaire can be used in a longitudinal follow-up study of the patients to determine their health history after discharge.

Factual questionnaires are perhaps the simplest type of data-collecting instrument to administer. Many factual questions are self-evident and require little interpretation. Assuming no major lapses in memory on the part of the respondent or a conscious determination to distort a reply, the precision of such questions is rather high. Questionnaires of this type can be distributed through the mails, enabling wide coverage at low cost. With appropriate controls over return of the questionnaires, such as follow-ups to delinquent respondents, a high response rate should be obtained, keeping the bias of a "voluntary" sample to a minimum.

Factual questionnaires are generally easy to process. The response categories for qualitative variables can be framed in such a way as to make the questionnaire "self-coding." A "self-coded" questionnaire is one in which the respondent replies to the items by checking the appropriate category. To tabulate the questionnaires the number of checks is counted to obtain the total frequency for the different classes of each question. A questionnaire is not self-coded if it requires open-ended, narrative responses to qualitative variables. These must be coded upon return, a process of categorizing the responses into various classes. One type of open-ended factual instrument is the so-called "diary" method, in which the subject makes a continuous narrative recording of events, impressions, or findings concerning the variables under study. These narrative data are then coded and tabulated. Some structure could be incorporated into the diary method by including questions or checklists to which the subjects regularly respond.

PSYCHOLOGICAL AND SOCIOLOGICAL PENCIL AND PAPER INSTRUMENTS

Many of these instruments have been mentioned previously in the discussion of measurement of variables. These instruments measure such variables as personality, intelligence, interest, motivation, attitudes, and perception. They are called "pencil-and-paper" instruments because the subjects respond by writing a narrative statement or making a check mark, or some other similar type of response. For a few psychological variables mechanical instruments can provide an indirect measure, but are not commonly used. As an example, anxiety might be measured in terms of blood pressure level, loudness of heartbeat, or amount of moisture on the skin.

Instruments to collect data on some psychological and sociological variables could be administered in the same way as factual questionnaires. Graphic rating scales as well as other types of sociological scales could be mailed to the study subjects. However, many psychological tests need to be highly controlled in their administration and require the presense of a member of the research team when they are being filled out by the subjects. One reason is that many of these instruments have to be regulated as to time permitted for reply. Also, there is need to insure that the respondent receives no assistance while replying to the instrument and is free from distractions and interruptions. For economy, study subjects are often assembled and the test administered to a group rather than an individual. Some tests require that an observer be assigned to one study subject during the entire course of the administration of the instrument, acting as an interviewer or nonparticipant observer. In such a situation, the instrument cannot be classified as self-recording but as one that employs an observer-recorder.

Psychological and sociological instruments are of two broad types—those that are direct and highly structured, and those that are less direct and unstructured. The latter are called nondirective or projective techniques and include such methods as the Rorschach test and thematic apperception test, which require a high degree of skill for proper administration and interpretation. Many instruments such as these are available for collecting data. To develop one especially for a study could be a formidable undertaking. However, this should not discourage the use of such instruments, since they can provide valuable criterion measures in studies of nursing and of patient care.

MECHANICAL INSTRUMENTS

Many instruments are now available that can provide quantitative measurements on a self-recording basis. For example, certain types of thermometers can be attached to a patient to provide a continuous temperature reading. A variety of electronic patient monitoring apparatus is available for diagnosis and therapy and can also be used as research instruments. Such instruments are useful because the observer is eliminated, removing one possible source of bias, and quantitative measurements are provided of a highly precise and sensitive nature. A question remains as to the validity of such measurements. A measurement can be precise and sensitive, but may not be valid because the variable being measured is not relevant to the research problem. Validity is the overriding consideration in the determination of the adequacy of a criterion measure.

An interesting example of a mechanical instrument used to obtain data without an observer is the equipment used in measurement of the size of the audience of television programs. This equipment is a monitoring device called an audimeter that is attached to the television receivers of sample viewers. When the TV is turned on, the monitoring device records the station to which it is turned and the amount of time it is in use. These recordings are collected routinely and the data tabulated to provide ratings for different programs.

One problem in the use of such devices is the lack of control over the data-collecting process. It is somewhat analogous to permitting a subject to take a test home and work on it at his leisure. The lack of validity of such audience measurement was underscored during a congressional investigation of TV ratings. One of the sample viewers was found to have a very high rate of viewing, much higher than would be expected of people with similar socioeconomic characteristics. Closer investigation revealed that this viewer owned a dog. When she left the house for an extended period of time, she turned the set on to keep the dog company. The monitoring device was indeed precise, but the data was not valid.

Combined Methods

Many studies employ not just a single method of data collection but a combination of methods. In experiments that test the effects of drugs on patients, data on the criterion measure are usually collected by an observer. Data on important organismic variables related to the patient are obtained through factual questionnaires, interviews, and existing records.

Sometimes two or more different methods of data collection are employed to gather data on the same variable. The separate approaches are used to reinforce the findings or as a means of elaborating the amount of information gathered on the explanatory variables. Thus a factual questionnaire may be filled out by the subjects and later an interviewer will repeat some of the questions to corroborate the replies as well as to obtain more depth.

Another combined approach, also used to enhance the precision of the data, is to give a factual questionnaire to a subject while an interviewer stands by to assist in clarifying the meaning of any questions that the subject does not fully comprehend.

HOW TO SELECT A DATA COLLECTION METHOD

The choice of methods to use in a study for collecting the data will depend on consideration of a number of elements:

- The research problem
- The design of the study—experimental or nonexperimental
- The variables being studied—how they are defined, how they are measured
- The sampling units to be included—their type, number, location
- The amount of time available in which to complete the study
- The amount of resources available to do the study

Often the nature of the variables will dictate the method to be used for data collection. A variable to be measured quantitatively may require the use of mechanical apparatus necessitating the use of observers to read the instruments. Variables that are essentially factual can be measured with questionnaires, while psychological and sociological measurements are usually in the form of pencil-and-paper tests, rating scales, questionnaires, or a projective design. Data to be collected longitudinally on ongoing phenomena may require observers or monitoring systems.

Highly controlled experimental studies usually require direct observation of phenomena being studied. In nonexperimental studies, particularly where the subjects are widely dispersed geographically, data are frequently collected with instruments that are distributed through the mails.

Where the measurements required are complex, difficult to make, and need considerable interpretation, the use of an observer to collect the data will be a greater necessity than where the variables are well-defined, specific, unidimensional, and easy to measure.

Importance of a Pretest

The adequacy of a data-collecting instrument can best be assessed by pretesting it before it is applied to the subjects in the actual study. The pretest should be done on subjects representative of the study subjects. Sufficient time should be allowed for the pretest to fully analyze the results so as to make all necessary changes in the data-collecting procedures.

A pretest can be used to validate the measures of the variables being studied by correlating them with outside criteria. It can also be used to check the reliability of the data-collecting instruments by such means as comparing responses to alternative ways of constructing the items relating to the same variable, by test-retest, and by comparison of independent observations of the same phenomena. The pretest also provides a "dry run" of the total administration of data collecting and processing phases of the research. It goes without saying that validity and reliability of the data-collecting instruments and procedures should be established by the pretest. The actual data collection phase should not begin until this has been achieved.

Criteria for Evaluating Data-Collecting Instruments

The criteria for evaluating data-collecting instruments are the same as those for assessing the quality of the measurement of variables:

- *Validity:* Does the data-collecting instrument yield data relevant to the problem being investigated? Does it measure what it is supposed to measure?
- *Reliability:* Are the data precise? Would two independent observers observing the same phenomena record comparable data? Would two independent interviewers asking the same questions elicit similar responses from the

same subject? Will identical responses to the same factual questionnaire be obtained if given to the same subject at short-spaced intervals? Will the subject respond to the same test or scale consistently on a retest?

- *Sensitivity:* Are the scales for different variables on which data are being collected of sufficient sensitivity to be discriminating and selective? Can they detect significant differences among the study subjects?
- *Meaningfulness:* What is the substantive significance of the differences found among the subjects from whom data are collected? What practical importance do the data possess?

PRECISION IN DATA COLLECTION

The precision of the data collected is influenced by various sources of error. Fortunately some errors that occur in data collection are random rather than systematic and as such can cancel each other out. This would tend to be more true as the number of subjects on whom data are being collected increases. An error arising from a subject who mistakenly checks her field of practice on a factual questionnaire as hospital nursing when it really is private duty nursing may be offset by another respondent checking private duty nursing when it should be hospital nursing.

However, some errors are systematic in nature and can reduce the precision of the data. Many studies have shown that a variable such as age is consistently underestimated. Also, there is a tendency to round off data reported for certain variables such as age. The U.S. Bureau of the Census finds, for example, in its decennial census, that there are more persons reported at ages such as twenty, twenty five, thirty, thirty five, etc., than at the in-between years.

Questions such as age can be independently verified by asking for the same information in two ways on a questionnaire. Thus, an early question might be: How old are you? A later one might ask: What is the date of your birth? Underestimation or rounding off is likely to be detected by the response to the latter question, since it is more difficult for the subject to either round off or underestimate his birth date than his age.

Systematic errors are troublesome when the criterion measure is to be assessed in terms of the absolute units of the scale of measurement. It is of less serious consequence if we are interested only in relative comparisons or trends. As Deming[7] remarked:

> When trends or proportions rather than absolute numbers are to be considered no harm is done if the figures to be compared are all in error by the same percentage. Moreover, in some problems an error of 100 percent or even more will not affect the decision one way or another.

For example, if our study is measuring the effects of teaching on the weight reduction of diabetic patients, we might be interested simply in the fact that the experimental group subjects weighed less than the control group at the end of the study. If there were a systematic bias in the weight scales that underestimated the weights of the subjects by about 5% on the average, the comparison would be unaffected by the error. If the average weight for both groups were the same at the beginning of the study, and if at the end of the study the control group averaged 150 pounds and the experimental group weighed 140 pounds, we still can make a valid interpretation of the data—weight loss was related to patient teaching—even though the true final weights were 160 pounds for the control group and 150 pounds for the experimental group.

Collection of data by observers can be fraught with both random errors, which hopefully will cancel themselves out, and systematic errors, which are more likely to reduce precision. A poorly trained observer can consistently make the same mistake in reading a mechanical instrument or in applying a rating scale to the events being observed. Psychological bias, too, can systematically distort data collected by an observer. In a study where the criterion measure is a rating of the quality of patient care, an observer, if a nurse, may unconsciously substitute her own values for the definitions of the scale categories established in the study.

The major sources of error in a study that can reduce the precision of the data can be summarized as follows:

SAMPLING ERROR

This error has been defined as the ratio of the variation of the values of the measurements among the sampling units of a target population to the square root of the number of sampling units in the sample. This is the only kind of error in data collection that is actually measurable by mathematical formulas. Of course, such errors should only be computed when the sampling units were randomly selected from some larger target population. If nonrandom sampling is used, or if the whole target population is studied, sampling error should not be computed with conventional formulas.

Sampling error is computed for the summary measures of a sample of measurements. Each summary measure has its own sampling error formula, called *standard errors*. The formula for the standard error of the mean in a simple random sample is identical with the one stated above. The numerator of the formula is the standard deviation of the values of the measurements among the sampling units of a target population. Since in most studies we do not know the standard deviation of the values of measurements for all sampling units in a target population, but only for those units actually in the sample, we use the standard deviation of the sample measurements in the computation of the standard error as the "best" estimate of the population standard deviation.

To illustrate the computation of the standard error of the mean, we can use the data presented in the next chapter on the blood pressure measurements for a sample of fifteen patients. For the Group A patients we found a mean of 133 and a standard deviation of 16. The standard error of the mean is therefore:

$$\frac{16}{\sqrt{15}} = \frac{16}{3.9} = 4.1$$

The standard error of a summary measure such as the mean is interpreted in the same way as a standard deviation of the values of the individual measurements. A standard error of a summary measure is, conceptually, the standard deviation of all the values of the summary measures that can be computed from successive samples drawn from the same target population. Thus, if our target population consisted of 100 patients (a very small target population indeed), we could sequentially draw samples of fifteen patients, compute the mean blood pressure for each sample, and return the fifteen patients to the target population. Each sample of fifteen would be randomly drawn from the population of 100 patients so that the same patients could appear over and over again in the different samples selected. However, each sample is likely to be a different set from every other sample set. Consider that although as many as fourteen of the sampling units may be the very same patients that composed another sample that was selected, the fifteenth may be an entirely new patient in the sample set. In fact, the number of different samples that could be drawn is astronomical. This is obvious if you consider the number of different bridge hands that can be drawn from a deck of fifty two playing cards—over 600 billion different combinations of thirteen cards. In mathematical terms the number of different samples that can be drawn from a population is: $\binom{n}{r}$, where $n =$ the total number of different sampling units in the population and $r =$ the number of sampling units in the sample. This is the well-known combination theorem that gives us the total number of combinations of n total units selected r at a time. Mathematically, $\binom{n}{r}$, which can also be stated as nCr, is equal to:

$$\frac{n!}{r!(n-r)!}$$

The exclamation point, !, designates the mathematical operation called "factorial," which means that the number preceding the factorial is multiplied by all the positive integers preceding it. Thus 15! would be equal to $15 \times 14 \times 13 \times 12 \times 11 \times 10 \times 9 \times 8 \times 7 \times 6 \times 5 \times 4 \times 3 \times 2 \times 1$.

Substituting our values we find that the number of different samples of fifteen patients that can be selected from a target population of 100 patients by simple random sampling is:

$$\frac{100!}{15! \, 85!} = 25{,}333{,}846 \times 10^{10}$$

After drawing successive samples of fifteen patients and computing the mean blood pressure for each sample, if we plotted the values of these means for all samples, we would find that they would form a normal curve, even if the actual blood pressures of the 100 patients in the target population did not. The mean of this distribution of means—called a sampling distribution—would be equal to the population mean, the mean for the 100 different blood pressures. The standard deviation of this sampling distribution is called the *standard error of the mean* and its value is estimated by the standard error of our sample mean. We can therefore interpret the value of a standard error in the same way as a standard deviation: ± 1 standard error would include 68 percent of the values of all the mean blood pressures that could be selected from the $25{,}333{,}846 \times 10^{10}$ means in the sampling distribution; ± 2 standard errors would include 95 percent of all the means; and so on.

The standard error of a sample statistic thus provides us with an estimate of the range within which the population parameter can be found at a stated level of probability. This range is called *confidence interval,* and the level of probability is called the *confidence coefficient.* Since our sample

of fifteen patients had a mean of 133 and a standard error of 4.1, we estimate, with a confidence coefficient of 95 percent, that the interval 124.8 to 141.2 embraces the true population mean: $133 \pm 2(4.1)$.

The size of the confidence interval around a summary measure is the measure of the sampling error of the statistic computed from the sample. It provides a measure of the precision of the statistic as an estimate of the value of the population parameter. For other types of summary measures the measure of the sampling error is analogous to that of the standard error of the mean. Sampling errors can be computed for data obtained from qualitative scales as well as from quantitative ones. Summary measures of the frequencies in each of the qualitative scale categories (e.g., the number of males, the number of females; or the number of patients who died, the number who recovered) are known as *rates* or *proportions.* For a simple random sample, the standard error of a proportion is the square root of the ratio of the proportion multiplied by its complement (1 minus the proportion) to the number of sampling units in the sample. The numerator in this case, although it seems far removed from the numerator of the standard error of the mean, is quite analogous to it, since it is also a measure of the variability of the measurements among the sampling units of the target population.

To illustrate the computation of a standard error of a percentage, assume we took a random sample of twenty five patients and wanted to estimate the percentage of patients in the target population who needed intensive care. If, among our sample of twenty five patients, 10 percent needed intensive care, our estimate of the population percentage would be 10 percent ± 12, a confidence interval of 0–22 percent with a level of confidence of 95 percent, since the standard error of our sampling percentage is:

$$\sqrt{\frac{(.10)\,(.90)}{25}} = 0.06 \text{ or } 6\%$$

OBSERVER ERROR

This type of error is either random or systematic. Random errors occurring more or less accidentally and with no particular pattern may offset each other, particularly when the number of measurements is very large. Systematic errors, arising from such causes as inadequate training or psychological biases, can reduce the precision of the data. One way to assess the extent of observer error is to have two observers independently measure the same phenomenon and compare the results.

RESPONSE ERROR

This error may also arise either randomly or systematically. It is more apt to be present where self-recording methods of data are employed and there is no observer to check the accuracy or completeness of responses. One type of response error is nonresponse. In mailed questionnaires some of the subjects selected for study may not reply. Those who do may not provide an adequate sample of the target population.

The various kinds of response errors can be controlled by making the instruments used as unambiguous and self-explanatory as possible and by making the aims of the study clearly known to the respondents. Also, the importance of submitting complete and accurate replies should be stressed.

PROCESSING ERRORS

This type of error should be under the complete control of the researcher and should therefore be kept to a minimum. With the availability of highly accurate computers there is little reason why any significant amount or error should occur during this phase. One possible source of processing errors is the translation of open-ended responses into categories in order to obtain the frequency of occurrence of the different categories. However, if the categories composing the scales for the vari-

ables are clearly defined there should be little difficulty in keeping the data free of errors during this stage of data processing.

SUMMARY

Data collection is frequently the most time-consuming and expensive stage in conducting research. A variety of ways exist to collect data. The method chosen depends on the research problem and purpose, the variables to be measured, and the hypotheses to be tested, if any. The method also depends on the population to be studied—its size, composition, location, and whether human or not. Data collection must be as free as possible of the various kinds of errors that can occur in order to yield valid, reliable, and usable information.

REFERENCES

1. Faye G. Abdellah and Eugene Levine, *Appraising the Clinical Resources in Small Hospitals.* U.S. Public Health Service Monograph No. 24. Washington, D.C., Government Printing Office, 1954.
2. Eugene Levine, "Turnover Among Nursing Personnel in General Hospitals." *Hospitals, J.A.H.A.,* **31:**50–53, 138, 140, September 1, 1957.
3. Marion J. Wright, *Improvement of Patient Care.* New York, G. P. Putnam's Sons, 1954.
4. Monroe Lerner and Odin W. Anderson, *Health Progress in the United States.* Chicago, University of Chicago Press, 1963.
5. W. Edwards Deming, *Some Theory of Sampling.* Mineola, NY, Dover, 1984.
6. Gladys L. Palmer, "Factors in Variability of Response in Enumerative Studies." *J. Am. Statistical A.,* **38:**148–152, 1943.
7. Deming, *op. cit.*

PROBLEMS AND SUGGESTIONS FOR FURTHER STUDY

1. Obtain a recent edition of *Facts About Nursing* (published by the American Nurses' Association, Kansas City, Missouri). Examine some of the data contained in this book. Discuss three studies that could be made that would be based wholly or in part on these

data, assuming, of course, that previous editions of *Facts* could be used for the study. (Example: a study to answer the question: Have the salaries of public health nurses kept pace with the rise in the cost of living over the past fifteen years?)

2. Design a factual questionnaire containing eight to twelve items to gather data on one of the following topics:

   a. To what extent do professional nurses marry physicians?

   b. The characteristics of patients in private psychiatric hospitals.

   c. Staffing patterns in intensive care units of hospitals.

   d. The family characteristics of patients receiving home nursing care from public health agencies.

   e. A comparison of reasons for turnover of nursing personnel employed by nongovernment hospitals and government hospitals.

   f. The amount of information patients possess about their illnesses.

   g. How do directors of nursing service evaluate recent graduates of collegiate programs in nursing?

   h. The work patterns of private duty nurses.

3. Read the article "Ranking the Nursing Schools" by Patricia A. Chamings (*Nursing Outlook,* **32:**238–239, September/October 1984). Comment on the author's use of the term "opinionnaire" to collect the data. Can you suggest the kinds of items included in the "opinionnaire"? Is an opinionnaire different from a questionnaire? Was a sample used in this study?

4. Describe what methods you would use to collect the data needed to test the hypotheses listed on pp. 115–116. What are some of the ways in which the costs of collecting the data for these studies could be kept as low as possible?

5. Comment on the following statement by Hyman in his *Survey Design and Analysis* (New York, The Free Press of Glencoe, 1955, p. 28), "There is the realization that the standardization of inquiry in large scale survey research, while making for efficiency and necessary to insure comparability among field workers, at the same time may impose some artificiality on the phenomenon studied, particularly when the analyst does his planning away from the live events."

6. Discuss the following statement by Walter I. Wardwell and Claus B. Bahnson ("Problems Encountered in Behavioral Science Research in Epidemiological Studies," *Am. J. Pub. Health,* **54:**972–981, June 1964): "A very great advantage of home interviewing is that the patient's home and often also his family can be observed as well as the patient's behavior in relation to them. In his natural habitat, as it were, a different quality of information may be obtained about the patient than would be possible in the more standardized and possibly threatening environment of the hospital or examination clinic" (p. 979). Are there any disadvantages in obtaining research data by interviewing the patient in his home? What are the advantages of conducting an interview study of institutionalized patients?

7. In the article "A Description of Participant Observation of Clinical Teaching" by Catherine M. Robertson (*J. Adv. Nursing,* **7:**549–554, 1982) several limitations of a participant observer are presented. While these are discussed in relation to evaluating clinical teaching, are they also relevant in research applications of participant observation? How can the Hawthorne effect be controlled when participant observation is used to collect data for a study? For what kinds of research problems is participant observation a desirable method for collecting data?

14

Process and Summarize the Data

OBJECTIVES

- To highlight the role of the computer in research.
- To explain how data are processed.
- To clarify the components of a statistical table.

THE ROLE OF COMPUTERS IN RESEARCH

Electronic computers are a fact of today's life. With the advent of relatively inexpensive "personal computers," these technological marvels are becoming as commonplace in the home as toasters or television sets.

Computers can perform a variety of useful functions quickly, accurately, and inexpensively. Perhaps nowhere is this so clear as in research. At least nine applications of computers in research can be performed, at least at a basic level, on the smallest computers—the microcomputer, also known as the personal computer (PC). The applications are:

1. *Review of the literature:* As discussed in Chapter 7, computerized document re-

trieval systems such as MEDLINE are an important resource in conducting a literature review.

2. *Collecting data:* Computers can be used as the means for gathering data for research. Used in this way a computer is a research instrument similar to the data collection instruments discussed in Chapter 13.

3. *Processing data:* Computers are used to summarize and store data.

4. *Analyzing data:* Computers can perform the most complex statistical analyses of research data, including some from the domain of multivariate analysis, that would be impossible to do otherwise.

5. *Preparing tabulations of data:* Computers can prepare statistical tabulations of data in a variety of ways. Statistical tables consisting of enumerations or of computed

measures can be prepared for single variables or for cross-tabulations of two or more variables.

6. *Assembling listings:* These can be used for a variety of research purposes including listings of the data for individual cases (showing the responses on a questionnaire, for example), lists of names and addresses of study participants, and an assembly of narrative information collected.

7. *Graphing and plotting data:* For visual display of data, as well as for analytical and interpretative purposes, computers can prepare many different types of charts and graphs, including histograms, scatter plots of correlated data, time series, and probability plots.

8. *Report writing:* A computer through its "word-processing" capability has become an indispensable tool in the preparation of research reports. Combined with the table- and graph-producing capabilities as well as its listing function, computers can make the preparation of the final report much less burdensome and more informative than previously.

9. *The computer as the heart of an information system:* Computers are increasingly being utilized in the health care industry in comprehensive and integrated systems.[1] For example, linking all units within a hospital, computers are used primarily for patient, personnel, and financial management. However, data gathered for management purposes can also be used for research purposes. For example, the diagnosis related group (DRG) to which a patient is assigned can be linked to a nursing intensity measure to see if the patient's needs for nursing care are related to the DRG. Another example: Using its computerized information system, a home health agency can relate what the nurse did in a home to a client's socioeconomic characteristics.

Components of a Computer System

Basically a computer consists of (1) "hardware" made up of several components for entering, storing, processing, and displaying information, (2) "software,"

called the program, that instructs the hardware what to do with the data and how, and (3) the actual data.[2] It is beyond the scope of this book to attempt to teach the reader how to operate a computer. Information abounds on this subject. Hardware comes in many different types and styles although all basically perform the same functions. Moreover, many statistical packages are available for summarizing and analyzing the kinds of data that are gathered in nursing research. To describe any one hardware or software system would invite quick obsolescence, since the computer field is constantly changing. On the horizon are intelligent computers that will be able to "think" for themselves. Also, while the trend in computers has been toward greater miniaturization, computers of the future may make the so-called personal computers of today look large.

While personal computers are the most widely used and the least expensive, large computers called mainframes have important applications in education and health care institutions, information systems, data management, and large data-processing and analysis applications. Microcomputers may be too slow or lack sufficient capability for some applications. Intermediate-sized computers, called minicomputers, span the gap between microcomputers and mainframes.

Understanding a Computer

Among the many trends in the development of the electronic computer has been simplification. To "program" the early computers esoteric languages had to be employed—Fortran, Cobol, etc.—which required lengthy study to understand their use. Microcomputers can be learned quickly. The statistical packages available today enable the user to engage in highly complex data analyses with minimal instruction and with little or no knowledge of the theoretical basis of the analysis used. However, doing statistical analyses without appreciation of rationale or purpose can lead to employing inappropriate or meaningless techniques. Also, the speed and ease with which the analyses can be performed leads to the overuse of certain statistical procedures. Statistical tests of significance, for example, if conducted on a "wholesale" basis can yield findings of statistical significance by chance alone. Also, applying techniques such as multiple regression that encompass a multitude of variables, some without logical or conceptual relationship, can produce meaningless conclusions from the data if little or no knowledge of the theoretical basis of the analysis used exists.

In the following chapter the role of the computer in the *analysis* of research data will be discussed. Suffice it to say that the computer cannot replace the human mind in making research decisions as to what analyses should be used and, most particularly, how to interpret the results.

Processing Data by Computer

The main steps in transforming the data from their raw state to a finished product include the following: editing the raw material; coding, scoring, and scaling the data; summarizing the data into statistical tables. These steps assume that the data are to be processed by a computer. In very small studies, which involve few variables and study subjects, it may not be advantageous to process the data electronically. Whenever feasible, computer processing should be used, as it is more precise, faster, and less burdensome, and can yield a greater amount of information per dollar spent on data processing. Moreover, the data can be permanently stored for reuse in the future if desired. A brief description of the major steps in data processing by computer follows:

1. *Edit the raw material:* This usually involves an examination to see that all the questions have been answered and to evaluate the reliability of the responses. If reliability questions are included—asking a person's age in two different ways—these can be compared

2. *Code, score, and scale the data:* In data processing by computers it is neces-

sary to transform data on qualitative variables into numerical codes that can be entered into the computer. If a questionnaire or checklist contains no open-ended items or if the responses are in terms of a number (How many years of schooling do you have?), the instrument is said to be "self-coded" and after editing the data can be entered into the computer.

When psychological tests are used, the responses have to be scored. It is advantageous in the use of such tests in research to employ a device such as "mark-sensing" in which the subject marks his reply on a specially prepared answer sheet that can be fed directly into an optical scan machine for scoring, a process similar to that of self-coding in the use of questionnaires and checklists. Projective tests in the psychological area present their own special problems. The scoring of these often has to be done by specially trained personnel. Sociological instruments may also have to be scaled if they are not of the self-scaling type, as are the graphic rating scales.

3. *Enter the data into the computer:* Data entry consists of transferring data from the basic document on which it was collected—a questionnaire, checklist, observer's record, or interviewer's schedule —to the computer. Data entry can be accomplished in various ways. Through optical scanning the data can be entered directly from the source document onto punched cards, magnetic tape, hard disks, floppy disks, or cartridges and then used as input to the computer. Or an operator can abstract the data from the document onto cards, tape, or disks, or directly into the computer through a keyboard. Data entry can also be accomplished from remote terminals, long distances away over telephone lines.

4. *Instruct the computer to tabulate and summarize the data:* The *program* of instructions may be from a statistical package and contained on cards, magnetic tape, disks, or cartridges. Programs can also be entered directly through a keyboard. While many statistical packages exist for microcomputers to summarize and tabulate data,

each has individual characteristics and advantages. A statistical package should be judged on its ability to manipulate data, the variety of statistical procedures it provides, the output quality produced, speed and accuracy, and ease of use.[3] For microcomputers the following are examples of statistical packages containing most data manipulation and statistical procedures that would be used in nursing research:

AbStat 3.3
Anderson-Bell
P.O. Box 191
Canon City, CO 81212
303/275-1661

Crisp 83.1
Crunch Software
1541 Ninth Ave.
San Francisco, CA 94122
415/564-7337

Microstat Release 4.0
Ecosoft, Inc.
P.O. Box 68602
Indianapolis, IN 46268
317/255-6476

SL-Micro
Questionnaire Service Company
P.O. Box 23056
Lansing, MI 48909
517/641-4428

Systat
Systat, Inc.
1127 Asbury Ave.
Evanston, IL 60202
312/864-5670

SPSS/PC
SPSS, Inc.
444 N. Michigan Ave.
Chicago, IL 60611
312/329-2400

5. *Tabulate the data:* The end product of descriptive studies is the computation of summary measures for the data that have been collected and the preparation of statistical tables that portray the data in summary form for the variables studied. If the data are based on samples, confidence intervals are computed for the various statistics.

In explanatory studies a procedure known as testing the significance of the data is performed. This procedure, to be discussed in the following chapter, is analogous to the computation of confidence intervals for sample estimates. It tests whether there is statistical significance in the differences between the values of the criterion measures for the alternative groups studied.

With appropriate programs computers can summarize data into tables, and compute the summary measures—means, medians, rates, standard deviations—and their confidence intervals. Computers can also easily perform tests of significance. In studies involving a large number of summary measures or employing more complicated tests of significance, the use of electronic computers is the most efficient way of processing data. As described by Rand:[4]

A Cambridge couple . . . have begun studying crime and juvenile delinquency by computer analysis of figures they have been collecting since the nineteen-thirties. Someone else has calculated word frequencies in twelve of the Federalist Papers as a means of assigning their authorship to either Madison or Hamilton; Madison was declared the winner. And last winter a visiting psychologist did a computer study of a nine-session psychotherapy undertaken by a psychiatrist several years ago and recorded by him verbatim in book form. In this study, the text was fed into a machine programmed to count various word usages of the patient and the psychiatrist throughout the nine sessions—and also to calculate changes in the frequency of these usages as the sessions progressed . . . the psychologist's work is typical of much that is being done in Cambridge today—by historians, anthropologists, public health experts, and many others. With the computer's help, they are paying profound attention to small, specific details that may mean little singly but when plotted in a big way are expected to reveal larger, less tangible truths.

Computers can be used not only to process great masses of data and to perform mathematical operations quickly, but also to solve problems in a manner analogous to the research process. One such technique, known as "simulation," is a method of programming a computer to imitate a real-life situation in terms of an abstract mathematical model. The purpose is to find out what could happen if certain variables included in the model were altered. Computer simulation has been used to predict nursing requirements under varying social and economic conditions.[5]

An electronic computer can thus be a most valuable aid to research, as a tool for processing data as well as a problem-solving instrument. For some studies, however, the amount of data collected may not warrant the expense involved in employing electronic computers. It is difficult to set forth generally applicable guidelines for determining when to consider the use of computers in a study. However, one should consider their use in any study with reasonably large data requirements.

PROCESSING DATA BY HAND

The steps in hand processing of the data are analogous to the use of computers. Briefly the steps are:

1. *Edit the raw data:* Review the data contained in the data-collecting instruments—questionnaires, checklists, observers, records, tests, scales, interviewers' records—for completeness and accuracy.

2. *Tally the data on worksheets:* Worksheets are a means of bringing together in one place the data collected on all study subjects. For each variable studied, the frequency with which each scale value was reported for the individual subjects can be recorded by means of tally marks:

Male	𝟕𝑯𝑳	𝟕𝑯𝑳	𝟕𝑯𝑳	/
Female	𝟕𝑯𝑳	𝟕𝑯𝑳	𝟕𝑯𝑳	𝟕𝑯𝑳 ///

Worksheets are so arranged as to permit the cross-tabulation of variables—the si-multaneous tallying of the scale values of two or more variables for each individual:

	IMPROVED	NOT IMPROVED
Male	𝟕𝑯𝑳 𝟕𝑯𝑳 //	𝟕𝑯𝑳
Female	𝟕𝑯𝑳 𝟕𝑯𝑳 𝟕𝑯𝑳 /	𝟕𝑯𝑳 //

3. *Tabulate the data:* This involves converting the tally marks to actual numbers, computing summary measures, preparing summary tabulations of the data, and if required by the study, computing confidence intervals for sample estimates. In explanatory studies this step frequently includes performing tests of statistical significance. For these activities a desk calculator is usually used.

Preparing Summary Measures and Tabulations of the Data

The main summary measures are:

- For qualitative data—rates, ratios, percentages
- For quantitative data—measures of central tendency: mean, median, mode; measures of variation: range, standard deviation

In addition to these, other types of summary measures can be computed. The decision concerning which to compute should be based on the nature of the variables studied—qualitative variables require one type while quantitative variables require another. The types of summary measures computed also depend on the nature of the distribution of the values of the measurements in the population—highly skewed distributions, for example, are better summarized by the median than the mean.

The end product in processing data is usually the preparation of statistical tables, which can take many different forms, but essentially contain the same basic ingredients. The preparation of statistical tables begins with the design of the outline of the table, called dummy or skeleton tables. In all studies it is highly advisable that skeleton tables be prepared before any data are collected, since they can be of great assistance in clarifying the variables being studied and in directing and focusing the analysis of the data, which in turn clarifies the focus of the total study.

Table 14-1 shows a skeleton outline of a table called an "explanatory table." Explanatory tables show the data for a dependent variable—in this case the average percentage of patients reporting dissatisfaction with length of time spent waiting for nursing service—in relationship to an independent variable. In Table 14-1 there are actually two independent variables: age of the patients and size of the room accommodations. Explanatory tables, thus, present data concerning the *relationship among the variables* studied. By contrast "descriptive tables" (below) usually present data for only one variable at a time:

Number of Patients by Size of Room Accommodations

SIZE OF ROOM	NUMBER OF PATIENTS
All room accommodations	227
Private	20
Two beds	94
3–6 beds	60
7 or more beds	53

The major components of an explanatory table are:

1. *Title:* Describes the data contained in the table—the variables for whom the data

TABLE 14-1.
A Skeleton Layout of a Statistical Table†

Average percentage of patients* reporting dissatisfaction with length of time spent waiting for nursing services, by age of patient and size of room accommodation, 60 general hospitals, 1956. } (1) **Title**

Percentages denote the percentage of the total number of patients in each age and accommodation group who reported dissatisfaction with length of time spent waiting for nursing services. } (2) **Headnote**

(6) **Column**

AGE OF PATIENTS*	ALL ROOM ACCOMMODATIONS	NUMBER OF BEDS IN ROOM			
		PRIVATE	2 BEDS	3–6 BEDS	7 OR MORE BEDS
All ages					
(5) Under 20 years					
20–29	(7) **Cell**				
30–39					
40–49					
50–59					
60 and over					

(4) **Box Head**

(5) **Line**

(3) **Stub**

(8) **Body**

*Nonobstetrical patients. } (9) **Footnote**

†*Source:* Questionnaires to patients in 60 general hospitals. For a complete report of the study see Faye G. Abdellah and Eugene Levine, *Effect of Nurse Staffing on Satisfactions with Nursing Care.* American Hospital Association, Monograph No. 4, 1958. } (10) **Source**

are presented, the study subjects, where the data were collected, and the time period to which they refer.

2. *Headnote:* Contains information pertaining to the table as a whole that would be unwieldy if placed in the title. Headnotes are used infrequently.

3. *Stub:* Contains the scale categories for one of the independent variables. If there is more than one independent variable, the main variable is usually shown in the stub.

4. *Box head:* Contains the scale categories for the second independent variable. If there is only one independent variable, it is shown in the stub and the box head is not used.

5. *Line:* Shows the data on the dependent variable for one scale category of the independent variable contained in the stub according to the scale categories of the independent variable contained in the box head.

6. *Column:* Shows the data on the dependent variable for one scale category of the independent variable contained in the box head according to the scale categories of the independent variable contained in the stub.

7. *Cell:* The intersection of a scale category of one variable with a scale category of the other variable.

8. *Body:* The aggregate of all the cells in the table.

9. *Footnote:* Provides additional information for a specific part of the table, if needed.

10. *Source:* Describes the origin of the data.

SUMMARIZING RESEARCH DATA

In research, measures for individual study subjects obtained through the use of qualitative or quantitative scales are frequently combined and a summary measure computed for the total group. Comparisons are then made of the summary measures for different study groups. Therefore, research usually deals with group measures rather than with measures of individuals, although occasionally data for individuals composing the different groups are compared individual by individual.

The following brief discussion of some of

the more common summary measures is not definitive. Excellent statistical textbooks provide a thorough explanation of these measures, some of which are cited in the bibliography. This discussion will provide some insight into how the individual measures made in a study can be summarized in a meaningful way.

Qualitative Scales

The summarization of data obtained from qualitative scales (nominal or ordinal) is not mathematically sophisticated as are summarizations of measurements obtained from quantitative scales. Qualitative scales produce counts of the number of study subjects in each scale category. One of the most effective ways of summarizing such data is in the form of percentages. For example, for a group of 275 hospitalized patients classified into three categories according to nursing care needs, the following distribution was found: intensive care 31, intermediate care 177, self-care 67. To convert these figures into percentages, each figure can be multiplied by 100 to move the decimal point two places to the right, which puts the data into manageable whole numbers, and each is then divided by the total, 275. The following percentage distribution is obtained:

	PERCENT
TOTAL	100*
Intensive care	11
Intermediate care	64
Self-care	24

*Note: adds to 99 because of the process of rounding off the figures

Percentages are a type of summary measure known as a *rate*. A rate expresses the relative frequency of occurrence of the particular scale value for which it is computed. For the 275 patients in the example cited, the relative frequency of occurrence of intensive care needs is 11 per 100 patients.

In a rate the denominator denotes the total "group at risk," so to speak, to exposure to the variable being studied. The notion of "at risk" comes from the field of vital statistics where such rates as death rates, case fatality rates, prevalence rates, provide a summary measure of the number of individuals enumerated in a specific class of the variable from the total group "exposed" to the variable.

In a death rate the denominator represents the total group exposed to the risk of dying. The scale for this variable consists of two alternative categories: died, did not die. The numerator expresses the number of the total who were exposed to death who actually died.

Suppose we are interested in computing the death rate among the patients composing the active case load during the year of a home nursing care program. We would multiply the number of deaths occurring among the total case load by 100 (or some multiple of 100) to have the resulting rate in a whole number, and then we would divide the figure by the total case load. If the total case load were 26,433 and the number of deaths 619, the death rate, called a case fatality rate, would be 2.3 per 100 cases ($619 \times 100 \div 26,433$), or in whole numbers, 23 per 1,000 cases. This rate could be refined even further. The total case load could be divided into specific disease categories—cardiovascular, cancer, communicable diseases, and so on—and the case fatality rate computed for each category by dividing the number of deaths occurring among patients having the specific disease by the total number of cases in the disease category.

A true rate (relative frequency) has the following basic formula:

$$\frac{a}{a + b}$$

Where:

a = Number of individuals in a specific category of the variable

b = Number of individuals in all other categories of the variable

In a true rate the numerator is included in the denominator. If the summary measure does not possess this property, it is not a true rate. The so-called sex ratio shows the number of males in the group for every 100 females. To illustrate, if the number of males in our total home care case load is 10,415, and the number of females is 16,018, the sex ratio is 65 males for every 100 females: $\frac{10,415 \times 100}{16,018}$. It is obvious that this is not a true relative frequency, since the numerator (number of males) is not part of the denominator. If it were we would have a true rate. Such a true rate would show the percentage of the total case load that consists of males:

$$\frac{10,415 \times 100}{26,433} = 39 \text{ percent.}$$

Table 14–2 contains some of the most widely used rates in the field of vital statistics. In these rates the total group at risk is usually the entire population of a community, city, state, or nation. However, the denominator could also consist of a selected group of study subjects (patients in a hospital, students in a school, residents of a housing development). The rates shown in Table 14–2 have been frequently used as criterion measures in research studies in the health field. Death rates have played important roles as criterion measures in research such as that linking smoking to cancer of the lung. Incidence rates are widely used in research on causes of cancer.

The use of rates as summary measures of qualitatively scaled variables has several important advantages in research:

1. They are true relative frequencies and can be subjected to statistical tests of significance (see Chapter 15). In experimental studies of the effects of different methods of treatment on the survival rates of patients (similar to death rates except the numerator consists of the group who lived rather than died), a test of the significance of differences in rates can be applied as in the following data:

TREATMENT GROUPS	TOTAL IN GROUP	NUMBER LIVING AFTER 1 YEAR	1-YEAR SURVIVAL RATES (IN PERCENT)
Group I	176	114	64.8
Group II	191	119	62.3
Group III	183	101	55.2
Group IV	166	113	68.1

2. Rates reduce large numbers which are difficult to interpret into simpler, more digestible data. In the following data the first column, showing the number of graduates from schools of nursing in the United States according to performance on state board exams, is much more difficult to interpret than the corresponding percentages:

	NUMBER OF GRADUATES	PERCENTAGES OF GRADUATES
TOTAL	(35,328)	(100.0)
Passed	29,647	83.9
Failed	5,681	16.1

3. Rates are especially advantageous as summary measures in comparing data for

TABLE 14–2.
Rates Used in Vital Statistics

NAME OF RATE	HOW COMPUTED
1. Prevalence rate	$\dfrac{\text{All cases of specific disease at given time} \times 1{,}000}{\text{Population at given time}}$
2. Case fatality rate	$\dfrac{\text{Deaths from specific disease in given period} \times 100}{\text{Cases of specific disease in given period}}$
3. Annual death rate	$\dfrac{\text{Deaths from all causes in calendar year} \times 1{,}000}{\text{Population of July 1}}$
4. Annual age-specific death rate	$\dfrac{\text{Death from all causes for given age group in year} \times 1{,}000}{\text{Population for given age group, July 1}}$
5. Annual death rate from specific cause	$\dfrac{\text{Deaths from specific cause in year} \times 100{,}000}{\text{Population of July 1}}$
6. Annual case incidence rate of a specific disease	$\dfrac{\text{New cases of specific disease in year} \times 1{,}000}{\text{Population of July 1}}$
7. Annual birth rate	$\dfrac{\text{Live births in year} \times 1{,}000}{\text{Population of July 1}}$
8. Stillbirth rate	$\dfrac{\text{Stillbirths in year} \times 100(\text{or } 1{,}000)}{\text{Total births in year}}$
9. Infant mortality rate	$\dfrac{\text{Deaths under one year of age in year} \times 1{,}000}{\text{Live births in year}}$
10. Neonatal mortality rate	$\dfrac{\text{Deaths under one month of age in year} \times 1{,}000 \text{ (or } 10{,}000)}{\text{Live births in year}}$
11. Maternal mortality rate	$\dfrac{\text{Maternal deaths in year} \times 1{,}000 \text{ (or } 10{,}000)}{\text{Live births in year}}$

different-sized groups. The rates, expressed in terms of per 100, per 1,000, or some other base, reduce the data to comparable units. Thus, a comparison of the number of deaths among the patients in two hospitals that differ greatly in size can give the misleading impression that the occurrence of death was greater in the larger hospital when in fact on a relative frequency basis the reverse was true:

	TOTAL NUMBER OF PATIENTS ADMITTED DURING THE YEAR	NUMBER OF DEATHS AMONG PATIENTS ADMITTED	DEATH RATE PER 1,000 PATIENTS
Hospital A	21,415	419	19.6
Hospital B	7,631	184	24.1

4. Rates are statements of probability of occurrence, and as such can be useful in making predictions.

Quantitative Scales

For many quantitatively scaled variables the values of measurements for the individual subjects follow what is known as a bell-shaped curve if plotted on a graph. In such a graph the vertical axis, known as the Y axis, represents the number of study subjects having the values measured, and the horizontal axis, the X axis, represents the values of the scale. The bell-shaped curve shows that the majority of the subjects cluster together and have about the same scale value, while fewer subjects are found at the extremes. The ideal *bell-shaped curve* is called the *normal curve*, the normal frequency distribution, or the *Gaussian curve,* after its discoverer the German mathematician Karl F. Gauss. Such a curve, shown in Figure 14–1, has a single peak where the majority of subjects cluster. As the values of the measures fan out symmetrically from the central peak, the curve tapers off to the extremes, where only a few subjects are found.

In actual studies the distributions of measurements do not precisely follow the shape of the normal curve. Measurements of some variables are better described by other types of curves. In general, though, these curves will also have the property of a single peak, and the values taper off at each side of the peak, but not so symmetrically.

For many quantitatively scaled variables, the normal curve provides a rough approximation of the distribution of the measurements of the variable. It can be used without violating statistical theory as the model for the analysis of many variables employed in research studies.

Distributions of measurements of variables having quantitative scales can be described by two summary measures. One, known as the *measure of central tendency,* or the *average, is the measure of the value that is most typical of the values of all the individual measurements.* In a normal curve it is the value on the X axis that lies beneath the peak of the curve (in Figure

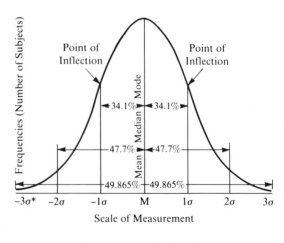

Figure 14–1 The normal, bell-shaped distribution.

KEY POINT

14–1, it is the value labeled M). The other summary measure is that of the variation of the values of the individual measurements around the average value. This is known as the *measure of the dispersion of the individual values.*

Theoretically, measures of central tendency and variation are applicable only to data obtained from quantitatively scaled variables. However, they are also used for qualitatively scaled variables. For example, achievement and other types of psychological tests, which usually yield ordinal-type data, are scored and analyzed, not by rates as for qualitatively scaled data, but by the measures of central tendency and variation for quantitatively scaled data. Teachers compute the average score and the variation of the scores for students on achievement tests.

In addition, the rates obtained for qualitatively scaled variables are often averaged. For example, the percentage of the population immunized against polio could be computed for each of the communities studied. The individual percentages can be combined in terms of a summary measure that expresses the average percentage of the population immunized in all communities studied. In a sense the individual percentages for each community are quantitative measures of the extent to which the members of each community are immunized. Therefore, they can be treated as values arising from a quantitative scale.

Measures of Central Tendency

The three main summary measures that describe the central tendency of a distribution of measures of a quantitative variable are the *mode, median,* and *mean* and are known as averages. When the individual measures form a normal curve, the values of the three summary measures are equal. In distributions that depart from normality the values are different.

To illustrate the differences in the three measures, assume we are experimentally testing the effects on their blood pressure of giving patients an extra amount of tender loving care. Our experimental group is labeled A and the control group receiving the usual amount of T.L.C. is labeled B. Randomly allocate thirty patients (and the personnel, too) to the two alternative groups, fifteen in each group. Then apply extra T.L.C. generously to Group A and after a suitable period of time measure the blood pressures for the fifteen patients in each group:

PATIENT NO.	BLOOD PRESSURE	
	GROUP A	GROUP B
1	130	161
2	139	112
3	149	155
4	120	101
5	118	176
6	130	97
7	138	137
8	160	128
9	110	185
10	145	248
11	148	133
12	123	129
13	105	114
14	155	179
15	130	104

MODE

The mode is the most common or typical value in a distribution of measurements. It is found by locating the value occurring most frequently. In Group A the most common value is 130, since it was recorded for three patients. For Group B no value appears more frequently than another; thus there is no modal value.

As a descriptive as well as an analytical summary measure the mode is less frequently used than the other two averages. One of its shortcomings is the fact that it is sometimes incalculable. Also it may be an arbitrary value. This is particularly true when the individual measurements are grouped into classes and the value of the mode is influenced by the grouping of values the researcher selects.

MEDIAN

When the values of the measurements are arranged in order of magnitude, the median is the value that is larger than half of the values and smaller than the other half —the middle value of a distribution. To determine the median blood pressure values for our two groups of fifteen patients first arrange the individual values in order of magnitude:

GROUP A	GROUP B
105	97
110	101
118	104
120	112
123	114
130	128
130	129
130	133
138	137
139	155
145	161
148	176
149	179
155	185
160	248

The median blood pressure reading for Group A is 130 and for Group B is 133. These values are the middle values among the groups of readings: they are the eighth values among the fifteen readings when they are arranged in order of magnitude. They are larger than seven of the values and smaller than the other seven. Thus in a series of measurements arranged in order of size consisting of an *odd* number of measurements, the median value is actually the middle value. If a series of measurements consists of an even number of items, the median would be found lying between the *two* middle values. For example, if Group B consisted of only 14 values (omit 248), the median would lie between 129 and 133. In practice these two values are added together and divided by 2 to obtain a single value for the median, which in this example would be 131: (129 + 133) /2.

The median is a very useful summary measure of central tendency, particularly where the distribution of measures departs significantly from the model of the normal curve. Such asymmetrical distributions are called *"skewed"* distributions. The median is simple to calculate only requiring the individual values to be arranged in order of magnitude.

MEAN

Unlike the two previous summary measures, which depend upon the most frequently occurring value (mode) or the value located in the middle when the values are arranged in order of magnitude (median), the mean is calculated by taking account of the actual value of each of the individual measurements. The mean is simply the sum of all the values divided by the number of values. For Group A the mean is 2,000/15 = 133. For Group B it is 2,159/15 = 144.

The mean is probably the most widely used measure of central tendency. One of the reasons is its mathematical properties, not possessed by the mode or median, which make it very valuable in statistical analysis of the data. These properties are:

1. If the value of each individual measurement is subtracted from the mean and the differences (deviations) are then added, with the plus and minus signs of the deviations considered, the sum of the deviations will always be zero.

2. If these deviations are squared (the value of each deviation multiplied by itself) and then summed up, the value of this sum will be smaller than the value of the sum of the squared deviations of each value from any quantity other than the mean.

Because of these properties, as well as the fact that the actual value of each measurement is considered in its calculation, the mean provides more information about a set of measurement values than do the other averages.

Measures of Variation

KEY POINT

The other important summary measure is the *measure of variation of the individual values*. This tells us how much the values for the subjects differ. Such a measure complements the measure of central tendency, since it is obvious that two sets of measurements could have identical values for their measures of central tendency, yet be very different in terms of the spread of the individual values. For simplicity, take two groups of five patients in which the following body temperatures are recorded:

GROUP A	GROUP B
98.6° F.	96.6° F.
98.6°	97.6°
98.6°	98.6°
98.6°	99.6°
98.6°	100.6°

The mean and median would be identical for both groups—98.6°F.—yet it is obvious that the two distributions of temperatures are very different. In Group A there is no variation among the patients whereas in Group B there is a considerable amount of difference in the temperatures recorded.

There are many summary measures of variation. Three will be briefly described: *range, percentile,* and *standard deviation.*

RANGE

This is the simplest measure of variation to compute. It consists of the lowest and highest values in the set of measurements. Sometimes the range is considered as the difference between the lowest and highest values. Thus in our blood pressure data (p. 256) the range is 105–160 for Group A. For Group B it is 97–248. This means that Group B's measurements have greater variation than do Group A's. A shortcoming of the range is that it is greatly influenced by extreme values. In Group B, the reading of 248 is considerably out of line with the rest of the measurements. If it

were excluded. the range would be 97–185, much closer to Group A's range.

PERCENTILE

The concept of percentiles, not to be confused with percentages, is an elaboration of the concept of median. A percentile is a positional value that is found by lining up the values in order of magnitude. The median is the fiftieth percentile. To find any other percentile we would follow the same procedure as in locating the median. To find the tenth percentile we find the value that is larger than 10 percent of the measurements and is smaller than 90 percent of them. Conversely, the ninetieth percentile is the value that is larger than 90 percent of the values and is smaller than 10 percent of them. For the blood pressure data it would be difficult to calculate percentiles, since there are so few values. Percentiles are most meaningful when the number of measurements is large, preferably in the hundreds. Roughly, the tenth percentile for Group A lies somewhere between 105 and 110 and for Group B is between 97 and 101.

Percentiles have many interesting uses both descriptively and analytically. They have been widely applied in the field of psychological tests and measurements. *As a measure of variation the percentile has an advantage over the range in that it tones down the effects of extreme values.* One such measure is called the interquartile range, the range between the twenty-fifth percentile (the first quartile) and the seventy-fifth percentile (the third quartile—the median is the second quartile). To illustrate how to find the first and third quartiles for our two groups of patients we would find the values that are higher than 25 percent of the values and are lower than 75 percent—the first quartile—and those that are higher than 75 percent of the values and are lower than 25 percent—the third quartile. For Group A the interquartile range is 120–148. And for Group B it is 112–176, indicating considerably greater variation of the values of individual measurements for this group of patients. In fact the interquartile range for Group B patients extends over twice the magnitude, 64, of the range for Group A, 28.

STANDARD DEVIATION

By far the most widely used measure of variation is the standard deviation. This measure complements the arithmetic mean. Briefly, the computation of the standard deviation is as follows: The difference between the values of each individual measurement and the mean is determined. Each deviation is then squared. The sum of all the squared deviations is divided by the number of measurements. The square root is then found of the resulting quotient (that number which when multiplied by itself will yield the quotient), which is the value of the standard deviation. For Group A the standard deviation is *16* and for Group B it is *40*.

It is obvious that the *value of a standard deviation provides a meaningful indication of the extent of variation among the values of the individual measurements*. If there were no differences among a set of measurements, the value of the standard deviation would be zero, as in the example of the five patients in Group A who had identical temperatures of 98.6°F. The greater the value of the standard deviation, the greater the variation among the values of the measurements.

Like the arithmetic mean, the standard deviation has several valuable mathematical properties. One is that in measurements distributed approximately like the normal curve, deviations of the value of the standard deviation from the arithmetic mean include the following percentage of all the values of the measurements found among the study subjects:

- Plus and minus one standard deviation from the mean = 68 percent of all the values
- Plus and minus two standard deviations from the mean = 95 percent of all the values
- Plus and minus three standard deviations from the mean = 100 percent of all the values

These ranges apply best where the number of measurements is large. In small groups of measures they are only approximate. To illustrate: in Group A the mean ±1 standard deviation gives the range 117–149 (133 ± 16). This range actually includes eleven of the fifteen values, or 73 percent of them. And ±3 standard deviations from the mean gives the range 85–181, which includes 100 percent of the fifteen values.

The various summary measures that we have computed for the quantitative measurements of the variable "blood pressure" for our two groups of fifteen patients are:

CENTRAL TENDENCY	GROUP A	GROUP B
Mode	130	Nonexistent
Median	130	133
Mean	133	144
VARIATION		
Range	105–160	97–248
Quartile range	120–148	112–176
Standard deviation	16	40

These summary measures provide a succinct and meaningful picture of the distribution of the individual measurements.

Grouped Data

When the number of individual measurements is large, it is best to group the measurements into a broader scale categories. From a descriptive standpoint grouped data are often more meaningful than ungrouped data. The detail provided by individual measurements may be unnecessary, since small differences in values may not indicate substantive differences in the variable measured. From an analytical viewpoint, grouping the data may reveal the shape of the distribution of measurements being analyzed. In grouping the data on the blood pressure measures we find that A patients appear to follow the pattern of the bell-shaped curve while the B patients' measurements can best be described by what is called a U-shaped curve.

BLOOD PRESSURE (GROUPED)	GROUP A	GROUP B
Total	15	15
Less than 120	3	5
120–139	7	4
140–159	4	1
160 and over	1	5

It is not difficult to compute summary measures from grouped measurements. When the number of measurements is very large, it is often faster to compute summary measures from grouped data than from individual measurements. Methods for such computations are contained in the statistical texts cited in the bibliography.

SUMMARY

The computer has made the processing and summarizing of statistical data in research fast, easy, and accurate. Inexpensive "personal" computers can be used for many research purposes in nursing. One danger is that the computer may replace the inquisitive, creative, and critical thinking that is necessary for fruitful research. It can also produce meaningless output that could mislead the data interpretation.

The main summary measures are the measures of central tendency and variation. These are important descriptive measures. Important, too, descriptively is the presentation of data in a statistical table. Summary measures and statistical tables can yield important interpretative information about research data.

REFERENCES

1. Study Group on Nursing Information Systems, "Computerized Nursing Information Systems: An Urgent Need." *Research in Nursing and Health*, 6:101–105, 1983.
2. Mary M. Ziemer, "Issues of Computer Literacy in Nursing Education." *Nursing and Health Care*, 5:537–542, December 1984.
3. Nancy Goodban and Kenji Hakuta, "Statistical Quintet." *PC World*, 2:186–195, September 1984.
4. Christopher Rand, "Center of a New World." *The New Yorker Magazine*, 58, 60, April 1964.
5. Massachusetts Area Health Education Center Program, *Nursing Manpower in Massachusetts: Projected Supply and Demand and Implications for Policy*. Worcester, MA, Massachusetts Area Health Education Center, July 1984.

PROBLEMS AND SUGGESTIONS FOR FURTHER STUDY

1. What does the term "computer literacy" mean? Describe the steps necessary in attaining computer literacy for the purposes of using computers in research. Note: Various articles in the December 1984 issue of *Nursing and Health Care* will be helpful in responding to this problem.
2. Computers are used for a variety of purposes including the statistical processing of data. Discuss the various applications of computers and indicate how these could be helpful in conducting research. In answering this question the following book could be helpful: Mary Ann Sweeney, *The Nurse's Guide to Computers*. New York, N.Y., Macmillan Publishing Co., 1985.
3. The following data are taken from a descriptive study reported in the *American Journal of Public Health* by Testoff and Levine on the characteristics of patients sixty five years of age and over who received public health nursing services in their homes on April 30, 1963.

Number of Patients Sixty Five Years of Age and Over Receiving Nursing Care at Home from Public Health Agencies, on April 30, 1963

AGE	NUMBER OF PATIENTS
Total all ages	17,501
65–69	3,400
70–74	4,148
75–79	3,776
80–84	3,376
85–89	1,825
90–94	770
95–99	170
100 and over	36

a. Convert the numbers into a percentage distribution.

b. What is the modal age group? What is the median age?

c. Would you say that this distribution is approximately a normal one? Is it symmetrical?

d. How would the arithmetic mean be computed from such data? The standard deviation?

4. Read the article by R. Cooper and others, "Is the Period of Rapidly Declining Adult Mortality in the United States Coming to an End?" *Am. J. Pub. Health,* **73:**1091–1093, September, 1983 and the Letter to the Editor "On Declining Adult Mortality in the U.S." *Am J. Pub. Health,* **74:**730–731, July 1984. What is meant by an age-standardized rate? What kind of summary measure is *life expectancy?* Why is a drop of 0.4 per 1,000 in the age-standardized mortality rate for adults important?

15

Data Analysis

OBJECTIVES

- **To describe the most commonly used techniques of statistical analysis.**
- **To explain the difference between techniques for quantitative and qualitative variables.**

- **To describe the application of techniques to the analyses of multiple variables.**

Most researchers are concerned with drawing inferences from sample data about populations. The two main purposes of statistical inference are to test statistical hypotheses and to estimate population parameters. In testing statistical hypotheses, we use information from a random sample to test preconceived ideas about the population from which our data are a sample. Statistical estimation deals with estimating values of parameters from observations of a random sample.

A single value, which is in a sense the best single guess as to the value of the parameter being estimated, is called a point estimate. Examples are: (1) measures of central tendency and (2) rates. However, the point estimate does not provide a measure of the degree of confidence we may place in the estimate; the sampling error is the measure of the precision of the estimate, expressed in terms of the confidence interval.

A fundamental purpose of statistical analysis is to determine the amount of sampling error in the data. In random sampling the sampling error arises from having randomly selected one set of sampling units from the many sets that could have been selected. As was shown in chapter 13, p. 242 the number of different samples of size 15 out of a target population of 100 is $\dfrac{100!}{15!\,85!}$

In random assignment of subjects to alternative groups the sampling error arises from having randomly allocated the subjects to certain groups from the many groups that could have been formed from the total number of subjects in the study.

The number of different groups (samples) of subjects that could be formed by randomly assigning thirty subjects to two equal-sized groups is $\frac{30!}{15!\ 15!}$, a huge number indeed.

In descriptive studies the sampling error is computed as a measure of the precision of the estimate obtained from the sample. This is done by computing confidence intervals around the sample estimates of the population parameters. The interpretation of the confidence interval is as follows: If we draw repeated samples of size n, and if for each of these samples we estimate the population parameter and its corresponding confidence interval, which is a random variable, then we may expect a certain percentage of these intervals, called the level of confidence, to include the population parameter. Thus, in the example of blood pressure measures, introduced in Chapter 14, the mean blood pressure for Group A patients was 133, and the sampling error (standard error) of the mean was computed to be 4.1. At a level of confidence of 95 percent the mean blood pressure for the population was estimated to lie within the range of 124.8–141.2. The mean blood pressure for Group B patients was 144, and with a standard error of 10.3 the 95 percent confidence interval is 123.4–164.6. Because the variability of the measurements among the Group B patients is considerably higher than for Group A—the standard deviation for Group B is 40 compared with 16 for Group A—the estimate of the population mean for Group A is more precise than for Group B.

KEY POINT In explanatory studies the purpose is to evaluate whether the values of the summary measures for the alternative groups are different. Such an evaluation is done through a technique known as a *test of significance*. The purpose of the test is to see whether the summary measures being compared, after making allowances for sampling error, could be independent estimates of the same population parameter.

It would be unwise to attempt to provide a detailed discussion of available statistical techniques in this book. Many excellent books exist that explain in detail the rationale and methodology for these techniques. Some books are even devoted to a single methodology, such as analysis of variance or multiple regression.

The purpose of this chapter is to present an overview of the most widely applicable techniques in nursing research. Deep understanding is not the intent since lengthy exposition would be required to do justice to this subject. The intention is to convey an appreciation of the rationale for the use of these techniques. It is hoped that an understanding will be gained of the conditions under which the techniques can be best applied as well as the appropriateness of the application.

As we indicated in the previous chapter, the advent of the computer has made it possible to apply the most advanced form of statistical analysis on even the smallest electronic computers without an in depth understanding of the techniques themselves. The danger in this is the possible misapplication of techniques. Also, excessive and unnecessary tests of significance can result in findings of statistical significance by chance along.

While care has to be taken not to "overanalyze," the availability of the computer for statistical analysis has been a boon to research. In the previous chapter mention was made of the "statistical packages" that can enable even the smallest computers to perform a variety of useful functions in research.

The use of computers in providing the summary descriptive measures of central tendency and variation was mentioned. In this chapter we move from descriptive statistics to inferential statistics in which we are essentially interested in drawing inferences about the relationships among our study variables. The computer and the statistical packages that are available to inform and direct the statistical analyses are ideally suited to analyze the relationships through a variety of statistical techniques.

Although sharp distinctions are often drawn between descriptive and inferential statistical techniques, the latter are frequently used for descriptive purposes. Multiple regression, for example, can be used as a descriptive tool to summarize the dependence of one variable on others. Correlation coefficients are often used to summarize the extent to which variables are related to each other.

The major techniques of statistical analysis can be classified several ways. First are the techniques that are primarily used when the dependent variable is quantitative— measured on at least an interval scale— —and those where the dependent variable is qualitatively scaled. Quantitatively scaled variables form distributions and yield parameters (summary measures) so that the techniques analyzing them are called parametric. Qualitatively scaled variables are essentially distribution-free, and the techniques for analyses are called nonparametric.

Techniques can also be divided according to the number of variables they analyze. Summary measures of single variables are labeled univariate statistics. Techniques to analyze the relationship between one dependent variable and one independent variable are called bivariate techniques, or, as in the case of analysis of variance, "one-way" techniques. Techniques to analyze a single dependent variable and two or more independent variables are called multivariate techniques, although that term is sometimes reserved for methods of analyzing the relationship among more than one *dependent* variable and multiple independent variables. A more detailed discussion of the most important statistical techniques follows.

TESTS OF SIGNIFICANCE FOR QUANTITATIVE VARIABLES

Variables that are measurable in terms of either interval or ratio scales are called *quantitative variables*. Such variables have a continuous numerical distribution and when used as criterion measures can provide refined distinctions among the sub-

jects. In explanatory studies the purpose is to assess the relationship between the independent variable, whose different levels or versions are represented by the different groups of subjects, and the dependent variable, measured by the criterion measure. When the criterion measure possesses a numerical scale, summary measures such as a mean and standard deviation are computed for the values of the measurements of the individuals composing the groups. *The test of significance evaluates the differences in the values of the summary measures for the groups to determine to what extent they could have arisen by random sampling.* In comparing two means, the *t* test is usually employed. In comparing more than two means, as in studies having more than two study groups or where more than one independent variable is being tested at the same time, the technique of *analysis of variance* is the most widely used method.

KEY POINT

Test of Significance of the Difference Between Two Means

In a test of the significance of the difference between the mean blood pressure readings for Group A patients of 133 and Group B of 144, the question is: considering the sampling error for these means, what is the probability that they could have come from the same population? That is, are the patients in the two groups really samples from the same population? For Group A patients the interval within which the population mean could be estimated to lie with 95 percent confidence is 124.8 to 141.2 and for Group B the interval is 123.4 to 164.6. The interval for B encompasses that for A, giving rise to the belief that the two sample estimates could have come from the same population. In other words, the difference between the means of the two samples, 133 and 144, may well be due to sampling error and not to the independent variable being tested.

Sampling error could have been generated in these data in two ways. In a nonexperimental explanatory study of the relationship between quality of nursing care provided and blood pressure levels of the patients, we could have selected a random sample of fifteen patients from one hospital known to provide high-quality care, called Group A, and another random sample of fifteen, called Group B, from a hospital known to provide lower-quality care. Or, in an experimental study we could have taken thirty patients, randomly assigned them to two groups, the A patients receiving high-quality nursing care (lots of reassurance, emotional support, T.L.C., etc.) and the B patients receiving minimal care. Then, after both groups have been suitably exposed to the independent variable we could measure their blood pressures. The hypothesis would be concerned with the relationship between quality of care and patients' blood pressure.

Instead of comparing the confidence intervals for the summary measures for the two groups, the usual procedure is to do a test of significance of the difference in the values of the summary measures. For a comparison of two means *computed from small samples* the test is called a *t* test. This test is based on Student's *t* distribution rather than the normal distribution that was discussed in Chapter 14. The *t* test is in the form of the following ratio:

$$t = \frac{\text{Difference in sample means minus difference in population means*}}{\text{Standard error of the difference in sample means}}$$

The denominator of this ratio, the standard error of the difference between two sample means, is directly analogous to the standard error of a sample mean. The standard error of a sample mean is the standard deviation of a sampling distribution of means—the distribution of the values of all the means that could be calculated from repeated samplings of a specified number of sampling units from the target population. The standard error of the dif-

ference between sample means is the standard deviation of a sampling distribution of differences between means—the distribution of the values of all *differences* between means that could be calculated from repeated samplings of a specified number of samplings units from two populations. And if the two population means have the same value—in essence, the two populations are the same population with respect to their mean values—the mean of the sampling distribution of differences between means would be equal to zero. Such a sampling distribution, with a mean equal to zero and a standard deviation equal to the standard error of the differences between two means, is the statistical model underlying tests of differences between two sample summary measures.

The standard error of the difference between two sample means is calculated from the following formula:

$$s_p\sqrt{\frac{1}{n_1} + \frac{1}{n_2}}$$

Where: s_p = a weighted average of the two sample standard deviations
n_1 = size of first sample
n_2 = size of second sample

Note that the denominator of the *t*-test is in terms of standard error units. Thus, the *t* ratio converts the numerator of the ratio—the difference in sample means—into standard error units. In interpreting the *t* ratio value, the size of sample upon which it is based must be considered. For example: in samples of size 5, ±2.6 standard errors include 95 percent of the values, and in samples of size 30 ±2.0 standard errors will include 95 percent of the values. Thus if our ratio exceeds 2.0—that is, the difference between the sample means is larger than twice the value of the standard error of the difference between the means —it has exceeded the 5 percent level of significance. In other words, the difference that we have found in the values of the summary measures for the alternative groups would occur less than five times out of 100 in repeated random samplings. Since such an occurrence is rare, we say

---

*In most applications of this test the difference in population means is hypothesized as being zero (null hypothesis), therefore, in the following discussion this term will be omitted from the formula.

that the difference between the sample measures is significantly greater than zero.

The normal distribution can be used to evaluate the differences between sample means where the samples are large, consisting of more than thirty sampling units; in smaller-sized samples the t distribution is used. From the properties of a normal distribution, we have seen that approximately ± 2 standard errors includes 95 percent of all the values in a distribution. Tests based on the normal distribution are called by some T tests and by others the K test or Z test. This test is identical with that of t, having the ratio:

$$T = \frac{\text{Difference in sample means}}{\substack{\text{Standard error of the} \\ \text{difference in sample means}}}$$

The 5 percent level has been traditionally accepted as a suitable level of significance for many studies, although other levels could be chosen. The 1 percent level—that of finding a difference in the sample summary measures that, in a sample of size 30, would be nearly three times larger than the value of the standard error of the difference between the sample measures—signifies that such a difference could occur by chance only 1 time in 100. This is a more stringent significance level than the 5 percent level because larger differences are required between the sample statistics before they are considered to be significantly greater than the value that could be attributable to random sampling error.

The levels of significance of the values of the t ratio for various-sized samples are as follows:

SIZE OF SAMPLE t TEST	LEVEL OF SIGNIFICANCE	
	5%	1%
5	2.57	4.03
10	2.23	3.17
15	2.13	2.95
20	2.09	2.84
25	2.06	2.79
30	2.04	2.75
T-test	1.96	2.58

Applying the t test to the data on the difference between the mean blood pressures for Groups A and B, we find that the value of this difference is $144 - 133 = 11$. The standard error of this difference, determined from the formula just provided, is 11.1, $(30.5 \sqrt{1/15 + 1/15})$, since Group A's standard deviation is 16 and Group B's is 40, and as both have sample sizes of 15 the weighted average of the two sample standard deviations (s_p) is 30.5. The t ratio value is, therefore, $11/11.1$ or 1, which is well below the 5 percent level and thus not considered statistically significant. This confirms the conclusions from the comparison of the confidence intervals for the means of the two groups where it was found that the interval for Group A fell within the interval for Group B. The conclusion is that both means come from the same population, and are therefore not considered significantly different. In terms of the hypothesis being tested there is no relationship between quality of nursing care and blood pressure levels of patients.

Analysis of Variance

Many explanatory studies are directed toward a comparison of the values of quantitative criterion measures for more than two groups. Instead of comparing the mean blood pressures for Groups A and B, more than two groups could have been set up in the experiment, each representing a different scale value of the independent variable, quality of nursing care. Moreover, many studies are concerned with the analysis of the effects of multiple independent variables, as in a factorial design. The method of statistical analysis of such data is called the *analysis of variance* (ANOVA). Originally conceived by the late R.A. Fisher and coworkers, this is a powerful statistical tool for analyzing multiple comparisons. It is intimately related to the design of experiments and is the analytical method for treating data obtained from such designs as the *latin square* and the *factorial design*.

The computational procedure for the

analysis of variance is contained in most texts on statistical methodology. This procedure is a rather straightforward and ingenious one. It consists in its simplest application, called one-way analysis of variance, in which there is only one independent variable, of computing two kinds of variances (the square of the standard deviation): The variance of the measurements within each of the alternative groups and the variance among the means of the alternative groups. The first measure of variation is called the "within-group" variation and the second the "among-group" variation. The within-group variation should reflect only the effects of chance—as a consequence of randomization—since theoretically all subjects within a group have been treated identically. The among-group variation, in addition to being influenced by chance, should also reflect the effects of the independent variable being tested. The test of significance is called the F test (for R.A. Fisher) and is the ratio:

$$\frac{\text{Variance among groups}}{\text{Variance within groups}}$$

KEY POINT If there were no difference in the measurements among the groups, except for chance variation attributable to randomization, the value of the numerator of the F ratio would be similar to that of the denominator. To the extent that the means of the groups differ significantly from each other, the numerator tends to be larger than the denominator and the value of the ratio increases. Tables are available by which the level of significance of the value of the F ratio can be assessed. Thus, the F test is analogous to the t test. It provides the relative frequency (5 times out of 100, 1 time out of 100, etc.) of obtaining a value as large as that computed from the ratio by random sampling (randomization). The higher the value of the F ratio for specified-size samples, the greater the probability that the means being compared are really different from each other.

More complex forms of analysis of variance are available than one-way ANOVA. In *two-way ANOVA* two independent variables are present. In *repeated-measures ANOVA* the same subjects are observed at several different times or under different treatment conditions. In multivariate analyses of variance (MANOVA) more than one dependent variable is analyzed, somewhat similar to repeated-measures ANOVA, except that in the latter the same dependent variable is repeatedly measured. In the analysis of covariance (ANOCOVA) the effect of initial differences among the study groups is adjusted for or eliminated.

The analysis of variance is an important technique because it provides more information in factorial experiments than just a test of the significance of differences among the means of the groups. It also yields an assessment of the effects of combinations of the variables included in the study, known as the interactions.

Regression Techniques

The statistical model underlying hypotheses that express a relationship between independent and dependent variables is called the general linear hypothesis. In its most basic form the formula $Y = a + (b)\,X$ states that Y, the dependent variable, is a function of X, the independent variable. In this equation a is called the *intercept* and (b) the *slope of the line*. The equation states that whenever X is changed Y also changes. In studies of independent and dependent variables that are both measurable in terms of quantitative scales, if there were a sufficiently large number of sampling units, it would be possible to fit a regression equation to the data that would precisely express the relationship between the two variables. The test of significance of the relationship between the two variables would be based on an evaluation of the slope of the line that is fitted to the data, called the *regression coefficient*. That is to say, if two variables are positively related, the line fitted to the data—assuming that the relationship is linear, e.g., in the form of a straight line—should look as

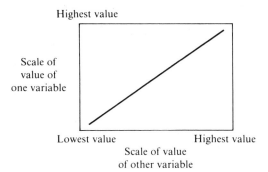

Figure 15–1 Positive relationship between two variables.

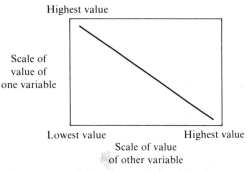

Figure 15–2 Negative relationship between two variables.

follows when plotted on a chart (see Figure 15–1:

Or, if the variables had a negative relationship, the chart would appear as follows (see Figure 15–2):

If there were no relationship between the variables, the slope of the line would be zero and the chart would appear as follows (see Figure 15–3):

The test of significance would be:

$$t = \frac{\text{Slope of the regression equation for sample data} \quad \text{minus} \quad \text{Slope of the regression equation for the population*}}{\text{Standard error of the slope}}$$

Regression analysis can be extended to include more than one independent variable. Known as multiple regression, the contribution (weight) of the values of each of the independent variables toward the value of the dependent variable can be assessed. Such an approach is analogous to a factorial design in which the data are analyzed by the method of analysis of variance.

An example of the use of multiple regression analysis in a study in nursing is reported in *Effect of Nurse Staffing on Satisfactions with Nursing Care.*[1] In this study, the dependent variable was a measure of the unfulfilled needs for nursing services as perceived by patients and personnel in sixty general hospitals. Four independent variables were included in the regression equation: total hours of nursing care provided per day, hours of professional nursing per day, size of hospital, and ownership of hospital. The equation for the regression analysis was:

$$Y = u + b_1X_1 + b_2X_2 + b_3X_3 + b_4X_4 + e$$

Where:
Y = satisfaction with care
X_1, X_2, X_3, X_4 = independent variables
b_1, b_2, b_3, b_4 = weights of independent variables
u = general mean
e = random error (due to random sampling)

Computationally the values of the b's were estimated by a mathematical procedure known as the method of least squares. The statistical significance of each of the

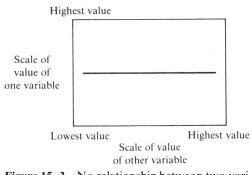

Figure 15–3 No relationship between two variables.

*Assumed to be zero (null hypothesis).

four factors in terms of their contribution to the value of Y was determined by the analysis of variance technique.

CORRELATION TECHNIQUES

A technique related to regression analysis is that of *correlation*. In some applications of statistical methods, particularly in the field of educational statistics, it is one of the most widely used techniques. In the correlation method a coefficient of correlation, called r, is computed. This coefficient varies between -1 and $+1$, and its value is a measure of the degree of association between the variables studied. The closer the computed value of the r is to $+1$ or -1, the higher is the degree of relationship between the variables studied.

The coefficient of correlation is essentially a summary measure, not a test of significance. For quantitative variables the coefficient of correlation is computed by a technique known as the product-moment method, which is essentially the ratio of two standard deviations. The numerator of the ratio is the standard deviation of the

values of the dependent variable *calculated* from the regression equation, and the denominator is the standard deviation of the *actual* values of the dependent variable that were obtained from the sample.

For qualitative variables, the coefficient of correlation can be estimated by a variety of techniques. One technique, known as *Yule's coefficient of association,* is applicable to data concerning two variables, each of which has only two scale values. To illustrate, Safford and Schlotfeldt[2] conducted a study a number of years ago in a general hospital to test the relationship between the number of patients assigned to a nursing team consisting of one registered and two practical nurses and the ratings of the quality of care provided by the team. The independent variable is the number of patients assigned to the team. In this comparison two groupings were used: thirteen and nineteen patients. The dependent variable is the rating of the care by patients and personnel. Here also, two groupings were used: "excellent" and "all other." The number of ratings in each category were as follows:

NUMBER OF PATIENTS ASSIGNED TO TEAM		RATING OF CARE		
		EXCELLENT	ALL OTHER	TOTAL
13		51	39	90
19		38	55	93
	Total	89	94	183

Yule's coefficient of association has the following formula:

$$A = \frac{ad - bc}{ad + bc}$$

A is equivalent to r, the coefficient of correlation, and also varies between ± 1. The letters in the formula represent the four cells in the table:

		RATING OF CARE	
		EXCELLENT	ALL OTHER
Number of patients	13	a	b
assigned to team	19	c	d

It is obvious that if all frequencies fall into the a and d cells and none in b and c or, conversely, all fall in b and c and none in a and d, there would be extremely high correlation between the variables and the value of A would be $+1$ or -1.

The value of A for the study of the work load of a nursing team and the rating of the care provided by the team is computed to be 0.31. Since a perfect correlation is designated by +1 or −1, and complete lack of correlation by zero, these variables can be interpreted to be mildly related.

TESTS OF SIGNIFICANCE FOR QUALITATIVE VARIABLES

Much of the data in nursing and patient care research are concerned with qualitative variables—those whose scales of measurement are either nominal or ordinal. Such scales yield counts of the frequency with which a scale value is recorded for the sampling units. When the dependent variable of an explanatory study is measured in terms of such a scale, tests like the ones just described—the difference between two means and the analysis of variance—cannot be used. However, other tests can be applied to the data to determine the probability (level of significance) that the differences in the criterion measures among the groups could have arisen from random sampling. In one of these tests we can evaluate the differences in the percentage of subjects in certain classes of the criterion measure, similar to the test of the difference between means. For example, the percentage of subjects in the experimental group who recovered after treatment can be compared with the percentage recovered in the control group. Such a test can use as its model the t or normal distributions previously described to evaluate the level of statistical significance of the difference in proportions. In another test, we can compare the numerical frequencies in each of the scale categories for the study groups and evaluate their differences by use of a test known as *chi square*.

Tests of Significance for Proportions

Many qualitative variables—those possessing nominal or ordinal scales—are often summarized into relative frequencies, called rates, such as the percentage of total number of subjects possessing each value of the scale. If the variable has only two values—sometimes called an all-or-nothing variable— and there are two groups being compared, a direct test can be made of the statistical significance of the difference between the percentages for the two groups. This test is analogous to the test of the difference between two means. The t ratio for small samples is computed from the following formula:

$$t = \frac{\text{Difference in sample percentages}}{\begin{array}{c}\text{Standard error of the difference} \\ \text{in sample percentages}\end{array}}$$

The formula for the standard error of the difference between two percentages is:

$$\sqrt{\frac{P(1-P)}{n_1} + \frac{P(1-P)}{n_2}}$$

Where: $P = \dfrac{n_1 p_1 + n_2 p_2}{n_1 + n_2}$, a weighted mean of the two sample percentages, n_1 = size of first sample, and n_2 = size of second sample. (For computational purposes the figures are expressed as proportions not percentages: e.g., 50 percent = 0.50).

To illustrate, assume that instead of recording *quantitative* blood pressure measurements on the two samples of fifteen patients each, we had simply recorded whether the patient's blood pressure was high or normal according to a qualitative scale. These data could be tabulated as follows:

	HIGH BLOOD PRESSURE		NORMAL BLOOD PRESSURE		TOTAL	
	NUMBER	PERCENT	NUMBER	PERCENT	NUMBER	PERCENT
Group A	7	47	8	53	15	100
Group B	13	87	2	13	15	100
Total	20	67	10	33	30	100

The t ratio would be:

$$t = \frac{(0.87 - 0.47)}{\sqrt{\frac{(0.67)(0.33)}{15} + \frac{(0.67)(0.33)}{15}}} = \frac{0.40}{0.1715} = 2.3$$

Thus, $t = 2.3$. This value exceeds the 5 percent level of significance but is below the 1 percent level. Since the sample size is small, the t rather than the normal distribution is used. In large-sized samples, the t test, based on the normal distribution, would be used to assess the difference between two percentages.

Chi-Square Tests

When the qualitative variable being studied has more than two categories, the chi-square test can be applied to analyze the significance of differences among the groups. The chi-square test is applied directly to the frequencies in the various categories of the variables and not to the percentages. In a sense chi-square is an extension of the tests of the significance of the difference between two percentages (or any other type of relative frequency) and is similar to the extension of the test of significance of differences between two means to differences among more than two means by the analysis of variance.

The chi-square test of signficance is analogous to the t or F tests in that it is computed from a test ratio. The value provided by the computation of this ratio is a measure of the probability of obtaining the value by random sampling. The higher the value of chi-square for specified-size samples, the greater the probability that the frequencies for the different groups being compared are really different from each other and not just the result of random sampling.

The computation of chi-square:

1. Determine the theoretical frequency for each of the cells in the table.
2. Subtract each theoretical frequency from the actual frequency in each cell.
3. Square the difference.
4. Divide by the theoretical frequency for each cell.
5. Total all the quotients.

The formula for chi-square is thus:

The sum for all cells of the table of: $\left(\dfrac{\text{The squared difference between sample and theoretical frequencies for a cell}}{\text{The theoretical frequency for the cell}} \right)$

Chi-square can also be applied to data in which the scale has only two categories. Although such data can also be analyzed by a test of significance of the difference between two percentages, the chi-square test is easier to compute. For the same data the level of significance of a chi-square test and a t test of applied to the differences between the percentages would be identical.

Using the data on blood pressure readings for the two groups of patients, we can calculate the chi-square value and compare it with the previously computed t test of the difference between the two percentages. The results of the two tests should be the same.

The frequencies in each of the cells are as follows:

	HIGH BLOOD PRESSURE	NORMAL BLOOD PRESSURE	TOTAL
Group A	7	8	15
Group B	13	2	15
Total	20	10	30

The first step is to calculate the theoretical frequencies for each cell. These are the frequencies that would be found if there were no difference in the distribution of blood pressure readings between the two study groups. If this were the case, the number of patients in each group with normal and high blood pressures would be the same as the distribution of all thirty patients—two-thirds (20/30) in the high blood pressure group and one-third (10/30) in the normal group:

	HIGH BLOOD PRESSURE	NORMAL BLOOD PRESSURE	TOTAL
Group A	10	5	15
Group B	10	5	15
Total	20	10	30

The actual frequency in each cell is subtracted from its theoretical frequency, the difference squared, and the result divided by the theoretical frequency.* The value of chi square is the sum of the quotients:

$$\frac{(7-10)^2}{10}+\frac{(8-5)^2}{5}+\frac{(13-10)^2}{10}+\frac{(2-5)^2}{5}=5.4$$

To determine the level of significance of the computed value of chi square we refer to the distribution of chi-square values. This distribution, as is the case for the normal t and F distributions, can be found in tabled form in the appendices of most statistical texts. The table shows, for different levels of *degrees of freedom*, the relative frequency (probability) of obtaining the value of chi square by random sampling as high as that computed for the data.

The value of chi-square for various degrees of freedom at the 5 and 1 percent levels of significance are as follows:

DEGREES OF FREEDOM	LEVEL OF SIGNIFICANCE 5%	1%
1	3.8	6.6
2	6.0	9.2
3	7.8	11.3
4	9.5	13.3
5	11.1	15.1
10	18.3	23.2
15	25.0	30.6
20	31.4	37.6
25	37.6	44.3
30	43.8	50.9

The degrees of freedom for the data in the above example are found by multiplying the number of scale values of one variable (the number of columns in the table) minus one by the number of scale values of the other variable (the number of rows in the table) minus one. For the blood pressure data there are two scale values for blood pressure and two for the groups representing different qualities of nursing care. The degrees of freedom, therefore, are: $(2-1) \times (2-1) = 1$. Thus, with one degree of freedom the value of chi-square of 5.4 exceeds the 5 percent level of significance, which is 3.8, but is below the 1 percent level, which is 6.6. This means that such a value of chi-square could be obtained by chance in less than five but more than one samplings out of 100. We would thus say that the relationship between quality of nursing care and the blood pressure of patients is significant at the 5 percent level. This conclusion is identical with that found when the test of the difference between the two percentages was used.

*A correction factor known as *Yate's correction for continuity* should be applied to these data. This correction is applied to data being tested by chi square when the scale of classification for each variable has only two discrete values, known as a 2 by 2 table, and where the expected frequencies are small. The correction, which involves reducing the absolute value of each difference between the actual and theoretical frequencies by one-half prior to squaring, is fully described by Allison.[3]

SHORT-CUT METHOD OF CALCULATION

A short-cut method is available for the calculation of chi-square for data in tables with two columns and two rows, the so-called 2 × 2 table just discussed. The formula for this short-cut is:

$$\frac{N(ad-bc)^2}{(a+b)(c+d)(a+c)(b+d)}$$

Where N = Total number of subjects in the study and a,b,c,d, the various cells in the fourfold table: $\frac{a\,|\,b}{c\,|\,d}$

Applying the short-cut method to the blood pressure data we compute the following value of chi-square:

$$\begin{aligned}
\text{chi-square} &= \frac{30(14-104)^2}{(15)(15)(10)(10)} \\
&= \frac{30(90)^2}{(15)(15)(20)(10)} \\
&= \frac{243{,}000}{45{,}000} = 5.4
\end{aligned}$$

This is a value identical with that obtained by the long method.

CHI-SQUARE FOR OTHER THAN 2 × 2 TABLES

To illustrate how the chi-square value would be computed from data containing variables having more than two scale categories we can assume the following study. Suppose we randomly assign 200 undergraduate nursing students to two groups, one in which the course in nursing arts is taught by conventional methods, and one in which programmed instruction is used.

At the end of the course we give an achievement exam to the students which grades them into three categories: low, medium, and high achievement. We then apply a chi-square test to the data to see if there is any relationship between teaching method and achievement score. The data are as follows:

Computation of Chi-Square for a 2 × 3 Table

METHOD	ACTUAL FREQUENCIES SCORE ON FINAL EXAM				THEORETICAL FREQUENCIES SCORE ON FINAL EXAM			
	LOW	MEDIUM	HIGH	TOTAL	LOW	MEDIUM	HIGH	TOTAL
Programmed instruction	a30	b 50	c20	100	a20	b 65	c15	100
Conventional instruction	d10	e 80	f10	100	d20	e 65	f15	100
	40	130	30	200	40	130	30	200

CELL	ACTUAL FREQUENCIES	THEORETICAL FREQUENCIES	DIFFERENCE	DIFFERENCE SQUARED	CHI-SQUARE RATIO
a	30	20	+10	100	100/20 = 5.000
b	50	65	−15	225	225/65 = 3.462
c	20	15	+ 5	25	25/15 = 1.667
d	10	20	−10	100	100/20 = 5.000
e	80	65	+15	225	225/65 = 3.464
f	10	15	− 5	25	25/15 = 1.667
					Chi-square = 20.260 or 20.3

The degrees of freedom of these data are 2: (3 − 1 columns × 2 − 1 rows). Since the calculated chi-square value, 20.3, is considerably larger than 6.0, the chi-square value at the 5 percent level with two degrees of freedom, we can say that there are significant differences among the two groups in terms of the achievement scores of the students on the final exams. In other words a value of chi-square of 20.3 can be expected to occur by chance alone considerably fewer times than 5 out of 100 samples —in fact fewer than 1 out of 1,000.

Distribution-Free Methods

With the exception of the chi-square test, all statistical tests thus far discussed have two features in common. First, they make an assumption about the form of the underlying distribution of the measurements in the target population—i.e., the values of measurements are normally distributed, or, that at least, the distribution is approximately symmetrical and has a single peak. Second, they focus upon testing hypotheses about *parameters* of the underlying distribution, as in testing the significance of differences in sample means or percentages.

For data where little is known about the underlying distribution of the measurements of the variable being studied, or where the distribution is not of the type required by the test of significance, certain tests can be employed that are valid regardless of the character of the distribution of the measurements in the target population. The only assumptions to be met are: that the samples were selected randomly and that the measurements made of the sampling units are independent of each other. Such tests of significance are called distribution-free or *nonparametric* tests in contrast to tests based on the normal, *t,* or *F* distributions, which are called *parametric* tests. A chi-square test is essentially a nonparametric test since its application is not restricted to variables whose measurements are normally distributed or to test or estimate means or standard deviations of these measurements, but rather it is applied to qualitative variables, where the measurements are in the form of frequency counts for the different categories of a qualitative scale.

Nonparametric tests have several useful features. First, they may provide the only way of testing the statistical significance of frequency data obtained through nominal or ordinal scales. By converting actual frequencies into relative frequencies, it is possible to apply a parametric test to data such as the *t* test of the difference between two proportions. Converting frequencies into rates transforms the data for the groups of subjects as a whole from a qualitative to a quantitative scale.

For example, when we calculate the percentage in a sample of patients recovered from an illness, the basic qualitative scale may consist of only two classes: recovered, died. By computing the rate of recovery we have substituted for this discrete scale a continuous numerical scale ranging from 0 to 100 which represents the degree to which patients, considered as a group, recover from their illnesses. Our sample percentage is an estimate of the population percentage of patients expected to recover from the illness. If we took a large number of samples, the values of the percentages computed from each sample should approximate the normal distribution, and the value of the standard deviation of the sampling distribution is estimated by the standard error of a sample percentage.

Second, nonparametric methods are generally quicker and easier to compute than parametric techniques. A method such as the analysis of variance can involve a great deal of computational work requiring the use of elaborate data-processing equipment. On the other hand, some nonparametric tests do not even require a desk calculator. Nonparametric techniques can be applied to quantitative data as short-cut substitutes for parametric techniques. For example a nonparametric analysis of variance tests is available that is faster than the parametric test, although, it is considerably less sensitive.

Third, most nonparametric tests provide an exact statement of the probability of obtaining test results for the sample irrespective of the shape of the distribution of the values of the measurements in the target population, i.e., the values do not have to be distributed normally.

A major limitation of nonparametric tests of significance is that they can be wasteful of information. This is particularly true if a nonparametric test is used as a substitute for a parametric test. The parametric test would have yielded a more sensitive, discriminating test of data. To illustrate this we can use the nonparametric test known as a *sign test* to evaluate the effect of an independent variable on a criterion measure. Assume that twenty newly born normal infants were paired according to a number of important characteristics, as birth weight, sex, race, etc. One of the pair is randomly assigned at birth to the experimental group, which receives a newly developed feeding formula while its mate is assigned to the control group and receives the standard formula. At discharge the weights of the two groups are compared. Since weights are quantitative measurements, the mean weight for each group can be computed and a *t* test applied to assess parametrically the significance of the difference in weights between the two groups.

In the nonparametric sign test, only the fact that the experimental infant's weight is higher (plus sign) or lower (minus sign) than his control is considered, not the extent to which the actual weights differ. The significance of the difference between the groups is evaluated by determining the probability of obtaining that number of plus signs by chance alone. Suppose the data in this experiment were:

INFANT PAIR NO.	WEIGHT AT DISCHARGE (IN GRAMS)		SIGN
	INFANTS FED ENRICHED FORMULA	INFANTS FED REGULAR FORMULA	
1	3,682	3,143	+
2	2,970	3,012	−
3	3,422	2,815	+
4	4,082	3,677	+
5	4,312	3,785	+
6	3,075	2,633	+
7	3,857	3,059	+
8	4,490	3,990	+
9	3,951	3,344	+
10	3,222	3,240	−

If the study showed that for eight of the paired infants, the experimental members weighed more at discharge than their con-

trols while in two pairs the reverse was true, the probability of getting such a result is the same as the probability of obtaining eight or more heads in ten tosses of a coin, where the chance of getting either a head or tail in one toss is $1/2$. This probability is found by the following formula:

$$P = (nCr)\, p^{n-r} \cdot q^r$$

Where n = total number of coins tossed (total number of pairs of infants)
r = number of heads (number of plus signs)
p = probability of obtaining a tail (minus sign)
q = probability of obtaining a head (plus sign)

For eight heads

$$_{10}C_8 \left(\frac{1}{2}\right)^2 \cdot \left(\frac{1}{2}\right)^8 = \frac{10!}{8!\,2!} \cdot \left(\frac{1}{2}\right)^{10} = \frac{45}{1024}$$

For nine heads

$$_{10}C_9 \left(\frac{1}{2}\right)^1 \cdot \left(\frac{1}{2}\right)^9 = \frac{10!}{9!\,1!} \cdot \left(\frac{1}{2}\right)^{10} = \frac{10}{1024}$$

For ten heads

$$_{10}C_{10} \left(\frac{1}{2}\right)^0 \cdot \left(\frac{1}{2}\right)^{10} = \frac{10!}{10!\,0!} \cdot \left(\frac{1}{2}\right)^{10} = \frac{1}{1024}$$

Thus

$$P = \frac{45}{1024} + \frac{10}{1024} + \frac{1}{1024} = \frac{56}{1024} = 0.54$$

According to this model, if we tossed ten coins many times and did nothing to influence the greater occurrence of either a head or tail, we would expect that eight or more heads would appear purely by chance in our random tossing (random sampling), slightly more than 5 times out of each 100 tossings of the ten coins.

In terms of our experimental data, this means that, by chance alone, we would expect that in a little more than 5 out of 100 samplings we would obtain at least eight plus signs in ten comparisons. Since this is greater than the 5 percent level, selected as our level of significance, we must say that there is no relationship between type of feeding and weight gain. Even though they were fed the enriched formula the performance of the experimental infants was not better than what could be expected by chance alone.

However, if we look at the actual weights we see that the infants fed the enriched formula did reach a substantially higher weight level than those fed conventional formula. For several pairs the infant fed the enriched formula weighed several hundred grams more than the control fed a regular diet. In pair number 7 the difference was nearly 800 grams, or over a pound and a half. In the two pairs where weights of the control infants were higher than the experimental infants—numbers 2 and 10—the difference was slight, less than 50 grams in both instances.

The mean weights for the two groups are:

Experimental group	3,706	grams
Control group	3,270	grams

When a *t* test is applied to these means in a test of the significance of the difference between means, the result is highly significant. The *t* ratio value is 2.88, which means that such a difference could occur by chance alone only 1 time in 100 samplings.

These data illustrate the loss of information that results from the use of a nonparametric tests for data that could be validly analyzed by a parametric method such as the *t* test of the difference between two means. The nonparametric sign test in this example took highly refined quantita-

tively scaled data—the actual weights of the infants—and converted them into a crude ordinal scale consisting of only two categories: more than (+) and less than (−). As a result there was much less sensitivity of the statistical test and differences in the weights of the infants in the two groups was nonsignificant. The only advantage in the use of the nonparametric test is that it provides a short-cut in computation, a slight advantage when compared to the great loss of sensitivity.

Nonparametric tests are most useful when the data cannot be treated by parametric tests. A nonparametric technique often used instead is the *rank correlation* method, a technique analogous to the product-moment coefficient of correlation computed from numerically scaled data. The rank correlation coefficient has the formula:

$$r_s = 1 - \frac{6(\text{sum of the squared differences in the ranking of the subject on the two variables})}{n(n+1)(n-1)}$$

Where n = number of subjects being ranked.

To illustrate: Assume we randomly selected ten freshman students in a school of nursing and ranked them from highest to lowest, 1 to 10, in terms of two ordinally scaled variables: (1) intelligence level as determined from preadmission test scores, and (2) the degree of interest showed in their education program. The rankings are:

STUDENT NO.	INTELLIGENCE LEVEL	INTEREST IN EDUCATIONAL PROGRAM	DIFFERENCE	DIFFERENCE SQUARED
1	1	1	0	0
2	5	4	1	1
3	3	5	−2	4
4	7	3	4	16
5	9	2	7	49
6	8	10	−2	4
7	2	8	−6	36
8	4	7	−3	9
9	6	6	0	0
10	10	9	1	1
Total				120

$$r_s = 1 - \frac{6 \times 120}{10 \times 11 \times 9} = 0.27$$

Since perfect correlation between the two variables would result in a value of $+1$ if the variables were positively associated and -1 if negatively associated, and 0 would mean no association at all, a value of 0.27 indicates a slight association.

It is possible to determine the probability of obtaining such a value of r_s by chance alone by reference to tables showing the level of significance of the values of r_s for different numbers of subjects:

SIZE OF SAMPLE	LEVEL OF SIGNIFICANCE	
	5%	1%
5	0.90	1.00
10	0.56	0.75
20	0.38	0.53
30	0.31	0.43

From these figures it can be seen that a value of r_s of 0.27 with ten subjects can be expected to occur by chance more frequently than 5 times in 100, since the 5 percent level value is 0.56. Even if the sample had included as many as thirty subjects such as value of r_s could not have exceeded the 5 percent level.

Nonparametric tests of significance are sometimes called *order statistics*. Many of these tests treat data in terms of ordinal rankings or comparisons, as in the rank correlation and the sign test techniques, as well as in other nonparametric methods such as the run test, median test, and the so-called Mann-Whitney U test. Thus, the designation, order statistics, is an apt description of their method as well as their purpose—to see whether the ordering of the data follows a random pattern or not.

Other Techniques

The discussion, thus far, has not by any means exhausted all the statistical techniques that can be applied to research data. As has been indicated, the advent of the computer has made available to everyone the application of what were previously esoteric techniques available only to specialists. Three of these techniques will be briefly discribed: discriminant analysis, path analysis, and factor analysis.

DISCRIMINANT ANALYSIS

The objective of discriminant analysis is to distinguish between two or more groups in terms of the characteristics that most clearly set them apart. The initial groups, for example, could be clusters of institutions with different levels of performance on an outcome variable of interest, such as graduates of diploma, associate degree and baccalaureate programs. The statistical aim of discriminant analysis is to select a collection of other variables about the groups that together, can accurately predict their classification on the output variable. The results indicate the relative importance of the discriminating variables. One possible application of the technique is to find the factors that most clearly distinguish between nursing schools with different levels of key outcome variables.

PATH ANALYSIS

Path analysis is essentially a tool for decomposing and interpreting linear relationships within a set of variables (VARs) by assuming that the causal order in which they affect one another is known (e.g., good nursing care reduces patients' length of stay in the hospital). It also assumes that relationships among the variables are causally closed, which to say that VAR1 is a cause of VAR2 if and only if VAR2 can be changed by VAR1 and by no other variable. The path diagram that charts out how the variables are related to each other is a useful descriptive device and provides a "model" of the phenomenon being analyzed. Path analysis is sometimes considered a "degenerate" version of multiple regression since it places many restrictions on the "model" and purports to deduce the model from the data rather than to develop the model from a knowledge of behavior and test its applicability to the real world. However, when the behavioral model is not well understood at the outset of analysis, it can be very helpful.

FACTOR ANALYSIS

Factor analysis is closely related to multiple correlation analysis. Its major use is as a data reduction tool. It rearranges a matrix of Pearson correlation coefficients among any subset or all of the variables used in a study to highlight the major patterns of interrelationship among them. This makes it possible to carry out the bulk of an analysis in terms of a few representative or "tracer" variables with confidence that the results truly reflect the patterns present in the full set of data.

SUMMARY

Powerful statistical techniques are available to analyze research data, e.g., to analyze the relationships among the variables studied in the research and to draw inferences from the analyses to the real world. Techniques are available for analyzing quantitative variables (parametric) and qualitative (nonparametric). There are techniques for analyzing a few variables and for multiple variables. Statistical packages that can be used on the smallest computers have been developed to perform analyses that until recently could only be done on "mainframes." The results of a statistical analysis can only be as good as the quality of the data that have been collected as well as other aspects of the research design.

REFERENCES

1. Faye G. Abdellah and Eugene Levine, *Effects of Nurse Staffing on Satisfactions with Nursing Care.*

Hospital Monograph Series No. 4 Chicago, The American Hospital Association, 1958.
2. Beverly J. Safford and Rozella M. Schlotfeldt, "Nursing Service Staffing and Quality of Nursing Care." *Nursing Res.,* 9:149–154, summer 1960.
3. Harry E. Allison, "Computational Forms of Chi Square." *Am. Statistician,* 18:17–18, February 1964.

PROBLEMS AND SUGGESTIONS FOR FURTHER STUDY

1. Discuss the comparative advantages and disadvantages of parametric and nonparametric tests of significance. Are there any assumptions at all that have to be met concerning the data before nonparametric tests can be applied? Why are nonparametric tests useful in research on nursing and patient care? Explain why there is a loss of information when a non-parametric test is used in place of a parametric test. Discuss the statement by Wallis and Roberts in their *Statistics: A New Approach* (New York, The Free Press of Glencoe, 1956) that "Not all non-parametric tests are quick and easy, by any means, even though most quick and easy methods are non-parametric" (p. 592).
2. For each of the following tests of significance describe a study in which the test would be used:
   a. A T test of the difference between two percentages
   b. A chi-square test
   c. A sign test
   d. A t test of the slope of a regression equation
   e. An F test
3. Why do you think the chi-square test is so popular in research on human beings as a test of significance of the data? What are the advantages in the use of this test? What are the disadvantages? Why is chi-square a more widely applicable test than the analysis of variance? But why is the analysis of variance a more powerful test than chi-square?
4. What is the relationship between regression analysis and the analysis of variance? Are the two techniques identical in that they are concerned with the relationship between dependent and independent variables? How

are they different? How does regression analysis differ from correlation analysis?

5. Discuss the following statement by E. J. G. Pitman, "Statistics and Science," (*J. Am. Statistical Assoc.*, **52:**322–330, September 1957), "The scientist with ideas frames his hypotheses and wishes to test them. He would be happy if he could devise a test which would decide with certainty whether a hypothesis is true or not. When he cannot do this, he must use a test which has only a certain probability of giving the right answer" (p.323).

6. Read the article by Gerri S. Lamb and Rudolph J. Napodano, "Physician-Nurse Interaction Patterns in Primary Care Practices." *Am. J. Pub. Health*, **74:**26–29, January 1984. How would you describe the variables in the study—quantitative, qualitative? What kind of statistical analysis would you apply to the data? What do the authors mean by "process analysis"?

7. Comment on the statistical analyses employed in the following studies. Are the applications appropriate? Could you suggest other approaches to statistical analysis?

a. Richard N. Winickoff, Susan Wilner, Ross Neisuler, and G. Otto Barnett, "Limitations of Provider Interventions in Hypertension Quality Assurance." *Am. J. Pub. Health*, **75:**43–46, January 1985.

b. Jacquelyn H. Flaskerud, "A Comparison of Perceptions of Problematic Behavior by Six Minority Groups and Mental Health Professionals." *Nursing Res.*, **33:**190–197, July/August 1984.

c. Evelyn Crumpton and Eileen P. Rogers, "Some Effects of Team Nursing on a Psychiatric Ward." *Nursing Res.*, **12:**181–182, summer 1963.

d. Judith T. Shuval, "Perceived Role Components of Nursing in Israel." *Am. Sociol. Rev.*, **28:**37–46, February 1963.

e. Margaret W. Linn, Lee Gurel and Bernard S. Linn, "Patient Outcome as a Measure of Quality of Nursing Home Care." *Am. J. Pub. Health*, **67:**44–77, April 1977.

f. Marlene Kramer and others, "Extra-Tactile Stimulation of the Premature Infant." *Nursing Res.*, **24:**324–334, September/October, 1975.

g. Jean Hayter, "Sleep Behaviors of Older Persons. "*Nursing Res.*, **32:**242–246, July/August 1983.

h. John A. Ward and John M. Griffin, "Improving Instruction Through Computer-Graded Examinations." *Nursing Outlook*, **25:**524–529, August 1977.

8. Read Chapter 7, "Some Fundamental Problems and Limitations to Study by Experimental Designs" in F. Stuart Chapin, *Experimental Designs in Sociological Research*, (1974 reprint of 1955 ed., Westport CN, Greenwood, pp. 165–190.). What are the various definitions of "probability" that are given by the author in this chapter? Explain what the author means in stating that probability tests (tests of significance) serve only as an "empirical safety device, and not to provide the basis for extensive generalizations" (p.185).

9. Read the article, "Increasing Efficiency and Precision of Data Analysis: Multivariate vs. Univariate Statistical Techniques." *Nursing Res.*, **33:**247–249, July/August 1984. Discuss the advantages of multivariate techniques stated by the author. How does the author define "multivariate" techniques? While the author says that multivariate statistical techniques should be used whenever possible, what are some disadvantages of these techniques?

10. Critique the use of one-way analysis of variance in the article by Rene Day and Louise Payne, "Comparison of Lecture Presentation Versus Computer Managed Instruction." *Computers in Nursing*, **2:**236–240, November/December 1984. Have all the conditions for the use of ANOVA been met? Would repeated measures ANOVA or MANOVA be applicable to these data?

11. Does all explanatory research require that the data be evaluated by tests of significance? What other ways are there of evaluating data in addition to tests of significance? What really does a test of significance do? Why, in looking at the process of research in its entirety as it is currently being applied to problems in nursing and patient care, might the process of applying tests of significance to the research data be of minor importance?

CHAPTER
16

Determine How
to Interpret the Data

OBJECTIVES

- To clarify the meaning of statistical significance.
- To describe the errors committed in the use of statistical significance.

- To show how to interpret data in statistical tables.
- To point out the pitfalls in interpreting data in tables.

THE MEANING OF STATISTICAL SIGNIFICANCE

Statistical tests of significance, whether parametric or nonparametric, are used to analyze research data where measurements of either quantitative or qualitative variables have been made of the study subjects selected through a random process. Randomization can enter into a research study in several ways. In nonexperimental studies the subjects may be randomly drawn from a larger target population. In an experimental study the subjects not only may have been drawn randomly from a larger population but also randomly assigned to alternative groups.

The function of the test of significance is to test whether two or more groups being compared in terms of a summary mea-

sure—a mean, standard deviation, a percentage, or nonparametrically as by rank order on a qualitative scale—could be considered to have come from the same target population or not—i.e., are they essentially two independent samples from the same population? In a nonexperimental study the target population could be all general hospitals in the United States. We group the hospitals into two subpopulations by amount of nursing care provided, high and low, which serve as the independent variable. We then draw random samples of hospitals from the two groups. For our dependent variable we measure the quality of care the patients receive in terms of a valid quantitative criterion measure. We then test the significance of the difference in the values of the summary measures for the two groups. If, at the level of significance chosen, the 5 percent level, we find that the difference is not statistically significant—the difference would occur more frequently than 5 times in 100 repeated samplings—we say that the hospitals belong to the same population in terms of the variable "quality of care provided." In other words, the distinguishing characteristic of the two subpopulations—the different amounts of care received by patients—is not significantly related to the dependent variable.

In an experimental study, patients would be randomly assigned to two groups, analogous to the subpopulations in the nonexperimental study—in one group more intensive nursing care would be provided. Here the subpopulations are formed by the experimenter, whereas in the nonexperimental approach they have already been formed. If the test of significance shows that the difference in the values of the summary measures is not significant, we say that the two groups are samples from the same population. If the difference in the values of the summary measures is statistically significant, we say that the groups represent different populations and that quality of care *is* related to the amount of care provided.

A test of significance, then, is basically a test of the extent to which random sampling error is the explanation for the difference in the summary measures. At the level of significance chosen, if sampling error explains all of the difference in the summary measures, we say that the difference is not significant and there is no relationship between the dependent variable and the variable that distinguishes the alternative groups. If sampling error does not explain all of the difference, we say that the summary measures are significantly different and there *is* a relationship between the dependent variable and the variable distinguishing the alternative groups.

If the subjects have not been randomly selected from the target population or randomly assigned to alternative groups, or both, a test of statistical significance should not be applied to the summary measures. In such cases any differences in the values of the summary measures could not be attributed to random sampling error. To apply a test of significance to such data, which is an evaluation of the extent to which the difference observed exceeds the amount attributable to random sampling, is not only inappropriate, but meaningless.

THE NULL HYPOTHESIS

In explanatory studies that employ tests of statistical significance to evaluate a difference in the values of summary measures for the alternative groups, the hypothesis being tested is that the population differences is really zero and any difference found in the sample values is due to the fact that we sampled. Thus, the null hypothesis says: (1) the alternative groups can be considered as independent samples from the same population and (2) their summary measures are independent estimates of the same population parameter. To the extent that the difference in sample summary measures does not exceed the value established in the test of the significance as attributable to random sampling error, we accept the null hypothesis as being true.

When we sample, we expect to obtain results that are not exactly the same as if we had studied the entire population. The smaller the sample, the greater is the possible deviation between sample value and actual population value. Conversely, the larger the sample the smaller is the sampling error. If we had a 100 percent sample—that is, if we had studied all the sampling units in the population—the sampling error would be zero, and the value of our sample statistic would be equal to the value of our population parameter.

As has been stated before, the basic model for most tests of significance is the following ratio:

$$\frac{\text{Difference in values of sample summary measures } \textit{minus} \text{ Difference in values of population summary measures}}{\text{Standard error (sampling error) of the difference in the values of sample summary measures}}$$

The hypothesis for a study describes the expected differences in the values of the population summary measures for the alternative groups. The way of stating the hypothesis for a statistical test of significance is the form of a *null hypothesis*—that there is no difference in the values of the population measures for the alternative groups. Examples of null hypotheses are:

- There is no relationship between smoking and lung cancer.
- The amount of nursing care provided is not related to the quality of care.
- A graduate of diploma program in nursing is as proficient as a graduate of collegiate program.
- There is no difference in the amount of nursing care required by patients in different age groups.
- Nurses do not have greater job mobility than members of other occupational groups.

Because a hypothesis is stated in the null form does not mean that the researcher expects that his data will support it. Generally, the opposite is true; the researcher expects that in the real world the alternative to the null hypothesis will be true—that smoking *is* related to lung cancer, that higher amounts of nursing care *will improve* the quality of care, and so on.

The use of the null form in stating hypotheses is dictated by the nature of statistical tests of significance. In a statistical test we are evaluating the extent to which the difference we have measured in the sample deviates from the difference that could be expected due to chance, as a result of random sampling.

When our study is based on a sample, we are uncertain about the realities in the total population. We can only estimate it based on data from our sample. In testing hypotheses in explanatory studies, we are estimating from our sample data whether or not there is a relationship between the variables. Since the data are based on only sample evidence, which may not correspond with the true state, there is the possibility that the sample could yield a result different from that found if we studied the total population. In other words, because

our sample can differ significantly from the population as a whole, we may find that a relationship exists between the variables in the sample, when in fact such a relationship does not hold for the entire population. Our level of significance tells us the probability of such an occurrence. By setting this level at a relatively rare frequency—5 times out of 100, or less—an erroneous interpretation becomes unlikely.

When the difference between the groups is statistically significant, we reject the null hypothesis and accept the alternative hypothesis—that there is a relationship between the independent and dependent variables. By rejecting the null hypothesis we have not *proved* that the alternative hypothesis is true with absolute certainty, just as when we accept it we have not proved that the null hypothesis is true with absolute certainty. We have only demonstrated that our difference exceeds or falls below the value that, with a certain relative frequency, called the level of significance, could be attributable to chance. If our difference can occur by chance fewer times than our level of significance, we are willing to accept the alternative hypothesis, knowing full well that there is a small possibility it may not be true.

Although the null hypothesis is meant to denote a hypothesis of zero difference between the summary measures, a more meaningful approach may be to test the differences for the study groups against some value greater than zero that is considered to be the minimum value of no importance. For example, if we are testing the effects of an educational program on weight reduction, we might establish our null difference not as zero but as 10 pounds, if this were considered to be the minimum weight loss of importance. An average weight loss of less than 10 pounds would not be significant. Our statistical test of significance would be:

$$\frac{\text{Difference in values of sample summary measures } \textit{minus } 10}{\text{Standard error (sampling error) of the difference in the values of sample measures}}$$

Thus, "null" really should mean a difference of no particular importance, not just a zero difference.

ALTERNATIVE HYPOTHESIS

The alternative hypothesis is the form of the statement of hypothesis that represents the expectation of the researcher. A researcher embarking on a study often expects, or at least is hopeful, that the independent variable he is manipulating is related to the dependent variable he is measuring. If he were certain that the variables were unrelated, he would most likely not undertake the research.

The alternative hypothesis to the null hypothesis may be either implicit or explicit. In many studies, the alternative hypothesis needs no explicit statement, since it is self-evident. In others it may be necessary to clearly spell out the alternative hypothesis, since it can be formulated in various ways. Broadly speaking, alternative hypotheses can state that:

1. The independent variable will have some effect, either positive or negative, on the dependent variable.
2. The independent variable will have a positive effect on the dependent variable.
3. The independent variable will have a negative effect on the dependent variable.

If we are studying the effect of a nursing procedure on a patient, we may be interested in any statistically significant effect produced, whether it be positive or negative. Or we may only be interested in whether we can produce a positive effect—a negative effect would be interpreted that the independent variable had produced no effect and would lead to acceptance of null hypothesis.

In assessing the effects of testing drugs on patients we would only accept the drug as being effective (reject the null hypothesis) if we would produce a positive effect on patients. However, we would also be interested in any significant negative results because this could have important implica-

tions for further development of therapy. Although in many nursing and patient care studies we are fundamentally interested in seeing whether the effect produced by the manipulation of our independent variable is positive, we are also interested in negative effects. We are interested in any effect produced.

Studies with alternative hypotheses directed toward any effect, regardless of direction, employ what is called two-sided or two-tailed tests of significance. Studies interested only in either a positive or a negative effect employ a one-sided or one-tailed tests.

We do not care whether sample A's sumary measure is higher than sample B's, or vice versa, but only that there is some difference between the two sample values. If we were interested only in a one-sided alternative—that is, we would consider our difference as statistically significant only if A were higher than B and not if B were higher than A—we would achieve a greater level of significance for the same difference in the values of the summary measures than for the two-sided alternative. In other words, for the same data we can reject the null hypothesis and accept the alternative hypothesis with lower values of t when a one-tailed test is used. To illustrate, if our level of significance is 5 percent we will reject the null hypothesis and accept the alternative hypothesis if our t ratios for various-sized samples are as follows:

SIZE OF SAMPLE	TWO-TAILED TEST	ONE-TAILED TEST
5	2.57	2.02
10	2.23	1.81
15	2.13	1.75
20	2.09	1.72

Level of Significance

A test of significance provides an evaluation of the extent to which data depart from what would be expected if only chance factors are affecting the data. For example, in the t ratio we divide our sample difference by the measure of random sampling error. The probability of getting such a t ratio value in repeated random sampling by chance alone is called the level of significance. The 0.05 (5 percent) level of significance is employed. This means that 5 times out of 100 such a difference in the summary measures found in the study can be attributable to chance factors arising from random sampling. There is nothing magical about the 0.05 level. Other levels can be used. The 0.01 (1 percent) level is more stringent because the chance of finding a difference in the summary measures attributable to random sampling rather than to the independent variable is 1 in 100, an even rarer occurrence.

If we want to be more certain that our results are not accidental, due to having selected an atypical sample, we choose a more stringent level of significance. If our study is concerned with matters of vital importance to the health and welfare of human beings, or if decisions based on the study would involve great expense, we want to be more certain in rejecting the null hypothesis and accepting the alternative that our results were not accidental, and we would then, select a 0.01 or even 0.001 level of significance. If we were less concerned about rejecting the null hypothesis when it were really true, we can select a less stringent level: 0.05 or even 0.10.

The level of significance tells us the risk of rejecting the null hypothesis and accepting the alternative hypothesis when in fact the null hypothesis is true. This risk is called the Type I error in applying tests of significance. Assuming sample size is not changed, the risk of committing a Type I error can be reduced by using a more stringent level of significance, say, 0.01 instead of 0.05. However, reducing a risk of Type I error increases the risk of a Type II error. The Type II error is incurred when we accept the null hypothesis and reject the alternative hypothesis when the alternative hypothesis is true.

There is an inverse relationship between the two types of errors, since if we decrease the probability that one will occur, we increase the probability that the other will occur. If we change our level of significance from 5 to 1 percent, we will reject the null hypothesis falsely only 1 time in 100 rather than 5 times in 100. However, by so doing we will increase the probability of rejecting the alternative hypothesis falsely.

For many studies the danger of a Type I error may be more serious than that of a Type II. If we are testing the effects of a drug to chance and thus conceal its true the effects really exceeded what would be expected to occur purely by chance.

We might select a 0.01 or 0.001 level of significance, even though we would be more likely to attribute real effects of the drug to chance and thus conceal its true value. In other words we would make the level of significnce more stringent, say, 0.01 instead of 0.05, in order to decrease the Type I error if the findings of our study can result in life or death of a patient and we want to be very sure that the differences are real. We could accept a higher level of significance, 0.05 instead of 0.01, if we were not so concerned with the consequences of falsely accepting the alternative hypothesis and wanted to decrease the chance of masking any real differences in data.

Each study must balance the risks in committing Type I and II errors. Usually a compromise is made which serves to optimize the balance between the two errors. In reaching this balance the *power* of the test is evaluated. The power of a test can be defined as the probability of rejecting the null hypothesis when it is actually false. The power is determined by the following formula:

1 minus probability of Type II error

The probability of committing a Type II error can be assessed by the computation of the power curve for the test, also known as the power function. By reducing the probability of committing a Type II error the power of the test is increased.

The power of a test is a measure of the sensitivity of the test—the extent to which it uncovers real differences among the groups studied. Power can be increased in several ways. First, it can be increased by employing the most powerful test of significance that the characteristics of the data will permit—an analysis of variance, for example, is more powerful than a nonparametric test. Second, the use of one-tailed tests, when warranted by the nature of the hypothesis being tested, will provide a more powerful test than a two-tailed one. Finally, the power of the test can be increased by enlarging the sample size, although unlike the other approaches to the increase of power, this can significantly add to the cost, time, and effort required to do the study.

Use of Prior Probabilities

In recent years, some research has begun to employ the "Bayesian inference" in the analysis and interpretation of statistical tests of significance. Traditional tests of significance, known as the Neyman-Pearson approach, are those in which the null hypothesis is formulated, the alternative hypothesis is explicitly or implicitly stated and the level of significance established *in advance* of data collection and kept fixed during the study. This procedure is more objective. The tests of significance employed essentially make no use of prior knowledge. In the Bayesian approach, so named because it derives from and employs Baye's probability theorem, the use of prior knowledge is employed in the test of significance. In this sense it is a subjective approach to significance testing. As described by Mosteller and others,[1] the Bayesian approach involves the following:

> An experimenter might assign probabilities that are in some way proportional to the "intensity of belief" he has in the various hypotheses. (Another investigator might assign quite different probabilities.) An experiment is performed, with the aim of discovering evidence to modify these prior probabilities. Such evidence may even assign such low posterior probabilities to some of the hypotheses as to eliminate them from further consideration. . . .
> Each new experiment can begin with *a*

priori probabilities of the remaining hypotheses proportional to the *a posteriori* probabilities that resulted from the previous experiments. In this way, scientific evidence accumulates and modifies our beliefs, weakening our intensity of belief in some hypotheses, strengthening it in others.

COMMON ERRORS

Statistical tests of significance in research studies[2-7] are frequently misused. It often seems that use of tests of significance have become a sort of ritualism in research. They are applied to data as window dressing to give a veneer of scientific authority. To avoid the mistaken use of tests of significance a clear understanding should be had of their purpose. Purely and simply, they are a means of testing whether the data gathered through a random process vary from what would be expected if the influences on the data were solely chance. In other words, a test of significance, like the determination of a confidence interval for a sampling estimate of a population parameter, is a measure of sample error around the estimate. For example, in a t test of the difference between two sample means, the sample estimate is the value of the difference between the means. The standard error of this difference is a measure of its sampling error and can serve as the value of the confidence interval around the estimate. The t ratio measures the probability that a confidence interval around the sample estimate of the difference will include the value of the hypothesized population difference. With the null hypothesis the population difference is hypothesized to be zero.

The misuses of tests of significance are numerous. The following are the most common ones:

1. *Inapplicability of tests of significance.* Not every study employs randomization either in the selection of subjects from the target population or in the assignment of subjects to alternative groups. Such studies do not involve sampling, but encompass a target population. For such

studies the use of tests of significance is inappropriate, since the data do not contain random sampling error. Of course, such data may contain other types of error, but these are not measurable by confidence intervals or significance tests.

The idea of a "hypothetical universe" has been advanced to provide a rationale for the use of significance tests in studies in which random sampling has not been employed. The rationale of a "hypothetical universe" is that every finite target population is in reality a subpopulation from some superpopulation. Therefore, data from such a subpopulation is a sample and, like a random sample, is subject to sampling error. If we conduct a study in one school of nursing, it can be considered to be a sample from the superpopulation of all nursing schools. Although this may well be true, the tests of significance and the formulas for calculating confidence intervals have been derived from models in which random sampling is an important, fundamental assumption. And in a study in which a school of nursing has been selected because of convenience and not by random methods, we do not have a *random* sample as technically defined. Consequently, we cannot apply conventional statistical tests to our data.

A clear distinction should be made between statistical and nonstatistical generalizations. A statistical generalization derives from the computation of a test of significance or confidence interval. We may say, "One hundred patients' records were selected randomly from the 10,000 records in the files of the agency to evaluate the completeness and usability of the information contained in the records. From these sample records we estimate that in 16 to 24 percent of all the agency's patients' records the information is poor."

A nonstatistical generalization does not derive from significance tests or confidence intervals but from the researcher's interpretation of the data collected. The quality of this interpretation will depend on many things, including expert knowledge of the subject matter to which the data pertain as well as ability to logically fathom the meaning of the data. When the data have been collected through a random process of some kind, both types of generalizations can be made. The statistical generalization is concerned with assessing the degree to which random error has influenced the data. The nonstatistical generalization is concerned with interpreting what the data mean, how they have contributed to the fund of accumulated knowledge in the field, and how they can be applied.

If the data collection has not involved a random process, only the latter type of generalization need be made, since the former would be superfluous and not add anything meaningful to an understanding of the data. And it is often this latter type of generalization that is the most important for a study, particularly where the data are not amendable to treatment by statistical analysis, as in nonquantified data.

2. *Significance and causal relationships.* In explanatory studies in which the relationship between the independent and dependent variables is assessed, a finding that is statistically significant is sometimes taken to mean that the dependent variable is *causally* related to the independent variable. This certainly is not the case. Significance of a statistical relationship among variables does not prove causation. Causal relationships are extremely difficult to establish, particularly in studies of human beings because the interconnection between a cause and an effect is very complex with many intervening variables. In highly controlled experimental research, we can hope to come closer to causal relationships than in nonexperimental studies. In the latter, the most we can often aim for is to demonstrate a clearly defined, stable association between the variables that can be useful for predictive purposes, even though it may not provide us with a basic explanation of phenomena.

The ability to establish cause and effect relationships is a function of the design of the research and is influenced by the degree to which intervening, extraneous variables can be kept under control. A test of significance in no way assesses this ability. However, to the extent that we define our variables precisely and meaningfully, sharpen our measuring instruments, employ designs that will sort out and control extraneous variables, and minimize the psychological biases that can distort data, the greater will be the likelihood that we will find statistically significant differences in the measures compared as well as produce findings that will be substantively significant.

3. *A finding of statistical significance is no indication of the quality of a study.* The fact that a statistical analysis reveals that our findings are statistically significant does not put a stamp of approval on the quality of the study design. A poor study can produce statistically significant findings, whereas a well-designed study may turn up nonsignificant results. Conversely, a poorly designed study may overlook significant results. Sometimes the poor quality of a study design is obscured, perhaps intentionally, in the reporting of results by the inclusion of page after page of esoteric mathematics. The mathematics prove nothing, but serve as a convenient smokescreen for the inadequacies of the study design. Some of the most significant —meaning *substantively* significant —research findings have been completely free of any mathematical manipulations.

Bear in mind that the determination of sampling error through the calculation of a standard error measures only one type of error. Actually this is not error in the common usage of the term—a mistake, something done wrong. The "error" of sampling is basically the consequence of the variability of the sampling units in the target population and the fact that we happened to select only a small number of these units to serve as subjects. If we included the whole population in the study, or if there was no variability among subjects, this source of error would be eliminated. But we do not want to include the whole popu-

lation because that would usually be too expensive. Moreover, in everything that is measured there is variability among sampling units. In research we must contend with sampling error.

Nonsampling errors are often caused by mistakes—mistakes in defining the problem or in the measuring instruments or in data collection procedures or in handling of the data after collection, or in interpreting the meaning of the data, or in providing sufficient control over extraneous factors. These errors are not assessed by tests of significance or by confidence intervals.

4. *Use of the wrong tests of significance.* In the discussion of the various types of random sampling methods it was pointed out that each method employs a different mathematical formula for the calculation of sampling error. The standard error of a mean for a sample selected by the cluster method has a more complicated formula than that for means based on a simple random sample, since the intercorrelations among the sampling units within a cluster must be considered. Quite often the simple random sampling standard error formula is used indiscriminately, regardless of the nature of the sampling method employed.

Moreover, each of the various tests of significance, particularly parametric tests, require that the data meet certain assumptions before the test can be applied. For example, in addition to the requirements that the measurements be obtained through a random process and that they be independent of each other (i.e., that the value of the measurement for sampling unit A should not be influenced by the value of the measurement for B), the analysis of variance test has certain other requirements. These include that the distribution of the values of the measurements in the population from which the sampling units were randomly selected be reasonably normal, that the scale underlying the measurements be a continuous one, and that the effects attributable to the independent variable(s) be additive. Frequently, tests of significance are employed for data that deviate widely from the assumptions underlying the tests. Nonparametric tests can provide a safeguard against this problem, although they may have drawbacks in the loss of information and decreased sensitivity that results from the use of such tests.

5. *Fishing for statistical significance.* Quite often the researcher may apply a number of statistical tests of significance to data after they have been tabulated. Every summary measure is compared in *t* tests with every other summary measure. New summary measures are often computed and tested by regrouping the scale values of the criterion measure. Tests of significance are applied on an ex post facto basis to differences in the values of summary measures even though no hypotheses concerning these comparisons were stated prior to data collection.

With such abundant significance testing, sooner or later *t* ratio values will be found that exceed the 5 percent level of significance, when perhaps no significance should really be attached to the differences. Significance levels state the risk of rejecting the null hypothesis when it is in fact true—the Type I error. If we were to run one hundred significance tests based on the same data—as in dividing our sample into smaller samples, computing the means of the measures for the subsamples, and running tests of significance on differences in the means—we would expect to commit the Type I error about 5 times in 100 tests at the 0.05 level of significance

Hypotheses that are formulated retrospectively, particularly if they are suggested by the data collected to test the original hypotheses, cannot be legitimately tested by traditional tests of significance. The Bayesian approach, with its use of prior information and the notion of "intensity of belief" the researcher has in various hypotheses about the subject being investigated, may appear as a modification of this rule. However, prior knowledge in this approach is used as a basis for formulation of a new hypothesis to guide the collection of new

data, not to suggest a new hypothesis to be tested by data already obtained.

6. *Impermanence of statistically significant results.* The fact that a test of significance has shown the data to be statistically significant does not mean that the research problem has been settled for all time. The finding of statistical significance today does not mean that we will find significance if we repeated the study a year from now or even next month. When the research is concerned with a complex set of variables operating in a fluid population, we cannot be sure how far into the future we can project the results of statistical significance tests. Even very significant findings may be transitory in nature. A study finding that primary Nursing yields a significantly higher quality of nursing care, even if based on a large, representative, and randomly selected sample, may only hold true for a limited time. There are many variables in this situation undergoing a continual change—the education of the Nursing staff is changing, the characteristics of patient care are being modified, attitudes toward care on the part of patients are changing, new facilities and new methods of patient care are being introduced, to name just a few of the dynamic ingredients.

The extent of statistical generalization is limited by the boundaries of the target population. One dimension of this boundary is the time period in which the population exists. Any generalization beyond this time period requires a nonstatistical generalization, and the scope of the generalization will depend on the researcher's assessment of the stability of the total situation with which the research is concerned.

Since one study will not answer a question for all time, the need for replication of studies cannot be stressed too strongly. By replication the stability of previous findings can be assessed.

7. *The level of significance does not necessarily denote the strength of a relationship.* In testing hypotheses concerning the relationship between independent and dependent variables the fact that the test

indicates significance well beyond the level chosen—say, at the 0.0001 level—does not necessarily indicate a stronger relationship than if the level turned out to be 0.01. For example, assume that our independent variable involved a comparison of two newly employed groups of public health nurses: those who had taken a course in public health nursing as part of their basic undergraduate prorgram and those who had not. The dependent variable is a measure of the ability of a nurse to adjust to a work situation in the field of public health nursing the first six months after graduation. If a comparison of the values of the summary measures of the dependent variable for the two groups shows a difference well beyond the level of significance adopted for the study—5 percent—we should not jump to the conclusion that the variables are strongly related—more strongly than if a lower level of significance were obtained.

We must bear in mind that the level of significance of the difference found is influenced not only by the effects of the independent variable but also by the homogeneity of the sampling units, and by the research design, which in essence is an artifact. We must consider that elements of the research design such as the sensitivity of measuring instruments, control over extraneous variables, and size of sample, to name just a few, can be greatly influenced by the researcher. For example, for a given difference in the values of the summary measures for the groups studied and a stated amount of variability of the values among the population, the significance of the findings can be increased by enlarging the size of the sample. This would not necessarily indicate a stronger relationship among the variables, but rather a more precise estimate of true difference among the groups.

8. *The use of a statistical significance test is not a guarantee of a good study.* Many excellently designed studies concerned with important research problems, do not employ tests of significance. This may be because the data do not warrant the use of tests—random sampling was not involved, or the study was concerned largely with nonquantitative data. The absence of tests of significance does not depreciate the findings of a study, just as the use of such tests does not necessarily raise the quality. Often the key interpretation of study results is made from analysis of tabulations of the data. Such interpretation of statistical tables, to be discussed shortly, can bring out the real meaning of the data.

Statistical analysis through significance testing should be placed in proper perspective. It is essentially a technique for evaluating the influence of sampling error and should not be regarded as the final step in determining what the data mean. We should not try to make these tests perform interpretative functions that they were not created to do.

9. *Insufficient time for significance to be revealed.* In some studies the time lag between the application of the independent variable and measurement of the effect in the dependent variable may be too short. As a result we do not observe any significant difference in the values of the summary measures. If we had waited longer—time for the "treatment to take," so to speak—significance may well have been obtained. In order to avoid the possible commitment of a Type II error—accepting the hypothesis of no difference when it is really false—the study should allow for a sufficient time to elapse before measurement of the dependent variable is made.

One of the factors in a study situation that could militate against obtaining short-run results in a study is resistance to change. Wallis and Roberts[8] give the following example:

A restaurant attempted to evaluate the effect on its cigarette business of changing from sales by cashier to sales by a coin-operated vending machine. The number of packages sold during the first month of machine sales was 51 per cent less than during the last month of cashier sales. As a basis of comparison sales for the same two months in two comparable restaurants were used. These showed decreases of 15 per cent and 3 per cent, respectively. As a result of this comparison, it was concluded that the "installation of the cigarette vending machine was detrimental to sales."

Perhaps if cigarette sales had been measured a year later when customers had adjusted to the change in the method of vending, the volume would have risen to a level at least as high as it was prior to the change.

10. *Overuse of the null hypothesis.* Many studies employ the null hypothesis as the model for the test of significance almost by rote. From a practical standpoint, a hypothesized zero difference frequently has no real meaning, and a positive value should be used instead. In other studies any difference, no matter how small, is important. If, for example, we are testing the effect of a drug on weight reduction, we might be interested only in differences between our experimental and control groups that significantly exceed a certain amount, say, a minimum of 10 to 20 pounds, before we accept a decision that the drug is effective. We would not just be interested that the difference was greater than zero. If, on the other hand, we are testing a drug in terms of its ability to reverse an incurable illness, we might use any amount greater than a zero difference as our standard of acceptance, since even one life saved would be significant.

11. *Confusion of statistical significance with practical significance.* One of the most common misuses of statistical significance is to confuse it with practical significance. A finding of statistical significance may in fact have little or no substantive meaning, particularly if based on the null hypothesis. Consider the fact that if our sample is large enough, even small differences not much greater than zero would be statistically significant regardless of how unimportant these differences may be. Moreover, artificial refinements in our measuring scale, such as dividing intervals into small segments, as in reading patients' temperatures

to one-hundredth of a degree, can yield statistically significant findings that would be meaningless. We must constantly remind ourselves that statistical significance means that the difference observed among sample subjects could only rarely have occurred by chance as a result of random sampling. It does not tell anything about the practical importance of this difference.

The substantive significance of a finding can only be assessed by the researcher's evaluation of its meaning within the subject matter framework of the area of research. In applied research this may be a pragmatic evaluation in terms of dollars and cents. If our study showed that raising salaries of the nursing staff by 10 percent resulted in a 10 percent reduction in turnover, the significance of this reduction can be appraised in a "balance sheet" type of analysis that weighs the cost of the salary increase against the monetary savings achieved by a turnover reduction as well as any nonmonetary gains such as higher morale and improved quality of performance.

In many studies, where the criterion measure cannot be correlated with some external pragmatic standard such as lives saved, improvement in services, or lowered costs, the practical significance of the findings is more difficult to assess. If our criterion measure is a subjective rating scale, how can we evaluate a statistically significant difference between an average rating of say, "excellent" and "very good," or "very satisfactory" and "satisfactory"? But even objective numerical measurement does not guarantee practical significance. How, for example, do we interpret the practical importance of small changes in blood pressure which might be statistically significant?

Until we can demonstrate that statistically significant findings also have substantive significance, our interpretation of the data is limited. This holds true for basic as well as so-called applied research. Application of results may well be the long-range objective of basic research. The findings of one basic study often serve to formulate problem and hypothesis for another study.

Each study, through its substantive contribution provides another step towards a meaningful contribution to the total research effort.

The significance of findings depends upon the quality of the measurement of the variables in the study. This quality is assessed by the criteria of validity, reliability, sensitivity, and meaningfulness. To the extent that the process of measurement in a study meets these criteria, the likelihood is increased that the findings will be not only stastically significant but substantively significant as well.

INTERPRETING DATA IN STATISTICAL TABLES

Perhaps the most useful approach to the interpretation of the statistical findings of a study is through organization of the data into statistical tables that help to focus attention on the practical meaning of the data in two important ways. First, since a table is a summarization of the data, the researcher must often regroup measurements into scale categories, called class intervals, that possess substantive meaning. Thus, if an independent variable is the age of a patient, recorded in years, the regrouping into class intervals will help to focus attention on the uses to which the data might be put. If the data are to serve in planning health programs for the elderly patient, perhaps two groupings will suffice: sixty five years of age and over, under sixty five years. If the study were concerned with health problems in each age group, a more refined grouping will be employed, such as under one year of age, 1–5, 6–20, 21–44, 45–64, 65 and over.

Second, the process of organizing data in tables enables the researcher to assess the relationship between the variables. Not only can the simple relationship between an independent and a dependent variable be studied, but the combined effects of several independent variables on the criterion measure can be assessed.

How the relationship between variables can be assessed through tabulation of the data is illustrated by the following study. A health department desired to evaluate the factors influencing people to be vaccinated against poliomyelitis. Over 600 people were interviewed to find out why they did or did not obtain immunization.

The most basic tabulation of data from a study is called a *univariate distribution.* Such a tabulation presents the data for only one variable at a time. For the immunization study a univariate distribution of the criterion variable—the extent of vaccine acceptance among the respondents—is presented in Table 16–1.

This table simply shows in percentage form the distribution of respondents according to one variable—their acceptance of the vaccine. The interpretation of the data is that nearly half of the respondents took both types of vaccine and less than one in five took neither.

In Table 16–2 another variable is introduced into the analysis: the educational level of the respondents. Such a table is called a *bivariate distribution.* In this table, vaccine acceptance is the dependent variable—the criterion measure of the success of the polio immunization program—while educational level—is an independent variable—a variable that may help explain the vaccine acceptance behavior of the respondents. As is seen in the table there is a

TABLE 16–1.
Percentage of Study Subjects Immunized Against Poliomyelitis

TOTAL	NONTAKERS	INJECTIONS ONLY	ORAL ONLY	BOTH VACCINES
100%	19	20	14	47

Source: A. L. Johnson, C. D. Jenkins, R. Patrick, and J. T. Northcutt, Jr., *Epidemology of Polio Vaccine.* Florida State Board of Health, Monograph No. 3, 1962, p. 35.

TABLE 16-2.
Percentage of Study Subjects Immunized Against Poliomyelitis by Educational Level

EDUCATIONAL LEVEL	NUMBER OF RESPONDENTS	TOTAL	NON-TAKERS	INJECTIONS ONLY	ORAL ONLY	BOTH VACCINES
All levels	624	100%	19	20	14	47
Fewer than eight grades	42	100%	52	7	24	17
Grade school gradate	43	100%	42	12	18	28
Some high school	133	100%	25	25	13	37
High school graduate	228	100%	16	21	15	48
Some college	128	100%	6	19	9	66
College graduate	50	100%	2	24	6	68

Source: as for Table 16-1.

direct relationship between the two variables: as educational level increases, so does acceptance of the vaccine. This suggests that the content of the program used to induce people to seek vaccination may have exceeded the understanding level of people with lesser education. The table demonstrates how the introduction of additional variables can provide meaningful insight into the behavior of the dependent variable.

Tables that contain more than two variables can be called *multivariate distribu-*tions; an example of such a table is Table 16-3 in the following section.

How to Interpret a Statistical Table

The elements of a statistical table provide the framework for the data incorporated into the table. There are many approaches to the interpretation of data contained in a table. Some direct their attention first to the body of the table and make a quick, overall evaluation of the data. Others take a more leisurely approach,

TABLE 16-3.
Average Percentage of Patients Reporting Dissatisfaction with Length of Time Spent Waiting for Nursing Services, by Age of Patients and Size of Room Accomodation (60 general hospitals, 1956)

AGE OF PATIENTS*	ALL ROOM ACCOMMODATIONS, AVERAGE	NUMBER OF BEDS IN ROOM			
		PRIVATE	2 BEDS	3-6 BEDS	7 OR MORE BEDS
All ages average	9.8	8.8	9.2	9.9	12.0
Under 20 years	14.9	12.8	13.0	12.9	18.8
20-29	12.5	14.1	12.1	12.3	12.7
30-39	9.9	9.0	8.2	10.2	8.1
40-49	9.3	9.0	8.2	9.5	9.3
50-59	8.0	7.1	8.7	7.7	8.6
60 and over	8.1	7.2	8.1	8.9	7.4

*Nonobstetrical patients. (Percentages denote the percentages of the total number of patients in each age and accommodation group who reported dissatisfaction with length of time spent waiting for nursing services).

Source: Questionnaires to patients in 60 general hospitals. For a complete report of the study see Faye G. Abdellah and Eugene Levine, *Effect of Nurse Staffing on Satisfactions with Nursing Care.* American Hospital Association, Monograph No. 4 (1958), 88 pp.

reading the title first, then the boxhead, stub, source, and even footnotes before studying the data. The following is a suggested step-by-step guide for interpreting the data in a statistical table, which, if followed in the sequence presented, should help the reader to derive the maximum amount of interpretative information.

The steps in interpreting a table are presented in the form of guide questions. The usefulness of these questions will be illustrated by applying them to a table containing findings from a study in which the relationship between the amount of nursing care provided and patient and personnel satisfaction with the care was explored. The design was nonexperimental. A sample of sixty general hospitals was selected according to the average daily amounts of nursing care provided to patients: high, medium, and low. The dependent variable, satisfaction with care, was assessed by checklists in which the patients and personnel in the sample hospitals reported omissions in nursing service. Table 16–3 is a by-product of this study. For this table a subscore of the dependent variable was computed showing dissatisfaction with the length of time spent waiting for services. This variable is analyzed in relation to two independent variables—the age of the patients and the size of their room accommodations.

Table 16–3, then, is a multivariate distribution. In such a table not only can the relationship between independent variables and the dependent variable be assessed, but the interactions between the independent variables can also be evaluated.

The guide questions for interpreting data in a table are:

1. What does the title of the table and other explanatory material tell us?
2. How were the data obtained?
3. What is being measured?
4. How much variation is there in the grand totals or averages for each variable?
5. How much variation is there within each of the scale values (classes) of the variables?
6. How are the variables related to each other?

7. Do the data reveal any unusual pattern?
8. What can be concluded from the interpretation of the data?

1. *What does the title of the table and other explanatory material tell us?* The title states that the purpose of the study is to determine whether age of patients or the size of their accommodations or a combination of the two variables is related to patients' dissatisfaction with nursing services in general hospitals. The data are classified according to two variables, age of patient and size of room accommodations. There is a third variable in the table. This is the dissatisfaction of patients with nursing services. Age of patients and room size are the independent variables. Dissatisfaction is the dependent variable. The table portrays the relationship between the independent variables, age of patient and size of his room accommodation, and the criterion measure, dissatisfaction with nursing service. The data were collected in only sixty general hospitals, a sample of the total population. The adequacy and scope of the sample can only be assessed by reference to the complete study. The headnote spells out specifically what the percentages in the table represent. The footnote limits the data to nonobstetrical patients.

2. *How were the data obtained?* The source tells us the data were collected by questionnaires filled out by patients. The data have come from an original source and not a secondary one.

3. *What is being measured?* The sampling unit in the study is a patient. Measurements have been made on three variables concerning each patient: size of room, age, and dissatisfaction with waiting for services. The table shows how these variables are related to each other.

4. *How much variation is there in the grand totals or averages for each variable?* There are two sets of overall averages in the table, one for each of the independent variables. These are the figures in the first column of the table under "All Room Accommodations, Average" and on the first line "All ages, average."

The figures on the line "All ages, average" indicate that as size of room increases, dissatisfaction with nursing services also increases. The percent of patients dissatisfied with nursing services in rooms with seven or more beds is nearly 50 percent greater than the percent dissatisfied in private rooms.

The figures in the column "All Room Accommodations, Average" show the following pattern: As age increases, percent of patients dissatisfied with nursing services decreases. The range of difference among the age groups is greater than for room size. The percentage of patients under twenty years of age dissatisfied with nursing services is nearly twice as high as the percentage of patients fifty years of age and over. This suggests age is more closely related to dissatisfaction than is size of room accommodation.

5. *How much variation is there within each of the scale values (classes) of the variables?* Data in each of the room size groups follow the same pattern as the overall average. In each of the different room accommodation groups, as age of patients increases, dissatisfaction decreases. The greatest variation is in the group "7 or More Beds," where the range is from 18.8

percent in the youngest group to 7.4 percent in the oldest.

The data behave differently for the age variable. Only in the youngest age groups is there an increase in dissatisfaction as room size increases, while among older patients there is no relationship at all between amount of dissatisfaction and room size.

6. *How are the variables related to each other?* The age of a patient has a considerably stronger relationship to dissatisfaction than size of room accommodation. While the average for all patients combined shows a rise in dissatisfaction as room size increases, only the youngest age group reveals this same pattern. Apparently, the pattern found in the youngest age group has a strong influence on the average for all ages combined.

7. *Do the data reveal any unusual pattern?* Why does the average for all patients combined show increasing dissatisfaction in waiting for nursing services as room size increases, when this pattern does not hold true for any age group except the youngest? The key to the answer to this question lies in Table 16–4, which gives the actual number of patients participating in the study for each cell. As can be seen from the table the largest proportion of younger pa-

TABLE 16–4.
Total Number of Patients in 60 General Hospitals Study, by Age of Patients and Size of Room Accommodations (1956)

AGE OF PATIENTS*	ALL ROOM ACCOMMODATIONS, TOTAL	PRIVATE	2 BED	3–6 BEDS	7 OR MORE BEDS
All ages, total	*7,024*	*1,330*	*2,425*	*2,408*	*861*
Under 20 years	720	63	162	249	246
20–29	846	107	285	315	139
30–39	1,057	159	364	411	123
40–49	1,264	255	481	412	116
50–59	1,333	285	498	430	120
60 and over	1,804	461	635	591	117

NUMBER OF BEDS IN ROOM

*Nonobstetrical patients.

Source: See Table 16–3.

tients are in the larger rooms, while the largest proportion of older patients are in private or semiprivate rooms. Since younger patients are more dissatisfied with nursing services than older patients regardless of room accommodation, the average percentages are weighted by the number of patients in different age groups who are in the various room size groups. Since there are more younger patients in larger rooms, and more older patients in smaller rooms, and since younger patients are more dissatisfied than older patients, the average for all patients combined shows an increasing dissatisfaction as room size increases. If considered by itself, this average is misleading, since it is distorted by the underlying disproportionate age distribution of patients in the different-sized rooms.

8. *What can be concluded from the interpretation of the data?* There is a strong relationship between the age of patient and dissatisfaction with time spent waiting for nursing services. As age increases, dissatisfaction decreases. Except for the youngest patients, there is no relationship between size of room accommodation and dissatisfaction with nursing services. Patients under twenty years in large rooms are more dissatisfied than patients under twenty in private rooms. The greatest range of dissatisfaction, according to age, is in the largest room accommodations. Patients under twenty are nearly two and a half times more dissatisfied with the amount of time they have to wait for nursing services than patients who are sixty years of age and over.

Some Pitfalls in Interpreting Data in Tables

There are a number of pitfalls in interpreting a table like the one just discussed. If they are not avoided, the interpretation of the data can be spurious. If an erroneous interpretation of data is used to guide action it can lead to costly wastes of effort, time, and money. A few of the major pitfalls will be discussed using the table just presented.

1. *Misinterpretation of cause and effect.*

Because a table reveals that the variables are related to each other does not by any means establish the fact that they are causally related. Particularly in nonexperimental studies, where many of the important extraneous variables may not be controlled, relationships between two variables shown in a table may actually reflect the influence of an extraneous variable. This point is demonstrated by the fact that the relationship between room size and patient satisfaction actually reflects the influence of patients' ages. When age is held constant, no important relationship can be seen between room size and satisfaction.

2. *Failure to consider variability around the measures of central tendency.* The figures shown in each cell of a table are summary measures around which may exist considerable variation of the individual values upon which they are based. The extent to which a summary measure, such as a mean, is a good descriptive measure of the individual values depends on how large the variation is. In interpreting data the fact that some summary measures may describe the individual values better than others should be kept in mind in evaluating differences between the values in different cells of the table. Suppose we had two samples, each consisting of five hospitals, for which the average percentage of patients reporting dissatisfaction with length of time spent in waiting for nursing services is computed as follows:

	SAMPLE 1	SAMPLE 2
	11.0	5.0
	11.0	7.0
	12.0	14.0
	13.0	14.0
	13.0	15.0
Mean	12.0	11.0

In sample 1 the individual values fall within a narrow range, whereas in sample 2 the values are highly variable. If we only examined the means it would appear that the hospitals in sample 2 had better satisfaction scores than those in sample 1. However, in sample 2 the scores of three of the hospitals indicate higher dissatisfaction than any of the hospitals in sample 1. This raises the question as to whether for a comparison of the two samples of hospitals the mean is a good summary measure of the average satisfaction level.

3. *Failure to account for the possibility of noncomparability of the groups included in the table.* In nonexperimental studies the comparison groups are usually not standardized by random assignment. Therefore, it is possible that the groups could differ in certain important characteristics that could affect the values of the criterion measures. One such characteristic is that for some of the very young patients, where highest dissatisfaction levels were found, it may have been the parent who responded to the checklist rather than the patient (the protocols for the study permitted this). In some cases, enough to influence the data significantly, the parents may have been more impatient with the length of time it took for a nursing service to be provided than the patients.

4. *Limitations of data due to possible inadequacies of measuring instruments.* In interpreting data in tables a skeptical attitude should be maintained concerning the quality of the measuring instruments employed, particularly their reliability and validity. This is particularly true in data such as those in these tables. The instrument used to collect these data was developed especially for the study and at the time of the study had not undergone extensive use, although it had received multiple pretests to check validity and reliability.

5. *Limitations of sample size in making generalizations.* Before any generalizations of the data can be made beyond the study setting, the method of selection of the sample as well as its size must be considered. In interpreting the data the following questions should be raised. Were the hospitals selected from a larger target population? If so, how was this population defined? Were the sample hospitals chosen randomly so that confidence intervals could

be computed for the summary measure? What kind of sample is this—if it is not a simple random sample, is it a cluster sample? If so, what formulas should be used in computing the sampling error? How many hospitals were included in the sample, and how many patients in each of the hospitals submitted checklists?

Answers to many such questions are not usually available just from inspection of a table. They can only be obtained by referring to the complete report of the study. If the data are to be definitively interpreted this must be done.

6. *In interpreting a statistical table it is important to consider all possible limitations of the data.* In addition to the limitations already mentioned—spurious relationships, possible weaknesses in the measurement process, lack of comparability of study groups, small size of sample, and its method of selection—all other limitations of the data should be weighed. These include the possible transient nature of the relationships found among the variables. What was found in this study would have to be corroborated by other studies to demonstrate stability and permanence of the findings.

7. *The substantive meaning of the data needs to be assessed.* Finally, the data must be evaluated in light of what substantive meaning they prossess. Are the data merely an interesting academic exercise, or do they offer any constructive suggestions, advice, or guidelines for pursuing a course of action in the real world?

REFERENCES

1. Frederick Mosteller, Robert E.K. Rourke, George B. Thomas, Jr., *Probability with Statistical Applications.* Reading, MA, Addison-Wesley Publishing Co., Inc., 1961, p. 146.
2. Hanan C. Selvin, "A Critique of Tests of Significance in Survey Research." *Am. Sociol. Rev.,* **22:**519–527, October 1957.
3. Robert McGinnis, "Randomization and Inference in Sociological Research." *Am. Sociol. Rev.,* **23:**408–414, August 1958.

4. Leslie Kish, "Some Statistical Problems in Research Design." *Am Sociol. Rev.*, **24**:328–338, June 1959.
5. Patricia L. Kendall, "Methodological Appendix," in Robert K. Merton, George G. Reader, and Patricia L. Kendall (eds.), *The Student Physician.* Cambridge, Harvard University Press, 1957.
6. Herman Wold, "Causal Inference from Observational Data." *J. Royal Statistical Soc.* (A), **119**:28–61, January 1956.
7. Lawrence M. Friedman, Curt D. Furberg and David L. De Mets, *Fundamentals of Clinical Trials.* Boston, John Wright, PSG Inc., 1984.
8. W. Allen Wallis and Harry V. Roberts, *Statistics: A New Approach.* New York, The Free Press of Glencoe, 1956, p.133.

PROBLEMS AND SUGGESTIONS FOR FURTHER STUDY

1. What is meant by interpreting the results of a study? Is this process different from analyzing the data from the study?
2. Read the article by Hanan C. Selvin, "A Critique of Tests of Significance in Survey Research," *(Am., Sociol. Rev.,* **22**:519–527, October 1957). Do you agree with the author's conclusions that "Statistical tests are unsatisfactory in nonexperimental research for two fundamental reasons. It is almost impossible to design studies that meet the conditions for using the tests, and the situations in which the tests are employed make it difficult do draw correct inferences" (p. 527). Also read the reply to this article by Leslie Kish, "Some Statistical Problems in Research Design," *(Am. Sociol. Rev.,* **24**:328–338, June 1959). Comment on this author's statement that "Selvin's logic and advice should lead not only to the rejection of statistical tests; it should lead one to refrain altogether from using survey results for the purposes of finding explanatory variables. In this sense, not only tests of significance, but any comparisons, any specific inquiry based on surveys, any scientific inquiry other than an 'ideal' experiment, is inapplicable. That advice is most unrealistic" (p. 331).
3. Evaluate the manner in which the data were interpreted in the following reported studies. Do you feel the authors provided sufficient data in their reports to enable the reader to verify the author's interpretation?

a. Joyce D. Sloane, "Bladder Atonia After Vaginal Delivery." *Nursing Res.,* **8**:26–32, winter 1959.
b. Richard M. Levinson, William L. Graves, Johnetta Holcombe, "Cross Cultural Variations in the Definition of Child Abuse: Nurses in the U.S. and the U.K." *Int. J. Nursing Stud.,* **21**:35–44, 1984.
c. Helene J. Krouse and John H. Krouse, "Cancer as Crisis: The Critical Elements of Adjustment." *Nursing Res.,* **31**:96–101, March/April 1982.
d. Peter Kong-Ming New and Gladys Nite, "Staffing and Interaction." *Nursing Outlook,* **8**:396–400, July 1960.
e. Beverly J. Volicer and Mary Wynne Bohannon, "A Hospital Stress Rating Scale," *Nursing Res.,* **24**:352–359, September/October 1975.
f. John A. Ward and John M. Griffin, "Improving Instruction Through Computer-Graded Examinations." *Nursing Outlook,* **25**:524–529, August 1977.
g. Alta Faye Woody *et al.,* "Do Patients Learn What Nurses Say They Teach?" *Nursing Manage.,* **15**:26–29, December 1984.
h. Noralou P. Roos, "Hysterectomies in One Canadian Province: A New Look at Risks and Benefits." *Am. J. Pub. Health.,* **74**:39–46, January 1984.
4. Read Chapter 14, "Probability and Induction," in Morris R. Cohen and Ernest Nagel. *An Introduction to Logic and Scientific Method* (1982 Reprint of 1934 edition, Darby, PA, Darby Books. pp. 273-288). How do the authors define inductive reasoning? Discuss the author's remarks that "an inductive argument, while it does not, in the strictest sense, demonstrate a universal proposition, may prove it to be the best evidenced of all suggested hypotheses" (p. 284).
5. Discuss the distinction between the following terms:
a. Practical significance of research findings and statistical significance of the findings
b. One-tailed and two-tailed tests of statistical significance.
c. The Neyman-Pearson method of statistical inference and Bayesian inference
d. Analysis of data and interpretation of findings

e. Random sampling and random assignment
f. Level of significance and confidence level
g. Statistics and parameters
h. Correlation and regression
i. Type I and Type II errors.

6. Obtain a copy of the latest edition of *Facts About Nursing* published by the American Nurses' Association (Kansas City, MO). Select five tables and apply the guidelines for interpreting data in tables contained in this chapter. Write a brief interpretation of the data they contain.

7. Discuss the following statement by E.J.G. Pitman, "Statistics and Science," (*J. Am. Statistical Assoc.*, **52**:322–330, September 1957), "The scientist with ideas frames his hypotheses and wishes to test them. He would be happy if he could devise a test which would decide with certainty whether a hypothesis is true or not. When he cannot do this, he must use a test which has only a certain probability of giving the right answer" (p. 323).

8. Comment on the following statement by Selltiz and others in *Research Methods in Social Relations* (New York, Holt, Rinehart and Winston, rev. ed., 1976). "If we want to make causal inferences—that is, to say that one variable or event has led to another—we must meet assumptions over and above those required for establishing the existence of a relationship" (p. 422). What are these assumptions?

9. Read Chapter 8, "How to Think," in Hans Selye, *From Dream to Discovery: On Being a Scientist* (New York, Arno, 1975). Discuss the following statement by the author:

> There is a great difference between a sterile theory and a wrong one. A sterile theory does not lend itself to experimental verification. Any number of them can be easily formulated, but they are perfectly useless. They could not possibly aid understanding; they lead only to futile verbiage. On the other hand, a wrong theory can still be highly useful, for, if it is well conceived, it may help to formulate experiments which will fill important gaps in our knowledge. Facts must be correct; theories must be fruitful. A "fact," if incorrect, is useless—it is not a fact—but an incorrect theory may be even more useful than a correct one if it is more fruitful in leading the way to new facts. (p.280.)

10. Comment on the following remarks by R.A. Fisher in his *The Design of Experiments* (New York, Hafner, 9th ed., 1974). " . . . it should be noted that the null hypothesis is never proved or established, but is possibly disproved in the course of experimentation. Every experiment may be said to exist only in order to give the facts a chance of disproving the null hypothesis."

CHAPTER 17

Communicating
and Utilizing Results

OBJECTIVES

- To describe the format and content of a research report.
- To explain how research is implemented.
- To provide guidelines for evaluating research.

Unless research findings are communicated, they have no benefit. The research investigator has an obligation to publish research to share the knowledge and subject the findings to testing by others. Some researchers view publication as only a scholarly achievement and do not feel obligated to publish. In such instances one can only wonder if the researcher fears exposure of inconsequential research and sanction by his colleagues. Some researchers, on the other hand, are perfectionists and never feel that their manuscripts are ready for publication. This attitude only delays the sharing of new knowledge that might be valuable to other researchers.

Many universities have now adopted the philosophy of "publish or perish." The intent here is to use one criterion—namely, publication—as a means of assessing the individual's readiness for promotion within the academic hierachy. This pressure often leads to publication of inconsequential research. This chapter presents some guidelines that the investigator may find helpful in thinking through the steps of preparing a manuscript for publication, as well as providing suggestions as to what to look for in published scientific papers.

RESEARCH UTILIZATION PROCESS

Research and research utilization may be considered as interdependent processes that move us closer to achieving a nursing science.[1] Together they comprise research activity. Nursing research may be viewed as identifying and refining solutions to problems through the generation of new scientific knowledge. Research utilization, on the other hand, is finding new solutions specifically for the purpose of improving nursing practice. Activities that comprise utilization include:[2]

• Identification and synthesis of multiple research studies in a common conceptual area.
• Transformation of the knowledge derived from a research base into a solution or clinical protocol.
• Transformation of the clinical protocol into specific nursing actions that improve nursing practice.
• A clinical evaluation of the new practice to determine whether the hypothesized results were achieved.

Communication of research findings requires a deliberate effort to bring about change to make the innovation acceptable. Basic to the communication process are a number of change components that interact over time:[3]

• *The change:* characteristics of the innovation.
• *The change agents:* those individuals and resources that will make the change possible.
• *The change targets:* the recipients of the change.
• *The change setting:* characteristics and resources of the setting where change will take place.
• *Rationale for the change:* costs and benefits resulting from the change or innovation.
• *The change strategies:* approaches to be used to achieve change.
• *The timing of the change:* other activities that can affect the change.

STEPS IN IMPLEMENTING RESEARCH FINDINGS[4]

1. Design the form the change or innovation will take in the particular setting (e.g., hospital; community-based agency; home).
2. Design an approach to evaluate the effects of the innovation and process for carrying it out.
3. Identify and delegate tasks to be accomplished in implementing and evaluating innovation.
4. Develop a realistic time table to achieve tasks.
5. Obtain formal (written) and informal approval to carry out tasks.
6. Introduce innovation on a trial basis on one unit or part of an agency.
7. Obtain necessary resources (e.g., personnel, budget).
8. Anticipate opposition to change and plan how to deal with the resistance.
9. Prepare for implementation (e.g., training of personnel).
10. Plan for evaluation of the innovation, making sure all biases are identified.
11. Seek assurance that all those involved in change are prepared and supportive.
12. Review the total plan prior to implementation.

PLANNING FOR PUBLICATION

The way in which research findings are communicated depends on how the original proposal was prepared. The type of thinking that has gone on initially is usually reflected in the final report. Therefore, it is important to consider early in the research process how the research findings are to be communicated.

Brockington[5] refers to the formative stage of writing as reflective thinking. Its quality is based on the clarity with which the research question is posed. If it is stated ambiguously, the entire report will reflect this confusion. Discussion of the research question with experts in the field will help to crystallize the problem.

When properly prepared, the research report can be a valuable research and educational resource. To be acceptable for publication in a scientific journal, the report should describe unusual or puzzling features (particularly clinical); should help clarify a new, little known, or rare syndrome; or should illustrate an unexpected favorable or adverse effect of an intervention (treatment; drug) not previously reported.[6]

The choice of journal is important, and the report should be directed to a specific audience. In selecting the journal, consider the scope, readership, prestige, and circulation of the journal; the quality of photographic reproduction; and the length of time before the report is published.

The principles of all good scientific writing include conciseness; restricting negative results to scientific significance; and deciding whether the report warrants publication.[7,8]

WRITING THE RESEARCH REPORT

Steps in the research process have been considered previously. These must be thought of within a framework of preparing the final report. Following is a checklist that summarizes important points.

Checklist for Planning a Research Report

☐ 1. *Statement of purpose*
State the specific aims of your research, limiting them to those that can be accomplished during the first two years of the proposed research. State the long-range goals indicating those goals you hope to achieve beyond the two-year period.

Provide the rationale or conceptual framework for your research, stating the operational definitions, concepts, and deductions or hypotheses related to your research.

☐ 2. *Methods to be used*
Provide the steps in the research plan indicating in detail methods to be used, why these were chosen and not others, what data you intend to obtain, how the data are to be obtained, how they will be analyzed. The latter should show skeleton tables with examples of data. Relate methods and findings to show that answers to specific aims will be provided.

☐ 3. *Significance of research*
Provide a justification for doing your research. Can any inferences be drawn from the findings?

☐ 4. *Research climate*
Describe the relationships worked out in the setting in which the research is to be undertaken and the facilities to which you have access.

Preparation of the Final Report

An aid in preparing the final report is the development of a skeleton outline specifying chapter titles, subheadings, table outlines, with examples of kinds of data you hope to find. This is more than a mental exercise and can save many months of pursuing an approach that does not answer the research question.

The selection of the title of the report should be given considerable thought. It should be stated concisely and communicate the central theme of the research. Following is a sample table of contents.

Sample Table of Contents

Foreword	ii
List of Tables (and or figures)	iv
Chapter	
I. STATEMENT AND ANALYSIS OF THE PROBLEM	1
Purpose	
History of the subject	
Past research on the subject	
Speculative analysis of the problem	
II. THE DATA AND THEIR TREATMENT	15
The procedure	
III. THE RESULTS SUMMARIZED	19
IV. THE GENERALIZED RESULTS AND THEIR INTERPRETATION	30
V. SUMMARY AND CONCLUSIONS	45
Review of the problem and procedure	
Limitations of the conclusions	
Conclusions	
Bibliography	49
Appendix	51

Source: Material prepared by Dorothy Sutherland for a Nursing Research Conference, Columbia Union College, Takoma Park, Maryland, November 1961.

List of Appendix Tables

1. A scxc cxcx cxcxc cxc.   xx
2. The vxczv vxvzuxvz vxv.   xx
3. Etc.   xx

Sample Arrangement of the Research Paper

1. *Title page:* title of project, author's name, date, location, and other pertinent identifying information.
2. *Preface or foreword* containing acknowledgments.
3. *Table of contents:*
   Chapter or other subheadings
   List of tables
   List of illustrations
   Bibliography
   Appendix
   Tables and graphs should be so clearly presented that they are self-explanatory: this means that headings and captions to figures and graphs must be complete.
4. *Introduction:*
   Should be included in the first section of the text. (Separate introduction not recommended. To many "forewords" slow down pace of getting into the substance of the report.) Note special limitations of report here. Mention special techniques employed in gathering and handling of material. Define terms used if unusual or "coined" for purposes of the study.
5. *The text:*
   Repeat title at top of first page, centered. Number pages consecutively.
   Begin each new section of the report on a new page.
6. *Bibliography:*
   List on separate page, with self-heading. Continue pagination of report.
7. *Appendix:*
   Material not legitimately a part of the text, but helpful to the reader; e.g., some tables, sample questionnaire forms, complete transcripts of documents or other reference materials, etc.
8. *Index:*
   An index can be an invaluable aid to the reader and should be included in a research report that is published as a monograph or book. Its value rests in the appropriateness of the classification of concepts that it uses.

Reviewing a Research Report

Hillway[9] cites four main purposes that a review of a research report should accomplish. First, the main thesis of the report should be stated. Were the research aims initially stated achieved? Were hypotheses formulated? Was there an original contribution to knowledge? Second, there should be a clear analysis and assessment of the data presented. What controls were identified and used? Third, has the author presented the ideas logically in understandable terms? Fourth, does the review contain a critique of the work presented in terms of its contribution to its field of knowledge?

Suggested Checklist for Reviewing a Research Report

1. Does the report clearly state the purpose of the study?
2. Is the methodology adequately described?
   a. Did the investigator use the method cited in his proposal, and if not, does his report explain his reason for deviating?
   b. Are the instruments fully explained and (when appropriate) included as figures in the text or as exhibits in an appendix?
3. Have raw data (source tables) been placed in an appendix? Are summary tables integrated into appropriate places in the text? Are the tables understandable? Does the text merely restate content of tables, or does it interpret and point out significant relationships?
4. Does the report plainly summarize the findings? Does it contain the investigator's conclusions? Interpretation of results?
5. Do the findings, as reported, suggest need for further research or recommendations for application of the new knowledge discovered (if the content is applied research)?
6. Does the report adequately credit all sources and resources tapped during the study? Are there an acceptable bibliography and index?

7. Was the report difficult to read? Did the language obscure the content and value of the research? Were you interested in the study, regardless of the manner in which the report was written, despite its style?
8. Does the report convey that the research was useful or important, even though the subject investigated might have been a small one? Or, conversely, is it so verbose that it suggests the entire investigation was "much ado about nothing"?
9. Is the report interesting?
10. Do you know what the investigator accomplished?
11. If human subjects are involved, have they been informed of their rights? Have appropriate steps taken to protect the subjects?

The importance of communicating research findings cannot be overemphasized. To be meaningful, research must be communicated. The writer has a responsibility of predigesting his material into clear, concise writing. It is not uncommon to find that a researcher has submitted a voluminous, unedited document to be published. Many of these reports are actually working papers from which the researcher has failed to extract the relevant material.

It is helpful to focus the report upon a central theme to provide continuity from chapter to chapter. Be sure to indicate the significance of your research and questions that still remain unanswered. Above all, write enthusiastically to express rather than impress. There is no substitute for simplicity and clarity in writing.

Selected Standard Abbreviations

anon., anonymous
bull., bulletin
c., copyright
ca., or c., (*circa*): about, approximately
cf. ante, (*confer-ante*): compare above
cf. post, (*confer-post*): compare below
chap(s). or ch., chapter(s)
col(s)., column(s)
ed., editor, edition, edited
ed. cit., edition cited; where specific reference is being made to one edition that has already been noted in the documentation

e.g., (*exempli gratia*): for example
et al., (*et alii*), (*et alibi*): and others, and elsewhere
et seq., (*et sequens*): and the following
fig(s)., figure(s)
ibid., (*ibidem*): in the same place. When two or more successive footnotes refer to the same work, use *ibid.* instead of repeating reference. If different pages are referred to, pagination reference must be shown
id., idem: the same
i.e.,(*id est*): that is
loc. cit., (*loco citato*): in the place cited
o.p., out of print
op. cit., (*opere citato*): in the work cited. If reference has been made to a work and new reference is to be made without intervening references to other works, ibid. may be used; if intervening reference has been made to different works, op. cit. must be used. The name of the author must precede.
q.v., (*quad vide*): which see
rev., revised
sic: thus; indicates an error of which you are aware, especially in matter
tr., trans., translator, translated, translation
vid. or vide: see, refer to
V. or Vol(s)., volume(s)

Implementation of Research Findings

Research findings will not be utilized unless they are appropriately communicated. Lelean questions whether the reason that nursing is not viewed as a research-based profession is lack of dissemination of research findings.[10]

EVALUATING RESEARCH

In their book *Summing Up: The Science of Reviewing Research*, Richard J. Light and David B. Pillemer stress the importance of evaluating completed research.[11] Evaluation takes several forms. In the early stages of our own research we initially review the literature to determine the existing state of knowledge. Then, at the other end, when research is complete, we evaluate a study as we prepare to apply the findings to nursing practice and education. The following questions can help the assessment of a research plan or a completed research project. They also serve as a summarization of the essential components of the research process.

Guide Questions for Evaluating a Research Plan or a Completed Research Project

1. *The problem:* Is it feasible to conduct research on the problem? Is the problem important? To what extent can the findings of the research be generalized? What will the solution of the problem achieve?

Is the researcher really interested in the problem? Is the researcher adequately competent to pursue the problem through research? Can the research best be labeled as basic or applied? If applied, what are the possible practical outcomes of the research?

2. *Review of the literature:* Have all possible sources of related literature been investigated? Are the findings of previous studies that are relevant to the research being considered? What practical problems have previous researchers encountered?

Does the review of the literature provide supporting evidence to show the need carrying out the research? In what ways does the research being considered go beyond what already has been found in previous studies? Does the research make provisions for consultation with experts in the field when they are needed?

3. *The framework of theory:* Does any applicable theory exist in the field of knowledge in which the research is being done? Can the problem area in which the research is being done be conceptualized in the form of a model of some kind? Is the model useful in clarifying concepts and relationships contained in the research?

If the research deals with statistical data, what is the statistical model for the analysis of the data? Are the theories or models used in the study meaningful and helpful to

the study, and not just used as window-dressing?

4. *Formulation of hypotheses:* Are the hypotheses stated clearly and unambiguously? Do they contain a statement of the dependent and independent variables and the target population to whom the findings will be generalized?

Do the hypotheses deal with causal or associative relationships? Is the study concerned with artificial relationships, and if so, are there dangers of inferring spurious relationships from the data?

Are the independent and dependent variables operationally defined?

Are these variables meaningful and realistic in terms of their possible application outside of the experimental situation?

Does the design recognize the extraneous variables that may affect the results of the study? How will these extraneous variables be controlled or eliminated? What are the major organismic and environmental variables that are involved in the study?

If the hypothesis is stated as a null hypothesis, what are the alternative hypotheses?

Are the major assumptions underlying the study stated explicitly or implicitly? Are the bases for these assumptions, theories, laws, common sense, generally accepted facts, or findings from previous research? Have they been documented by references in the literature?

5. *Definition of the variables:* What is the scale of classification for the explanatory variables? Do valid scales or instruments already exist for measuring the variables? Are the variables defined clearly and concretely enough so that they are readily understood?

6. *Quantification of the variables:* Are the variables to be studied capable of being quantified? Is the quantification meaningful, valid, reliable? Has the quantification of variables been established in previous studies, or does the research establish original quantifications of the variables? Does the research deal with any variables that can

not be quantified, and if so, how are these handled in the analysis? Are expert consultants needed to develop variables that can be quantified?

Do the measures of the variables have a practical application in the real world?

7. *The research design:* Is the choice of the design—experimental or nonexperimental—appropriate for the research problem? Is the setting for the study natural or artificial?

What controls over possible hidden biases have been set up for the study? If appropriate, will random assignment procedures be used to allocate the sampling units to the different groups under study?

If an experiment is conducted, is the length of the experiment adequate for drawing valid conclusions?

Can the data from the experimental setting be generalized to other settings?

8. *The target population:* Has the target population been clearly designated by the research? Is the target population reasonable, or is it too ambitious?

What type of sampling units does the target population consist of—people, things, ideas, etc?

Can an appropriate sample be drawn of the target population? Will it be possible to draw a valid sample of the target population that is representative of the population?

9. *Collecting and analyzing data:* Is the target population to be sampled randomly? Will the size of the study population be adequate for drawing valid generalizations?

Are the methods that will be used to collect the data and the measures that will be derived from them valid and reliable? Do these measures have any practical application in the real world?

Have the data-collecting instruments been carefully pretested? Have they been used in previous research, or have they been developed purposely for the research?

Does the study clearly indicate the ways in which the data will be tabulated? Will the tabulations permit a meaningful and comprehensive interpretation to be made of the data?

Has sufficient time been allowed for the period of data collection? Have provisions been made to ensure completeness of data?

If needed, have provisions been made to hire sufficient personnel (field interviewers, observers) to assist in the collection of data? Is specialized equipment needed to tabulate the data, and are provisions made to obtain it?

Is the budget allowed for the study adequate for the amounts and kinds of data to be collected, for the method of collecting the data, and for the time allowed to do the research?

Are the statistical methods that will be used to analyze the data clearly indicated? Are these methods appropriate to the kinds of variables that will be studied, the kinds of data that will be collected concerning these variables, the methods of collecting these data, and the nature of the study population? Does the analysis of the data relate in a relevant way to the research problem and to the hypotheses under study?

Are the data analyzed in such a way as to yield maximum information from the findings?

10. *Interpretation of the data:* If tests of statistical significance are included in the design, what levels of significance are being used? Are these appropriate to the kinds of data with which the study is concerned?

Apart from a statistical significance that might be obtained from the study data, what might be the practical significance of the findings?

What is the scope of the generalizations that can be made from the data—as to length of time for which this generalization might apply, the nature of the applicable population, geographic coverage?

Does interpretation of the data lead back to the hypotheses, theoretical framework, research problem? Does the interpretation relate the findings to the general body of knowledge in the field? Does it show what the study has contributed to the advancement of knowledge in the field?

11. *Communicating the research:* Have adequate provisions been made to com-

municate the method and findings of the research to the audience most likely to be interested in and concerned with the research? Is the format for reporting the research appropriate to the content of the study? Does the researcher convey any sense of interest and enthusiasm in pursuing his research study?

Does the report contain a clear statement of the problem and purpose of the research and the framework of theory? Is the methodology adequately described?

Have the limitations of the study been carefully spelled out in the report? Does the report contain appropriate cautions in interpreting the data?

In the presentation of the statistical data, are detailed source tables placed in the appendix or some other part of the report where they will not interfere with the flow of the reading? Are the findings clearly presented?

REFERENCES

1. Jo Anne Horsley, Joyce Crane, *et al.*, *Using Research to Improve Nursing Practice: A Guide.* CURN Project. New York, Grune & Stratton, Inc. 1983.
2. *Ibid.*, p. 2.
3. *Ibid.*, p. 3.
4. *Ibid.*, p. 6.
5. Fraser Brockington, "Preparation of a Research Proposal and Preparation of the Final Report," in Margaret G. Arnstein and Ellen Broe (eds.), *International Conference on the Planning of Nursing Studies.* London, International Council of Nurses, 1956, pp. 44–50.
6. Lois DeBakey and Selma DeBakey, "Medical Writing. The Case Report. I. Guidelines for Preparation," *Int. J. Cardio.* **4**:358, 1983.
7. *Ibid.*, p. 363.
8. Lois DeBakey and Selma DeBakey, "Medical Writing. II. Style and Form," *Int. J. Cardio.,* **6**:247–254, 1984.
9. Tyrus Hillway, *Introduction to Research.* Boston, Houghton Mifflin Co., 1956, pp.261–262.
10. Sylvia R. Lelean, "The Implementation of Research Findings into Nursing Practice," *Int. J. Nursing Stud.*, **19**:223–230, 1982.
11. Richard J. Light and David B. Pillemer, *Summing Up: The Science of Reviewing Research.* Cambridge, MA, Harvard University Press, 1984.

PROBLEMS AND SUGGESTIONS FOR FURTHER STUDY

1. Read the report, *Delphi Survey of Clinical Nursing Researh Priorities.* Western Interstate Commission for Higher Education, Boulder, Colorado, The Commission, August 1974. Does the absence of tests of significance of the data detract from the report? Applying the Checklist for Reviewing a Research Report, write a review of this report.

2. Summarize the major points in the article "Strategies for Publishing Research," by Elizabeth M. Tornquist (*Nurs. Outlook,* **31**:180–183, May/June 1983). List some of the different publications that publish nursing research (e.g., books, journals, newsletters).

3. What are some obstacles to implementing nursing research? How can these be overcome? Can you give some practical applications of nursing research?

4. Read Chapter 11, "The Evaluation Report: How to Get It Read," in Emil J. Posavac and Raymond G. Carey, *Program Evaluation Methods and Case Studies* (Englewood Cliffs, NJ, Prentice-Hall, 1980, pp. 273–321). Can the pitfalls in reporting discussed by the authors be applied to nursing research?

5. How can the organizational model for research utilization, presented by Holly S. Wilson in "Organizational Approaches to Bridging the Research-Practice Gap" (*J. Nursing Admin.* **14**:7–8, September 1984) be helpful in implementing the findings of nursing research?

THREE

STRATEGIES AND FUTURE DIRECTIONS FOR NURSING RESEARCH

18

Research Tactics

OBJECTIVES

- To learn how to secure and organize adequate staff for the research.
- To understand how to obtain a site in which to conduct the research.
- To be aware of the responsibilities of the researcher for protecting human subjects.
- To learn where to go to seek financial support for research.
- To learn how to develop a research protocol.

The preceding chapters have been concerned with the technical side of conducting a research project. In addition, every researcher is confronted with administrative problems in attempting to pursue the research efficiently and expeditiously. This chapter will briefly touch on the more important of these problems. The decisions a researcher makes in solving them are called research tactics or strategy.

The major administrative problems include those related to securing and maintaining adequate resources to conduct the study. These include staffing, facilities, study subjects, and financial support.

Research as an Organized Activity

It is rare today for a research project to be conducted by a lone investigator. In many areas of research the solo researcher has disappeared. This does not mean that useful research cannot be pursued individually. Research conducted for a doctoral dissertation is an example of research still being undertaken solo, although some dissertation topics are better accomplished as a group activity. In nursing and patient care a number of important research problems are sufficiently delimited to be conducted by a single investigator with assistance from others in the more routine aspects of data collection and processing. Many valuable contributions have been made in nursing by small, modestly financed studies.

However, many of the research problems in patient care are too complex to be approached through a small study. When a research project requires the attention of more than one full-time professional person and a supporting staff of technical and clerical workers, it is called collaborative re-

KEY
POINT

search. If the professional persons are members of different speciality fields—for example, a nurse researcher and a psychologist—the effort is called interdisciplinary research. Some interdisciplinary research projects involve specialists from a variety of professional fields.

Considerable criticism has been directed at interdisciplinary research. It has been said that the total research effort can become, when pursued by a team, too fragmented and can result in a deterioration of interest among members and a failure to reach the objectives of the research. On the other hand, the benefits of team research include greater efficiency in the conduct of a study as well as the capability to investigate broad, complicated problems.

When a research project is large enough to require a team, the administrative problems of securing adequate resources and maintaining cohesiveness and productivity of the group are multiplied. Projects needing a large research staff are essentially autonomous organizational entities, often managed by an administrative staff and a project director who devotes much of his time to the administrative rather than the technical problems. Such large-scale research efforts often become institutionalized, pursuing an organized program of research studies and engaging in more than one study at the same time.

There is some question as to whether research should be pursued as a full-time, specialized activity or combined with other functions. Some advocate that teaching and research should be combined and carried on either simultaneously or as consecutive activities. Some faculty members engage in research in the summer and teach the rest of the year. Some administrators do research during their spare time.

Although there is great value in combining the functions of teaching and research, many research problems require the continuing full-time attention of a team. If an organization with the primary objective of teaching or service wishes to pursue research on a large scale, this function must be conducted by a specialized unit. This is essential not only to provide sufficient resources for the effort but to create a proper climate for the careful, unhurried pursuit of the study free from the possible disturbing influences of the workaday world. In a service agency, research should be separated from the agency's primary objective in order to avoid biases that could affect the research and distort the findings when the two activities are intermixed.

SECURING ADEQUATE STAFF FOR THE RESEARCH

When a research project becomes too large for one investigator to manage, the services of other workers must be enlisted. These may be either professional staff, such as biologists and social scientists, industrial and systems engineers, statisticians and mathematicians, or personnel such as statistical clerks, electronic data-processing technicians, interviewers, and typists. These personnel can be employed on either a full or part-time basis depending on the requirements of the study. One type of part-time professional research staff member is the consultant, generally a specialist in an aspect of the problem who can be called upon as needed. Consultants can play a valuable role in a project, particularly in the more technical phases for which it would be impractical to employ a full-time team member. Such methodological problems as development of measuring instruments, selection of sampling units, and processing of data can be solved by a consultant.

Another way to obtain services other than hiring a full-time staff is to contract with specialized service agencies for certain parts of the study. For example, if the data are to be collected by mailed questionnaires from a large number of sampling units, the mailing can be handled by an appropriate organization. Also, there are available, even in the smallest community, agencies devoted to the processing of statistical data. Such agencies usually maintain data-processing equipment and have electronic computers available.

In team research, one person is designated as the principal investigator, assuming major responsibility for the administration of the research. The principal investigator is generally the individual who originated the study, developed the initial research plan, is mainly responsible for its execution, and may write the final report. In large projects the principal investigator may devote a major portion of time to administrative problems associated with the research, leaving the supervision of technical aspects to a project director or research associate.

In order to determine the staffing requirements the research plan must be well developed so that the demands for personnel can be assessed. Development of the plan should not be the sole responsibility of the principal investigator and/or the project director but should involve other members of the team. In addition to a financial budget, the research plan should include a staffing budget, formulated on the basis of an assessment of the staff requirements for each phase of the study. Heaviest requirements often arise during the data-collecting phase. This is particularly true when the data are to be collected by direct observation or interviewing with multiple observers.

It is advisable that all professional personnel involved in the study, even those on a part-time or consultative basis, be given an opportunity to become familiar with and offer suggestions about the research plan before it is completed and data collected. Early involvement of all members can lead to constructive suggestions for the improvement of the design, promote a sense of participation among members of the research team and stimulate a coordinated effort toward the accomplishment of the research aims.

The value of early participation in the development of the plan by all team members is illustrated by the role of the statistician who is often called in after the data have been collected and asked to make sense of them. If a statistician is involved before the data are collected, constructive advice can be obtained on the entire process of data collection and analysis as well on the total design. If these suggestions are implemented before the data are gathered, they can significantly improve the quality of the research.

It is helpful in executing a research plan, to set up an advisory committee consisting of people who are not full-time members of the research team. The committee can include consultants to the project, administrators in the service agency where the study is done, or faculty members if the study is being done in a university. These people can provide overall guidance and can serve as a sounding board to clarify objectives, concepts, and approaches.

Motivation of Research Team

During execution of the study the principal investigator and/or project director must be concerned with motivating and stimulating the team members toward the attainment of the research objectives. Ways of keeping the interest of the team high, of overcoming frustrations and disappointments that accompany any research effort, must be found. Some phases of nearly all research projects are repetitious and dull. It is essential, particularly in the data-collecting stage, for the project director to see that team members are sufficiently motivated to sustain them over these less exciting but essential phases.

Turnover in any organized enterprise can be deleterious, but in a research project it can be especially harmful. Because the reliability of the data collected depends on minimizing errors through appropriate training of investigators, loss of personnel through attrition can slow the project down because new personnel must be sufficiently oriented to the methods used in the study. For example, the introduction of a new person into the data collection process increases the risk that unconscious psychological bias will be introduced. For this reason the morale of the team members must be kept as high as possible. One way in which this can be achieved is to assure that the research team understand the research objectives and are kept informed about progress made. Opportunity should be provided for members to participate in discussions concerning the research, changes occurring in design of the study, and accomplishments achieved.

The Written Report

The product of many studies is a written report, hopefully one that is published. A boost to the morale of team members is appropriate recognition of their contributions. If possible, they should participate in the writing of the report with due credit for authorship. Members should be strongly encouraged to publish separately whenever they can report on a selected aspect of the research for which they had special responsibility. Publication should be planned for at all stages. It is particularly important for researchers to publish their studies in scientific and professional periodicals where peers can challenge their findings.

A useful device for keeping members fully informed of progress, as well as providing material that can serve as the foundation for the final report, is the preparation of periodic progress notes in the form of working papers. These should be more than just a "news item" type of informational release and should contain preliminary analysis of data, discussions of problem areas encountered in implementing the research design, and elaborations of the conceptual model underlying the research. Such reports, or working papers, can serve as stimulants for discussion and for critical examination and refinement of the entire effort. They can also be useful as historical documents concerning the development and progress of the research and as sources of ideas and guidance in the development of further research.

Guidelines for Attaining Effective Communication and Collaboration[1]

KEY POINT

1. Achieving an optimal initial orientation and realistic level of expectation.

2. Achieving maximum assimilation of "professional subcultural values" such as ideologies, technologies, and the language.
3. Making certain that the organizational structure in which the social scientist has to work permits him to fit into an appropriate postion.
4. Specific understanding and clarification of the roles involved in collaborative research.
5. Improving the "interpersonal skills" of the participants.

Following the above guidelines does not assure effective collaboration, but achieving some of these objectives is essential. Orientation efforts probably will have to be continuous. A systematic effort on the part of a discipline to assimilate a working knowledge of other fields is crucial. For example, key professional staff involved may exchange courses for which they are responsible for teaching.

The nursing profession has adopted a feverish pace in carrying out research endeavors. This, too, contributes to the shortening of the period of survival for the "change agent," who is caught up in this haste and is pressured to produce.

Strong administrative backing and support as well as a climate conducive to research contribute to a longer survival period. A built-in safety valve, such as permitting the researcher to return to the discipline or specialty periodically, is also crucial. This might be achieved by initially planning to have the researcher spend part time in the discipline—teaching, consulting, and/or doing research. Without this mechanism, within as little time as one year the researcher may find it impossible to withdraw intellectually and emotionally from the situation.

Another survival feature is the researcher's awareness of strategy essential to survive—i.e., knowledge of where to avoid existing cross-factions that may block any attempt at communication. Prior knowledge of the adopted profession and the health field in general can help to avoid errors of communication and the lack of identity of problems crucial to nursing.

As long as professional practitioners and researchers find themselves in interactive situations, hopefully there will be mutual learning and tolerance of viewpoints, if not acceptance.

The nurse as researcher faces many struggles similar to the scientist's. Main-taining one's identity is important. The choice at times can be a lonely one. Major barriers to collaborative effort often find their basis in the ways in which research is perceived by the practitioner and the scientist. This may be summarized as follows:

KEY POINT

PRACTITIONER	SCIENTIST
CLINICAL NURSE SPECIALIST OR NURSE PRACTITIONER	SOCIAL, PHYSICAL, OR BIOLOGICAL SCIENTIST (THIS MAY BE A NURSE SCIENTIST)
1. Problems selected for study are operational, requiring immediate solution and have practical application.	1. Problem selected for study may or may not have immediate relevance to the real world. (Research is both basic and applied.)
2. Conceptualization of research is empirical and pragmatic.	2. Theoretical framework for research stems from literature, previous research, and basic postulates.
3. A practical plan of action is outlined.	3. Operational definitions are spelled out and hypotheses formulated.
4. Methods are selected and adopted from other fields rather than developing new methods.	4. Methods may need to be developed. Other disciplines may provide models and methods.
5. She observes the consequences of her action in light of the total program goals.	5. Criteria to evaluate the results of the project, particularly those dependent variables that are observable, are determined.
6. Analysis of the results is often based on subjective judgments.	6. The research design is set up in a way to permit an objective analysis of the data as they are obtained. This would permit modification or changing of the hypothesis(es). (Serendipity.)
7. Weighs the results of action as they affect individual patients or groups of patients. Is slow to initiate change and may not do so if the patient(s) is not ready to accept the change.	7. Evaluation is based on criteria which are checked consistently for their validity and reliability. The theoretical framework provides the source to which the results of the experiment are directed.
8. Results of actions are limited to one situation and cannot be generalized.	8. Inferences can be drawn from the findings that can be related to other situations.
9. She uses the results of action to add to her experience to resolve similar problems.	9. New hypotheses are identified for future study.
10. Results of action are communicated immediately to permit solution of the problem. Experiences may be reported in professional journals as descriptive reports of one situation.	10. Research findings are reported to a body of scientists and practitioners through scientific and professional journals, papers, and conferences.

As nurses become increasingly oriented to the basic science disciplines and are able to direct their own research projects, it is hoped that more collaborative research can be achieved.

KEY POINT ## SECURING FACILITIES

Obtaining a site in which to conduct research is particularly important in experimental research. Experimental design requires that the setting in which the research is conducted be highly controlled. Often, a specially devised setting is necessary, such as an experimental unit or a laboratory with specially constructed facilities, equipment, and layout. In experimental studies the problem of securing facilties is usually greater than in research conducted in a natural or partially controlled setting. In studies conducted in natural settings, however, there may not be a clear separation between research setting and work situation. As a consequence, a problem often encountered is interference with the work being performed. If our study requires that we observe the delivery of infants on an obstetrical unit in a hospital, we must make sure that the process of observation will not disturb the functioning of the delivery room.

Where the data are to be collected by indirect means, as by a questionnaire, the interference problem is less obvious to the researcher but can raise havoc in an institution or agency when multiple questionnaires are received. It is the responsibility of the researcher, or the adviser of graduate students, to clear with the institution before questionnaires are sent out. Researchers and student advisers must assume greater responsibility in screening all questionnaires.

KEY POINT A research unit that is part of an operating agency, such as a school, public health department, or a hospital, has fewer problems in securing a setting than does an independent research agency that may have to depend on the cooperation of others. Ex-

perimental studies involving radical modifcations of existing facilities require detailed planning. Securing facilities for non-experimental research is largely a matter of having office space for the team members and facilities where the data can be processed.

THE RIGHTS OF HUMAN SUBJECTS

As nurse investigators seek to develop and refine scientific knowledge and theory in nursing through clinical investigations, increasing emphasis is being placed upon the protection of human subjects.

Nurse practitioners involved in data collection for other investigators are equally involved and also must be concerned about the protection of human subjects, particularly when the outcomes are not known.

The American Nurses' Association as part of the activity of the ANA Commission on Nursing Research has developed a useful document for human rights guidelines for nurses in clinical and other research.*
It is suggested that:

• All proposals, investigative instruments, protocols, and techniques to be used be specified and discussed with prospective subjects and other participating workers.
• Safeguards be developed to assure that no unanticipated physical, psychological, or social disadvantage accrues to subjects either during the investigation or as a result of dissemination of findings.
• Protection of the subjects' anonymity be assured.
• Confidentiality of information be assured when not under control of the investigator.
• Consent to participate in research or clincial activities be obtained from the prospective subject. Such consent is expected to cover an explanation of the study, the procedures to be followed, their purposes, a description of phys-

---

*American Nurses' Association. *Human Rights Guidelines for Nurses in Clinical and Other Research.* ANA Publication No. D-465M, February 1985.

ical risk or discomfort, any invasion of privacy, and threat to dignity and the methods used to protect anonymity and ensure confidentiality.

Institutional Review Board (IRB)

The IRB in most institutions usually includes a committee to review proposed studies and the progress of ongoing studies annually. Health care professionals and community representatives comprise such a board. It is most important that there be a nurse researcher represented on the IRB to have some input in the decision-making process. The research protocol and consent forms are reviewed by the IRB.*

Sponsorship

Most research proposals are submitted through a university or institution that serves as a sponsor. Sponsorship implies a commitment and endorsement of the proposed research and assurances that all appropriate clearances have been obtained.

The DHHS regulations for the protection of human subjects, 45 CFR 46, (revised March 8, 1983) are available from the Office for Protection from Research Risks, National Institutes of Health, Bethesda, MD 20205. The regulations provide a systematic means, based on established ethical principles, to safeguard the rights and welfare of individuals who participate as subjects in research activities supported or conducted by the DHHS.

The regulations define "human subject" as a "living individual about whom an investigator (whether professional or student) conducting research obtains (1) data through intervention or interaction with the individual, or (2) identifiable private information." The regulations extend to the use of human organs, tissues, and body fluids from individually identifiable human subjects as well as to graphic, written, or recorded information derived from individually identifiable human subjects. The use of autopsy materials is governed by applicable state and local law and is not directly regulated by 45 CFR 46. The regulations also specify additional protections for certain classes of human research involving fetuses, pregnant women, *in vitro* fertilization, or prisoners. The regulations require that all nonexempt research activities involving human subjects be reviewed and approved by an institutional review board.

Exempt from coverage by the regulations are activities in which the only involvement of human subjects will be in one or more of the following five categories:

1. Research conducted in established or commonly accepted educational settings, involving normal educational practices, such as (i) research on regular and special education instructional strategies, or (ii) research on the effectiveness of or the comparison among instructional techniques, curricula, or classroom management methods.
2. Research involving the use of educational tests (cognitive, diagnostic, aptitude, achievement), if information taken from these sources is recorded in such a manner that subjects cannot be identified, directly or through identifiers linked to the subjects.
3. Research involving survey or interview procedures, except where all the following conditions exist: (i) responses are recorded in such a manner that the human subjects can be identified, directly or through identifiers linked to the subjects; (ii) the subject's responses, if they became known outside the research, could reasonably place the subject at risk of criminal or civil liability or be damaging to the subject's financial standing or employability; and (iii) the research deals with sensitive aspects of the subject's own behavior, such as illegal conduct, drug use, sexual behavior, or use of alcohol. All research involving survey or interview procedures is exempt, without exception, when the respondents are elected or appointed public officials or candidates for public office.
4. Research involving the observation (in-

* ANA, *Human Rights Guidelines for Nurses in Clinical and Other Research.* ANA Publication No. D-465M, 2/85, p. 9.

cluding observation by participants) of public behavior, except where all of the following conditions exist: (i) observations are recorded in such a manner that the human subjects can be identified, directly or through identifiers linked to the subjects; (ii) the observations recorded about the individual, if they became known outside the research, could reasonably place the subject at risk of criminal or civil liability or be damaging to the subject's financial standing or employability; and (iii) the research deals with sensitive aspects of the subject's own behavior such as illegal conduct, drug use, sexual behavior, or use of alcohol.

5. Research involving the collection or study of existing data, documents, records, pathological specimens, or diagnostic specimens, if these sources are publicly available or if the information is recorded by the investigator in such a manner that subjects cannot be identified, directly or through identifiers linked to the subjects.

KEY POINT The Privacy Act (Public Law 93-579), effective on September 27, 1975, states that its primary purpose is to safeguard individuals against invasions of personal privacy. The Act requires federal agencies and federal contractors to:

- Permit individuals to determine what records pertaining to themselves the agency collects, maintains, uses, or disseminates.
- Permit individuals to prevent records pertaining to themselves obtained for a particular purpose from being used or made available for another purpose without their consent.
- Permit individuals to gain access to information pertaining to themselves in federal agency records, to have a copy made of their records, and to correct or amend their records.
- Collect, maintain, use, or disseminate records of identifiable personal information in a manner that assures that such action is for a necessary and lawful purpose, that the information is current and accurate for its intended use, and that adequate safeguards are provided to prevent misuse of information.
- Be subject to civil suit for damages which occur as a result of willful or intentional actions that violate any individual's rights under the Act.

In addition, subsection (i) of section 3 of the Act states that employees of an agency maintaining a system of records shall be subject to criminal penalties for willful or intentional actions that violate any individual's rights under the Act.

Comprehensive guidelines for ethical standards have also been issued by the American Psychological Association.*

Research subjects may take a variety of forms. If the subjects are inanimate, as in a study of the cost of different types of disposable syringes, or animals, as in a study of the effect of sensory deprivation on monkeys, the problems are few in obtaining cooperation. Where human beings are the subjects, problems of cooperation may be formidable, particularly where the research involves unpleasantness.

An important requisite in obtaining the cooperation of human research subjects is to explain fully the purpose of the study and to impress the subject with the importance of their participation. Sometimes an inducement, such as a promise to make the report of the study available to the subject, will help. Or where the study requires a large expenditure of time, an incentive as tangible as providing the subject with a free physical examination, free drugs, or services, or even the payment of money may help to offset any unpleasantness or bother. In any event, written permission from the patient to participate as a study subject is a *must*.

In studies involving cluster sampling, in which random samples are drawn at several stages—say, first a sample of schools is drawn, then a sample of students—the cooperation of two groups must be obtained. Random sampling, even at one stage, presents special problems. Theoretically each unit selected for study by the random process must be included. Failure to secure

---

* Ad hoc Committee on Ethical Standards in Psychological Research; *Ethical Principles in the Conduct of Research with Human Participants.* Washtington, D.C., American Psychological Association, Inc., 1973, 104 pp.

cooperation of a sampling unit that has been selected can bias results. In studies using mailed questionnaires such bias is called the error of nonresponse. To reduce this error various techniques can be employed, including sending follow-up questionnaires to those not returning the original and including a strong appeal for cooperation.

In prospective longitudinal studies where contact with study subjects often extends over a lengthy period, the problem of maintaining cooperation of the subjects throughout the study can be formidable. Attrition from such a study can seriously harm its validity. In developing the plan for a longitudinal study, safeguards must be provided to keep attrition of subjects to a minimum.

One way of increasing the likelihood that the cooperation of subjects will be secured and maintained is to assure confidentiality of data. This is particularly important where the study deals with matters of a personal nature. Assurance that the data collected from the subject will be kept strictly anonymous and that they will be used only for research purposes will help to alleviate any fears the subjects may have in this regard.

Ethics in Research

The nurse researcher frequently is faced with choosing between conflicting options in which there is no right or wrong. Ethical decisions usually are based on moral judgments. "Ethics involve the free, rational assessment, based on moral conscience, of courses of action."[2]

Ethical dilemmas faced by the nurse researcher focus on two issues: (1) weighing the potential risks to patients/clients participating against the potential benefits, and (2) protecting the patients'/clients' right to decide through a procedure of informed consent.

The researcher (usually the principal investigator) has the responsibility to obtain the informed consent of research subjects.

Consent forms are based on agreement that basic human rights will be respected and that no risk, discomfort, or inconvenience beyond what has been stated will be imposed without further permission.[3,4]

Misconduct in Scientific Activities

Instances of misconduct in scientific activities are rare. When such instances do occur, however, they present a serious threat to continued public confidence in the integrity of the scientific process. Misconduct is defined as (1) fraudulent or highly irregular practices in carrying out research or in reporting the results of such research; (2) material failure to comply with requirements affecting specific aspects of the conduct of research, e.g., the protection of human subjects and the welfare of laboratory animals; and (3) serious misappropriation of research funds, e.g., diversion of funds for personal use.

It is the responsibility of the university or agency sponsoring the research to ensure the implementation of policies and procedures for the fair and prompt handling of any alleged or apparent misconduct in science.

SEEKING FINANCIAL SUPPORT FOR RESEARCH

"Grantsmanship" is something that is learned empirically. (see Bibliography on Grantsmanship, p. 352 and Individual Reference Guide to Research Grant Support, p. 353). Some researchers have this skill and some don't. While most researchers express dislike for this aspect of research, it is a fact of life that cannot be ignored. One is well advised to understand its rules and consequences. Grantsmanship has a negative connotation and is not to be confused with the necessary, open, and straightforward application for research grants that is a legitimate function of qualified investigators.

University Research Versus Federal Research

The question must be faced as to the role of universities and the federal government in research. Universities provide a major site for research and the major source for the preparation of scientists. It is in the university setting that man's freedom to seek knowledge as well as to challenge our cultural and political systems can be safeguarded. For this reason universities must remain the most suitable milieu for research.

The federal government, on the other hand, cannot ignore its responsibility for research. Maintaining the national defense and safeguarding its people's welfare necessitates that the federal government be involved in scientific research whether conducted in federal laboratories or financed in other laboratories with federal funds.

The university system depends on the federal government for support, in spite of the generous contributions of foundations and private philanthropies, and, in turn, the federal government depends on the university for human resources.

Approximately 90 percent of all federal funds for research and development (training) and 99 percent of federal funds for research activities are provided under the statutory research charters of five agencies: the Department of Agriculture, the Public Health Service, the National Science Foundation, the Department of Energy, and the Department of Defense. (Most of the federally financed research is administered by operating organizations whose primary function is not research.)

The federal government's objective in supporting research in universities is to ensure that an activity vital to the national defense and/or welfare of people is carried out. This is achieved through contract research in which research services are purchased or through research supported by a grant to a nonprofit, nonfederal university, institution, or agency.

Each federal agency is an autonomous unit. Controls are exercised through Congress and the appropriations process. Each agency has its own review mechanism. For example, the Public Health Service's Division of Research Grants has many study sections made up of scientists qualified to review specific projects. One of the first reviewing groups, for example, is the Nursing Research Study group made up of nurse scientists, social scientists, physicians, hospital administrators, and biostatisticians, which meets three times a year to review research applications for scientific merit. Applications receive a second review by an appropriate council—for nursing, it is the National Advisory Council on Nurse Training, which reviews all applications for significance and determines which priority level of payment is possible in view of available funds.

The role of the university is the preservation, the transmission, and the creation of knowledge in a climate that provides a high degree of freedom for the investigator. It is committed to teaching, research, and service.

The role of the federal government is to encourage and support the endeavors of scientists and researchers to enlarge the understanding of the natural world in all its aspects, with federal oversight of taxpayer funds, but without control of the investigator's creativity, initiative, and imagination.

ROLES OF THE FEDERAL GOVERNMENT IN FURTHERING NURSING RESEARCH

The evolution of nursing research must be viewed in context with the evolution of medical research. The contribution of the federal government to medical research in the early 1900s was negligible, but today the federal government is the largest source of financial support for nursing research. Figure 18–1 is an organizational chart that

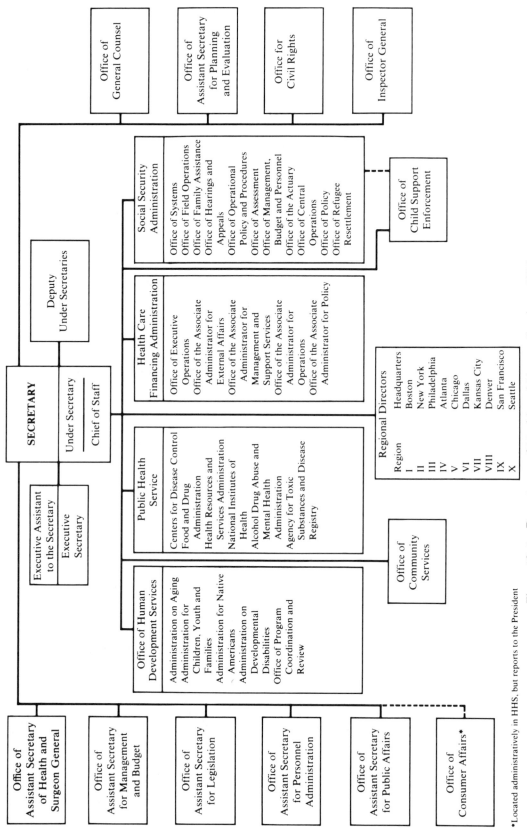

Figure 18-1 Department of Health and Human Services, 1986.

*Located administratively in HHS, but reports to the President

shows the relationships among several sources of federal funds for nursing research.

The federal government's participation traces back to only 1887 when a Laboratory of Hygiene was established at the Staten Island Marine Hospital (now the United States Public Health Service Hospital).[5-7] Emphasis was placed upon the study of bacteriological diseases brought back by merchant seamen, such as cholera, tuberculosis, diphtheria, typhoid fever. In 1891 the laboratory was moved to Washington, D.C., where it was known as the Hygienic Laboratory. In 1930 it was renamed the National Institute of Health—a name changed in 1948 to the National Institutes of Health.

The role of the federal government in supporting medical research became significant in 1938 through the establishment of grants-in-aid to universities and research institutions through a research grants program.

The Public Health Service Act of 1944 provided the Surgeon General with broad authority for the conduct and support of all kinds of medical research. The act provided that:

. . . The Surgeon General shall encourage, cooperate with and render assistance to appropriate public authorities, scientific institutions and scientists in the conduct and coordination of research, investigations, experiments, demonstrations and studies relating to the cause, diagnosis, treatment, control and prevention of the physical and mental diseases and impairments of man.

Chronological List of Dates in the Development of United States Public Health Service Programs Affecting Medical and Health-Related Research

1887 First research laboratory supported by federal government established at the Marine Hospital, Staten Island, New York.

1891 Hygienic Laboratory moved from Staten Island to Washington, D.C.

1902 First Advisory Board for Hygienic Laboratory formed. This was later renamed the National Advisory Health Council.

1912 Public Health and Marine Hospital Service renamed Public Health Service.

1930 Hygienic Laboratory renamed National Institute of Health.

1937 National Cancer Institute authorized by Congress.

1938 National Institute of Health establishes headquarters at Bethesda, Maryland. First research fellowships authorized.

1944 Public Health Service Act, giving Surgeon General broad research authority.

1945 First research grants awarded.

1946 First training grants awarded. Mental Health Act passed by Congress.

1947 Division of Research Grants established.

1948 National Institute of Health renamed National Institutes of Health. National Heart Institute and National Institute for Dental Research authorized by Congress. Other existing laboratories were reorganized to form Microbiological Institute, and Experimental Biology and Medicine Institute.

1949 Mental hygiene program expanded and organized as the National Institute of Mental Health.

1950 Two new institutes established: National Institute of Neurological Diseases and Blindness and National Institute of Arthritis and Metabolic Diseases (which included the former Experimental Biology and Medicine Institute).

1953 Federal Security Agency becomes Department of Health, Education, and Welfare. The Public Health Service represents the Health component of the new department. Clinical Center opened as first federal clinical research laboratory.

1955 Nursing Research Grants and Fellowship Program of the Division of Nursing established.
National Microbiological Institute renamed National Institute of Allergy and Infectious Diseases.

1957   Health Research Facilities Act passed by Congress, authorizing matching grants for research construction in non-federal institutions.

1958   Division of General Medical Sciences established, responsible for providing the scientific review processes for all noncategorical grants, including nursing.

1960   Public Health Service Act (1944) amended to provide for general support of research and research training programs in universities, hospitals, and other nonprofit institutions.
International Health Research Act passed by Congress permitting the expansion of NIH international programs.

1961   The Bureau of States Services–Community Health, Office of Research Grants was established and given primary responsibility at the bureau level, for leadership, coordination, and assistance in extramural research grants and research training grants. The office was responsible for: (1) the creation of national participation by competent scientists, state and local public health agencies, practitioners, and educators in research and training for research in community health; (2) the establishment of policies, organization, procedures, budget, reporting and control techniques, and effective project review and grants administration within Divisions, Bureaus, and in relation to P.H.S. and departmental systems; (3) the analysis of scope and content of research and research training, progress toward defined goals, and utilization of findings in Bureau, State, and local health programs; (4) assistance to regional offices in program promotion and grants management for research and research training; (5) the representation of BSS–Community Health program in operating relationships with NIH, other service and departmental components. The office also had continuing responsibilities for staff services to the National Advisory Community Health Committee in connection with its review of research and research training grants applications.

1962   Public Health Service Act amended to provide the establishment of two new institutes (Public Law 87-838, 87th Congress, H.R. 11099).
Establishment of the Institute of Child Health and Human Development for the conduct and support of research and training relating to maternal health, child health, and human development, including research and training in the special health problems and requirements of mothers and children and in the basic sciences relating to the processes of human growth and development, including prenatal development. Establishment of the Institute of General Medical Sciences for the conduct and support of research and research training in the general or basic medical sciences and natural or behavioral sciences that have significance for two or more other institutes, or are outside the general area of responsibility of any other institute, established under or by this act.

1962   Division of Research Facilities and Resources established to assume reponsibility for activities authorized under the Health Research Facilities Act.

1963   Transfer of Division of Nursing, Extramural Research Program from the Institute of General Medical Sciences to the Bureau of States Services–Community Health.

1967   Division of Nursing became part of the Bureau of Health Manpower.

1968   Division of Nursing, Bureau of Health Manpower transferred to The National Institutes of Health.

1969   Bureau of Health Manpower renamed Bureau of Health Professions Education and Manpower Training.

1973   Division of Nursing moved to the Bureau of Health Resources Development, Health Resources Administration, which also included the National Center for Health Statistics and Bureau of Health Services Research and Evaluation (now the National Center for Health Services Research).

1975   Bureau of Health Resources Development reorganized into the Bureau of Health Manpower and Bureau of

Health Planning and Resource Development, Health Resources Administration (HRA).

1978 Health Resources Administration reorganized into three Bureaus: (1) Planning, (2) Health Facilities Financing, Compliance, and Conversion; (3) Health Manpower with Division of Nursing in the Bureau of Health Manpower. A Division of Manpower Analysis was established in this Bureau to conduct manpower research.

1982 Public Health Service reorganized into five agencies: including the Health Resources and Services Administration in which the Division of Nursing is located.

1985 Congress authorizes a center for nursing research to be located at the National Institutes of Health.

PEER REVIEW OF FEDERAL GOVERNMENT SUPPORTED RESEARCH

Before describing the major federal agencies that support medical and nursing research, the NIH peer review process for evaluating submitted proposals will be described.

The NIH peer review system is based on two sequential levels of review, referred to as the "dual review system." Both levels have statutory bases. The first level of review is performed by scientific review groups that are established, in general, along lines of scientific disciplines and consist of experts in relevant research fields. The scientific review groups managed by the Division of Research Grants are referred to as Study Sections. The Study Sections usually consist of twelve to twenty members each and have as their primary function the review and evaluation for scientific merit of research grant applications. Other scientific review groups are managed by the Bureaus, Institutes, and Divisions

(BIDs) and have diverse review responsibilities, such as multidisciplinary research requests and a variety of other specialized proposals, including research contract proposals.

The second level of review for research grant applications is performed by a national advisory council or board (hereinafter referred to as council) for each BID which supports extramural research.

Scientific Review Groups

Each scientific review group is composed primarily of nonfederal scientists selected by the NIH for their competence in the particular scientific areas for which that group has review responsibilities. Review groups usually meet three times yearly. Each meeting generally requires two or three days of intensive review of research proposals. Six to eight weeks before the meeting date, the Executive Secretary, who is an NIH health scientist administrator, assigns specific applications to each member who prepares written detailed critiques prior to the meeting and leads the discussion on these applications at the meeting. In addition, every member is expected to read and be prepared to contribute to the discussion of all other applications to be reviewed at the meeting. Members also participate in project site visits when these are deemed necessary for an adequate review of a specific application. They survey, as scientific leaders, the status of research in their fields.

These groups review applications on the basis of scientific merit and scientific significance, including such considerations as (1) an assessment of the importance of the proposed research problem; (2) the novelty and originality of the approach; (3) the training, experience, and research competence or promise of the investigator(s); (4) the adequacy of the experimental design; (5) the suitability of the facilities; and (6) the appropriateness of the requested budget relative to the work proposed.

Recommendations of the scientific review groups are made by majority vote of the members. If recommended for approval, applications are assigned a technical merit priority rating by each individual scientific review group member, "1" being the most meritorious and "5" the least. The arithmetic average becomes the committee's priority score. Scientific review groups may also vote to recommend disapproval of applications or deferral for further information and later recommendation. Following the meeting, a summary statement is prepared by the Executive Secretary for each application reviewed. The summary contains the recommendation, the priority score for applications recommended for approval, and a summation of the reasons for the recommendation. This statement is forwarded to the appropriate BID for the next level of review—consideration by that unit's council.

The summary statement is automatically sent to the applicant following council review.

NIH research and development *contract projects* generally are subjected to a many-stage review process prior to any awards. For solicited contracts, program advisory committees, composed largely of non-Government experts, suggest types of projects which should be undertaken by the NIH programs to which they relate. Such recommendations are provided also through workshops, conferences, and similar advisory groups. The ideas are then translated by program staff into specific requests for proposals which define the program requirements and describe the criteria by which the proposals will be evaluated. Proposals received following such announcements are evaluated by additional technical review groups, again composed largely of nonfederal advisors. Recommendations from these groups, together with the results of separate business evaluations of the proposals are then reviewed further by appropriate NIH staff groups with out-side consultation as needed, who provide final recommendations to the directors of those Bureaus, Institutes, or Divisions.

National Advisory Councils and Boards

These groups are comprised of both scientists and non-scientists and have broader responsibilities. The mix of members brings to bear on the grant review and award process knowledge in each of the relevant programmatic areas, familiarity with NIH procedures as well as awareness of the roles of the diverse institutions in biomedical research and of the health needs of the American people. The councils and boards also offer advice and make recommendations on policy and matters of significance to the mission and goals of the BIDs they serve. The second level of review for contract proposals is conducted by an executive staff committee of each of the BIDs. The number of members is set by law, usually twelve or more, and include both scientists and others who are lay community leaders with a demonstrated interest in health areas relevant to the program areas of the particular BID. In general, the councils meet three times yearly for approximately three days.

Each council member receives in advance copies of the recommendations of the scientific review groups on applications for grants assigned to the BID to which the council is advisory and reviews them against a broad background of responsibilities that include, in part, a determination of the total pattern of research in universities and other institutions; the need for the initiation of research in new areas; the degree of relevance of the proposed research to the missions of the BIDs; and other matters of policy. The councils usually concur with the appraisal of the scientific review groups in regard to scientific merit, but they may have occasion to modify the recommendations in consideration of one or more of the factors mentioned above.

Nurse researchers should aggressively seek appointments to scientific review groups. Participation in such groups can help nonnurses understand what nursing research is and how it differs from biomedical research.

The primary requirement for serving on a scientific review group is competence as an independent investigator in a basic scientific or clinical discipline or research specialty. Assessment of such competence is based on the quality of research accomplished, publications in refereed scientific journals, and other significant scientific activities, achievements, and honors. Usually a doctoral degree or its equivalent is required. Service also requires mature judgment, balanced perspective, objectivity, ability to work effectively in a group context, commitment to complete work assignments, and assurance that the confidentiality of applications will be protected.

In addition to the individual characteristics outlined above, such factors as geographic distribution and adequate representation of younger, ethnic minority, female, and handicapped scientists must be considered. Further, no two members from the same institution may be appointed to the same advisory group, an interval of one year must occur before reappointment to an NIH committee, and no member may be appointed to serve simultaneously on two chartered committees of the Department of Health and Human Services. Exceptions to these restrictions are rare and must be approved by the Department Committee Management Officer.

In the next section the major agencies supporting medical and nursing research will be described. These include the various agencies of the public health service, primarily the National Institutes of Health and the Division of Nursing and includes the Health Care Financing Administration of the Department of Health and Human Services which supports a large grants and contracts program.

National Institutes of Health (NIH)

Initiated as a one-room laboratory of Hygiene in 1887, the National Institutes of Health today is the principal biomedical research agency of the federal government and one of the world's foremost medical research centers.

NIH's mission is to uncover new knowledge that will lead to

- Better understanding of the fundamental life processes, and
- Better means to prevent, detect, diagnose, and treat disease.

NIH works toward these goals by

- Conducting research in its own laboratories;
- Supporting the research of nonfederal scientists in universities, medical hospitals, and research institutions throughout the United States and abroad;
- Supporting the training of promising new researchers; and
- Fostering and supporting biomedical communication.

NIH COMPONENTS

Headquarters for the National Institutes of Health is a 310-acre reservation in Bethesda, Maryland. In this campuslike setting, NIH maintains hundreds of research laboratories; office facilities for staff attached to NIH Director's office and to individual research Institutes and Divisions; a 1050-bed research hospital, the Warren G. Magnuson Clinical Center, and its adjoining Abulatory Care Research Facility; the National Library of Medicine (the world's largest repository of biomedical information, and the Lister Hill Center, a national center for biomedical communications); and the Fogarty International Center, which fosters international research cooperation and provides facilities for foreign scholars-in-residence.

The NIH research institutes are:

- National Cancer Institute
- National Heart, Lung, and Blood Institute
- Nation Institute of Dental Research
- National Institute of Neurological and Communicative Disorders and Stroke

- National Institute of Arthritis, Diabetes, and Digestive and Kidney Diseases
- National Institute of Allergy and Infectious Diseases
- National Institute of General Medical Sciences
- National Eye Institute
- National Institute of Child Health and Human Development
- National Institute of Environmental Health Sciences (the only major NIH component located outside Bethesda, with headquarters at Research Triangle Park, North Carolina)
- National Institute on Aging

Other major components are the Divisions of Computer Research and Technology; Research Grants; Research Resources; and Research Services. Institute programs are described on pp 333–341.

Division of Nursing (DN) (Health Resources and Services Administration, U.S. Public Health Service)

Under the authorization of the Public Health Service Act, Sec. 301, the Division of Nursing, Bureau of Health Professions, Health Resources and Services Administration supports several types of grants. These grants are intended to enlarge the body of scientific knowledge that underlies nursing practice, nursing education, and nursing services administration, and to strengthen these areas through the utilization of such knowledge.

On January 14, 1985, the Department of Health and Human Services (DHHS) established a new Center for Nursing Research within the Division of Nursing. In November 1985 it was proposed that the center become part of the National Institutes of Health. However, the Office of Management and Budget (OMB) deleted the budget item from the 1987 budget and beyond.

Nursing research includes study of health promotion and the influence of social and physical environments on health. The research also investigates nursing needs for care of patients who are acutely or chronically ill, disabled or dying, as well as the needs of their families. Other emphases for nursing research include generation of knowledge about health care delivery systems and ethical guidelines for nursing services.

The primary criterion for assignment to the Division of Nursing is that the proposed research or program be designed, participated in actively, administered, or supervised primarily by nurse scientists or nursing personnel, or involve the development of knowledge and procedures that may have an impact on nursing practice and patient care, on nursing education, or on the delivery of nursing services.

Nursing Research Grants of Division of Nursing Program

Types of Grants
- *Nursing research project grants* support discrete, specified, circumscribed projects in an area representing the investigator's interest and competencies.
- *Nursing research program grants* support clusters of at least three studies focused upon a single theme.
- *New investigator nursing research awards (NINRA)* support small studies of high quality carried out by new investigators, up to three years.
- *Utilization of research in nursing awards (URNA)* support projects to bridge the gap between the generation of knowledge through research and the utilization of such knowledge in nursing practice, nursing education, or nursing services administration.
- *Nursing research emphasis grants for doctoral programs in nursing (NRE/DPN)* stimulate nursing research in areas that emphasize special health needs of the Nation, and advance the research efforts and resources of faculty in schools of nursing offering doctoral programs. Awards are for three years and renewal for an additional two years.

Guidelines
- Upon request, specific guidelines are available for all programs except Nursing Research Project Grants.

Eligibility
- Any individual, corporation, public or private institution or agency, or other legal entity. Principal investigators of NINRA projects must be first-time principal investigators for a Public Health Service-supported research project. Applicants should consult with Division of Nursing staff concerning the choice of application best suited to their needs. NRE/DPN projects are specifically designed for schools of nursing that offer doctoral programs.

Period of support
- One to five years
- NINRA Awards are limited to periods up to three years.
- NRE/DPN projects are also limited to three years, but additional support may be awarded to applicants for renewal of funded projects for periods not to exceed five years of total support.

Application Procedure
- Research grant application kits (PHS 398, Rev. 5/82) are available through the research offices of most institutions.
- Early in the process of developing an application, prospective applicants should contact the Nursing Research Support Section, Division of Nursing, to discuss plans. Section staff provide technical advice, and sometimes review drafts of proposals in advance of submission. Prospective applicants are advised to consider review of their proposals by local scientists or other experts.
- Before submitting an application, all applicants should provide the Nursing Research Support Section with the following information: title of proposal, name of principal investigator, applicant institution, and expected date of submission.
- Applications are submitted to a clearinghouse, the Division of Research Grants, National Institutes of Health, rather than to the Nursing Research Support Section. Address labels are included in application kits. Applications are assigned to the Division of Nursing on the basis of nursing relevance.
- Applications are accepted at any time. See application receipt deadline dates on p. 341. They should be submitted to the Division of Research Grants, National Institutes of Health, Room 240, Westwood Building, 5333 Westbard Avenue, Bethesda, MD 20205.

Review Process
- Applications assigned to the Division of Nursing are subject to peer review for scientific merit by an interdisciplinary group of sicentists. Recommendations of this group are forwarded to the National Advisory Council on Nurse Training for final recommendations.

Further Information
- Nursing Research Support Section
  Nursing Research and Analysis Branch
  Division of Nursing, BHPr, HRSA
  Parklawn Building, Room 5C-09
  5600 Fishers Lane
  Rockville, Maryland 20857
  Telephone: (301) 443-6315

Health Care Financing Administration (HCFA)

The Health Care Financing Administration administers a grants and contracts program for research and demonstration projects through the Office of Research and Demonstrations. Examples of projects supported follow:

HCFA funds are available for certain priority research and demonstration cooperative agreements and grants. HCFA makes funds available for activities that will help to resolve major health care financing issues or to develop innovative methods for the administration of Medicare and Medicaid. Most awards range from $35,000 to $275,000 per year. Projects are funded for a period of one year at a time and many continue funding on a non-competitive basis, generally for up to three years.

The HCFA cooperative agreement and grants program focuses primarily on analyses, experiments, pilot projects and demonstrations that provide information useful for the Medicare and Medicaid programs.

The principal purpose of the cooperative agreements and grants program is to stimulate and support statutorily authorized research and demonstrations projects. Cooperative agreements will generally be awarded when *substantial involvement* is anticipated between HCFA and the awardee during performance of the contemplated activity, whereas grants will normally be awarded whenever no substantial involvement is anticipated with the awardee. HCFA will decide which award instrument, cooperative agreement or grant, is appropriate for each project.

The office of Research and Demonstrations is composed of three distinct but highly interrelated plans for the short-term, mid-term, and long-term goals. In the short term, efforts are directed toward impact analysis and further refinement and extension of the Medicare hospital prospective payment system as well as development of the data bases which will enable HCFA to reform payment methods for physician, skilled nursing facility, home health and other services.

SHORT-TERM GOALS

Short-term goals are to analyze the Medicare and Medicaid programs. Major initiatives include ongoing studies of beneficiary access and utilization, examination of recent changes in Medicaid legislation, monitoring and refinement of the hospital prospective payment system, and study of alternative physician payment methodologies. In addition, demonstrations designed to enhance health maintenance organization (HMO) provisions of the Tax Equity and Fiscal Responsibility Act of 1982 (Pub. L. 97-248) (TEFRA) are included.

MID-TERM GOALS

Mid-term efforts are directed toward further development of innovative reimbursement methodologies for both institutional and physician providers, exploring alternatives to long-term care and assessment of the impact of emerging technologies. An important part of this research includes the development and testing of alternative prospective payment systems for other parts of the Medicare program (e.g., long-term care, clinical laboratory services, ESRD services, home health services and

durable medical equipment). These systems will be structured in a way to maximize the positive effects of introducing competition into the health care marketplace.

LONG-TERM GOALS

The potential conversion of the Medicare and Medicaid programs from a reimburser of health services to an agency which would purchase health services or encourage beneficiaries to shop for high quality health services is anticipated. The aim would be to maximize the government's ability to define its financial obligation and the beneficiaries' freedom of choice among health care options, while minimizing the size of the government bureaucracy necessary to manage the program.

EXAMPLES OF PROJECTS

- Projects that will gain a better understanding of whether and how patients treated in physician offices are medically different from patients treated in hospital outpatient or ambulatory settings, and whether the care which medically-similar patients receive differs by setting.
- Projects to gain a better understanding of the specific features of the hospital environment. The subject of these projects should include the characteristics of major types of hospitals, such as teaching institutions, regional referral centers, inner-city institutions, publicly-owned hospitals, sole-community hospitals, etc. Of special interest would be projects which seek to determine how voucher systems might be established and what impact these systems might have on hospital efficiency, solvency, capital formation, and outpatient access.
- Projects that would develop, refine, test, and evaluate new payment approaches for acute and subacute care episodes and which would involve one payment for most or all services utilized by patients during these episodes.
- Projects that examine the effect of hospital prospective payment on all providers, especially how PPS affects utilization of skilled nursing facility benefits, home health benefits, and rehabilitation services. Related to this are

projects which focus on acute care utilization, physicians, hospital, and other services furnished to nursing home patients.

- State and locality-developed projects that test alternative financing schemes for LTC services, including patient-related or case-mix based prospective payment and competitive bidding systems for skilled nursing facility and intermediate care facility levels of care; State and locality-developed projects which demonstrate the integration of payment for the continuation of services; and approaches which expand private risk-sharing for LTC costs, such as private LTC health insurance models, reverse annuity programs, life care centers, and various State tax incentive programs.
- State and locality-developed projects that assess the effects of innovative State, local, and private programs to promote home care by the family or by other community support arrangements, e.g., Alzheimer's patients.
- Projects that study the extent of the problem and alternative solutions as to why Medicaid patients in the absence of medical need, continue to stay in institutions.
- State and locality-developed projects that design and test criteria to identify institutionalized individuals who are potential candidates for noninstitutional care, and noninstitutionalized persons who are at risk of institutionalization.
- State and locality-developed projects that demonstrate and evaluate the effects of a single payment system on LTC institutions and networks.
- Projects that examine the characteristics of the Medicaid spenddown population (its size and rate of spenddown) and its impact in the provision, delivery, and utilization of LTC services, and states' ability to finance acute care services.
- Projects that focus on fundamental issues which relate to meeting program objectives, including:
  a. Determining effectiveness and efficiency in the provision of services funded by Medicare and Medicaid;
  b. Describing and interpreting differences in patterns of care, particularly geographic variations and measurable quality differences attendant to geographic variations.
  c. Measuring access to care, equity in the use of and expenditures for resources, and the barriers to the receipt of needed services; and

  d. Developing information about beneficiary knowledge of the programs, the deterrence of overutilization, and the encouragement of cost-effective preventive, and wellness care.
- Projects that develop, demonstrate, and evaluate quality of care measures for nursing homes and home health agencies, and refined quality of care and outcome measures for inpatient hospital services as well as the development and demonstration of monitoring systems for quality of care (particularly in the capitated environment).
- Research and demonstration projects that assess the cost-effectiveness and benefits of new procedures, treatments, and services, particularly in high cost areas.
- Projects that investigate the complex issues surrounding the development, adoption, and diffusion of new medical technologies and their relationship to programmatic issues involved in making eligibility, reimbursement, and coverage decisions. Concerns range from identifying emerging technologies to analyzing the costs and benefits of specific procedures, technologies, and treatment protocols.
- Projects concerning the impact of the prospective payment system on the introduction of new technologies and approaches to the integration of these technologies into DRGs or the addition of new DRGs when necessary.
- Projects that compare the costs and effectiveness of diagnostic imaging modalities such as conventional X-ray, CT scanners, nuclear magnetic resonance imaging, etc.
- Projects concerning the long-term costs, and effectiveness of kidney, bone marrow, and other organ transplantation.
- Projects to determine the desirability, feasibility, and cost of the reuse of so-called disposable medical devices; as well as projects that would give a better understanding of what items are currently being reused, the methods of preparation for reuse, and the extent of the practice. Such projects would include issues of safety, cost-effectiveness of sterilizing medical devices.
- Projects concerning the impact of new technologies of intermittent and continuous monitoring devices in the ambulatory center and home settings, including the use of home blood pressure devices, EKGs, EEGs, parenteral nutrition, and blood-sugar monitoring devices.
- Projects concerning other coverage issues including: hip replacement, pacemakers, in-

traocular lens replacement, alcoholism and mental illness treatment services, palliative and supportive therapy for catastrophic illness patients, and provision of low cost therapies.

- Projects on the extent to which preventive services and patient education or behavior modification efforts prevent, control, delay or reduce morbidity from chronic diseases, and reduce the overall cost of health care in the Medicare and Medicaid programs.
- Projects that address the effectiveness of self-care training for patients and their partners.
- Projects that develop, demonstrate, and evaluate systems which promote cost effectiveness through health education and behavior modification.
- Projects concerning the financial incentives, cost effectiveness, and other economic aspects of various preventive services, including Medicaid coverage of prenatal care and preventive services for children, and either Medicare or Medicaid coverage or both of preventive services for adults.

Application Kits

Standard application forms and guidance for the completion of the forms are available from:

Health Care Financing Administration
Office of Management and Budget
Projects Grants Branch
Room 389 East High Rise
6325 Security Boulevard
Baltimore, Maryland 21207-5187
(301)-594-3333

As projects are completed the reports are placed with the National Technical Information Service (NITS), Document Sales, 5285 Port Royal Road, Springfield, Virginia 22151, (703) 487-4650.

Alcohol, Drug Abuse, and Mental Health Administration (ADAMHA)

The major effort of ADAMHA is to understand and address alcohol abuse, alcoholism, drug abuse, and mental illness. The agency conducts clinical and biochemical research; funds extramural research, research training, and prevention programs through grants and contracts; provides technical assistance to states and communities to help them establish and operate alcohol, drug abuse, and mental health programs; and disseminates information about the major health problems it addresses to health professionals and the public.

ADAMHA's responsibilities are shared among three component institutes—the National Institute on Alcohol Abuse and Alcoholism, the National Institute on Drug Abuse, and the National Institute of Mental Health.

National Institute on Alcohol Abuse and Alcoholism (NIAAA)

The National Institute on Alcohol Abuse and Alcoholism—one of three institutes that comprise the Alcohol, Drug Abuse, and Mental Health Administration—heads the Federal effort to combat harmful use of alcohol. In carrying out its mission, NIAAA:

- Conducts and supports research on alcoholism and alcohol-related problems;
- Funds training for promising new alcohol researchers;
- Gives technical assistance to alcohol research, services, and prevention personnel in the field;
- Disseminates information on alcohol to researchers, health professionals, and the public.

National Institute on Drug Abuse (NIDA)

The National Institute on Drug Abuse is the second of three institutes that make up the Alcohol, Drug Abuse, and Mental Health Administration. NIDA's mission is to reduce the incidence, prevalence, and harmful health and social consequences of drug abuse through drug abuse research, information dissemination, and technical assistance for state and local drug abuse efforts.

National Institute of Mental Health (NIMH)

The National Institute of Mental Health—the third of the institutes forming the Alcohol, Drug Abuse, and Mental Health Administration—provides leadership for the federal effort to promote mental health, prevent and treat mental illness, and rehabilitate those who suffer from mental disorders.

The institute:

- Conducts and supports research on the biological, psychological, behavioral, and epidemiological aspects of mental health and illness;
- Funds training for promising new mental health researchers;
- Gives technical assistance to agencies and organizations working to establish mental health programs;
- Supports a National Clearinghouse for Mental Health Information, serving researchers, health professionals, and the public;
- Oversees operation of St. Elizabeth's Hospital, a facility in the District of Columbia for care and treatment of the mentally ill.

Centers for Disease Control (CDC)

The Centers for Disease Control directs a broad range of programs designed to safeguard and improve the health of Americans. CDC works to prevent the control infectious and chronic diseases; to prevent disease, disability, and death associated with environmental and workplace hazards; and to promote health and reduce health risks through education and information. The agency also provides support, in the basic areas of epidemiology, disease surveillance, laboratory science, and training, to local, state, national, and international disease prevention efforts.

CDC comprises six operating units responsible for agency efforts in the areas their names suggest:

- Center for Environmental Health
- Center for Health Promotion and Education
- Center for Infectious Diseases
- Center for Prevention Services
- Center for Professional Development and Training
- National Institute for Occupational Safety and Health (NIOSH)

The only Public Health Service agency with headquarters outside the Washington, D.C., metropolitan area, CDC is located in Atlanta, Georgia, with the exception of NIOSH, which is located in Rockville, Maryland.

CDC carries out a great variety of activities. The agency:

- Tracks disease incidence and trends. Exchanges epidemiological information with health authorities throughout the world, to enable them to take quick action as problems are identified.
- Works with governments of other nations and with international health organizations to help control the spread of diseases from one country to another. Provides epidemic assistance and consultation as requested.
- Administers a national quarantine program, carried out at U.S. ports of entry and at strategic locations overseas, to protect the United States from introduction of diseases from abroad.
- Assists state health departments in investigating outbreaks of disease. Examples in recent years are legionnaires' disease, toxic shock syndrome, and AIDS.
- Provides laboratory diagnostic services for unusual problems. Supplies rare vaccines, immune globulins, and therapeutic drugs not otherwise available for preventing or treating unusual diseases.
- Works with state and local health departments in developing and operating programs for venereal disease control and for childhood immunization against measles, mumps, rubella, whooping cough, tetanus, diphtheria, and polio.
- Assesses impact of environmental problems on health. CDC has been active in evaluating the health implications of the eruption of Mount St. Helens, the nuclear accident at Three Mile Island, and emergencies associated with toxic waste disposal.
- Conducts epidemiological studies and laboratory research to identify hazards in the workplace and determine steps that should be taken to eliminate them.
- Recommends acceptable exposure limits for toxic substances and harmful agents. Evaluates health conditions at work sites on request by employer or employee.
- Monitors licensing and certification of clinical laboratories and administers a comprehensive program to improve laboratory services.
- Trains some twenty thousand health workers each year.

• Works through school systems, health care providers, community organizations, and other channels to educate Americans about ways they can promote their own health and reduce health risks.

Food and Drug Administration (FDA)

The programs of the Food and Drug Administration have a single overall objective: consumer protection. As a regulatory agency, FDA works to ensure that:

• The nation's foods are safe and wholesome;
• Drugs, biological products, and medical devices are safe and effective;
• Cosmetics are properly manufactured;
• Products regulated by the FDA are accurately labeled and honestly packaged;
• Consumers are protected from unnecessary exposure to radiation from electronic products.

When hazardous products are identified, the FDA issues public warnings. The agency can initiate removal of a product from the market when new scientific evidence reveals unacceptable or unexpected risks. It can go to court to seize illegal products and to prosecute the manufacturer, packer, or shipper of adulterated or mislabeled products. It can take legal action against false or misleading labeling of products.

The FDA carries out its activities through a National Center for Drugs and Biologics, four bureaus, a toxicological research center, and a field staff of investigators, scientists, and consumer affairs officers located in 150 cities.

Health Resources and Services Administration (HRSA)

The Health Resources and Services Administration (HRSA), organized September 1, 1982, combines the programs of the former Health Resources Administration, Health Services Administration, and the Office of Health Maintenance Organizations.

The Agency directs programs and activities designed to improve health services and to develop health care and maintenance systems that are adequately financed, comprehensive, interrelated, and responsive to the needs of citizens..

The HRSA supports efforts to integrate health services delivery programs with public and private health financing programs, including health maintenance organizations; administers the health services block grants, categorical grants, and formula grant-supported programs; provides or arranges for personal health services—both hospital and outpatient care—to designated beneficiaries, including American Indians and Alaska Natives; administers programs to improve the utilization of health resources through health planning; provides technical assistance for modernizing or replacing health care facilities; provides leadership to improve the education, training, distribution, supply, use, and quality of health personnel; and provides advice and support to the Assistant Secretary for Health in the formulation of health policies.

HRSA Major Components

INDIAN HEALTH SERVICE (IHS)

The Indian Health Service assures a comprehensive health services delivery system for American Indians and Alaska Natives, with sufficient options for maximum tribal involvement. The IHS goal is to raise the health level of the Indian and Alaska Native people.

Bureau of Health Maintenance Organizations and Resources Development (BHMORD)

This bureau has responsibility for federal policies and programs pertaining to health planning and resources allocation for health care systems and organizations, including financial, capital, organizational, and physical matters. It administers grant, loan, loan guarantee, and interest subsidy programs relating to the construction, modernization, conversion, or closure of health and health care facilities and organizations; it plans, directs, administers, and evaluates national health planning and resources development program activities; it is responsible for the grant, contract, and loan aspects of the Public Health Service Act relating to Health Maintenance Organization (HMOs), and for other aspects of the federal HMO activities, including planning, development, regulations compliance, and qualification; and it coordinates and maintains liaison with both federal and nonfederal public and private entities.

Bureau of Health Professions (BHPr)

This bureau coordinates, evaluates, and supports the development and utilization of health personnel. It assesses and forecasts health personnel supply and requirements. It collects and analyzes data and disseminates information on the characteristics and capacities of health personnel production systems; develops, tests, and demonstrates new and improved approaches to the training and utilization of health personnel within various patterns of health care delivery and financing systems; provides financial support to institutions and individuals for health professions educational programs; administers federal programs for targeted health personnel development and utilization (such as primary care practitioners); and provides leadership and technical assistance for assuring equity in access to health services and health careers for the disadvantaged, as well as to national, state, and local agencies, organizations, agencies, and institutions for the development, production, utilization, and evaluation of health personnel. The Division of Nursing, described on pp 325–326, is included in this bureau.

Bureau of Health Care Delivery and Assistance (BHCDA)

This Bureau is the focus for efforts to assure the availability and delivery of health

care services in medically underserved areas and to special populations. It assists, through program and clinical efforts, in providing health care to underserved populations through the Primary Health Care and Maternal and Child Health Block Grants, which provide a principal means of support in maintaining and improving the health of mothers and children; it provides, through project grants to state, local, voluntary, public, and private entities, funds to help meet the health needs of special populations such as migrants and victims of black lung disease; it administers the National Health Service Corps program, which currently has over 2,000 health professionals in medically underserved communities; it directs the Bureau of Prisons' medical program, the National Hansen's Disease Program, and support for the Federal Employees Occupational Health Program, the CHAMPUS Program, and the Cuban and Haitian Refugee programs; and it administers a health program for designated PHS beneficiaries, including active duty members of the Coast Guard, PHS, and the National Oceanic and Atmospheric Administration.

National Center for Health Services Research (NCHSR)

The National Center for Health Services Research is the primary source of federal support for research on problems related to the quality and delivery of health services. Nursing is a major component of health services delivery and NCHSR is a very viable alternative for research funding by nurses who want to look at nursing and nurses in the context of the delivery system. An example of such research is a study of the cost effectiveness of primary versus team nursing.

National Institutes of Health (NIH)

The Public Health Service's National Institutes of Health (NIH) provides the largest support for biomedical research projects, including nursing research.[8] Projects are selected for scientific merit and relevance to health problems. The NIH draws for assistance on a national pool of scientists actively engaged in research. These scientists select the meritorious research projects of the highest quality to implement the research grant programs.

National Cancer Institute (NCI)

The National Cancer Institute was established in 1937 and became a component of what was then the National *Institute* of Health in 1944.

The National Cancer Act of 1971 greatly expanded NCI's responsibilities by creating the National Cancer Program. This nationwide effort against cancer made NCI the primary federal agency in cancer research, leading and coordinating all federal activities in this area and providing support to state and local governments, industries, voluntary health agencies, and other organizations. In addition, the Institute:

• Conducts cancer research in its own laboratories;
• Supports cancer research and a cancer control program through research grants and contracts;
• Supports training of new cancer researchers; and
• Collects and disseminates information on cancer to researchers, health professionals, and the public.

Approved and funded research of nurse principal investigators includes such projects as ameliorating the stresses of radiation therapy; counseling intervention for chemotherapy side effects; behavioral treatment for children receiving cancer therapy; postdischarge crisis in cancer patients; and relaxation training in reducing aversion to chemotherapy. NCI and the Division of Nursing are jointly supporting a project entitled, "Psychosocial Intervention for Radiation Therapy." Nursing care research where nurses are involved but not as principal investigators include dental compliance of irradiated cancer patients; behavioral aspects in cancer incidence and mortality; reducing adverse reaction to cancer chemotherapy; psychosocial correlates of survival; alternate cancer treatment—active noncompliance; neuropsychological assessment of children with cancer; breast cancer detection by breast self-examination; assessing the effects of counseling cancer patients; multidisciplinary approach to psychosocial cancer care; depression in cancer patients; patient education to reduce distress during chemotherapy; assessment of sleep in patients with neoplastic disease; patient and staff compliance with cancer therapy and primary prevention of cancer in childhood.

NCI activities related to support of nursing education are to:

• Initiate or expand curricula for nursing students and nurses in the areas of prevention, epidemiology, cancer patient nutrition, control and rehabilitation;
• Conduct seminars or workshops on current trends in oncology nursing;
• Provide student assistantships' support for short-term active participation in cancer research or service projects under a preceptor;
• Implement or expand continuing education acitivities; and
• Increase participation of nurses in interschool cancer activities.

Another major program of the NCI that involves nursing research activity is the Clinical Cooperative Group Program. Many of the fifteen cooperative groups support either an oncology nursing or a nursing research subcommittee. The nurses' activities in the clinical research efforts include participation in protocol development, with particular emphasis on the potential impact of different treatment options on patient compliance; facilitation of the informed consent process; development of nursing care and patient education approaches to deal with side effects of therapy; data management; attendance at scientific meetings; and presentation and publication of research results.

National Heart, Lung, and Blood Institute (NHLBI)

Established in 1948, the National Heart, Lung, and Blood Institute plans, conducts, and supports a coordinated program of research, investigations, clinical trials, and demonstrations relating to the causes, prevention, methods of diagnosis, and treatment of cardiovascular diseases.

- A Division of Heart and Vascular Diseases plans and directs NHLBI's grant, contract, and training programs concerned with atherosclerosis (including coronary heart disease); hypertension and kidney disease; and cardiac disorders such as congenital heart disease; rheumatic heart disease, heart failure, and shock.
- The Division of Lung Diseases guides and supports research in lung disorders, encompassing basic and targeted research, national pulmonary centers, technological development, and application of research findings.
- The Blood Diseases and Resources Division, through grants, contracts, and training programs, supports and directs research to improve the diagnosis, prevention, and treatment of blood diseases to assure the efficient and safe use of an adequate supply of high-quality blood and blood products.
- The seventeen Bethesda-based laboratories and branches of the Division of Intramural Research conduct basic and clinical studies on the cardiopulmonary, blood, and endocrine systems in health and disease.

NHLBI supports a nurse principal investigator and focuses on consolidating and strengthening programs that provide screening, education, counseling, and patient care to persons with sickle cell anemia. Projects in which a nurse is not the principal investigator include education and compliance in asthmatics; health education in self-management of childhood asthma; smoking cessation during obstetrical care; smoking cessation during comprehensive health care; the effectiveness of nurse practitioners as primary care providers for sickle cell anemia patients; and two projects on the education, testing, counseling, and supportive services on sickle cell anemia patients. In addition, there are projects with physician principal investigators, directed to the clinical training of nurses. Two projects are concerned with sickle cell anemia, specifically genetic counseling and education of nursing personnel in the disease syndrome, and another in transfusion medicine and education of students and staff nurses.

National institute of Dental Research (NIDR)

Established as a Dental Hygiene Unit under Dr. H. Trendly Dean in 1931, its primary function was to apply principles of epidemiology to a series of community studies on the oral disease known as "mottled enamel." Dr. Dean's research on flouride showed not only its relation to mottled enamel, but also its influence on tooth decay. The Dental Hygiene Unit was formally established in 1948 as an institute to conduct, foster, and coordinate research into the causes, prevention, diagnosis, and treatment of oral and dental diseases and condtions.

NIDR is the principal sponsor of dental research and research training in the United States through six categorical programs: periodontal diseases; craniofacial anomalies; restorative materials; soft tissue stomatology and nutrition; pain control and behavioral studies; and dental research centers.

The National Caries Program, begun in 1972, was charged to eliminate dental caries as a public health problem and to promote cost-effective agents and techniques to prevent caries. The program conducts research in four areas: combating caries-inducing microorganisms; increasing the resistance of teeth; modifying the diet; and improving delivery and acceptance of carries-preventive methods.

The institute also conducts related research in its own laboratories. Programs are directed toward the acquisition of fundamental knowledge about orofacial diseases and disorders and the development of treatment, control, and preventive measures. Areas of concern include dental caries, periodontal disease, congenital and acquired defects, benign and malignant soft tissues lesions of the oral cavity, and orofacial pain.

National Institute of Neurological and Communicative Disorders and Stroke (NINCDS)

The National Institute of Neurological and Communicative Disorders and Stroke, through its intramural and extramural programs, conducts research in fundamental neurosciences, communicative disorders, neurological disorders, and stroke and trauma. The institute, established in 1950, conducts, fosters, coordinates and guides research on the causes, prevention, diagnosis, and treatment of the above-mentioned disorders.

Areas of research under NINCDS's purview encompass:

- Disorders of early life such as cerebral palsy, hereditary metabolic diseases, autism, and dyslexia;
- Disorders of adult life including Parkinson's disease, Huntington's disease, and the dementias;
- Demyelinating disorders such as multiple and amyotrophic lateral sclerosis;
- Convulsive and paroxysmal disorders including epilepsy and narcolepsy;
- Neuromuscular disorders such as muscular dystrophy, myasthenia gravis, and the peripheral diseases of nerves; and
- Infectious diseases including slow viruses, encephalitis, and meningitis.

The institute is involved in the development of new diagnostic techniques, particularly computerized axial tomography, or CAT; positron emission tomography, or PET; and ultrasonic scanning.

Nurses participate in the research process. In the Anti-Epileptic Drug Development Program, Technical Information Section, Epilepsy Branch, under the Convulsive, Developmental and Neuromuscular Disorders Program (clinical trials by contract), nurses are an integral involved component of the research team directly involved in the research process. The research tasks include designing protocols and forms, monitoring data collection, site-visiting research centers to assess compliance of all research teams with established research procedures, editing and coding data as collected, review literature, and preparing manuscripts for publication.

In the Stroke and Coma Data Bank Centers centrally operated by contract under the auspices of the Biometry and Field Studies Branch, nurses carry out similar functions.

NINCDS and the Division of Nursing (DN) have a memorandum of agreement to support contract costs reimbursed by NINCDS to DN to foster nurses training in research and teaching at the Magnuson Center, NIH, and at academic institutions.

National Institute of Arthritis, Diabetes, and Digestive and Kidney Diseases (NIADDK)

The National Institute of Arthritis, Diabetes, and Digestive and Kidney Diseases, established in 1950, conducts and supports basic and clinical research into arthritis and connective tissue diseases; skin diseases; disorders of the bone and muscles; diabetes and other metabolic and endocrine disorders; digestive and nutritional diseases; kidney and urinary tract disorders; and blood abnormalities.

NIADDK's intramural research organization conducts studies in endocrinology; chemistry; biochemistry; metabolism; physical, chemical, and molecular biology; physics; pharmacology; and pathology. Institute scientists guide clinical research and treatment programs on arthritis, diabetes, and other metabolic diseases, cystic fibrosis, gastroenterology (including liver disease), and hematology.

The institute's extramural program is organized into four areas; arthritis, musculoskeletal, and skin diseases; diabetes, endocrinology, and metabolic diseases; digestive diseases and nutrition; and kidney, urologic, and blood diseases.

NIADDK supports nursing research activities through two major programs: the Diabetes Research and Training Centers and the Multipurpose Arthritis Centers.

The projects supported through the Arthritis Centers address both education and health services research. Examples include evaluation of current nursing curriculum from the standpoint of rheumatology needs, development of curriculum and implementation of the changed curriculum; and a project to provide a consumer guide to arthritis patients based on the perceived needs of a sample of 150 patients selected from the Visting Nurses Association and community health centers. Some of the projects are nursing specific, i.e., nursing management of diabetes, theory and practice, while others are interdisciplinary, i.e., symposium and preceptorship in diabetes care.

NIADDK also collects, prepares, and disseminates information on research progress within its general disease areas. The institute communicates with scientists, health professionals, and the public and maintains contact with professional associations and voluntary organizations.

National Institute of Allergy and Infectious Diseases (NIAID)

Beginning as the National Microbiological Institute in 1948, the name was officially changed to the National Institute of Allergy and Infectious Diseases seven years later.

NIAID conducts and supports research in allergic, immunological, and infectious diseases on a national, as well as international, scale.

To develop a better means of preventing, diagnosing, and treating illness, NIAID conducts studies on the following:

- The immune system—its genetic control, maturation, characteristics, and manipulation.
- Disorders and derangements of the immune system including asthma, immune deficiency states, and autoimmunity.
- The role of the immune system in chronic diseases such as arthritis, chronic glomerulonephritis, and lupus erythematosus.
- The etiology, epidemiology, and pathogenesis

of infections caused by viruses, mycoplasma, bacteria, fungi, and parasites, covering many organ systems.
- The diagnosis, treatment, and prevention of infections including research on antibiotics; antimicrobial, antifungal, and antiviral therapy; and vaccines.
- The role of nucleic acid recombination in microbial agents; the manipulation of nucleic acid recombination to produce medically or technologically useful by-products; and the assessment and control of risks involved with this type research.

NIAID supports nursing care research through its specialized center grants. Principal investigators of the center grants tend to be physicians, but nurse researchers manage the nursing research components of the subprojects. Nursing research is directed to developing and implementing a Spanish language program for self-management of asthma and epilepsy, assessing health status of subjects in self-management of asthma in an urban ghetto, and piloting a continuing education course for community-based nurses for care of patients with chronic disease.

National Institute of General Medical Sciences (NIGMS)

Established in 1963, the National Institute of General Medical Sciences, through support of research and research training in the basic biomedical sciences, seeks to expand knowledge about the fundamental life processes. NIGMS conducts studies on the following:

- Cellular and molecular basis of disease;
- Genetics;
- Pharmacological sciences;
- Physiology and biomedical engineering; and
- Intramural research.

While fundamental studies funded by NIGMS usually are not obviously related to a particular disease at the time they are being carried out, they lay the groundwork for important clinical advances. The most striking illustration lies in the dramatic strides being made in medicine and other areas using recombinant DNA technology. This technology was developed by scientists carrying out basic studies in genetics—the majority with NIGMS support.

NIGMS does not support nursing research as defined by the Task Force. However, nurses are involved in research projects that include: sample collection; recording of basic data; chart review; implementating the protocol treatments and tests; instructing patients in the protocol; obtaining patient permission for participation; coordinating clinical studies and laboratory scheduling; and training research nurses.

NIGMS supports research training through individual fellowships and institutional training grants. Efforts include a Minority Access to Research Careers Program designed to provide special training opportunities to minority students with research career potential, and to strengthen the research and teaching capabilities of schools with significant minority enrollment.

National Eye Institute (NEI)

The National Eye Institute became a component of NIH in 1968. The institute fosters research to gain knowledge and understanding of the normal function of the eye and visual system, the pathology of visual disorders, and the basic science underlying vision.

- Supports—through grants, fellowships, and contracts to medical schools and research institutions—research and research training aimed at improving the prevention, diagnosis, and treatment of visual disorders;
- Conducts laboratory and clinical research in its own facilities and fosters statistical and epidemiological studies of visual disorders in human populations;
- Promotes research to rehabilitate the visually handicapped;
- Encourages application of research discoveries to clinical practice;
- Heightens public awareness of vision problems; and

- Cooperates with voluntary organizations.

National Institute of Child Health and Human Development (NICHD)

The National Institute of Child Health and Human Development established in 1962 conducts and supports research on the reproductive, developmental, and behavioral processes that determine the health of children, adults, families, and populations. The Institute administers a multidisciplinary program of research, research training, and public information.

NICHD has four major components that engage in biomedical and behavioral projects and fundamental and clinical studies: the Center for Research for Mothers and Children, Center for Population Research, Intramural Research Program, and Epidemiology and Biometry Research.

The Institute supports research in the reproductive sciences to develop knowledge enabling men and women to regulate their fertility with methods that are safe, effective, and acceptable to various population groups, and to overcome problems of infertility.

In population, social, and behavioral sciences, the purpose of Institute-sponsored research is to understand the causes and consequences of population change.

Research for mothers, children, and families is designed to advance knowledge of fetal development, pregnancy, and birth; to identify the prerequisites of optimal growth through infancy, childhood, and adolescence; and to contribute to the prevention and treatment of mental retardation.

Examples of studies in which nurse researchers are involved are: comparison of methods used for multiple venous sampling; incidence of microbial contamination and blood loss; body-image, global self-esteem, perceived competence in school-age children and adolescents with alterations in growth and development; an exploratory study to identify selected behavioral expressions of children undergoing a painful experience; and relationship between growth hormone dose and ulnar growth velocity in patients with gonadal dysgensis.

National Institute of Environmental Health Sciences (NIEHS)

The only categorical component of NIH not located in Bethesda, the National Institute of Environmental Health Sciences established in 1969 is located at Research Triangle Park, North Carolina. The institute's goal is to provide the scientific information base, advanced methodology, and trained manpower to understand and prevent adverse effects of environmental factors, physical, chemical, and biological, on human health.

The institute supports training in environmental toxicology, pathology, mutagenesis, and epidemiology. NIEHS also funds basic and applied research on the exposure of man and other biological systems to potentially toxic or harmful environmental agents.

In its research, the institute attempts to learn:

- How and where potentially harmful agents, particularly toxic chemicals, are released;
- How these agents move, and possibly change as they move;
- The extent of exposure of various population groups;
- What effects these agents cause, by themselves and in combination with other environmental factors;
- What happens in biological systems after exposure to hazardous agents; and
- What diseases are caused or aggravated by environmental factors.

NIEHS supports efforts to identify hazardous agents before they are released into the environment. These include developing, testing, and validating biological assay systems to predict the toxic effects that may occur in humans. Program output is intended to aid agencies and organizations, public and private, responsible for developing and instituting regulations, policies, and procedures to prevent and reduce the incidence of environmentally induced diseases.

National Institute on Aging (NIA)

The National Institute on Aging was established by Congress in 1971 and given responsibility for "biomedical, social, and behavioral research and training related to the aging process and diseases and other special problems and needs of aged."

The Institute's extramural program supports biomedical and clinical studies through grants and contracts. Primary areas of emphasis include molecular and cellular biology, physiology of aging, geriatrics, and behavioral sciences research.

The bulk of the Institute's intramural research is conducted at the Gerontology Research Center in Baltimore, Maryland. Via the NIH associate, staff fellowship, and visiting programs, scientists at various stages of their careers gain sophisticated experience at the center. Areas studied include the relationship between aging and nutrition in animal populations —specifically, the effects of age on absorption, distribution, and utilization of known nutrients and mechanisms responsible for increased life-span associated with dietary restriction. Other special fields of interest include senile dementia of the Alzheimer's type; concern about how and where people spend their dying days (relevant to hospice planning); congestive heart disease; minor health problems such as headaches; and the changes that occur with aging.

Nurse principal investigators are studying: urine incontinency in older women and nursing interventions; social support processes in well-being in the bereaved; and the families' response to the mentally impaired aged person. Projects that address nursing care problems of the elderly, not directed by nurse investigators, are primarily broad-based research efforts that include nursing because of the nature of the care of the elderly rather than the specific research objectives. These projects include multiple subprojects through the Teaching Nursing Home Program supported by the NIA. Examples of areas being investigated are: home-based behavioral treatment of the elderly; incontinence in the elderly; social networks and the care of the frail elderly; the epidemiology of urinary tract infections in elderly institutionalized patients; stroke rehabilitation; diagnosis and assessment of senile dementia; the differential effects of drugs on the cardiovascular system; falls; monitoring behavioral toxicity of drugs in nursing homes; management of chronic urinary catheters in the elderly; identification of persons at risk of institutional placement; metabolic regulation; physical fitness of the elderly; and sleep-disordered breathing.

A primary and unique source of these investigations is the Baltimore Longitudinal Study on Aging. Men and women ranging in age from twenty to ninety six come to the center every one to two years to undergo 2-1/2 days of extensive clinical, biochemical, and psychological testing. Through this research project, scientists are learning about the normal process of aging.

In addition to nursing-care oriented projects, the NIA supports geriatric medicine academic awards that incorporate clinical training of geriatric nurse practitioners.

The NIA and DN have a cooperative agreement with the issuance of a request for applications on clinical trials of behavioral therapies for urinary incontinence in the elderly. Thirteen applications have been received. The applications are reviewed by both Councils. Funding decisions are made by both the Director, NIA, and the Director, BHPr.

Division of Research Resources (DRR)

The Division of Research Resources administers programs that develop and ensure the availability of resources essential to the efficient and effective conduct of human health research. The DRR supports nursing research activities through

two mechanisms: General Clinical Research Center Grants and Biomedical Research Support Grants.

A General Clinical Research Center is a miniature hospital-within-a-hospital with sophisticated equipment and expert personnel to provide a multidisciplinary clinical research environment. The nursing staff is highly trained not only to provide exemplary patient care, but also to make complex, detailed research observations and precise collections of specimens. The nursing density required in a Center is primarily determined by the number of research patient days and the complexity of the research and medical care being conducted at the Center. Nurses work in collaboration with physicians in these centers.

The objectives of the Biomedical Research Support Grant is to strengthen and enhance the research environment of institutions heavily engaged in health-related research. Through the use of flexible funds and local decision making, researchers are better able to conduct their research programs.

The major focus of this research is the behavioral aspects of disease and treatment. The behavioral subprojects include studies of adolescents, women and infertility, pregnancy, childhood problems, depression, and cardiovascular disease. Other nursing subprojects include monamine oxidase inhibitors and sleep, activity and intracranial pressure, surgical wound healing, health status of rheumatoid arthritis patients, mental health screening of preschoolers, falls in the elderly, glucocorticoids and gastrointestinal neurotransmitter enzyme activity, memory improvement in the aged, and vitamin D metabolic assay studies.

The General Clinical Research Centers Program supported studies, not headed by a nurse investigator, concerning failure to thrive in infants, renal transport in vitamin D metabolism in end-stage renal disease, use of sodium fluoride in coherence therapy of osteoporosis, alpha-2 interferon and psoriasis, and treatment of periodontal disease.

National Library of Medicine (NLM)

The National Library of Medicine is the world's largest research library in a single scientific and professional field. A statutory mandate from Congress directs the library to apply its resources broadly to the advancement of medical and health-related sciences.

An amendment in 1956 to Title III of the Public Health Service Act—the National Library of Medicine Act—placed the Armed Forces Medical Library (originally the Library of the Office of the Surgeon General of the Army in 1836) under the Public Health Service, giving the library its present name. The library collects, organizes, and makes available biomedical information to investigators, educators, and practitioners, and carries out programs designed to strengthen existing and to develop new medical library services in the United States. NLM was funded in fiscal year 1982 at nearly $44 million.

The Medical Literature Analysis and Retrieval System, or MEDLARS, was established in 1964 to gain rapid bibliographical access to NLM's store of biomedical information. The principal objective of MEDLARS is to provide references to the biomedical literature for researchers, clinicians, and other health professionals. This is accomplished through:

- Preparation of citations for publication in *Index Medicus,* a comprehensive subject-author index to articles from approximately 2,500 of the world's biomedical journals, and the NLM *Current Catalog*—a bibliographical listing of citations to publications cataloged by the Library.
- Compilation of other recurring bibliographies on specialized subjects of wide interest.
- Provision of online search services.

Through bibliographical citations yielded by MEDLARS databases, nurse researchers can identify relevant source material in nursing and related disciplines to review research project background information and theory, to assist in formulating project methodology, and to facilitate analysis and interpretation of project outcomes.

Other services offered by NLM include online databases (bibliographical searching through terminals in libraries at medical schools and hospitals), Regional Medical Library services (for efficient use of interlibrary loans), the toxicology information program (computer-based toxicology data banks), and grants.

The History of Medicine Division provides researchers of nursing history access to a variety of materials of interest.

NLM also comprises the Lister Hill National Center for Biomedical Communications (LHNCBC). The LHNCBC (and prior to its 1983 merger with the LHNCBC, the National Medical Audiovisual Center) has given educational support to nursing research. Audiovisual materials have been developed intramurally and extramurally to teach basic scientific concepts and practices of nursing care, while disseminating the findings of nursing and other health science research. The most extensive project, the Human Physiology Series, is targeted at graduate-level nursing students. A collaborative activity conducted by the LHNCBC is producing a series of videotaped educational programs on the protection of human subjects from research risks. Contemporary and historical materials of interest to nursing are being produced as the Distinguished Leaders in Nursing series, a videotaped educational program documenting the contributions of nurses and nursing to the USPHS from 1914 to present. All major nursing components of PHS are collaborating in this effort. LHNCBC also conducts a vigorous workshop and consultation program that promotes development, use, and evaluation of instructional materials, which, indirectly, supports nursing educational research. Audiovisual materials are made available to nurses through videotape loan programs and the General Services Administration and National Technical Information Service sales programs. Citations to these and audiovisuals produced by others are made available to nurses and through AVLINE, a database of MEDLARS.

Nurses are also eligible to participate in the NLM Medical Informatics postdoctoral research training program. NLM supports research training in medical informatics for persons who have earned doctorates in nursing, other health sciences, biological sciences, and computer science.

Application Procedure for All Agencies of the Public Health Service (PHS)

Grant applications (PHS 398, Rev. 5/82) are available through research offices of most institutions. Applications are submitted to the Division of Research Grants, National Institutes of Health, Room 240, Westwood Bldg., 5333 Westbard Avenue, Bethesda, Maryland, 20205, for assignment to the Division of Nursing or to another Institute if more appropriate.

Responsibilities of Universities and Health Agencies in Conducting Research

What are the responsibilities of universities and health agencies in conducting research? It is generally agreed that the goals of a university are teaching, research, and service. Teaching hospitals have similar goals. State universities, particularly land grant institutions, and hospitals must of necessity give more attention to service.

Many universities lack the organizational structure to facilitate interdisciplinary research. Departmental barriers inhibit rather than facilitate interdisciplinary research. In an attempt to solve this problem, universities have set up centers, institutes, and laboratories that provide a research climate where interdisciplinary research can be conducted.

In nursing, as well as in other fields of knowledge, the quality and volume of research can have a direct influence upon

Application Receipt Deadline Dates

PROGRAM AND URNA APPLICATIONS	PROJECT, NINRA AND NRE/DPN APPLICATIONS	RENEWAL SUPPLEMENTAL APPLICATIONS	REVIEW COMPLETED	EARLIEST POSSIBLE FUNDING
Feb. 1	Mar. 1	Feb. 1	Sept./Oct.	Dec.
June 1	July 1	June 1	Jan./Feb.	Apr.
Oct. 1	Nov. 1	Oct. 1	May	July

PREPARATION OF THE RESEARCH PROPOSAL IN APPLYING FOR FINANCIAL SUPPORT, AND RESPONSIBILITIES OF THE ADMINISTRATOR AND RESEARCHER

The following discussion is intended to provide guidelines for researchers in developing research proposals for which financial support may be sought. Because the administrator of a university, hospital, or health agency has an important role if the research is to be conducted successfully by these institutions, the responsibilities of the administrator and researcher will be discussed first.

the caliber of education provided by the university. If the research being conducted is pedestrian, the quality of teaching can suffer. To obtain a balance between research and teaching, the dean, director, or department head of the school must decide how much and what kind of research can be conducted within the school of nursing as well as in the clinical divisions of the associated hospital or health agencies. Too often administrators force research upon staff who have no training or talent for it. How much research and what kind, as well as the need for interdisciplinary research, must be determined by the dean, the faculty, and appropriate representatives of other departments (including hospital and nursing service administration) prior to initiating specific research projects.

KEY POINT Many difficulties in conducting research stem from the way in which the institution administers its research grants program. The following guidelines can help those responsible for administering such a program.

1. No research grant or contract should be secured and then assigned to someone to carry out who has not been involved in the research design.

2. The university or health agency concerned should support and encourage principal investigators to apply for and secure financing for their research projects.

3. Whenever possible, graduate and undergraduate students should be involved in the research program.

4. A research contingency fund should be set up by the institution to handle research expenses not chargeable elsewhere. Such expenses include support for time to develop a research proposal, travel to institutions conducting related research and for conducting small pilot studies.

5. Research activities that utilize space of the university or health agency should administer funds through that agency.

6. The institution administering the research should have prior publication and patent rights. Any royalties resulting should be shared by the institution and the investigator.

7. Salary supplements and consultant fees for those within the university or health agency should be prohibited. Those participating in research activities should be permitted to do so only on a released time basis.

8. Membership on the graduate faculty should include active participation in a research program that would justify a reduced teaching load.

9. Research proposals in departments of arts and sciences that relate to a particular profession such as nursing or public health should be reviewed by the professional school in that university or one within the immediate vicinity. Likewise, proposals developed in professional schools that utilize the research tools and/or resources of university departments should be reviewed by the chairman of the department. Some universities have found it helpful to set up specific procedures regarding clearance of research proposals before they are submitted for support.

10. The principal investigator should be a member of the university faculty or institution receiving the grant. This permits the administrator of the institution to achieve a proper balance between research and teaching and/or research and service.

11. To deal with the complex problems of grants management, some institutions, particularly universities, have employed a grants management officer. A scientist administrator would be an ideal person for this position. The grants associate program at the National Institutes of Health provides a twelve-month training program for this specialty.

Preparing a Research Proposal in Applying for Financial Support

In the preparation and review of research proposals it is wise to give equal consideration to the substantive and methodological aspects of the study of the administrative problems in carrying it out. The scientific substance of the plan is the responsibility of those who will execute it. The principal investigator should be given every opportunity to maintain scientific freedom in carrying out research objectives. However, once the plan has been approved and receives financial support, the investigator should be allowed to make only those changes in methodology, approach, or other aspects of the project that would expedite achievement of the objectives.

When support is requested from an outside agency it becomes all the more important for the institution in which the research is initiated to carry out its own preliminary review process before the application is submitted. Use of an internal advisory committee, previously discussed, is useful for this purpose.

The large amounts of federal funds being expended for medical research have brought external control by panels representing the special interests of particular fields of science. These panels review research proposals submitted for grant support and pass on their scientific merits and worthiness to receive financial backing.

WRITING A RESEARCH PROPOSAL

The following pages contain a suggested outline* of a research proposal that might be used in applying for financial support. Although the immediate purpose of such a proposal is to convince the money-granting authority of the merits of the project and secure their financial backing, it can serve as the plan for study and used to guide its execution. A proposal contains not only a description of the design of the research, it also provides a financial budget and a staffing plan that can be most useful in administering the project efficiently and economically.

Part I—Preplanning

1. ABSTRACT OF RESEARCH

In approximately 250 words state long-term objectives and specific aims making reference to the health/nursing relatedness of the project. Describe the methodology for achieving goals.

2. BIOGRAPHICAL SKETCHES

Provide a curriculum vitae for each key member of the research team. See suggested format in Figure 18-2.

*Adapted from U.S. Public Health Service Research Grant Application. PHS 398 (Rev. May 1982).

3. DETAILED BUDGET FOR FIRST TWELVE MONTHS

See suggested format in Figure 18-3.

PERSONNEL

List all professional (these should be named), technical, secretarial personnel on the research team, even if salary is not requested. For professional staff, indicate per cent of work effort on the project as averaged out over the year. For other staff, state the number of hours per week on the project. Separate out any deductions for social security, retirement, etc., and state as a separate amount for each member of the research team. On a separate page state the functions of key members of the research team.

CONSULTANTS

If needed, list consultants to the project. These should be named and their contribution indicated. Include fees, travel and per diem costs.

EQUIPMENT

List all large items of equipment separately. Small items may be grouped. Indicate which items are available at the institution and which ones will have to be purchased. Equipment items should be grouped into scientific equipment (e.g., tape recorder) and other equipment (e.g., desk, etc.).

SUPPLIES

List major items, such as tapes, office supplies, etc. Separate materials for scientific purposes (e.g., animals), from other supplies.

TRAVEL

Travel of the research team to related projects, professional meetings and patient

BIOGRAPHICAL SKETCH

Give the following information for key professional personnel, beginning with the
Principal Investigator / Program Director.

NAME	TITLE	BIRTHDATE *(Mo., Day, Yr.)*

EDUCATION *(Begin with baccalaureate or other initial professional education and include postdoctoral training)*

INSTITUTION AND LOCATION	DEGREE *(circle highest degree)*	YEAR CONFERRED	FIELD OF STUDY

RESEARCH AND/OR PROFESSIONAL EXPERIENCE: Concluding with present position, list in chronological order previous employment, experience, and honors. Include present membership on any Federal Government Public Advisory Committee. List, in chronological order, the titles and complete refernces, to all publications during the past three years and to representative earlier publications pertinent to this application. (Two pages.)

Figure 18-2

travel costs essential to the project are examples.

PATIENT COSTS

It may be necessary to cover the hospitalization costs for patients for study purposes. (The institution should be able to supply average per diem costs for patients to help you arrive at an estimate.)

ALTERATION AND RENOVATION

Any proposed changes should be detailed with justification. (Granting agencies usually set ceilings for this category.)

PUBLICATION

Specify any publication costs, reprints, etc.

OTHER COSTS

Machine tabulation, rental, and maintenance costs are examples that might be specified.

INDIRECT COSTS

Each institution or agency usually has a set indirect cost allowance. This amount usually goes to the institution to help to defray the costs of building maintenance, rent, etc. The amount of indirect cost allowance may vary from 50 to 100 percent.

TOTAL, ALL CATEGORIES

This should represent the total costs for the *first* twelve months of the project.

Part II—Research Plan

RESEARCH AIMS

State concisely and realistically what the research described will accomplish. Specify immediate aims (those to be accomplished the first two years) and long-range goals. Include hypothesis to be tested. (One page).

SIGNIFICANCE

Present the rationale for your research, giving particular attention to the theoretical basis for your research and its significance. Include background of proposal; critique of existing knowledge; and identify gaps that project is intended to fill. (Three pages).

PROGRESS REPORT/PRELIMINARY STUDIES

State any previous work that you and/or members of the research team have completed that would have bearing on the present research. Include relevant background graphs, diagrams, tables, and charts. (Eight pages).

EXPERIMENTAL DESIGN AND METHODS

Provide a statement of the nature of your proposed research—i.e., is it descriptive (experimental or nonexperimental), explanatory (experimental or nonexperimental), methodological, or a combination of these.

Describe your research plan, detailing the steps in methodology, relating each step to the specific aims stated under Research Aims. If you are testing hypotheses, state these concisely, providing operational definitions and relating the hypotheses to concepts that led you to make these deductions.

Specify what data you need to collect, relating it to the research question(s) posed, and how the data are to be collected, tabulated, and analyzed. Whenever possible provide examples of data to be collected, sample work sheets, and skeleton table outlines. If the research is experimental in nature, show how you propose to control for any biases—e.g., observer bias, contamination between control and experimental groups. Include a time table for the investigation. If methodology is new, state advantages over existing methodologies.

BUDGET FOR ENTIRE PROPOSED PROJECT PERIOD
DIRECT COSTS ONLY

BUDGET CATEGORY TOTALS		1st BUDGET PERIOD (from page 4)	ADDITIONAL YEARS SUPPORT REQUESTED			
			2nd	3rd	4th	5th
PERSONNEL (Salary and fringe benefits.)						
CONSULTANT COSTS						
EQUIPMENT						
SUPPLIES						
TRAVEL	DOMESTIC					
	FOREIGN					
PATIENT CARE COSTS	INPATIENT					
	OUTPATIENT					
ALTERATIONS AND RENOVATIONS						
CONSORTIUM/ CONTRACTUAL COSTS						
OTHER EXPENSES						
TOTAL DIRECT COSTS						

TOTAL FOR ENTIRE PROPOSED PROJECT PERIOD ⟶ $

JUSTIFICATION: Describe specific functions of personnel and consultants. Include justification for any costs that may not be apparent (e.g. equipment, foreign travel, alterations and renovations.

Figure 18-3

DETAILED BUDGET FOR FIRST 12 MONTH BUDGET PERIOD DIRECT COSTS ONLY		FROM		THROUGH	
		DOLLAR AMOUNT REQUESTED (Omit cents)			

PERSONNEL		TIME/EFFORT		SALARY	FRINGE BENEFITS	TOTALS
NAME	POSITION TITLE	%	Hours per Week			
	Principal Investigator					
	SUBTOTALS ——→					

CONSULTANT COSTS

EQUIPMENT (Itemize)

SUPPLIES (Itemize by category)

TRAVEL	DOMESTIC	
	FOREIGN	
PATIENT CARE COSTS	INPATIENT	
	OUTPATIENT	

ALTERATIONS AND RENOVATIONS (Itemize by category)

CONSORTIUM/CONTRACTUAL COSTS

OTHER EXPENSES (Itemize by category)

TOTAL DIRECT COSTS ——————————→ $

DEPARTMENT OF HEALTH AND HUMAN SERVICES

PROTECTION OF HUMAN SUBJECTS
ASSURANCE/CERTIFICATION/DECLARATION

☐ ORIGINAL ☐ FOLLOWUP ☐ REVISION

☐ GRANT ☐ CONTRACT ☐ FELLOW ☐ OTHER

☐ NEW ☐ RENEWAL ☐ CONTINUATION

APPLICATION IDENTIFICATION NUMBER *(If known)*

STATEMENT OF POLICY: Safeguarding the rights and welfare of subjects at risk in activities supported under grants and contracts from DHHS is primarily the responsibility of the institution which receives or is accountable to DHHS for the funds awarded for the support of the activity. In order to provide for the adequate discharge of this institutional responsibility, it is the policy of DHHS that no activity involving human subjects to be supported by DHHS grants or contracts shall be undertaken unless the Institutional Review Board has reviewed and approved such activity, and the institution has submitted to DHHS a certification of such review and approval, in accordance with the requirements of Public Law 93-348, as implemented by Part 46 of Title 45 of the Code of Federal Regulations, as amended, (45 CFR 46). Administration of the DHHS policy and regulation is the responsibility of the Office for Protection from Research Risks, National Institutes of Health, Bethesda, MD 20205.

1. TITLE OF PROPOSAL OR ACTIVITY

2. PRINCIPAL INVESTIGATOR/ACTIVITY DIRECTOR/FELLOW

3. DECLARATION THAT HUMAN SUBJECTS EITHER WOULD OR WOULD NOT BE INVOLVED

☐ A. NO INDIVIDUALS WHO MIGHT BE CONSIDERED HUMAN SUBJECTS, INCLUDING THOSE FROM WHOM ORGANS, TISSUES, FLUIDS, OR OTHER MATERIALS WOULD BE DERIVED, OR WHO COULD BE IDENTIFIED BY PERSONAL DATA, WOULD BE INVOLVED IN THE PROPOSED ACTIVITY. (IF NO HUMAN SUBJECTS WOULD BE INVOLVED, CHECK THIS BOX AND PROCEED TO ITEM 7. PROPOSALS DETERMINED BY THE AGENCY TO INVOLVE HUMAN SUBJECTS WILL BE RETURNED.)

☐ B. HUMAN SUBJECTS WOULD BE INVOLVED IN THE PROPOSED ACTIVITY AS EITHER: ☐ NONE OF THE FOLLOWING, OR INCLUDING: ☐ MINORS, ☐ FETUSES, ☐ ABORTUSES, ☐ PREGNANT WOMEN, ☐ PRISONERS, ☐ MENTALLY RETARDED, ☐ MENTALLY DISABLED. UNDER SECTION 6. COOPERATING INSTITUTIONS, ON REVERSE OF THIS FORM, GIVE NAME OF INSTITUTION AND NAME AND ADDRESS OF OFFICIAL(S) AUTHORIZING ACCESS TO ANY SUBJECTS IN FACILITIES NOT UNDER DIRECT CONTROL OF THE APPLICANT OR OFFERING INSTITUTION.

4. DECLARATION OF ASSURANCE STATUS/CERTIFICATION OF REVIEW

☐ A. THIS INSTITUTION HAS NOT PREVIOUSLY FILED AN ASSURANCE AND ASSURANCE IMPLEMENTING PROCEDURES FOR THE PROTECTION OF HUMAN SUBJECTS WITH THE DHHS THAT APPLIES TO THIS APPLICATION OR ACTIVITY. ASSURANCE IS HEREBY GIVEN THAT THIS INSTITUTION WILL COMPLY WITH REQUIREMENTS OF *DHHS Regulation 45 CFR 46*, THAT IT HAS ESTABLISHED AN INSTITUTIONAL REVIEW BOARD FOR THE PROTECTION OF HUMAN SUBJECTS AND, WHEN REQUESTED, WILL SUBMIT TO DHHS DOCUMENTATION AND CERTIFICATION OF SUCH REVIEWS AND PROCEDURES AS MAY BE REQUIRED FOR IMPLEMENTATION OF THIS ASSURANCE FOR THE PROPOSED PROJECT OR ACTIVITY.

☐ B. THIS INSTITUTION HAS AN APPROVED GENERAL ASSURANCE (DHHS ASSURANCE NUMBER _____) OR AN ACTIVE SPECIAL ASSURANCE FOR THIS ONGOING ACTIVITY, ON FILE WITH DHHS. THE SIGNER CERTIFIES THAT ALL ACTIVITIES IN THIS APPLICATION PROPOSING TO INVOLVE HUMAN SUBJECTS HAVE BEEN REVIEWED AND APPROVED BY THIS INSTITUTION'S INSTITUTIONAL REVIEW BOARD IN A CONVENED MEETING ON THE DATE OF_____ IN ACCORDANCE WITH THE REQUIREMENTS OF THE *Code of Federal Regulations on Protection of Human Subjects (45 CFR 46).* THIS CERTIFICATION INCLUDES, WHEN APPLICABLE, REQUIREMENTS FOR CERTIFYING FDA STATUS FOR EACH INVESTIGATIONAL NEW DRUG TO BE USED (SEE REVERSE SIDE OF THIS FORM).

THE INSTITUTIONAL REVIEW BOARD HAS DETERMINED, AND THE INSTITUTIONAL OFFICIAL SIGNING BELOW CONCURS THAT:

EITHER ☐ HUMAN SUBJECTS WILL NOT BE AT RISK; OR ☐ HUMAN SUBJECTS WILL BE AT RISK.

5. AND 6. SEE REVERSE SIDE

7. NAME AND ADDRESS OF INSTITUTION

8. TITLE OF INSTITUTIONAL OFFICIAL	TELEPHONE NUMBER
SIGNATURE OF INSTITUTIONAL OFFICIAL	DATE

HHS-596 (Rev. 5-80)

Figure 18–4 Sample form used by DHHS

5. INVESTIGATIONAL NEW DRUGS - ADDITIONAL CERTIFICATION REQUIREMENT

SECTION 46.17 OF TITLE 45 OF THE Code of Federal Regulations states, "Where an organization is required to prepare or to submit a certification . . . and the proposal involves an investigational new drug within the meaning of The Food, Drug, and Cosmetic Act, the drug shall be identified in the certification together with a statement that the 30-day delay required by 21 CFR 130.3(a)(2) has elapsed and the Food and Drug Administration has not, prior to expiration of such 30-day interval, requested that the sponsor continue to withhold or to restrict use of the drug in human subjects, or that the Food and Drug Administration has waived the 30-day delay requirement; provided, however, that in those cases in which the 30-day delay interval has neither expired nor been waived, a statement shall be forwarded to DHHS upon such expiration or upon receipt of a waiver. No certification shall be considered acceptable until such statement has been received."

INVESTIGATIONAL NEW DRUG CERTIFICATION

TO CERTIFY COMPLIANCE WITH FDA REQUIREMENTS FOR PROPOSED USE OF INVESTIGATIONAL NEW DRUGS IN ADDITION TO CERTIFICATION OF INSTITUTIONAL REVIEW BOARD APPROVAL, THE FOLLOWING REPORT FORMAT SHOULD BE USED FOR EACH IND: (ATTACH ADDITIONAL IND CERTIFICATIONS AS NECESSARY).

— IND FORMS FILED: ☐ FDA 1571, ☐ FDA 1572, ☐ FDA 1573

— NAME OF IND AND SPONSOR _____

— DATE OF 30-DAY EXPIRATION OR FDA WAIVER

(FUTURE DATE REQUIRES FOLLOWUP REPORT TO AGENCY) _____

— FDA RESTRICTION _____

— SIGNATURE OF INVESTIGATOR _____ DATE _____

6. COOPERATING INSTITUTIONS - ADDITIONAL REPORTING REQUIREMENT

SECTION 46.16 OF TITLE 45 OF THE *Code of Federal Regulations* IMPOSES SPECIAL REQUIREMENTS ON THE CONDUCT OF STUDIES OR ACTIVITIES IN WHICH THE GRANTEE OR PRIME CONTRACTOR OBTAINS ACCESS TO ALL OR SOME OF THE SUBJECTS THROUGH COOPERATING INSTITUTIONS NOT UNDER ITS CONTROL. IN ORDER THAT THE DHHS BE FULLY INFORMED, THE FOLLOWING REPORT IS REQUESTED WHEN APPLICABLE.

USE FOLLOWING REPORT FORMAT FOR EACH INSTITUTION OTHER THAN GRANTEE OR CONTRACTING INSTITUTION WITH RESPONSIBILITY FOR HUMAN SUBJECTS PARTICIPATING IN THIS ACTIVITY: (ATTACH ADDITIONAL REPORT SHEETS AS NECESSARY).

INSTITUTIONAL AUTHORIZATION FOR ACCESS TO SUBJECTS

— SUBJECTS: STATUS (WARDS, RESIDENTS, EMPLOYEES, PATIENTS, ETC.) _____

NUMBER _____ AGE RANGE _____

NAME OF OFFICIAL (PLEASE PRINT) _____

TITLE _____ TELEPHONE _____

NAME AND ADDRESS OF
COOPERATING INSTITUTION _____

— OFFICIAL SIGNATURE _____

NOTES: *(e.g., report of modification in proposal as submitted to agency affecting human subjects involvement)*

HUMAN SUBJECTS

If human subjects are used, review and approval by an institutional review board are required. See suggested format in Figure 18-4. In addition:

- Describe the characteristics of the subject population, such as their anticipated number, age ranges, sex, ethnic background, and health status. Identify the criteria for inclusion or exclusion. Explain the rationale for the use of special classes of subjects, such as fetuses, pregnant women, children, institutionalized mentally disabled, prisoners, or others who are likely to be vulnerable.
- Identify the sources of research material obtained from individually identifiable living human subjects in the form of specimens, records, or data. Indicate whether the material or data will be obtained specifically for research purposes or whether use will be made of existing specimens, records, or data.
- Describe plans for the recruitment of subjects and the consent procedures to be followed, including the circumstances under which consent will be sought and obtained, who will seek it, the nature of the information to be provided to prospective subjects and the method of documenting consent. State if the institutional review board has authorized a modification or waiver of the elements of consent or the requirement for documentation of consent. The consent form should have institutional review board approval.
- Describe any potential risks—physical, psychological, social, legal, or other—and assess their likelihood and seriousness. Where appropriate, describe alternative treatments and procedures that might be advantageous to the subjects.
- Describe the procedures for protecting against or minimizing any potential risks, including risks to confidentiality, and assess their likely effectiveness. Where appropriate, discuss provisions for insuring necessary medical or professional intervention in the event of adverse effects to the subjects. Also, where appropriate, describe the provisions for monitoring the data collected to insure the safety of subjects.
- Discuss why the risks to subjects are reasonable in relation to the anticipated benefits to subjects and in relation to the importance of the knowledge that may reasonably be expected to result.

CONSULTANTS

If consultants are used, confirm their participation in writing specifying role in the project.

LITERATURE CITATIONS

List at end of research plan.

SOME MAJOR DETERRENTS TO RESEARCH

Insufficient time and funds are cited by researchers as main deterrents to research. To counteract this there is an attempt now in many universities to establish research career award positions to provide sustaining support for investigators solely dependent upon research grant funds who have a distinguished record in research. Appointing researchers to faculty positions with tenure also helps provide the researcher with security regarding future assignments.

Another deterrent is lack of information on important areas of research.

Researchers have expressed a need for the following information:

1. Sources of financial support
2. Current research
3. Research personnel and consultants in the field
4. New innovations in equipment and techniques
5. Resources available on the campus or in the community

Another major deterrent to research is the lack of clarity with which a researcher prepares the protocol. In a study conducted by the National Institutes of Health, it was found that over half (58 percent) of the research proposals were disapproved because of weaknesses in the statement of the problem—for example, the proposed problem was scientifically premature and based on unsound hypotheses. In 73 percent of the applications disapproved, it was felt that the proposed research would not yield any useful data; and in 55 percent the research team did not give evidence of sufficient competencies to carry out the research.

The American Nurses' Association in cooperation with several agencies of the U.S. Public Health Service implemented a project during 1981–1983 to facilitate the review of draft research proposals written by nurse researchers.[9] The project was directed at recent doctoral graduates who could qualify as new investigators. Opportunity was provided for their research ideas to be reviewed by agency staff prior to submitting a formal application. Common criticisms identified were:

- Lack of pilot or preliminary studies that would lend credence to the significance of the proposed study.
- Orientation of the proposals toward improving one profession (nursing) rather than toward building general knowledge for all health fields.
- Methodological weaknesses, especially small sample size for the number of variables, convenience samples, failure to provide power calculations, unproven measuring instruments, inadequate definition of the variables, and inattention to the data analysis plan.
- Focus on measurement of outcomes rather than on discovering the fundamental mechanisms which produce the outcomes.
- Failure to collect a team (coinvestigators and/or consultants) to cover the range of expertise necessary to conduct the study properly.

A critique from federal grants is provided in the form of a "pink sheet" and contains decisions about funding and the scientific review of the proposal.[10] Such a critique can be very helpful and can guide the investigator if the proposal is submitted. (Incidentally, proposals are rarely approved with only one submission.) Reaffirmation of the research aims and reviewing the critique for factual information, identified problems, and possible solutions can be helpful.

Common Characteristics of Successful Award Recipients

- Senior leadership commitment.
- Institution-wide involvement.
- Perceived opportunity for organizational change.
- Experience in technological innovation.
- Fundamental resource commitment to project.

SUMMARY

A scientifically sound research plan does not guarantee that the research itself will be successfully executed. The plan must be soundly managed, which includes securing and maintaining adequate resources for the conduct of the research. Among the resources for a research project are personnel, money, a site to conduct the research, and study subjects from whom the data will be collected.

Administering a research project is similar to the management of any organized enterprise. Its quality can be improved by the use of such techniques as a financial and personnel budget, incentives for staff productivity, and the use of labor-saving devices.

REFERENCES

1. Russell Sage Foundation, *Annual Report 1959–1960*, New York, Russell Sage Foundation, pp. 8–9.
2. Reuben B. Bowie, "Research Ethics for the Clinical Nurse," *AORN J.*, **31**(6):1016, May 1980.
3. *Ibid.*
4. Anne J. Davis, "Why Nursing Law and Ethics?" Three Perspectives: A Nurse's View," *Nursing Law and Ethics 1*, **1**:5, January 1980
5. Dale R. Lindsay and Ernest M. Allen, "Medical Research: Past Support, Future Support, Future

Directions." *Science,* **134**:2017–2024, December 22, 1961.
6. Charles V. Kidd, "The Effect of Research Emphasis on Research Itself," in *Research and Medical Education,* Julius H. Comroe, Jr. (ed.) *J. Med. Ed.,* **73**:95–100, December 1962, Part II.
7. Jerome B. Wiesner, "Federal Research and Development: Policies and Prospects." *Am. Psychologist,* **19**:90–101, February 1964.
8. DHHS, PHS, *NIH Public Advisory Groups.* Authority Structure Functions Members. Bethesda, MD, NIH, NIH Publication No. 84011, January 1984.
9. Joanne Sabol Stevenson, *New Investigator Federal Sector Grantsmanship Project, Final Report.* Kansas City, MO, American Nurses' Association, Cabinet on Nursing Research, 1983.
10. Ellen O. Fuller, "The Pink Sheet Syndrome." *Nursing Res.* **31**(3):185–186, May/June 1982.

BIBLIOGRAPHY ON GRANTSMANSHIP*

Allen, E.M., "Why Are Research Grant Applications Disapproved?" *Science,* **132**(3439):1532–1534, November 25, 1960.
Berthold, J.S., "Nursing Research Grant Proposals; What Influenced Their Approval or Disapproval in Two National Granting Agencies." *Nursing Res.,* **22**(4):292–299, July-August 1973.
Bloch, D., Gortner, S.R., and Sturdivant, L.W., "The Nursing Research Grants Program of the Division of Nursing, United States Public Health Serivce." *J. Nursing Admin.,* **7**:40–45, March 1978.
Campos, R.G., "Securing Information on Funding Sources for Nursing Research." *J. Nursing Admin.,* **6**:16–18,54, October 1976.
Catalogue of Federal Domestic Assistance, Washington, DC, Superintendent of Documents, Government Printing Office.
Debakey, L., "The Persuasive Proposal," *J. Technical Writing Communication,* **6**:5–25, 1976.
Debakey, L., and DeBakey, S., "The Art of Persuasion: Logic and Language in Proposal Writing." *Grants Magazine,* **1**:43–60, March 1978.
Eaves, G.N., "A Successful Grant Application to the National Institutes of Health: Case History." *Grants Magazine,* **1**:263–286, 1978.
  Contents
  Schubert, D.R., "A Proposal to Study the Differentiation and Physiology of a Neuroblastoma: A Successful Research Grant Application Submitted to the National Institutes of Health."
  Pike, J.M., and Bernard, S.C., "The Research Grant Budget: Preparation and Justification in Relation to the Proposed Research."
Eaves, G.N., "Who Reads Your Project-Grant Application in the National Institutes of Health." *Fed. Proc.,* **31**:2–9, January-February 1972.
Fuller, E.O., "The Pink Sheet Syndrome." *Nursing Res.,* **31**:185–186, 1982.
Gortner, S R., "Research Grant Applications: What They Are Not and Should Be." *Nursing Res.,* **30**:292–295, July-August 1971.
Henley, C., "Peer Review of Research, Grant Applications at the National Institutes of Health." *Fed. Proc.,* **36**:2066–2068, July 1977; **36**:2186–2190, August 1977; **36**:2335–2338, September 1977.
Kaiser, L. R., "Grantsmanship in Continuing Education." *J. Nursing Education,* **12**:12–20, January 1973.
Krathwohl, D.R., *How to Prepare a Research Proposal* (2nd ed.). Syracuse, NY, Syracuse University Bookstore, 1977.
Merritt, D.H., and Eaves, G.N., "Site Visits for the Review of Grant Applications to the National Institutes of Health; Views of an Applicant and a Scientist Administrator." *Fed. Proc.,* **34**:131–136, February 1975.
Phillips, T.P., "What Is the Difference Between a Research Grant and a Research Contract . . . ?" *Nursing Res.,* **24**:388–389, September- October 1975.
"The Project-Grant Application of the National Institutes of Health." *Fed. Proc.,* **32**:1541–1550, 1973.
  Contents
  • Eaves, G.N., "Introduction."
  • Eaves, G.N., "The Grant Application: An Exercise in Scientific Writing."
  • Rifkin, D.B., "A Beginning Scientist's First Project-Grant Application."
  • Gee, H.H., "Preparation of the Project-Grant Application: Assistance from the Administrator in Charge of a Study Section."
  • Malone, T.E., "Preparation of the Project-Grant Application: Assistance from the Institutes and Other Awarding Units."
  • Ross, R., "Participation of the Administration of the Grantee Institution in the Preparation and Transmission of a Project- Grant Application."
  • Schimke, R.T., "Preparation of the Project-Grant Application: Assistance from the Grantee Institution's Experienced Investigators."
U.S. Department of Health and Human Services', Public Health Service, National Institutes of Health, *NIH Public Advisory Groups: Authority, Structure, Functions, Members.* Bethesda, MD, Committee Management Office, National Institutes of Health, 1986.

*Division of Nursing, Health Resources and Services Administration, Public Health Service, DHHS.

INDIVIDUAL REFERENCE GUIDE TO RESEARCH GRANT SUPPORT

Research Grants

American Nurses' Foundation 2420 Pershing Road, Kansas City MO 64108. *The Competitive Extramural Grants Program.*

Annual Register of Grant Support, 1983-84. 17th ed. Marquis Who's Who, Inc., Chicago, IL.

Catalog of Federal Domestic Assistance, 1983. Executive Office of the President, Office of Management and Budget. Orders: U.S. Government Printing Office, Washington, DC 20402.

DHHS/PHS. Division of Nursing, Bureau of Health Professions, Health Resources and Services Administration, (Program Announcement), 5600 Fishers Lane, Rockville, MD 20857.

DHHS. Health Care and Financing Administration, 200 Independence Ave., S.W. Washington, DC 20201.

Directory of Research Grants, 1983. 8th ed. Ed. by W. K. Wilson and B. L. Wilson. Oryx Press, AZ, 1983.

The Foundation Directory. 8th ed. Foundation Center, New York. 1981.

Foundation Grants Index. 12th ed. Foundation Center, New York, 1983.

Foundation Grants to Individuals. 3rd ed. Foundation Center, New York, 1981.

Grantsmanship: Money and How to Get It. 2nd ed. Marquis Academic Media, Chicago, 1978.

Grants Register, 1983-85. 8th ed. St. Martin's Press, New York, 1982.

International Council of Nurses. 3M-ICN Nursing Fellowship Program. Geneva, Switzerland.

Lauffer, Armand. Grantsmanship, Sage Publications, Beverly Hills, CA, 1977

Lee, Lawrence. The Grants Game: *How to Get Free Money.* Harbor Publications, CA, 1981.

Margolin, J. B. The Individual's Guide to Grants. Plenum Publishing. New York, 1983.

Nurses' Educational Funds, Inc., 555 W. 57th Street, New York, NY 10019.

Research Centers Directory. 7th ed. Ed. by R. C. Thomas and A. Ruffner. Gale Research Company, Detroit, MI, 1982.

Sigma Theta Tau (National Honor Society of Nursing, Inc.) 1100 West Michigan, Indianapolis, IN 46223. *Research Grants.*

Smith, C. W., and Skuei, E. W. Getting Grants. Harper and Row, New York, 1980.

Spiva, U. U. How to Get a Grant for Your Own Special Project. TIT Inc., Bloomington, IN, 1980.

Sultz, H. A., and Sherwin , F. S. Grant Writing for Health Professionals. Little, Brown and Co., MA, 1981.

Williams, C. H. The Complete Grants Reference Book: Writing the Proposal, Getting the Money and Managing the Project. Prentice Hall, NJ, 1984.

Writers' Manuals

Campbell, W. G., et al. Form and Style: Theses, Reports, Term Papers. 6th ed. Houghton Mifflin, Boston, 1981.

The Chicago Manual of Style. 13th ed., rev. University of Chicago Press, Chicago, 1982.

Mirin, Susan K. The Nurse's Guide to Writing for Publication. Nursing Resources, Wakefield, MA, 1981.

Robinson, Alice M., and Notter, Lucille E. Clinical Writing for Health Professionals. Robert J. Brady Co., Bowie, MD, 1981.

Schneller, Trudy. Writing Skills for Nurses. Reston Publishing Co., Reston, VA, 1983.

Strunk, W., Jr., and White, E. B. The Elements of Style. 3rd ed. Macmillan, New York, 1979.

PROBLEMS AND SUGGESTIONS FOR FURTHER STUDY

1. Make an analysis of university, hospital, or health agency policies regarding the use of grant funds for travel, equipment, and the use of consultants. Develop proposed policies that your institution might consider regarding these categories.

2. Prepare a budget page for a three-year research project relating it to the stated specific aims of your research. Develop a time schedule for your proposed research indicating which phases of the research will be covered.

3. What are some guidelines for determining when the services of a consultant are needed? How would you go about obtaining the services of a consultant for a research project?

4. Read the article by Lois DeBakey and Selma DeBakey, "The Case Report I Guidelines for Preparation," *Int. J. Cardiol.,* 4:357–364, 1983. Prepare a sample case report adhering to the three primary principles cited.

5. Indicate some of the practical problems that might be encountered in undertaking research on the following problems:

a. The "real" reasons why student nurses drop out of school.

b. What is the best way of teaching family members of patients in home care programs when there are difficulties in communication (language barriers, illiteracy, etc.)?

c. The role of the nursing aide in the care of emotionally disturbed patients in the short-term general hospital.

d. Developing a tool to measure the quality of performance of the staff nurse in a public health agency.

e. Is private duty nursing no longer necessary?

f. The use of television in monitoring patients.

h. What is the independent role of the professional nurse in patient care?

h. How can errors in the provision of patient care be controlled?

6. What are some of the benefits to be gained from the use of an advisory committee for a research study? Are there any problems that can arise from the use of such committees? What are some ways in which advisory committees can be utilized most effectively?

7. From an administrative standpoint how might the following situations that can arise in executing a research project be dealt with?

a. A hospital administrator refuses to participate in a study even though his institution was selected in the random sample drawn for the study.

b. During the processing of the data it is discovered that the original estimate for the cost of data processing was much too low. There is no money available in the budget to pay for the increased costs.

c. In a study that involves the direct observation of nursing personnel as they perform their tasks during the regular workday it appears that the personnel are not behaving naturally. Aware of being observed, they have altered their normal routines and are performing atypically.

d. A key research assistant has been offered a higher paying, more responsible position during the data-collecting phase of the study. If he leaves, the study will suffer a serious setback.

e. The research project was the joint effort of several investigators. Each contributed equally to its development and execution. Questions concerning who shall write the report, how shall credit be assigned, who is the senior author have arisen.

f. In collecting data on hospitalized patients by direct interviewing of the patients, the researcher notices a number of instances of poor practice in the provision of care to the patients. The interviewer does not know whether to communicate this to the nursing service administrator or not.

8. Describe a study involving patients in which you must collect clinical data directly from the patients. Specify the procedures to be followed, their purposes, describe any physical risk or discomfort; any invasion of privacy, and how you propose to handle the data to assure anonymity.

9. Review the following article: Ida Martinson, "Funding for Research." *J. Gerontol. Nursing*, 9(7):378–383,397, July 1983. Develop an outline of a research proposal and submit the outline to one of the funding agencies mentioned for review and critique.

10. Review the following article: Elizabeth A. Rimm, "Funding for Nursing Research." *AORN J.*, 34(1):56–63, July 1981. Determine what funds are available for nursing research through your own university, agency, or hospital. Prepare a summary of funding sources.

11. Review the following article: Susanna Garver Cunningham and Pamela H. Mitchell, "The Use of Animals in Nursing Research." *Advances in Nursing Science*, 4(4):72–84, July 1982.

12. Review the following report: President's Commission for the Study of Ethical Problems in Medicine and Biomedical and Behavioral Research, *Defining Death*. Washington, DC, U.S. Government Printing Office, July 1981. Identify the ethical issues related to defining death that the nurse researcher needs to understand.

CHAPTER 19

Future Directions of Research in Nursing

OBJECTIVES

- To identify nursing research priorities.
- To become familiar with possible research areas to further the evolution and improvement of nursing practice.
- To identify high-priority areas in long-term care research.
- To identify high-priority areas in health promotion and disease prevention.
- To understand the impact of technology on nursing research.
- To understand the potential of computers as tools for the nurse researcher.

Much has changed in the world of health care in the past two decades; some things have changed little or not at all. While there have been some remarkable advances in the physical and the more difficult biological sciences, the advances have been less striking in the infinitely more complex nebulous fields of the social sciences, one of which encompasses nursing practice. These areas, though they are also a part of the "hard" sciences in certain practices and usages, are more intimately involved with the most difficult of societal problems— human-to-human contact, interpersonal relationships, measurements of and judgments about the effects of one individual's actions toward another. Problems are difficult to formulate, describe, solve, and resolve in terms of principles and guidelines for prediction and action. Richard Leakey, the eminent natural historian and anthro-

pologist, believes that human beings increased their brain and thinking abilities, not because they learned to use tools, but because they began to live in groups and had to accommodate and deal with the subtleties of diverse types of personalities and behaviors.

In nursing research, which deals with both "hard" and "soft" sciences, much intensive work has been done, but much of the development and organization of the knowledge necessary to major advances in nursing practice remains to be done.

Nursing education, occupational orientation, and career dynamics have been undertaken in major studies. Less attention has been given to studies classified as patient care research or clinical research.

If existing biomedical knowledge does affect nursing practice, what are some areas that might be rewarding to explore? What are some of the research questions that need in-depth study? The authors discuss some of these research opportunities with no attempt at complete coverage but to raise questions and to stimulate thought.

NURSING RESEARCH PRIORITIES

The setting of priorities is necessary to the ordering of nursing research topics, problems, or events to be studied. Particularly important in view of the overall reduction of resources and shortage of qualified nurse researchers, the final setting of priorities should provide the maximum nursing research effort to achieve improved quality of care.

Nurse researchers should seek opportunities to gain input into the decision process of setting priorities. Determination of nursing research priorities should be made at three levels: personal priorities at the individual level based on the nurse researcher's interests, education, capabilities, and personal goals; priorities at organizational or institutional levels by mutual consent of individual researchers; and priorities determined at the level of the nursing profession based on the overall goals of the profession.[1] Nurse researchers have an obligation to set priorities that serve choices made by individuals, organizations, and the nursing profession.

Lindeman used the Delphi technique to identify fifteen high-priority areas for clinical nursing research.[2] Priorities will change in response to new development in health care, legislation, public perception of health needs, education of professionals, and increased scientific knowledge and technological advances. Following are some research priorities in nursing. Individuals, organizations, and the nursing profession may choose to set their own.

Research Priorities in Nursing[3,4]

- Studies in long-term care of the elderly, mentally retarded, and developmentally disabled with particular attention to the design of quality assessment tools that will take into account functional status and the limited patient outcome goals and complex treatment processes characteristic of much long-term care.
- Studies of clinical problems related to nursing practice, especially descriptive studies of physiological and behavioral responses of patients with various diagnoses in varied settings, both institutional and noninstitutional.
- Studies to develop instruments to measure patient care directly.
- Studies to identify the criterion measures needed to study the effect of nursing care.
- Studies to develop models and theories of nursing practice.
- Studies of effects of technological advances on the functions of nursing service personnel.
- Studies of the organization of patient care systems; health services delivery systems that maintain quality of care and are cost effective.
- Studies to develop tools to measure effectiveness of health services.
- Studies in preventive health care to determine how best to change individuals' behavior and attitudes.
- Studies in nutrition to determine how healthful food consumption practices can be fostered.
- Studies of genetics of human diseases to prevent and better understand the degree to which genetic factors underlie susceptibility to such diseases as psychoses, diabetes, high blood pressure, coronary heart disease, and lung cancer.
- Studies to improve the outlook of high-risk parents and high-risk infants.
- Studies of life-threatening situations, anxiety, pain, and stress.
- Studies of manpower for nursing education, practice, and research.
- Studies of contraceptive and social science research to explore ways to prevent unplanned pregnancies and to develop a systems approach to strengthen comprehensive health, education, and social services.
- Studies in mental health to determine ways of preventing psychosocial disabilities.
- Studies using epidemiologic techniques to understand the mechanisms and sites of action as a result of toxic substances.
- Historical research in nursing using the vast number of primary resources maintained in individual schools of nursing, universities, the Library of Congress, the National League for

Nursing, historical documents at the National Library of Medicine in Bethesda, Maryland, and the U.S. Archives.

- Studies of ways to standardize medical and nursing records for computerization.
- Studies of patient care using monitoring systems and computer-aided diagnosis.
- Studies of communication of nursing information in relation to organization patterns of nursing service in the hospital, home, and community.
- Studies of methods of incorporating new scientific and technological advances into the nursing curriculum.
- Studies to develop criteria of job performance and measures for evaluation.
- Studies to define success in nursing and to develop tools to measure this.

Research priorities identified by the Commission on Nursing Research of the American Nurses' Association[5] include:

Priority should be given to nursing research that would generate knowledge to guide practice in:

1. Promoting health, well-being, and competency for personal care among all age groups;
2. Preventing health problems throughout life that have the potential to reduce productivity and satisfaction;
3. Decreasing the negative impact of health problems on coping abilities, productivity, and life satisfaction of individuals and families;
4. Ensuring that care needs of particularly vulnerable groups are met through appropriate stategies;
5. Designing the developing health care systems that are cost- effective in meeting the nursing needs of the population.

Examples

Examples of research consistent with these priorities include the following:

1. Identification of determinants (personal and environmental, including social support networks) of wellness and health functioning in individuals and families, e.g., avoidance of abusive behaviors such as alcoholism and drug use, successful adapation to chronic illness, and coping with the last days of life.
2. Identification of phenomena that negatively influence the course of recovery and that may be alleviated by nursing practice, such as anorexia, diarrhea, sleep deprivation, deficiencies in nutrients, electrolyte imbalances, and infections.
3. Development and testing of care strategies to do the following:
   a. Facilitate individual's ability to adopt and maintain health enhancing behaviors (e.g., alterations in diet and exercise).
   b. Enhance patients' ability to manage acute and chronic illness in such a way as to minimize or eliminate the necessity of institutionalization and to maximize well-being.
   c. Reduce stressful responses associated with the medical management of patients (e.g., surgical procedures, intrusive examination procedures, or use of extensive monitoring devices).
   d. Provide more effective care to high-risk populations (e.g., maternal and child care service to vulnerable mothers and infants, family planning services to young teenagers, services designed to enhance self-care in the chronically ill and the very old).
   e. Enhance the care of clients culturally different from the majority (e.g., black Americans, Mexican-Americans, Native Americans) and clients with special problems (e.g., teenagers, prisoners, and the mentally ill), and the underserved (the elderly, the poor, and the rural).
4. Design and assessment, in terms of effectiveness and cost, of models for delivering nursing care strategies found to be effective in clinical studies.

The foregoing priorities are directly related to developing the knowledge and information needed for improvement of the practice of nursing. While priority should be given to this form of clinical research, there is no intent to discourage other forms of nursing research. Such investigations would include utilizing historical and philosophical modes of inquiry, and studies of nursepower for education, practice, and research, as well as studies of quality assurance for nursing and those for establishment of criterion measures for practice and education.[6]

Areas identified for research needs in the twenty first century by ANA's Cabinet on Nursing Research include:

- Aging populations
- Life-style and environment
- Mental health
- Poverty
- Alcoholism/drug abuse
- Children with catastrophic illnesses and anomolies
- Technology and transplants
- Use of complex health care technology in homes
- Chronic illness (e.g., Alzheimer's disease)
- Self-care and greater responsibility of consumers for their own health
- Quality of life
- Cost containment
- Extended life-span
- Families' increased responsibility
- Health promotion in the workplace, schools, community nursing centers, and home care
- Regional tertiary treatment centers
- Resources that would complement existing family resources
- Collaborative research centers
- Emphasis on graduate education for health promotion and health maintenance

Priorities include:

- Promotion of health and well-being and the ability to care for oneself.
- Prevention of health problems.
- Minimizing the negative effects of acute and chronic health problems.
- Ensuring that those needing care receive that care.
- Evaluation of effectiveness of nursing education.

Historical Research

A much neglected area is historical research—the systematic collection and critical evaluation of data, preferably from primary sources. Historians may undertake research to test hypotheses; to answer questions; to determine cause-effect relationships; or to identify trends. Historical research is particularly useful in tracing the development of nursing theories.

An example of how historical research can help to clarify present concepts is the one of quality in nursing care.

Quality in nursing care has been talked about for a long time, initially mentioned in the Goldmark report in 1923. That report concluded that in the United States nursing was deficient in quality of care. This led to improvements in nursing education beginning in the 1930s. Measurement of quality of care research was not undertaken intensively until the 1950s. Margaret Arnstein, former director of the Division of Nursing Resources in the Public Health Service, was deeply interested in the relationship between nursing care and patient welfare. One of the earliest of the Division's research grants was to the University of Ohio in which an industrial engineer, Daniel Howland, and others investigated the relationship of quality of care to patient care. Another early effort in this area was that of Aydelotte at the University of Iowa, who looked at outcome measures (effect or dependent variables) as indicators of quality of nursing care in hospitals. Abdellah and Levine used patient and personnel satisfaction with care to evaluate staffing patterns at hospitals in the 1950s and 1960s. All these major studies were supported by the federal government. Also, the early studies on quality used patient outcome measures as indicators of quality.

In the 1970s focus was on the quality of the nursing process. Medicus, Wayne State University, and the work of Mabel Wandelt at the University of Texas are examples. Current research is shifting back to the study of outcomes, but nothing definitive has been developed as yet.

DRGs and Their Impact on Quality of Care—Another Historical Perspective

On April 20, 1983 President Reagan signed into law P.L. 98-21, the Social Security amendments of 1983. This milestone legislation was the most dramatic health care legislation since the passage of Medicare in 1965. The new law focuses on prospective reimbursement policies for hospitals by establishing a payment schedule based on diagnosis related groups (DRGs).

Why Did DRGs Come About?

Concern over rising health care costs (population changes—rapid increase of elderly population, effects of supply and demand, new technologies, intensity of services) contributed to the need for some form of change in the way health care was delivered. There was also concern about the danger of insolvency of the Medicare trust fund system. DRGs are used to determine a flat amount paid for each Medicare patient discharge. All discharges must fit into one of 467 DRGs.[7]

Contrary to current belief, DRGs are not new. A rudimentary classification system of diseases can be identified as early as 3000 B.C.[8] Galen, who influenced the course of medicine up to the Middle Ages, practiced in Rome in the last half of the second century A.D. and used a primitive classification of diseases. The first systematic attempt to classify diseases was found in John Graunt's, *Natural and Political Observations upon the Bills of Mortality,* published in London in 1662. The father of the international classification of diseases—the basis for DRG methodology—was Jacques Bertillon. He headed a committee in 1891 charged with the preparation of classification of causes of death. The system was adopted in Vienna in 1893. In the 1930s the first important use of disease classification for other than statistical studies was by the Committee on the Costs of Medical Care, later published in the United States in 1933 and entitled *The Fundamentals of Good Medical Care,* by Lee and Jones.[9] In 1934 the classic study of Johns and Pfefferkorn, *An Activity Analysis of Nursing,* developed a list of diseases called conditions.[10] In 1954, *Appraising the Clinical Resources in Small*

Hospitals (Abdellah/Levine) developed a tool with which hospitals could provide clinical experiences for students.[11] The methodology used in that study provided a system of coding 1,915 coded discharges into fifty-eight groups representing nursing problems that were related to physical needs of the patient, emotional problems, the need for rehabilitative measures, or the unique problem or characteristic of the disease requiring a special nursing problem category. The Abdellah/Levine work was used primarily for diagnostic data for resource management and planning. The methodology closely followed the Lee/Jones methodology. In 1954 *Patient Centered Approaches to Nursing* (Abdellah *et al.*) focused specifically on those diagnostic categories requiring nursing intervention for resolution of the patient's problem. This methodology was further expanded by the introduction of the progressive patient care concept in 1957, which provided a methodology for classifying and assigning patients by their medical and nursing needs.[12]

In 1972, Schonfeld and Thompson at Yale University School of Medicine reported a replication of the Lee/Jones study. In 1975 the General Medical Education National Advisory Committee (GMENAC) utilized disease-oriented data based on the International Classification of Diseases to forecast physician requirements. Thus, DRGs date back fifty years in the United States to the Lee/Jones Study.

Steps Involved in Historical Research

The steps involved are similar to those taken for other types of research described previously. The key difference is that historical research is nonexperimental and is based on events that occurred in the past. There are obvious restrictions in that the research cannot manipulate the variables, but there are opportunities to construct or select the data collection tool.[13] There are also constraints regarding sampling.

The researcher should not equate the step of literature review with historical research. The purpose of historical research needs to be clear—namely, to explain the present or to anticipate future events. The goal is similar to other research—the discovery of new knowledge.

The formulation of hypotheses is difficult as the researcher can only conjecture what happened among historical events, trends, and phenomena. The historian has a wide choice for sources of data that go beyond records and reports. Oral histories, films, photographs, audiovisual materials, and tapes provide rich sources of data.

The experienced historian will seek out primary sources such as original documents, thus maintaining a high degree of reliability. In this way the biases of multiple interpreters can be minimized. On the other hand, secondary sources such as reference books may be all that is accessible. Evaluation of historical data requires special attention. External criticism is concerned with the authenticity and genuineness of data.[14] Internal criticism of historical data is concerned with the validity of the data. Analysis of data from historical research requires sophistication in that one is tempted to be overly subjective. In spite of the limitations, historical research in nursing needs to be given high priority lest we repeat the mistakes of the past.

Research in Health Policy

Nursing research can contribute to the field of policy studies. "Policy is a governmental statement that defines a course of action which will attain or preserve some desired or acceptable state of affairs."[15] Its purpose is to alter what would occur otherwise. If policy impacts on peoples' health, it is called public policy. In nursing it implies health services policy.

The necessity for policy-relevant research is increasing and will continue to increase. There is a full spectrum of policy-relevant research—for example, policy analysis research; more focused program-evaluating policy research; theoretical or experimental disciplinary research. All policy-relevent research may contribute in one or more ways to the policy development process. The process includes:[16]

• Monitoring the course of events that might be relevant to policy.
• Forecasting emergent problems prior to their recognition.
• Identifying and analyzing problem-raising situations.
• Critiquing current policies that are based on poor understanding of the problem.
• Redefining the problem.
• Analyzing the policy-making process itself (including initiations, development, implementation, outcome, and feedback).

Policy analysis research is done to help policymakers make choices and guide action.

Policy research is an empirical investigation of the application of a policy in specific situations in order to uncover some of its effects. The scope is limited and focuses on past events. There is greater use of primary data and less reliance on value judgments.

Evaluative research is sometimes considered policy research—for example, a study of the cost-effectiveness of increased Medicare coverage of in-home services in a sample of home health agencies. The policy analyst could use these findings to help answer a policy question concerning whether Medicare should cover more in-home services.

One has only to read a sample of professional journals to be aware of the increased attention being given to policy issues. There is, however, a dearth of policy analysis research and little done by nurses. A significant example of policy-relevant research involving nurses was Aiken, Blendon, and Rogers' (1981) study of the hospital nursing shortage. The study contributed to a restatement of a national policy problem, i.e., the maintenance of adequate hospital nursing staff. The policy research question was: How may nurses' salaries be maintained adequately, instead of, how can the supply of nurses be increased? The revised policy problem statement invited the exploration of new policy solutions.

Most policy-analysis studies in nursing are limited to defining, analyzing, or redefining the policy issue. What is needed is the systematic analysis of explicit policy proposals either in their application in limited settings (policy research) or in terms of broad, clearly defined health, economic, fiscal, and political consequences (policy analysis research).[17] The most common form of health policy research (studying the efficacy, safety, effectiveness, or efficiency of particular health improvement techniques) is increasing. Limitations on use of the findings in health policy analysis include the assumptions inherent in methods of measurement, and their focus on single hardware and postprevention technologies rather than on software and primary prevention strategies.[18]

The field of health policy is considered relatively new, thus providing nurse researchers special opportunities to collaborate with other disciplines, especially in methodological areas.

NEW HORIZONS IN NURSING RESEARCH

Evaluation and Improvement of Nursing Practice

Improvement of nursing practice will come from research in the biological sciences and social sciences. Studies concerned with gross physical and psychological signs directly relevant to nursing practice are needed, as are descriptive and analytical studies of characteristics of gross behavior in relation to the nature and stages of illness; assessment of the value of visual and other sensory observations and prodromal signs (cues to impending disaster for the patient); and studies of the relative reliability and risks of automated instrumental monitoring as compared to monitoring by a nurse.

A major focus of the nursing research effort should be on the studies concerned with patient care.[19] The evaluation of patient

care should be based on nurse actions. Observations of nursing practice must be based on scientific inquiry and concepts founded on physiological, biological, and psychological principles.

In the area of patient care, criteria are needed that measure the effects of nurse actions on physical and emotional care, teaching of patients, observation and communication of observations to nurses and others, teaching and supervision of nursing personnel, and participation with health team members in planning community health programs.[10]

Measurement of patient care is a difficult problem. Instrumentation that can read and measure a greater variety of things more accurately and automatically should provide some answers. If research in nursing is to advance scientifically, measurements must be precise, not based solely on subjective observations. A major breakthrough in medical research is the electron microscope, which has brought about many advances in the field of cell biology.[21] Electronic computers have proven their value in medical research and opened many avenues for the correlation of complex physiological data. Instrumentation that permits continuous measurement of body processes concurrently can help in the understanding of such phenomena as stress and pain.

Possible Research to Further the Evaluation and Improvement of Nursing Practice

1. Identification of criterion measures of nursing practices that are both physiological and psychological
2. Establishment of the scientific bases for nursing practices
3. Description of behavior patterns of patients with different types of diagnoses in different settings
4. Assessment of the nurse's observational power to predict prodromal signs
5. Adaptation of instrumental monitoring devices in furthering analyses of patient care data important to predicting nurse actions
6. Adaptation and development of instruments to measure the effects of nurse actions upon patient welfare.

ORGANIZATION AND DELIVERY OF NURSING SERVICES

Crucial problems plague nursing practice. Some progress has been made on problems of nurse utilization and facilities. Problems basic to nursing resources and logistics fundamental to patient care, problems of communication of nursing information about the patient's progress, and problems of the organizational patterns of nursing services in the hospital, home, and community require further study.

In the area of demand for service and utilization of facilities Flagle[22] emphasizes the need to study the incidence of illness and accidents and the intensity and duration of need for hospitalization or occupancy of clinical facilities. Included here are studies of the phenomena of expressed need for service and the duration of service.

Much work remains on problems dealing with the creation and distribution of resources to meet demands.[23] How can patients be moved from one area to another? How can supplies such as drugs and blood reach the right area when they are needed?

Instrumentation, including the use of computers, promises many changes in the area of organization and delivery of nursing services—for example, computer-aided diagnosis and electronic monitoring of patient's physiological changes. As progress is made in the storage, retrieval, and analyses of complex medical data, new avenues to the communication of vital information important to patient care should become available.

"Adequacy" of nursing care has yet to be defined. How much and what level of nursing care should specific types of patients receive?

Possible Research to Further the Organization and Delivery of Nursing Services

1. What elements of patient care (in this case, organization and delivery of nursing services) have an effect upon patient care?
2. What are optimal and minimal levels of nursing care services for different types of patients in different settings?
3. How can the methods of operations research be used in the decision making problems related to establishing the upper limits of capacity of facilities?
4. What are the common nursing needs of patients for care, regardless of diagnosis?
5. How can completed research be replicated and applied to other test situations?
6. What communication channels are necessary for planning patient care? How can effective communication essential to patient well-being and personnel satisfaction be achieved?
7. How can experimental changes employing or utilizing social facilities in the physical planning and arrangements in the hospital be measured?

Nursing as an Occupation

Promising areas for studies are the ecology of the nurse; longitudinal studies of career patterns that seem to be the most promising for success in nursing; studies of competing occupations when men and women have equal opportunities; studies of why nursing as a career is not selected by more men; and studies of the public image of nursing and ways in which it might be changed.

Little is known about the impact of research upon students and curriculum. Research in nursing schools should deal with broad questions of health that are patient-centered and not disease-oriented. One needs to look for the results of this experience upon students rather than the kinds of experiences to which they should be exposed. Exposure to research in the undegraduate curriculum can help the student develop an approach to dealing with the unknown or with the unfamiliar.

Research is needed to find out why students possessing the high qualities apparently important for success in nursing find nursing schools less challenging and satisfying than do students of lesser talent. Why do nursing schools continue to ignore independent study programs that have proved highly successful in many liberal arts colleges, and some high schools? Are we deliberately ignoring the highly qualified students? Why do so many of these students withdraw from nursing schools for nonacademic reasons? One possible solution to this problem is to offer a minor or a second major for selective students in a science area. A combined experimental R.N.-doctoral program at the undergraduate level should also be explored.

A crucial area for research is to find ways in which nursing students can be motivated to exercise critical faculties and problem-solving skills. It is easy to say that the good nurse practitioner should solve nursing problems presented by the patient in a scientific way, but what does this mean and how can it be taught? Research is needed to show how the scientific method can be applied to the kinds of difficult problems with which the nurse must deal.

Nurse educators agree that the student must acquire a certain minimum of information and skills. If the nursing school is to play an important part in the education of nurses for services to the individual and the community, it must provide the student with a core of basic knowledge and skills in the biological, behavioral, and social sciences, as it relates to the effective nurse practitioner.

The application of television, teaching machines, and other automated devices as laboratory tools in the classroom and clinical situation offers fruitful exploration. How much of present teaching methods are outmoded? How best can the new technology be used in the nursing school, postgraduate and continuing education?

Research in the educational processes of nursing provides a fertile field for investigation. In the area of graduate education, one can find tenets that need explanation. Why, for example, do we compare educational qualifications of faculty in nursing programs with each other instead of with faculty members in nonnursing programs at a similar level? Why in graduate education do we tolerate those without research training guiding those seeking this training? Why is a common yardstick used to measure those who receive professional and technical education? Why is the R.N. student exempt from certain course requirements in the baccalaureate program that the basic student in other programs is not?

Much research has already been done on problems related to the role of the professional nurse. What steps must be taken to resolve the problems of role conflict?

Possible Research to Further Clarify Nursing as an Occupation

1. In order for television, teaching machines and other automated devices to serve nursing education and nursing practice with maximum effectiveness in teaching-learning, how can interaction between teacher and student be achieved?
2. Is there a concept of nursing that can be clearly defined? What are the essential learnings that must be communicated to students?
3. What are the role conflicts faced by nurses? What are their consequences in institutional practices?
4. What conflicts exist between role expectations and role performance?
5. What are the conflicting role expectations held by nurse educators and nurse practitioners? In what ways can they be resolved?
6. As the nurse becomes a contributing member of the health/or research team the role conflicts she must face are maximized. How can the nurse deal with these conflicts? What research needs to be undertaken?

Development of Theories in Nursing and a Nursing Science

Why should we be so concerned about the development of theories in nursing? Theories form the basis of nursing practice and contribute to the formulation of a nursing science. "Nursing science is a body of scientific knowledge characterized by descriptive, explanatory, and predictive principles about the life process in man."[24] Typologies of nursing problems and nursing treatments are the principles of practice and constitute the unique body of knowledge that is a nursing science.[25]

Professionalization of nursing requires that nurses identify those problems that depend for their solution upon the nurse's use of her capacities to conceptualize events and make judgments about them. Nurses must become skilled in recognizing nursing problems, analyzing them, and working out courses of action by applying principles of nursing practice.

Rogers[26] describes the professional practice of nursing as the process by which this body of scientific knowledge is used to assist human beings achieve maximum health. It is evaluative and diagnostic as well as interventive.

There are five elements of nursing practice that are dependent upon a nursing science.[27] First: continuous mastery of human relations, including technical and managerial skills needed to take care of patients. Second: ability to observe and report with clarity the signs and symptoms and deviation from normal behavior that a patient presents. Third: ability to interpret the signs and symptoms that comprise the deviation from health and constitute nursing problems. Fourth: analysis of nursing problems that will guide the nurse in carrying out nursing functions, and the selection of the necessary course of action that will help the patient attain a realistic goal. Fifth: organization of efforts to assure the desired outcome. Nursing practice may be considered to be effective when the nurse is able to help the patient return to health or what can approximate health for him.

Konlande[28] describes a patient with hyperthyroidism as an example of the importance of utilizing the biological sciences in the treatment of this patient. The nurse must know how the body responds to excess thyroxin in order to provide effective nursing care. For example, large quantities of thyroxin may increase the metabolic rate as much as two to two and a half times. The patient loses weight in spite of a hearty appetite, feels uncomfortably warm because of increased heat production, and is more excitable because of increased activity of the nervous system. With this knowledge in mind, the nurse is better able to develop and carry out an effective nursing care plan.

Basic concepts in physics are frequently applied to nursing care[29]—for example, gravity effects on the circulation of the blood. In shock this concept comes into play when the patient is placed in a Trendelenburg position. Patients with edema of the extremities can be relieved considerably by elevating the extremities. Reduced or impaired circulation in the extremities can be improved by changing the position of the patient. Patients following surgery are placed in a position to maintain a patent airway. In each instance knowledge of the principles of gravity is necessary in planning nursing care for the patient. Scientific principles related to fluid and electrolyte balance are basic to maintaining a state of homeostasis.

Possible Research to Further the Development of Theories in Nursing and a Nursing Science

1. Development of a typology of scientific principles to coincide with the typology of nursing problems already developed to comprise a body of scientific knowledge
2. Development of theories in nursing that have a specific effect upon nursing practice
3. Evolvement of a nursing science based upon a scientific body of knowledge

International Health Research

Research in nursing in the international field is much to be desired. Much can be learned about practice and nursing education from other countries where the development is not as complex as in this country. Many of the knotty problems plaguing nursing, such as patterns of nursing education, ratio of nurses to patients, and role image of the nurse, have so many intervening variables that these problems should be studied in a setting where fewer variables affect a given situation.

Glaser[30,31] has shown how the nonmedical culture and social structure of a country affect its medical services. Patterns of hospital and nursing administration in other countries compared to ours can provide many valuable insights.

Possible Research to Further the Development of International Health Research

1. Why do American hospitals have more nursing employees per patient than foreign hospitals? Can the effects of nursing care upon patients show differences in the varied patterns in different countries?
2. American hospitals have many more categories and levels of nursing personnel than foreign countries. What effect does this have on patient care? Have American hospitals succumbed to Parkinson's law? Are so many categories needed? Does the delegation of tasks in American hospitals contribute to role conflicts nonexistent in foreign hospitals?
3. The cost of nursing services far exceeds other personnel services' costs in both American and foreign hospitals. Do these costs truly reflect nursing services to patients? Is this a catchall category for related hospital services such as housekeeping, dietary, messenger services?
4. Nurses perform many more activities for patients in American hospitals as compared to foreign hospitals. This contributes to higher operating costs, but most important, do the increased activities for patients result in improved patient care?
5. What is the role of the director of nurses in American hospitals as compared to other countries? Is the lay nurse administrator an emerging concept of nursing service?
6. Nursing education in some foreign countries, particularly England, is changing slowly from an apprentice-type training to an educational program. How are these changes brought about? Will more than one pattern of nursing education emerge? How can American nursing schools consolidate existing patterns? What can be learned from developing patterns in other countries?
7. The hierarchical structure of hospitals in America and foreign countries differs markedly. What is the role of the nurse in these various hospitals? What are the role relationships of the nurse to her peers, to her supervisors, to physicians?
8. Recruitment, career development, and job satisfaction are complex problems facing American nursing, which if studied in foreign countries might provide a better understanding of contributing factors that bring about desirable and undesirable effects. The role of women in American and foreign cultures warrants study and could form the basis of many fruitful studies in human ecology.
9. Catholic hospitals compose approximately two-thirds of general hospitals in Latin American countries. Professional nurses are unhappy that nursing nuns are sometimes placed into top supervisory positions in preference to equally qualified nurses who are nonnuns. It would be helpful to study this problem in countries with a high percentage of church hospitals to determine the contributing factors to this dissatisfaction and to find appropriate ways to resolve this problem.
10. Nurses in America have greater opportunity for decision-making, as the nurse is the only member on the health team who is continuously with the patient. Nurse action in dealing with the patient's problems is crucial and is one of the decisive differing factors between American and foreign nursing. Therefore, when one speaks of professional nursing, is the conceptual basis for nursing practice closer to that of a nursing science as practiced in America as compared to foreign countries?

Patient Care Research

The preceding pages have described some of the new horizons for nursing research that directly or indirectly affect patient care. Freeman[32] in a report of a symposium of patient care research has described patient care as varied phenomena that are interrelated and refer to a wide range of objectives, events, and people that have to do with health and illness behavior.

Patient care [is] regarded as a process which involves recognizing actual and potential health problems, delineating possible courses of action, deciding what should be done, providing personal health services built around an individual, and assessing the impact of these activities upon the public health. It represents a synthesis of three components: (1) the way in which people cope with their actual and potential health problems—what happens to them when they become patients, receive care, and relinquish their patient status; (2) the patterns of practice followed by the health professions singly and together; and (3) the ways in which the values, perceptions, and skills of patients and health personnel affect one another.[33]

The seven broad classes of patient care problems that were identified in which nursing research plays a key role provide a summary of needed research in patient care:[34]

I. Sociocultural Contexts of Patient Care

A. Concepts of wellness and their relation to cultural patterns.

B. Cultural and social factors in perception of changes in physiological, personal, or social functioning as symptoms of illness. This includes differences between lay people and members of the health professions in the way they define illness.

C. The types of sick roles and well roles which the culture makes available.

D. The kinds of arrangements for care defined by the culture and provided by the society, such as scientific and lay medicine, the variety of practitioners and agencies giving care and the conditions governing access to them and their use.

E. The assumptions and value systems of the health professions and the lay public as they impinge on matters of health, other than their concepts of health and illness per se.

II. Dynamics of Patient Care Systems

A. The process by which people come to be defined as sick, to select from among alternative sick roles, and to secure endorsement of the role selected.

B. The influence of symptoms and other factors on the process whereby sick people become patients and select a source of care.

C. The kinds of health problems patients bring to family physicians, to internists, to gynecologists, to pediatricians, to public health nurses, to pharmacists, to chiropractors, and so on, and how these practitioners perceive the problems and what they do about them. (This would be the beginning of a descriptive classification of illness and disordered behavior based on patients' symptoms, patients' folklore, assumptions, values, and language, as a supplement to the nosology developed by contemporary Western health professions.)

D. How people move through the patient care system and how they are separated, by themselves and others, from the sick role.

E. Longitudinal, or natural history, studies of medical and patient care could determine what happens to cohorts of patients with particular problems or living in particular social environments in terms of seeking or not seeking help, and the results of this behavior, expressed in terms of "health," or "social productivity," or "dollars." Such studies eventually could contribute to the development of criteria for measuring the quality and efficacy of the work of the health professions for both communities and individuals.

F. Cross-cultural, cross-national, and historical comparisons of the routes people take to obtain health services, and the factors which influence this.

III. Communication

A. The language of patient care: symptoms as the language of illness, professional students' jargon, and so on.

B. The influence of health education and other channels of formal and informal communication from health personnel to patients upon patients' behavior—their use of patient care facilities, compliance with medical advice, and so forth.

C. Interprofessional communication, both formal and informal—the effects on professional practice of the form and content of personal, institutional, and mass communication among members of different professions.

D. Intraprofessional communication, both formal and informal—the effects on professional practice of the forms and content of personal, institutional, and mass communication among members of the same profession.

IV. **The Diagnostic Process**

A. Fashions in diagnoses—individual, professional, and cultural—and the diffusion of knowledge problem. (A patient cannot have a disease, let alone die of it, unless his physician or someone else can name it.)

B. The relation between the purpose or the purposes for which a diagnosis is made and the way diagnosis proceeds, the procedures undertaken, and so on. (A diagnosis for purposes of prevention is quite a different process from a diagnosis for therapeutic purposes. This again is a different process from a diagnosis for restorative purposes or rehabilitation. In addition, there is the traditional investigative "medical" diagnosis of the type conducted in many university hospitals where the object frequently is to satisfy the clinical investigators' curiosity and to improve the long-range health of society, not necessarily that of the particular patient undergoing investigational diagnosis. A program of therapy of course, generally is initiated on the basis of the investigative diagnosis. All four are different processes and involve personnel.)

C. What conditions influence the usefulness of different types of diagnosis? Prediction of future performance, identification of genetic, dynamic, predisposing, precipitating, perpetuating, and/or ameliorating factors, and so on?

D. Evaluation of the patient's total problems: the multiprofessional aspects of diagnosis; the social diagnosis; the evaluation of the patient's health problems in the context of his life situation.

E. The involvement of the patient in the diagnostic process. The influence of his expectations of different sources of care upon their participation in the process.

F. The determination of the level of personal and social competence which is maximal for the patient and the selection of a course of action which will help him to achieve and maintain this level of competence.

V. **Quality of Patient Care**

A. Perspectives of the different health professions regarding the quality of patient care.

B. How can the quality of care be measured? "Best practice" is one approach to measurement, but it is important to know what some, or all, professional people think should be done, and to know which of the alternatives is thought to be best practice, and who says so. Other approaches include prerequisites of care, elements of performance, and end results.

C. How can scientific advances in understanding disease processes be translated into practice? What is the influence of communication and values in motivating lay individuals, professional people, and the community to adopt innovations?

E. How can patient factors, professional factors, and the interactions between them be identified and manipulated to produce better outcomes for patients and greater satisfaction for members of the health professions?

F. How do a patient's expectations of a source of care and the professional's approach to him influence the outcome of care?

VI. **Influence of Various Characteristics of Patient Care Organizations upon Professional Practice**

A. The effect on professional practice of the policy of the organization regarding the type of job specification used—whether job assignments provide for differentiation of functions or overlap of functions.

B. The effect on professional practice of formal and informal specialization among personnel.

C. The effect on professional practice of the form and content of personal, institutional, and mass communication among personnel in the organization.

VII. **Influence of Organizational Characteristics upon the Movement of Patients into and Through the Organization**

A. How do the assumptions of health personnel regarding health, disease, and patient care affect the movement of patients into and through organizations providing care?

B. The consequences for patient movement of variations in the role of members of the patient care team.

C. The effects on patient movement of the form and content of personal, institutional, and mass communication among personnel of the organization.

D. The effects on patient movement of the complexity of the way in which the work of patient care is organized and of the diversity and specialization of occupational roles.

E. For what categories of personnel is the patient the desired, reluctant, or abhorred focus of work, and what are the consequences of this combination of circumstances for the patient?

F. How does the coordination of activities of the patient care agency with those of other groups in the community affect patient movement?

G. How is the utilization of the care provided by one agency influenced by the functions which other community agencies perform?

Two other classes of patient care problems were identified, but not further developed. They are the *economic aspects of patient care* and the *design of facilities for patient care*.

Future Directions

LONG-TERM CARE[35]

Nurse researchers can make tremendous strides in the area of long-term care. Although researchers do not ordinarily choose to do research in this area, long-term care—which includes the needs of the elderly, developmentally disabled, physically handicapped, and mentally retarded—represents opportunities for nurses to have a direct effect upon improving practice.

The older population has been increasing at a far more rapid rate than the rest of the population for most of this century. In the last two decades the sixty-five plus population has grown twice as fast as the rest of the population. The number and proportion of older persons will continue to grow more rapidly than the general population. At the beginning of the century less than 10 percent of the total population, about 7.1 million persons, were aged fifty-five and over. In 1982, over one-fifth of the American population was fifty-five years or over, an estimated 48.9 million persons. This trend is expected to continue well into the next century. According to U.S. Bureau of the Census projections, while the total U.S. population is expected to increase by a third between 1982 and 2050, the fifty-five plus group is expected to grow at the rate of 113 percent.

Long-term care is the provision of services—physical, psychological, spiritual, social, and environmental, including economic—that help people attain, maintain, or regain their optimum level of functioning. It includes health maintenance throughout life as well as care during acute and protracted illness and disability. In long-term care, patients often experience overwhelming effects of disease, residual pathology, and irreversible disability, and this affects patients, residents, families, and communities.

Until individuals everywhere are convinced that helping people maintain optimum health takes precedence over other types of care, the country will continue to be faced with expensive illness and disability that could have been prevented. Until we accept that, long-term care at best is a catchup effort rather than a direct attack on the problems. What are some of these problems that need to be studied?

Health care assessment efforts should address the needs of the chronically ill. Many individuals, particularly the aged, have several chronic conditions. Thus, health care assessment must not be limited to only diagnostic—specific criteria—but must use functional status as a measure. The long-term nature of the patient's condition and frequent fluctuations in physical and mental states requires that treatment and care plans vary. Patients/residents may require differing levels of care within a short period of time, ranging from acute hospital care, skilled nursing services, intermediate care services, home health services to periodic office visits. Health care assessment needs to include all sources of care and should consider the impact of care on the patients'/residents' expected and actual ability to function in daily life.

One way of improving patient care is to obtain and refine a mechanism by which an individual patient's care outcome can be measured systematically. This would provide a method for determining the allocation of resources and whether those services provided are needed by the patient. A patient appraisal, care-planning, and evaluation (PACE) system is one such approach. The patient appraisal system has important implications for care in long-term care facilities, hospitals, home health agencies, and ambulatory care settings. There must be linkage between levels of care, both institutional and noninstitutional, to assure readily accessible services.

It is necessary to link nursing homes with home-care programs, day care centers and congregate living facilities into an integrated program that assesses the quality of care provided by the total health system, so that there is an integrated review of the total range of services. Anything less than this will be based on evaluation of care

from the fragmented view of individual facilities or programs that perpetuate the current inefficient and costly services. Health care assessment is based on health outcomes despite the limitations of current measures of which patient satisfaction is one indicator.

Health care assessment uses a multidisciplinary approach in which several disciplines, such as physicians, nurses, pharmacists, therapists, nutritionists, and social workers, join with their patients/residents in establishing realistic time-limited outcome objectives and examining reasons for success or failure to meet them.

Rehabilitation Services for Elderly Increases

From 1970 to 1979, there was a 67% increase in people over eighty-five years of age. For the next twenty years, the overall percentage of the elderly proportion of the population will remain relatively stable. However, the proportion of the old-old (i.e., over seventy-five years of age) will double. This is the group whose use of medical and health resources are disproportionate to their numbers.

The demographic phenomenon of a large aged and aging population is reflected increasingly in the bed utilization in acute care hospitals. An expected outcome of this change in hospital population is the shift upward in the age of patients admitted to physical medicine and rehabilitation services.

It is assumed that resultant health needs of the old-old population represented by this second demographic revolution may be met by the Tax Equity and Fiscal Responsibility Act (TEFRA) of 1982 (P.L. 97-258). The onset of prospective reimbursement under the TEFRA requirements will exacerbate the demand for inpatient rehabilitation beds for the aged. The mandate of the diagnosis-related groups (DRGs) inpatient length of stay limitation is already forcing acute-care hospitals to participate actively in the continuity of care needs of chronic elderly patients.[36] Acute-care hospitals are developing stepdown treatment modalities to ease the return of these patients to the community. Two major stepdown methods are inpatient rehabilitation beds and day rehabilitation hospitals. As a result, the demand for rehabilitation services for the aged will become a dominant feature.

CONTROLLING THE SYSTEM

Coordinated management and improvement of institutional and noninstitutional long-term care services are essential if the needs of the elderly and developmentally disabled are to be met.

Control of the system needs to be shared by providers, consumers, and state and federal agencies. Particularly needed is increased consumer involvement in the planning, management, and evaluation of health care programs.

The delivery of long-term care services must fit within a range of services provided by hospitals, nursing homes, home health care programs, community mental health centers, day care centers, health maintenance organizations— all linked together. This requires that long-term care services be managed efficiently and that patients/residents be appropriately placed within the system.

Federal and state barriers have to be removed to permit integrated management of long-term care services. Attention also must be given to:

- Alternatives to institutional care such as home care, day care centers, community mental health centers;
- Increased effectiveness of medical review (MR), independent professional review (IPR), and utilization review (UR) to assess patient/resident needs to assure proper placement;
- Inclusion of long-term care facilities (institutional and noninstitutional) in the activities of PSRO;
- Activating nationwide the patient appraisal, care-planning, and evaluation (PACE) system and extend it to all health care facilities both institutional and noninstitutional.

PREVENTIVE HEALTH CARE

The nation's health care system has grown in response to acute needs of the sick. Manpower and education in the health field is oriented toward illness. Major expenditures at all levels of public and private interest are made to support the provision of acute care. Health insurance plans tend to cover costs only after a well-defined illness. Industrialization and urbanization frequently create unhealthy and unsafe living and working conditions. The rural population is also more at risk than previously thought. Similarly, the demands and expectations of our social system create a stressful environment.

Prevention is clearly the number one priority for a future health care system. Although much is known about the cause of diseases, the scientific and technological capacity to prevent major diseases is limited because of lack of knowledge and in most cases have not reached full potential. However, some educative efforts in recent years have been quite successful, and it appears that more people are increasingly aware of their own roles in maintaining good health through proper diet and exercise and refraining from practices detrimental to health.

Public health programs have not been able to keep pace with the risks created by the newer technologies and altered lifestyles in the United States. For example, hypertension can now be controlled by antihypertensive drugs. Cancer of the lung is a preventable disease with cigarette smoking identified as a leading cause. The total number of people smoking continues to rise as the population increases, with the largest increase among women and young people. The increase in smoking among women began during World War II, peaked in the midsixties and now shows a slight decline. However, the scare of a "cancer epidemic" in the late seventies was due to the large increase in lung cancer in women. Because of the long latent period of lung cancer, these cancers were found in older women who had begun smoking during and after World War II. The bill is not yet in for the younger women. At present, and at today's level of scientific knowledge, technologies for the prevention of most cases of heart disease, cancer, and stroke are lacking. Nurse researchers can contribute greatly by undertaking studies to learn how to influence individuals and institutions to change to more healthful behavior.

The ever-increasing American expenditures on health care could be controlled by giving greater attention to the prevention of the major chronic and disabling diseases.

Health education activities have often followed the same disease orientation approach. Information is dispensed through public media, community meetings, and in publications of many agencies and special interest groups, on the impact of disease on various human biological systems. In recent years, patient education programs have been developed to provide specific information to patients afflicted with a specific disease.

Community health education programs operated by public health agencies, for example, often are not integrated with school health education programs. Patient education is sometimes disregarded by community health educators but quite often is considered to be the only health education of importance by disease-oriented health service providers.

Teenage pregnancies continue to increase with the added problems of damaged babies, not only because of low weight, but because of drug addiction of the infant from the parent's addiction. Taking drugs has become socially acceptable in some segments of society. Obesity, even in very young children, will lead to hypertension and cardiovascular disease. Increasing numbers of young people are suffering hearing loss from the high-decibel electronic music.

The Public Health Service has made significant progress in recent years in formulating an agenda for the nation in health promotion, health protection, and disease prevention. *Healthy People: The Surgeon General's Report on Health Promotion and Disease Prevention 1979*, published in 1979,[37] introduced a set of major goals for improving the health of the American people through the 1980s. That report also called attention to fifteen areas within which more specific programmatic achievements could contribute to attainment of the stated goals.

In 1980, the Public Health Service published a report entitled *Promoting Health/Preventing Disease: Objectives for the Nation*.[38] Fifteen specific priority areas were used to formulate a framework for presenting 226 objectives, the attainment of which will contribute to improving the health of the American people. The objectives selected were chosen because of the potential contribution their attainment could make to realization of the major goals in *Healthy People*. In 1983 PHS published *Implementation Plans for Attaining the Objectives for the Nation*, an important companion to the reports issued in 1979 and 1980.[39] In it, the PHS presents a series of implementation plans that embody the steps to be taken by agencies of the federal government in pursuit of the "Objectives for the Nation."

In considering the major health problems confronting Americans today, especially chronic degenerative disease and traumatic injury, the Surgeon General's report noted that many of them are rooted in lifestyle or environmental factors that are amenable to change. Health promotion and disease prevention, therefore, would appear to hold the key to further improvements in the health status of the American people. The major goals, one for each of the five stages of life, are as follows:

- To continue to improve infant health, and, by 1990, to reduce infant mortality by at least 35 percent, to fewer than 9 deaths per 1,000 live births.
- To improve child health, foster, optimal childhood development, and, by 1990, reduce deaths among children aged one to fourteen

years by at least 20 percent, to fewer than 34 per 100,000.

- To improve the health and habits of adolescents and young adults, and, by 1990, to reduce deaths among people aged fifteen to twenty-four by at least 20 percent, to fewer than 93 per 100,000
- To improve the health of adults, and, by 1990, to reduce deaths among people aged twenty-five to sixty-four by at least 25 percent to fewer than 400 per 100,000
- To improve the health and quality of life for older adults and, by 1990, to reduce the average annual number of days of restricted activity due to acute and chronic conditions by 20 percent, to fewer than thirty days per year for people aged sixty-five and older.

The fifteen priority areas are: high blood pressure control; family planning; pregnancy and infant health; immunization; sexually transmitted disease control; toxic agent and radiation control; occupational safety and health; accident prevention and injury control; fluoridation and dental health; surveillance and control of infectious diseases; smoking and health; prevention of misuse of alcohol and drugs; improved nutrition; physical fitness and exercise; and control of stress and violent behavior.[40,41]

RESEARCH ON AGING

The Research on Aging Act (May 31, 1974) authorized the establishment of the National Institute on Aging (NIA) for the conduct and support of biomedical, social, and behavioral research and training related to the aging process and the diseases and other problems and needs of the aged.

The NIA conducts laboratory and clinical research at its Gerontology Research Center (GRC) in Baltimore. Such research includes the Baltimore Longitudinal Study of Aging initiated in 1958. Repeated observations of the same individuals are made over a long period of time to learn what happens to people as they age. The GRC Laboratory of Behavioral Sciences uses behavioral and psychological techniques such as biofeedback to control or modify physiological responses in adults of all ages. In a clinical setting, a number of individuals are being treated for urinary and/or fecal incontinence. Other areas under investigation include Alzheimer's disease; hip fractures and osteoporosis; heart disease and digitalis; sleep disturbances; and the relationship between cancer and aging.

Another major effort includes support of the Teaching Nursing Home Program, which supports research on health problems, therapies, and health maintenance strategies for older persons in nursing homes and other clinical settings.

Other areas affording research opportunities in the elderly population include:

- *Nutrition*: to understand the role of nutrition in diseases associated with old age.
- *Neuroscience*: to understand the normal and abnormal changes in the nervous system resulting from age, affecting hearing, vision, sleep, and emotional disturbances.
- *Endocrinology*: to understand endocrine function and its relationship to age with regard to the secretion, metabolism, and biological actions of hormones.
- *Exercise physiology*: to determine the relationship of exercise to changes with age in various organ systems.
- *Immunology*: to understand the relationship of altered immune system function to the aging process.
- *Pharmacology*: to understand altered drug responses in the elderly so that more reliable prescription guidelines for geriatric patients can be developed.

RURAL HEALTH SERVICES FOR THE LONG-TERM-CARE PATIENT/RESIDENT

The provision of the full range of preventive health service to migrants and seasonal farm workers and their families, including the elderly and disabled, is a continuing lack in the American medical system. The success of these and other rural programs is too often contingent on the ability of nonphysician providers to generate income from third-party reimbursement.

In the field of rural health, nonphysician providers are trained with federal funds and utilized, and yet Medicare, which is federally administered, does not recognize such personnel as eligible for reimbursement as does Medicaid.

HEALTH CARE SYSTEMS RESEARCH

Equity of access to health care services of a high quality necessitates that research be undertaken to develop health care delivery systems that provide a full range of health services; ability to serve a population defined by geography and enrollment; a built-in capability that assures that the system has a corporate identity; a unit record system that is a family-linked system; capability of providing twenty-four hour accessible services; and transportation and linkage with an emergency health services system.

A health care system having these characteristics will require major changes in what we now consider appropriate facilities in which health services are to be provided. Major structural reforms of traditional patterns of providing health services are needed. Most health services need to be extended into the community through Health Maintenance Organizations (HMOs), neighborhood health centers, home health agencies, day care centers, and so forth.

Health Care Training

Research must determine whether the American health economy will support a growing array of health specialists needed for a variety of health care delivery systems. How should they be educated? The growth of health and medical manpower has risen rapidly during this decade.

There are major areas that impact on new roles in nursing that need to evolve if we are to meet the health needs of Americans and develop necessary strategies to meet these needs.

As we view the impact of new roles in nursing, can we in all good conscience believe that health is a right of every American? A "right" is more than just an interest that an individual might have or a state of being that an individual might prefer. A "right" refers to entitlements—not those things that would be nice but rather those things they are *entitled* to have. The term "right" is often confused with the concept of equality and this is particularly true when we speak of rights to health care and equality in respect to health care. The right to health care for every American is an idealistic goal, but equality of health care in terms of access, provision of services, and costs may not be attainable. Therefore, nurses need to look at new roles in nursing and develop strategies that are based on an optimum level of health services to be provided rather than upon a maximum level. For example, more than ten million Americans could benefit from renal dialysis, but neither the persons nor the facilities are available to provide the services. Another example is the need to activate a national program of home health services to the one-third of long-term-care patients who do not belong in institutions such as nursing homes. There is now no national community network to provide the needed backup services. Fifty percent of visiting nurses' associations have only two or fewer nurses on their staffs.

If health care is a right, we must recognize that medical care with its emphasis upon "curing" rather than "caring" represents only a very small if not marginal contribution of health care services. It has been stated that 80 percent of illness is functional and can be effectively treated by any talented healer who displays warmth, interest, and compassion. Another 10 percent of illness is wholly incurable and only in the remaining 10 percent does scientific medicine—at considerable cost—have any value. Our dilemma is that not only is the number of unoccupied beds growing but that our present costly institutional facilities are designed predominantly to meet the requirements of the 10 percent of sick people.

The Recipient of Services

The client, that is, patient, resident, or individual recipient of health services, is a part of a delivery system of health. Such a health care delivery system must:

- Provide a full range of medical and health services;
- Have the capability of serving a population defined by geography and enrollment;
- Provide a unit record system that is family-oriented system;
- Provide an organization and a system of accountability;
- Have the capability of providing twenty-four hour accessible services; and
- Provide transportation and linkage with an emergency health services system.

An integral part of the health care delivery system is *primary* care, presently unavailable to many people. Primary care is a continuous source of care to which an individual or family first must turn for help in each episode of illness. Primary care must also". . . educate clients to preventive measures and offer them regularly, whether these are immunization of a child, antepartal care, or alcohol and drug preventive." Six stages of primary care have been described:

- *1st stage*: purely preventive—the preservation of existing health both physical and mental.
- *2nd stage*: also preventive but addressed particularly to those individuals at special risk for a variety of reasons, e.g., genetic (sickle cell anemia), poverty, lack of motivation.
- *3rd stage*: early detection of existing problems both physical and mental.
- *4th stage*: manifest illness—the acute stage to which the present health system directs its greatest effort.
- *5th stage*: rehabilitation needs to be activated from the time the individual is identified as a patient.

- *6th stage*: those persons for whom care is also concerned with monitoring to alleviate unnecessary suffering and prevent crippling complications, according to Virginia Henderson, "letting the chronically ill person die as he would want to die if he had the strength and the will and the knowledge to control the circumstances for himself."

Providers of Services

The roles of nurses are continually undergoing changes. As licensed nurse practitioners increase substantially, they become more independent in their practice. The Montana, ruling* concerning the firing of physician assistants for practicing nursing without a license is a significant legal decision, supporting the right of only *licensed* nurses to function as independent nurse practitioners and practice nursing. New types of nurses will appear in response to new technology in addition to those now highly specialized in acute care—the family nurse practitioner who can deal with major health problems, particularly those that are preventable (e.g., smoking, alcoholism, drug addiction, stress problems, child abuse, mental illness). Multiple health care delivery systems will require nurses to assume leadership roles in administering them, e.g., HMOs, ambulatory clinics, planning for health services, and delivery of health services. Direct reimbursement covering payment for nursing services provided in community settings and homes is now a fact.

Research in nursing practice will be key to identifying strategies to cope with health problems and outcome measures to assess the services provided. Some of the problems basic to nursing that must be addressed are:

1. Paucity of nurses prepared and functioning as nurse researchers.
2. Lack of financial support for nursing research.

* State of Montana, Office of the Attorney General, State Capitol, Helena, Montana, August 28, 1975, Volume 36, Opinion No. 18.

3. Lack of incorporation of research findings into practice.
4. Lack of integration of researcher role into the employment situation.
5. Dearth of good clinical studies.
6. Need for instruments and criterion measures to evaluate effects of nursing care.

Educating Providers of Health Care Services

Many changes in the systems of nursing education are required if the strategies outlined previously are to be achieved, and if health care services are to be related to those who need these services. Primary health care practitioners and gerontological nurse practitioners are needed in greater numbers. Both undergraduate and graduate nursing programs need to be redesigned to prepare these people. Preparation in leadership and decision-making skills is paramount. We no longer can afford the proliferation of nursing schools. Educational efforts, due to limited economic resources, will have to be accountable to society and consumer demands. Hospital-based programs will decrease. Baccalaureate and higher degree programs will undergo major changes in order to adapt to the demands of health care delivery systems. Clinical practice will shift drastically to community health settings and long-term care facilities. The shift of the base of employment away from acute care setting to community-based settings will occur. An increasing number of surgical procedures are carried out on an outpatient basis requiring the increased skills of the surgical nurse practitioner.

TECHNOLOGICAL ADVANCES AND THEIR IMPACT ON NURSING RESEARCH

We are in the midst of a technological revolution. The critical care unit symbolizes the impact of this technological revolution on health care. This revolution has increased the diagnostic and therapeutic re-

sponsibilities of the nurse, who must use physiological data provided by instrumentation to make critical judgments and to manage the machines.[42]

High technology is an essential component that the nurse researcher must become aware of in planning and conducting research. Appropriately used it may enable a diagnosis to be made quickly and completely with less discomfort and danger to the patient. One must also be aware of the high costs related to the introduction of new technologies. A serious analysis of costs needs to be undertaken to weigh the cost-effectiveness with the cost-benefits.[43]

Nurses are the chief users of health care technology. They need to have the skills to manage that technology. Electronic devices can instantly inform the nurse about the patients' vital signs. It is now possible to monitor the patient's response to therapy through instrumentation. Interpretation of this new data requires acquisition of new skills. No single area of nursing practice is unaffected by advances in health care technology.[44]

The triad of issues related to technology include cost, continuity care, and comprehensive health care for chronic illness. They are also interwoven with the issues of safety, morality, and equity raised by technology.[45]

Computers can handle the quantity and complexity of data generated by nursing systems. The use of computers requires nursing to translate goals into quantifiable standards.[46] Learning to be comfortable with a computerized medical information systems (MIS) is a goal to be achieved by every nurse researcher.

The researcher might ask, "How can theory be translated with computerized content?" Carlson[47] approached this by first accepting the nursing process as a problem-solving approach. Assessment provided the structure to describe the factors drawn from abstract theory. Basic and sociopsychological needs or factors were expressed in terms of characteristics, if present or absent, and their influence on the patients' coping behavior. Translation of the abstract theory into concrete documentation screens was facilitated by the learning methods of group interaction, peer presentations, and expert consultation. Computers do not necessarily change information but allow us to enhance the data and manage it and summarize it in ways that cannot be done by a manual system. In some aspects of care planning computers can provide protocols for care to see what should be done with a given diagnosis and what the follow-up should be for a given patient problem. The most important way that the research can be helped with the computer is with accuracy.

Thus, an entire nursing subsystem was constructed that permitted the comprehensive documentation of dependent, independent, and interdependent functions of nurses. The goal was to achieve a theory-based documentation process that was the outcome of an application of the way adults are motivated and self-directed in the learning process for the specific aim of solving problems in their everyday work.

The Computer as a Tool

A machine is characterized by sustained, autonomous action. It is set up by human hands and then is set loose from human control. The computer is a language machine, but if treated as a language tool, the computer can serve as an ideal dictionary and reference grammar, for it can provide definitions and rules. The principle to remember is to build into the program a place for the human operator. By promoting the computer as a tool, there could be a synthesis of man and computer, rather than the replacement of man by a machine.[48]

The development of computer application in health care has accelerated at a rapid rate. The computer is transforming how the researcher conducts research. The computer today has become the *sine qua non* of effective research. The distinction between the computer and the scientific instrument is rapidly disappearing. The computer is particularly useful for clinical research where the researcher is dependent on patient data that must be accessed to deduce logical conclusions from common presentations and responses to care, or induce principles from clinical observations. The clinical research of the future will require that systems designed for research be able to interface with systems storing patient-related data.

The proliferation of personal and microcomputers will revolutionize the information access and retrieval field. The technolological and telecommunication developments have brought about major changes in the publishing world with electronics emerging as a means of controlling information.[49,50] It is not necessary to be a genius to use computers. One must, however, be knowledgeable regarding the state of the art in order to define how computers can best be used in nursing research.[51]

A central problem of health care is how to marshal the expertise of the array of technology and people to meet the needs of individuals not only efficiently, but humanely. The changing role of hospitals is inevitable. The proliferation of HMOs, home health care agencies, will eventually shift the arena of health care services away from the hospital limiting the latter to acute critical care. One can easily envision specialized health professional teams that can evaluate and respond as consultants to monitored information and wired medical data relayed from the bedside of a distant patient to the office of a distant health care provider.

The development of better computer tools and the more widespread use of computerized data and records are crucial if the technological possibilities of decentralization are to be realized and hospital staff are to keep pace with the growing number of medical interventions performed.[52]

The technological revolution in health care is a significant component of everyday life. It offers the means to improve dramatically the patient's quality of life and to sustain life under conditions of great suffering. Thus, the ethical and economic issues must also be considered by the researcher in using these tools.

The computer has altered the status of the nurse and the nurse researcher in that the nurse using the computer acquires greater responsibilities for developing and interpreting the clinical database. Researchers will have at their disposal machines programmed to question patients about their illnesses, monitor physiological functions, and analyze data generated. Machines can supplement or replace human analyses of facts and simplify or automate therapeutic actions.[53] Emerging technologies will include devices useful to the researcher such as ambulatory cardiac monitoring, communicative devices for nonspeaking patients, circulatory assist devices, and infusion pumps to regulate insulin, electrolytes, anticoagulants, tranquilizers, and pain medications.

Core knowledge needed by nurses to make the best use of emerging technologies includes:[54]

• *Science*: knowledge of empirical relationships governed by scientific laws.
• *Remedial and therapeutic healing arts*: knowledge of remedies and prescriptions as well as therapies and procedures for health and disease prevention.
• *Focus/direction of knowledge from cell to society*: specialization cores include genetics, cell morphology, and cell functions.
• *Professional conditions and controls*: includes code of ethics, attributes of education, regulation, and licensure. High technology demands the need for high touch and concentrated controls. "History has provided evidence that the society needs competent, knowledgeable practitioners who appropriately apply and interpret technology in delivering nursing care."[55]

Science and Technology

Scientists have been slow to leave the protective isolation of the laboratory and to involve themselves in the public policy process. This has resulted in a gap between the technological sophistication of our tools and our social ability to manage them.

Freedom and creativity are linked with the scientific outlook. The popular image of the computer is a dramatic symbol of this shift. The computer is no longer seen as dehumanizing and depersonalizing. Instead, it is the very expression of freedom and autonomy.

Henderson points out that humane service from all health workers is dependent upon what societies value. Nurses are a part of those societies and can influence the public to support a health service that supplies humanistic care as generously as it supplies technologically sound treatment. Henderson identifies the following characteristics of administration that might encourage holistic or humanistic nursing care:[56]

1. A democratic pattern that encourages group decisions and individual initiative in both health care providers and consumers.
2. Decentralization of authority with creation of small clinical units to allow patients/clients and families to get to know those caring for them.
3. The assignment of patients/clients to nurses.
4. An organizational structure that gives nurses the same professional responsibility and accountability for patient care as other health care providers.
5. A system of joint appointments permitting those wishing to give nursing service also opportunities to teach and do research.

In nursing education include the development of habits and skills of inquiry, the problem-solving approach, and the value of scientific investigation while recognizing the value of authority as a basis for action.[57]

How can research preserve the essence of nursing in a technological age?[58]

1. Research on basic human needs as related to health.
2. Research on problems in basic nursing care.
3. Research that if applied, would influence the effectiveness of basic nursing.
4. Research on nursing problems that recognizes the value of related studies.

Computerized Nursing Information Systems Needed

A system of information consists of data that nurses collect, transmit, store, and use, as well as data entry, processing, and retrieval. The identification of meaningful categories or sets of data is an essential first step.[59] A computerized nursing information system is needed for the following functions:[60]

1. Patient care
2. Resource allocation
3. Personnel management
4. Education
5. Planning and policy making
6. Investigations (both clinical evaluation and nursing research)

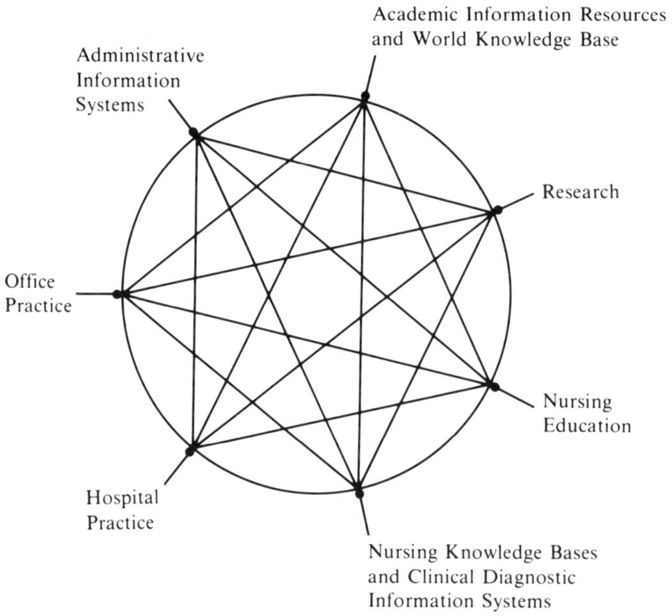

Figure 19–1   Nursing Information Systems

Council on Computer Applications in Nursing Established

The American Nurses' Association (ANA) Council on Computer Applications in Nursing was established in 1984 for the benefit of nurses in the various clinical and functional areas of nursing (practice, education, administration, and research), who are involved in the development and use of computerized information systems for the improvement of professional practice. It is a multiple-area council. This council will provide opportunities for nurses to: keep abreast of advances in computer technology that are pertinent to nursing practice, education, administration, and research; learn about and use computerized telecommunication systems; encourage research on and development of computer use in nursing; assume responsibility for development and management of information that affects practice in all areas; identify, explore, and make recommendations on issues pertinent to computer use in nursing; enhance patient monitoring systems; develop standards for computer applications in the various aspects of nursing; explore ways in which computers can be of help in effective, efficient nursing education, for example, computer-assisted instruction; use the computer as a tool in nursing quality assessment work and allocation of nursing resources; monitor cost-effectiveness of nursing services; develop networks pertinent to communication and dissemination of information relevent to computer applications in nursing; conduct meetings to share developments and progress in computer use in nursing; establish various types of media (e.g., newsletters, reports, monographs) for communicating intra- and extra-nursing; and establish/maintain liaison among nurses from the various areas of nursing and between nurses and other professionals working in, and contributing to, the advancement and use of computer technology.

Information Resources in Clinical Care Research

Computer applications in clinical care provide a bridge between traditional teaching and research that uses clinical databases. Although fewer than half of the teaching hospitals have a hospital information system, the trend is rapidly changing to build in systems that would make clinical investigations feasible. Characteristics of a hospital information system (HIS) include:

- Medical records are automated.
- Laboratory and pharmacy orders are automated and transmitted quickly and accurately.
- Procedures and pharmaceutical and laboratory orders can be converted to charges by the financial management system.
- Reports of tests can be reported promptly.
- Concurrent record review is possible as well as retrospective review for use by epidemiologists and researchers.
- Electronic bulletin board facilitates communication between health professionals.[61]

Knowledge required of a computer user involves learning about system design and recognizing the capabilities and constraints of a computer system.

A computer system consists of four essential hardware components and software known as:

- Input device(s)
- Central processing unit(s)
- Output device(s)
- External storage device(s)
- Software (directs the operation of the hardware and its processing of the data)[62]

When planning and selecting your system take time to analyze what you wish to accomplish with the computer system. Microcomputer comparison charts are available to help you choose the system that best suits your needs.[63] Also, there are a number of automated hospital system vendors who can help you.[64]

REFERENCES

1. Dorothy L. McLeod, "Nursing Research Priorities: Choice or Chance," in *Communicating Nursing Research, Nursing Research Priorities: Choice or Chance*, Vol. 8. Boulder, CO., Western Interstate Commission for Higher Education, March 1977.
2. Carol A. Lindeman, "Delphi Survey of Priorities in Clinical Nursing Research." *Nursing Res.,* **24:**439, November-December 1975.
3. National Institutes of Health, NIH Task Force on Nursing Research. Report to the Director 1984. NIH, Beth. Md., December, 1984.
4. American Nurses' Association, *Priorities for Research in Nursing* (Publication No. D-51) Kansas City, MO, ANA, May 1976.
5. American Nurses Association, *Research Priorities for the 1980s: Generating a Scientific Basis for Nursing Practice.* (Publication No. D-68), Kansas City, MO, ANA, 1981.
6. *Ibid.*
7. A full description of the DRG methodology is contained in the Sept. 1, 1983 edition of the *Federal Register*, Part IV, DHHS, "HCFA Medicare Program: Prospective Payments for Medicare Inpatient Hospital Services." Vol. 48, No. 171, pp. 39752–39890. Also see *Case Mix Systems: Development, Description and Testing.* Chicago, Hospital Research and Educational Trust, 1983.
8. Eugene Levine and Faye G. Abdellah, "DRGs: A Recent Refinement to an Old Method," *Inquiry,* **21:**105–112, summer 1984.
9. Roger I. Lee and Lewis W. Jones, *The Fundamentals of Good Medical Care*, Committee on the Costs of Medical Care, Publication 22: Chicago, University of Chicago Press, 1933.
10. Ethel Johns and Blanche Pfefferkorn, *An Activity Analysis of Nursing.* New York, Committee on the Grading of Nursing Schools, 1934.
11. Faye G. Abdellah and Eugene Levine, *Appraising the Clinical Resources in Small Hospitals*, Public Health Monograph 24. Washington, DC, Government Printing Office, 1954.
12. Faye G. Abdellah and Eugene Levine, *Better Pa-*

tient Care Through Nursing Research (2nd ed.). New York, Macmillan Publishing Co., Inc., 1979, pp. 473–496, for a historical development of patient classification systems.

13. Denise Polit and Bernadette Hungler, *Nursing Research. Principles and Methods* (2nd ed.). Philadelphia, J.B. Lippincott Co., 1983, p. 202.

14. *Ibid.*, p. 205.

15. Nancy Milio, "Nursing Research and the Study of Health Policy," in Harriet H. Werley and Joyce J. Fitzpatrick, *Annual Review of Nursing, 1984.* New York, Springer Publishing Co., 1984, Vol. 2, p. 291.

16. *Ibid.*, p. 293.

17. *Ibid.*, p. 298.

18. *Ibid.*, p. 300.

19. Rozella M. Schlotfeldt, "Summaries of Workshop Group Discussions, Conferences and Workshop on Research in Nursing." Cleveland, OH, American Nurses' Foundation, Inc., September 14–17, 1958.

20. *Ibid.*, p. 4

21. Dale R. Lindsay and Ernest M. Allen, "Medical Research: Past Support, Future Directions." *Science*, **134**:2017–2024, December 22, 1961.

22. Charles D. Flagle, "Operational Research in the Health Services," *Research Methodology and Potential in Community Health and Preventive Medicine. Ann. New York Acad. Sci.*, **107**:752, May 22, 1963.

23. *Ibid.*

24. Martha E. Rogers, "Some Comments on the Theoretical Basis of Nursing Practice." *Nursing Sci.*, **1**:11, April-May 1963.

25. Faye G. Abdellah *et al.*, *Patient-Centered Approaches to Nursing.* New York, Macmillan Publishing Co., Inc., 1960, p. 12.

26. Martha E. Rogers, *loc. sit.*

27. Faye G. Abdellah, *op. cit.*, p. 27.

28. Mildred Konlande, "Nursing Care Based Upon Selected Concepts from Biological Sciences." Report of the Conference of the Council of Member Agencies of the Department of Baccalaureate and Higher Degree Programs, Kansas City, KS, National League for Nursing, Department of Baccalaureate and Higher Degree Programs, November 8–10, 1961, pp. 39–40.

29. Rhoda Bowen, "Nursing Care Based Upon Selected Concepts from Physics." Report of the Conference of the Council of Member Agencies of the Department of Baccalaureate and Higher Degree Programs, Kansas City, KS, National League for Nursing, Department of Baccalaureate and Higher Degree Programs, November 8–10, 1961, pp. 41–44.

30. William A. Glaser, "Hospital Organization—A Comparison of American and Foreign Systems." Paper presented at the Advanced Institute of American College Administrators, The Roosevelt Hospital, New York, April 4, 1963, unpublished.

31. William A. Glaser, "American and Foreign Hospitals—Some Sociological Comparisons," Eliot Freidsen (ed.), *The Hospital.* New York, The Free Press of Glencoe, 1963.

32. Ruth Freeman *et al.*, "Patient Care Research: Report of a Symposium." *Am. J. Pub. Health*, **56**:965–969, June 1963.

33. *Ibid.*, p. 966.

34. *Ibid.*, pp. 966–968.

35. American Academy of Nursing, "Long-Term Care in Perspective: Past, Present, and Future Directions for Nursing." (ANA Publ. G-120) Kansas City, MO, The Academy, 1976.

36. Eugene Levine and Faye G. Abdellah, op. cit.

37. U.S. Public Health Service, *Healthy People: The Surgeon General's Report on Health Promotion and Disease Prevention 1979,* DHEW Publication No. 79-55071 Washington, DC, Government Printing Office, 1979.

38. U.S. Public Health Service, *Promoting Health/Preventing Disease, Objectives for the Nation,* fall 1980. Washington, DC, DHHS/PHS, Government Printing Office, 1980.

39. U.S. Public Health Service, *Promoting Health/Preventing Disease. Public Health Service Implementation Plans for Attaining the Objectives for the Nation.* DHHS/PHS, *Public Health Reports,* Supplement to September-October 1983 Issue, Washington, DC, Government Printing Office, 1983.

40. U.S. Public Health Service, *Staying Healthy,* A Bibliography of *Health Promotion Materials,* DHHS/PHS, Government Printing Office, November 1984.

41. Rebecca S. Parkinson *et al.*, *Managing Health Promotion in the Workplace,* Palo Alto, CA, Mayfield Publishing Co., 1982.

42. Gail Laing, "The Impact of Technology on Nursing," *Med. Instrumentation,* **16**(5):241–242, September-October, 1982.

43. Bryan Jennett, *High Technology Medicine.* London, Nuffield Provincial Hosptial Trust, 1984.

44. Janet K. Schultz, "Nursing and Technology." *Med. Instrumentation,* **14**(4):211–214, July-August, 1980.

45. Shizuko Fagerhaugh *et al.*, "The Impact of Technology on Patients, Providers, and Care Patterns," *Nursing Outlook,* **28**(11):666–672, November, 1980.

46. Rebecca Clark Culpepper, "Computers for Quality Care. What Can They Do?" *Computers in Nursing,* **2**(3):85–87, May/June 1984.

47. DHHS, PHS. *2nd National Conference. Computer Technology and Nursing.* Bethesda, MD,

NIH Publication No. 84-2623, September 1984, p. 15.

48. J. David Bolter, *Turing's Man. Western Culture in the Computer Age*. Chapel Hill, the University of North Carolina Press, 1984, p. 238.

49. Joyce C. Loepprich and Julie L. Smith, "Can Computers Solve Nursing's Information Overload?" *Imprint*, 30(5):49–58, December-January, 1984.

50. Kathleen J. Sofaly, "The Nurse and Electronic Data Processing." *Med. Instrumentation*, 14(3):169–170, May-June 1981.

51. Marion J. Ball and Kathryn J. Hannak, *Using Computers in Nursing*. Reston, VA, Reston Publishing Co., Inc., 1984.

52. Stanley J. Reiser and Michael Anbar (eds.), *The Machine at the Bedside. Strategies for using Technology in Patient Care*. Cambridge, MA, Cambridge University Press, 1984, p. 12.

53. *Ibid.*, p. 18.

54. Kathleen A. McCormick, "Preparing Nurses for the Technologic Future." *Nursing and Health Care*, 7:381, September 1983.

55. *Ibid.*, p. 382.

56. Virginia A. Henderson, "Preserving the Essence of Nursing in a Technological Age." *J. Advanced Nursing*, 5(3):248, May 1980.

57. *Ibid.*, p. 252.

58. *Ibid.*, p. 255.

59. Study Group on Nursing Information Systems, "Special Report. Computerized Nursing Information Systems: An Urgent Need," *Research in Nursing and Health*, 6(3):101–105, September 1983.

60. *Ibid.*, p. 104

61. Association of Academic Health Centers, *Executive Management of Computer Resources in the Academic Health Center. A Staff Report*. Washington, DC, Association of Academic Health Centers, 1984, pp. 21–22.

62. Susan J. Grobe, *Computer Primer and Resource Guide for Nurses*. Philadelphia, J.B. Lippincott Co., 1984.

63. *Ibid.*, p. 45.

64. *Ibid.*, p. 61.

SUGGESTIONS FOR FURTHER READING

1. American Nurses' Association, *New Directions for Nursing in the'80s*. Kansas City, MO, American Nurses' Association, 1980.

2. Susan R. Gortner, "Nursing Research Out of the Past and Into the Future." *Nursing Res.*, 29(4):204–207, July-August 1980.

3. Harriet R. Feldman, "Nursing Research in the 1980s: Issues and Implications." *ANS/Advances in Nursing Science*, 3(1):85–92, October 1980.

4. Maria C. Phaneuf, "Future Direction for Evaluation and Evaluation Research in Health Care: The Nursing Perspective." *Nursing Res.*, 29(2):123–126, March-April 1980.

5. Kathryn E. Barnard," Knowledge for Practice: Directions for the Future." *Nursing Res.*, 29(4):208–212, July-August, 1980.

6. Eli Ginzberg, "Predictions and Options for Nursing and Health Care." *NLN Publication*, 52(1815):9–17, 1980.

7. Eunice King, "Health and Nursing Issues in the Eighties." *NLN Publication*, 16(1839):1–9, 1980.

8. Gloria R. Smith, "Nursing Beyond the Crossroads." *Nursing Outlook*, 28(9);540–545, September 1980.

9. Rozella M. Schlotfeldt, "Nursing in the Future." *Nursing Outlook*, 29(5):295–301, May 1981.

10. National Commission for the Protection of Human Subjects of Biomedical and Behavioral Research, *Special Study. Implications of Advances in Biomedical and Behavioral Research*. Washington, DC, DHEW Publication No. (OS) 78-0015, September 30, 1978.

11. DHEW, PHS, *National Conference on Health Promotion Programs in Occupational Settings. The Proceedings*. Washington, DC, DHEW Publication, Office of Health Information and Health Promotion, January 17–19, 1979.

12. Eugene Levine, "Nursing in the UK and the USA," *Nursing Times* 79(51):35–38, December 21, 1983.

13. Ann Marriner, *Nurse Theorists and their work*. Princeton, N.J., Mosby, 1986.

Glossary

algorithm: A name that is sometimes used for iterative solution procedures. It is a common name for solution procedures used in obtaining an optimal integer linear programing model.

analysis of covariance (ANOCOVA): A statistical procedure for adjusting the data to equalize the groups studied in terms of important extraneous variables (covariables) after the independent variable has been applied to the subjects and measurements have been made of the dependent variable. Combines the two techniques of analysis of variance and regression analysis.

analysis of variance: A statistical test of significance of the results of a study in which the effects on the dependent variable of more than two alternatives of an independent variable (or more than one independent variable) are being tested simultaneously. In testing multiple independent variables this procedure can provide valuable information on the effects of not only each independent variable, but also of combinations of these variables. In the test of significance the F-test is employed. Analysis of variance (ANOVA) is the analytical method for treating data obtained from such experimental designs as the latin square and the factorial. When the analysis of variance is applied to data on *one* independent and *one* dependent variable, it is called one-way analysis of variance. In two-way analyses of variance the effects of two independent variables are tested on one dependent variable. Three-way ANOVA has three independent variables, etc. If the analysis of variance is to be made of multiple *dependent* variables, it is called multivariate analysis of variance (MANOVA). If the same dependent variable is measured at successive time periods, *repeated-measures* analysis of variance can be applied. Many statistical packages are available to perform analyses of variance on microcomputers.

associative relationships: A change in the dependent variable is related to a change in the independent variable, but we cannot with certainty say that the effect on the dependent variable was directly caused by the independent variable.

assumption: A statement whose correctness or validity is taken for granted.

balancing: A procedure for equating the subjects in the experimental and control groups of an experiment in terms of important organismic variables by matching the groups as a whole in terms of these variables rather than by matching the individuals composing the groups, as in pairing.

Bayesian statistics: An approach to statistical inference that employs Baye's probability theorem. Since prior knowledge is used in testing the significance of the results of a study, Bayesian inference is considered to be a subjective approach to statistical inference.

bimodal: A frequency distribution in which the values of the measurements that have been made for a group of study subjects form two peaks (modes).

binary: Composed of two elements or parts—e.g., binary logarithm or binary number system. As compared with the decimal system, the binary number system is composed of only zero and 1. This system is used in electronic computers and in information theory.

calibration: The marking off of the intervals that make up the scale of a measuring instrument.

canonical correlation: A technique of multivariate statistical analysis has as its basic input two *sets* of variables, each having a theoretical meaning as set. The goal of canonical correlation is to determine a linear combination from each of the sets of variables that maximizes the correlation between the two sets. Analogous to principal components analysis.

case study: A detailed, factual, largely narrative description and analysis of individuals, institutions, communities, whole societies, incidents, situations, inanimate objects, plants or animals.

causation: The process whereby a given event or phenomenon, called the cause, invariably precedes a certain other event, called the effect.

cause and effect: The cause of a certain effect is some appropriate factor that is invariably related to the effect.

central limit theorem: *The sampling distribution* of a mean approaches the normal distribution as the number of random samples becomes very large, even if the values that comprise the sample means and the population from which the random samples are drawn do not form a normal distribution.

chi-square test: A nonparametric statistical test of significance based on the chi-square distribution. It can be used to analyze the significance of differences among groups that are being compared in terms of qualitative variables. The data, called frequency distributions, consist of counts of the number of study subjects in each group found to possess each of the scale values of the variables measured. The test is performed by calculating theoretical frequencies for each scale value (i.e., for each cell of the table into which the frequencies are tabulated), subtracting the theoretical from the actual frequencies, squaring the differences, dividing by the theoretical frequency, and then summing up all the quotients. This sum is the computed value of chi-square for the sample data. The larger the computed value of chi-square, for specified-size samples, the smaller is the probability that the differences in the frequency distributions being compared are due to random sampling.

class interval: Subdivision of a quantitative *variable* into groups, called class intervals, for purposes of data presentation and analysis.

cluster: A subgroup of variables each of which is more closely correlated with other members of the subgroup than with the other variables in the larger group.

cluster analysis: A technique for determining clusters. It is analogous to the technique of factor analysis.

cluster sampling: See **sampling.**

coefficient of correlation: A summary measure called r that varies between -1 and $+1$. Its value is a measure of the degree of relationship between the variables studied. The closer the computed value of r is to $+1$ or -1, the higher is the degree of relationship among the variables studied.

cohort: A set of study subjects who are grouped together according to certain characteristics and observed longitudinally. In explanatory studies these characteristics would be the independent variables. Cohort studies are essentially repeated cross-sectional studies that involve the same subjects.

comparative experiments: Explanatory experiments in which the effects produced by the application of alternative values of the independent variable to different groups of study subjects are compared in terms of some criterion measure to find out which alternative produces the most desirable effect.

computer: Refers to the electronic device that stores, summarizes, and analyzes research data. Consists of input, program, processor, and output. Large centralized computers operated by remote terminals are called mainframes. Desktop computers, having many research applications, are called micro- or personal computers. Statistical packages are available for performing many statistical analyses.

conceptual framework: A theoretical approach to the study of problems that are scientifically based which emphasizes the selection, arrangement, and clarification of its concepts. A conceptual framework states functional relationships between events and is not limited to statistical relationships.

conceptualization: The ordering of data by means of concepts (general meanings, ideas, properties)—i.e., the appropriate concepts that will put a group of facts into a rational or useful order.

concomitant variation: Whenever two phenomena vary together in a consistent and persistent manner either the variations represent a direct causal connection between the two phenomena, or else both are being affected by some common causal factor.

confidence interval: A measure of the precision with which a sample statistic (summary measure) estimates the parameter of the population from which the sample was randomly selected. Determined from the standard error of the statistic, the confidence interval provides a range within which we estimate that the true value of the population parameter lies at a stated level of probability (confidence coefficient). Thus, for example, the 95 percent confidence interval—the value of the sample statistic ±2 standard errors—tells us that the probability that the interval embraces the true parameter value is nineteen to one.

consensual validation: The determination that something is real by the fact of agreement between the perceiving of several persons.

constellation: Any inclusive and organized grouping of phenomena.

construct: An abstraction from reality that focuses on selected aspects of reality and ignores others. It is a *heuristic assumption* designed to guide and suggest fruitful areas of investigation, not a literal description of concrete phenomena.

content analysis: A systematic method for coding, quantifying, and interpreting verbal communications.

continuum: Describes the scale for a variable in which within the interval between any two values it is always possible to have a third value.

control: Any operation that is designed to test or limit any of the conceivable sources of error and distortion in knowledge. In research, experimental control refers to the manipulation or modification of the conditions under which the observations are to be made. Statistical control involves the treatment of the data to remove the effects of extraneous factors.

control group: Subjects who are as closely as possible equivalent to an experimental group and exposed to all the conditions of the investigation except the experimental (treatment, stimulus) variable.

correlation: The relationship of two or more variables so that an increase in the magnitude of one of the variables is associated with an increase or decrease in the magnitude of the other. Thus when two variables are highly correlated it is possible to predict with reasonable accuracy the magnitude of the other. The correlation may be positive or negative. When the magnitudes of the variables are in the same direction, it is positive; when they vary in the opposite direction, it is negative.

criterion measure: A measure of the dependent variable that serves to indicate the effect of the independent variable upon the subjects being studied.

criterion measures (evaluation of):

meaningfulness: Pragmatic test of the measure as a whole. Does the measure have any practical, real-life meaning and application?

reliability: The consistency or precision of the measure. A measure is considered reliable if it is consistently reproducible.

sensitivity: Ability of the measure to detect fine differences among the subjects being studied.

validity: Does the measure actually measure what it is supposed to measure? Also referred to as relevance.

cross-sectional design: A type of research design in which data from a specific point in time are collected and analyzed, as in a descriptive survey.

cross-tabulation: A summarization of research data in statistical tables in which two or more variables are presented in relation to each other.

cybernetics: The scientific study of messages and of regulatory or control mechanisms whether found in machines, persons, social groups, or institutions (e.g., communication theory, information theory).

decision-making research: A study conducted for the purpose of selecting a course of action from several alternative cources of action that could be taken.

deduction: A process of reasoning that starts with given premises and attempts to derive valid conclusions. Reasoning from the general to the particular.

Delphi technique: A consensus-generating technique that can be used to obtain research data from a group of subjects that cannot be acquired in other ways. The data are considered subjective and judgmental.

demography: The study of population size, composition, and distribution, and their patterns of change. Population composition and distribution include not only such variables as fertility, mortality, age and sex, but also marriage, divorce, family size, race, education, illiteracy, unemployment, distribution of wealth, occupational distribution, crime rates, and migration.

demonstration: The aim of a demonstration is to show how a particular research finding can be applied to a specific situation. A demonstration differs from research in that it does not seek answers to questions nor does it require a tight research design.

discriminant analysis: A statistical technique for distinguishing among two or more groups in terms of the characteristics that most clearly set them apart. A collection of variables about the groups are selected that, together, can accurately predict their classification of the output variable. The statistical analysis indicates the relative importance of the discriminating variables.

double blind: A control technique in an experiment in which neither the investigator nor the study subject knows which subject receives the placebo and which the actual treatment. It is employed to provide additional assurance that the experimental and control groups are identical in every way except in terms of the independent variable that is being tested.

ecology: The study of organisms in reference to their physical environment—i.e., the ways in which humans adapt to an environment and the resulting geographic distribution. An attempt to determine which parts of the physical and social environment (for a specific period) are transformed into goals, barriers, boundaries, and other psychological factors that constitute an individual's *life space.*

effect: An event or phenomenon that follows another phenomenon; a result as manifested in an effect (dependent) variable.

empirical: Based on factual investigation, experience, or observation.

empirical law: A law based on facts or observations and expressing in general form the relationships between two or more sets of data.

empirical test: A test of a hypothesis in which the investigator observes the phenomena in question (either under experimental or 'natural' conditions) to determine whether the hypothesis is supported or contradicted by the observations. Other qualified investigators following the specified procedure should reach the same conclusion about a hypothesis as the original investigator.

empiricism (scientific): A philosophical movement in which the instruments of all sciences are the experience of the scientist himself.

epistemology: Philosophical study of the origin, nature, and limits of knowledge.

equal-appearing-intervals method: A method of scaling variables developed by L. Thurstone that is an adaptation of the logical principles of the equal sense differences method to the task of scaling judgements of any kind, such as attitudes and opinions.

errors in research: In addition to sampling error, the following are the three major sources of error in research:

observer error: These may be random or systematic. The latter can result from inadequate training or psychological biases of the observer.

processing error: A type of error resulting from faulty data processing such as the errors in translation of open-ended responses, arithmetical mistakes.

response error: May also be random or systematic (bias) and arise where there is no observer to check the accuracy or completeness of responses.

experiment: An arrangement of conditions under which the phenomenon to be observed shall take place. In explanatory experiments the aim is to determine for that phenomenon the causal influences of these conditions.

experimental design: The step-by step plan of an experiment, including the determination of the conceptual basis for the research, the selection of study subjects, the specification of instruments for data collection, and the determination of the analysis and interpretation of the findings. Experimental designs set forth the conduct of the research under highly controlled conditions. In explanatory experiments subjects are randomly assigned to the alternative groups being studied.

experimental group: Subjects who are exposed to the experimental (treatment, stimulus) variable and whose reactions will reflect the *effect*, if any, of that variable.

explanatory research: The purpose of this type of research is to seek answers to questions concerned with "Why does something happen?" "What would happen if . . . ?" Explanatory research is essentially concerned with studying the relationship among two or more variables. Explanatory research can be employed to discover causal relationships, to establish predictive relationships or to evaluate a method, program, or procedure.

exploratory study: A preliminary study using a small sample to become familiar with the phenomenon that is to be investigated, so that the study to follow may be designed with more understanding and precision.

extrapolation: Estimating values of a function beyond the range of available data. The extension may be done mathematically by fitting a curve to the data or graphic methods.

fact: An event, a phenomenon; something that has actually happened.

factor: In psychological research, a factor is considered to be any one of several conditions that together may be the cause of an event or phenomenon.

factor analysis: A statistical technique for interpreting scores and correlations among scores from a number of tests. It attempts to find functionally unitary traits in two or more correlated variables but does not distinguish between dependent and independent variables.

factorial design: This design tests the simultaneous effects of several independent variables on a dependent variable. The design may also involve multiple alternatives for each of the independent variables.

field surveys: The gathering of statistical data from the study subjects in their natural habitat. Data are collected either directly as in an interview or indirectly as in a mailed questionnaire.

frequency distribution: A grouping of data collected in a study that indicates the number of study subjects possessing the different values of the scale of the variable measured.

F test: A test of the significance of differences in the values of summary measures, based on the F distribution. It is employed in such statistical procedures as the analysis of variance. The F test, which is the ratio of:

$$\frac{\text{Variance among groups}}{\text{Variance within groups}}$$

provides the relative frequency (5 times out of 100, 1 time out of 100, etc.) of obtaining by randomization a value as large as that computed by the ratio. The higher the value of the F ratio, for specified-size samples, the greater is the probability that the summary measures being compared are significantly different from each other rather than their differences being attributable to random sampling. A parametric test.

generalization: Application of a general concept or idea to a relatively new object or situation.

general linear hypothesis: The statistical model underlying many hypotheses tested in explanatory research, such as comparative experiments. It expresses the statistical relationship between independent and dependent variables. In its most elementary form it can be stated as: $Y = a + (b)X$ in which Y, the dependent variable, is a function of X, the independent variable.

Hawthorne effect: A term used to describe the way people who are put in a specialized research setting tend to respond psychologically to the conditions of the study—i.e., to the novelty of the situation or to the fact of having been treated in a special way. It was first described in the classic experiments at the Hawthorne plant of the Western Electric Company in Chicago during the late 1920's and early 1930's. The psychological reaction to the study conditions can be mistaken for the effect of the explanatory independent variable manipulated by the experimenter and can lead to spurious inferences.

historical method: A study of persons by tracing the events in their life history.

hypothesis(es): Statement(s) of the expected relationship(s) among the phenomena being studied; tentative explanation of a complex set of data not yet proved; a tentative deduction; usually the first step in problem solving.

induction: A process of reasoning that starts with facts about specific situations and attempts to establish general propositions. Reasoning from the particular to the general.

inference: A judgment based on other information rather than on direct observation. Statistical inference is the process by which one is able to make generalizations from the data. The process consists of conducting an experiment in such a way that it is possible to replicate the exact experiment in other situations or groups. Statistical methods make it possible to determine to what extent the new averages, measures of variation, and relationships differ from those obtained by prior experiments.

interviewing: A process by which the observer gathers data by verbal questioning of the study subjects to elicit data on the variables being studied.

investigation: The systematic examination of phenomena to describe or explain them.

Kolmogorov-Simirnov D test: A nonparametric statistical test designed to measure the significance of the difference between two frequency distributions. The distributions being compared may be from two independent samples or the distribution of one sample and a theoretical distribution.

Kuder-Richardson formula: Provides estimates of test reliability.

latin-square design: A type of experimental design involving multiple comparisons that was developed to make efficient use of the study subjects. In this design the number of times each alternative of the independent variable is replicated is equal to the number of different comparison groups.

level of significance: States the risk of rejecting the null hypothesis and accepting the alternative hypothesis when in fact the null hypothesis is true.

Mann-Whitney U test: When data from two samples are in the form of ranks, or relative position in terms of magnitude, this nonparametric test may be used to determine whether one sample has significantly higher ranks than the other sample.

matching: A method for matching pairs of subjects on relevant variables and assigning one pair member to the control group and the other to the experimental group.

measure of central tendency: A summary measure of the values of the measurements of a particular variable that represents the most typical, common, central, or average value for all the subjects studied. The three most frequently employed measures of central tendency are the mean, median, and mode. In a normal distribution of measurement values the mean, median, and mode are identical in value.

mean: The sum of all the values in the distribution divided by the number of values.

median: When the values of the measurements are arranged in order of magnitude the median is the value that is larger then half of the values and smaller than the other half. It is the middle value of a distribution—the fiftieth percentile.

mode: The most common value in a distribution of measurements.

measure of variation: A summary measure of the dispersion of the values of the measurements of a particular variable among the study subjects. Common measures of variation are: range, standard deviation, and variance.

range: The lowest and the highest values in the set of measurements. Sometimes considered as the difference between the lowest and highest values.

standard deviation: The most widely used measure of variation. It is computed as follows: the difference between the value of each individual measurement and the mean is determined and each deviation is squared. The sum of all the squared deviations is divided by the number of measurements, and the square root of this quotient is obtained.

variance: The square of the standard deviation.

MEDLARS: Medical Literature Analysis and Retrieval System is a computer-based bibliographic system making possible the publication of an index to the published medical and related literature and the retrieval of specialized bibliographic information on both recurring and demand bases.

Meta analysis: A technique of multivariate analysis for synthesizing and summarizing multiple variables in research data.

method of agreement: If the circumstances that lead up to the ocurrence of a given event, *B*, have during every occurrence of the event only one factor in common. *A*, then *A* is probably the cause of *B*.

method of difference: If two or more sets of circumstances are different in respect to only one factor, *A*, and if a given event, *B*; occurs only when *A* is present, then *A* is likely to be the cause of *B*.

method of residues: When the factors that are known to cause a part of some phenomenon are isolated, the remaining part of the phenomenon is the effect of the residual factors.

model, conceptual: A diagrammatic representation of a postulate or concept. A model in research is a symbolic or physical visualization of a theory, law, or other abstract construct. It is an analogy of the actual phenomenon expressed in a format that is more readily grasped and understood than the abstract conceptual scheme it is used to describe. Models can either be physical or symbolic. Physical models include life-like physical representations, abstract physical representations, and schematic and other diagrams. Symbolic models include mathematical and statistical models in which letters of the alphabet are used to represent the various elements included in the model, while especially devised symbols are used to indicate the mathematical operations designated by the model. Mathematical models are an exact quantitative formulation of the relationship among the variables they include. A statistical model states the quantitative relationship among the variables in probabilistic terms.

Multivariate analysis: A term applied to statistical techniques that analyze the relationships among variables such as analysis of variance and multiple regression. In a more restrictive sense the term is sometimes applied to techniques in which multiple dependent variables are analyzed such as discriminant analysis, multivariate analysis of variance, and canonical correlation.

Neyman-Pearson approach to statistical inference: This approach uses traditional tests of significance in which all elements of the research design—the null hypothesis, the alternative hypotheses, and the level of significance —are established in advance of the actual data collection and kept fixed during the course of the study. An objective approach to significance testing as compared to the personalistic approach of Bayesian inference.

normal curve: A bell-shaped curve that indicates that the majority of the values of the measurements of a variable for a group of study subjects cluster together and possess about the same scale value while fewer and fewer subjects possess the more extreme values—those away from the values held by the majority of subjects. Also called the gaussian curve after its discoverer, the German mathematician, Karl F. Gauss. The properties of the normal curve are very valuable in statistical analysis of data. In a normal curve:

± 1 standard deviations from the mean = 68 percent of all the values.
± 2 standard deviations from the mean = 95 percent of all the values.
± 3 standard deviations from the mean = 100 percent of all the values.

norms: A set of scores on a test derived from a representative group of respondents. Norms are used as standards for evaluating the scores obtained by users of the test.

null hypothesis: When we are studying the differences between experimental and control groups, or in any research in which we are comparing summary measures determined from samples, we usually wish to test some hypothesis about the nature of the true difference between the populations represented by the samples. Most commonly, the statistical analysis is directed toward testing the *null hypothesis*, which states that the obtained differences in the values of the summary measures between the groups being compared could have occurred by chance alone, because of being sampled, and there really is no difference between the groups. This means that if we repeated our experiment many times and calculated the differences in the values of the criterion measures between the experimental and the control groups for each experiment, the average difference would be zero. (We add the positive differences together and subtract the negative differences, and divide by the number of differences we have measured.)

If our statistical analysis (called the statistical test of significance) leads us to the conclusion that the observed differences in our samples could have arisen by chance *only* a small percentage of times in the absence of true differences between the populations represented by our samples, we reject the null hypothesis; that is, we conclude that there probably is a genuine difference between the two populations. In the social sciences, it is more or less conventional to reject the null hypothesis when the statistical analysis indicates that the observed difference would not occur by chance alone more often than 5 times out of 100 repeated experiments (called the .05 level of significance).

In addition to the null hypothesis every explanatory study also includes *alternative hypotheses*. These may express the expectation of the researcher—that there is a genuine difference between the groups he is studying. If on the basis of the study findings we reject the null hypothesis, we have thus accepted the alternative hypothesis. Conversely, when we accept the null hypothesis, we reject the alternative hypothesis.

nursing: It is a service to individuals and to families, therefore to society. It is based on an art and science that mold the attitudes, intellectual competencies, and technical skills of the individual nurse into the desire and ability to help people, sick or well, cope with their health needs.

nursing diagnosis: Determination of the nature and extent of nursing problems presented by individual patients receiving nursing care and their families.

nursing research: A systematic, detailed attempt to discover or confirm the facts that relate to a specific problem or problems in the field of nursing. It has as its goal the provision of scientific knowledge in nursing. Research in nursing is primarily interdisciplinary.

nursing science: A body of scientific knowledge from the physical, biological, and social sciences that is uniquely nursing.

observers: Research personnel who collect the data.
   nonparticipant observer: Serves as the recorder of the data, but is not one of the study subjects.
   participant observer: Collects the required data while taking part in the activity being studied.

operational definition: A series of words that clearly designate performable and observable acts or operations that can be verified by others.

optimum allocation: A technical procedure to determine the best possible allocation of the sampling units into strata. Can tell the researcher what is the most efficient size sample for each stratum.

pairing: A method of matching the individual members of the experimental and control samples with respect to relevant organismic covariables. Helps to equate the groups more closely than what can be achieved by randomization alone.

panel design: A technique in which a selected sample of subjects is interviewed, usually about the same variable (e.g., income), recurrently over an extended period of time to study the change that has taken place.

parameters: Summary measures, such as means and standard deviations, that are computed from data obtained from all the sampling units in the target population.

path analysis: A method of tracing out the implications of a set of causal assumptions on a system of linear relationships.

percentage: A type of summary measure known as a rate. A rate expresses the relative frequency of occurrence of the particular scale value for which it is computed among the subjects studied. (See page 253 for definitions and types of rates commonly used in the health field.)

percentile (P): The point in a cumulative percentage distribution below which the percent of cases indicated by the given percentile falls.

phenomenon: That which is open to observation; an event; a fact.

pilot study: A study carried out before a research design is completely formulated to assist in (a) the formulation of the problem, or (b) the development of hypotheses, or (c) the establishment of priorities for further research. Also called an exploratory study.

placebo (Latin—"I will please."): Term used in clinical trials of drugs to describe an inert capsule, tablet or injection given to members of the control group that is disguised to serve as an imitation of the drug actually being tested among the experimental subjects. It is used to control psychological bias by matching the experimental and control groups in terms of equivalent exposure to the process of drug administration.

poisson distribution: A binomial distribution where the probability of occurrence of a defined event is extremely small.

prediction: A statement about an event not yet observed detailing what will be found when it is observed.

premise: A proposition stated or assumed as leading to a conclusion. Something taken for granted.

pretest: This test takes place after the research

design has been formulated (a) to develop the procedures for applying the research instruments, or (b) to test the wording of questions, or (c) to ensure, as far as practical, that the specific questions or observations are relevant and precise.

product-moment method: A technique used to compute the coefficient of correlation (r) for quantitative variables. It is the ratio of two standard deviations. The numerator of the ratio is the standard deviation of the values of the dependent variable calculated from the regresson equation, and the denominator is the standard deviation of the actual values of the dependent variable that were obtained from the sample. Also known as the Pearsonian r.

projective techniques: A method for collecting data in which the subjects are asked to respond to nonstructured or ambiguous stimuli—an ambiguity that the investigator may make no attempt to conceal. Examples of projective techniques are the Rorschach test, the thematic apperception test, and the word association test.

prospective design: A type of research design, also known as a longitudinal study, in which the collection of data proceeds forward in time. It includes such studies as an experiment in which the study begins with alternative groups of study subjects who are exposed to the independent variable and then followed up over a period of time and compared in terms of some criterion measure. Prospective designs are also used in nonexperimental research.

A *cohort* study is a type of prospective nonexperimental study in which the same group of subjects—e.g., all graduates from a school of nursing in a certain year are followed up over a period of years, and data are periodically gathered from them on variables of interest to the researcher.

Q sort: A technique originally developed to explore the personality of individuals. Provides a method for deriving an ordinal scale for measuring certain kinds of variables. A sorting process is employed in which the rater is given a collection of items to sort into a number of piles to determine the rater's own attitudes toward the object being rated (e.g., satisfaction with nursing care). It is a *forced choice* method of scaling a variable in that the number of items that can be sorted into any one pile is predetermined. In the Q-sort the number of items that can be placed in each pile follows the pattern of the normal curve. It is also known as a probability sample.

random sample: A sample of the members of a population drawn in such a way that every member of the population has a known chance of being included—that is, drawn in a way that precludes the operation of bias or purposive selection. An advantage of random samples is that formulas are available for estimating the expected variation of the sample statistics from their true values in the total population, known as the sampling error.

random start: In systematic sampling, as in sampling from names on a list, the first name is chosen randomly from among the first n names, and after that every nth name is selected for the sample.

randomization: A technique in experimental research to equalize the composition of the various groups under study so that they are identical in respect to all pertinent organismic variables. Subjects are allocated to the different study groups according to the laws of chance. The procedure of randomization is known as random assignment or allocation.

regression analysis: In studies of independent and dependent variables that are both measurable in terms of quantitative scales, if a sufficiently large number of measurements were obtained, it would be possible to fit an equation, called a regression equation, to the data which would express the relationship between the variables. The test of significance between the variables is an evaluation of the slope of the line that is fitted to the data, called the regression coefficient.

reliability: A criterion for assessing the quality of data. Data are reliable if they are consistent, accurate, and precise. Another term for reliability is precision.

replication: The subdividing of an experiment into a number of parts—the replicas—each of which contains all the essential elements with which the experiment is concerned. The term is also applied to a repetition of the identical study design among a different set of study subjects.

research: An activity whose purpose is to find a valid answer to some question that has been raised. The answers provide new knowledge to the world at large. It is a purposeful activity.

applied research: To obtain new facts and/or identify relationships among facts that are intended to be used in a real-life situation. Specifically, applied research is intended to solve a problem, make a decision, or develop or evaluate a program, procedure, process, or product.

basic or pure research: To establish fundamental theories, facts and/or statements of relationships among facts in some area of knowledge that are *not* intended for immediate use in some real-life situation. The aim of basic research is to advance scientific knowledge and to facilitate further research in the area of knowledge.

descriptive research: The research is primarily concerned with obtaining accurate and meaningful descriptions of the phenomena under study. "Absolute" research is sometimes used as a designation of a descriptive study.

developmental research: The aim of this research is to develop a new procedure, program, or product.

evaluative research: A program, method, procedure, or product is tested to assess the quality, applicability, feasibility, desirability, or worth in terms of some meaningful criterion measure.

experimental and nonexperimental research: In experimental research all elements of the research are under control of the investigator, and it is often conducted in a specialized research setting: laboratory, experimental unit, or research center. This type of research is prospective. In nonexperimental research all elements of the research are not under direct control of the investigator, and it is conducted in a natural setting such as a school, a public health agency, a hospital, or a patient's home. This type of research is frequently retrospective.

explanatory research: The aim of this type of research is to test a hypothesis about a relationship between an independent variable (causal, treatment, stimulus variable) and a dependent variable (effect, response, or criterion variable). The independent variable is manipulated by the researcher.

historical research: Examines the past not as a fragmented collection of facts and dates, but to analyze the relationship of facts and events to the past and current trends and issues.

longitudinal research: A study in which data are collected on the same subjects at various points in time, in contrast to a *cross-sectional* study, which is conducted at one point in time.

Also known as *cohort* research. Generally prospective but can be conducted retrospectively as in historical research. Can be experimental or nonexperimental.

methodological research: To develop methods, tools, products, or procedures for conducting further research or for use in practice; to develop theories and models.

research design: Plan of the research that is developed prior to the actual launching of the study. It is part of a number of steps beginning with the formulation of the problem and ending with a report of the findings of the study. Sometimes referred to as the research protocol. Research designs may be experimental or nonexperimental, prospective or retrospective, longitudinal or cross-sectional.

research personnel:

principal investigator: One designated as assuming major responsibility for the administration of the research. The individual who originated the study, developed the initial research plan, and is responsible for the scientific merit of the research.

project director: An individual who is designated to work under the direction of the principal investigator and is responsible for the technical aspects of the research, such as data collection. Some studies designate only a project director, in which case the individual carries out the functions of both the principal investigator and the project director.

research associate or assistant: A junior investigator who works under the direction of the project director.

research problem: The motivation for undertaking a study that consists of a definition of concepts and terms narrowed down from a broadly stated question into one more restricted in scope and related to research findings that have been obtained by others.

research proposal: The written plan and justification for a research project, prepared before the project begins. A proposal is prepared when applying for financial support to do the research. A proposal consists of a description of the following components:

1. The aims of the research
2. Gaps in existing knowledge and the importance of the research proposal
3. Any preliminary work that has been done

4. The research design
5. Protection of human subjects
6. Project budget
7. Description of research setting
8. Project personnel
9. Gantt chart showing project scheduling of major tasks to be performed and level of effort of project personnel

retrospective design: In nonexperimental explanatory studies it is the type of design in which the dependent variable is observed first and the data are traced back and related to possible relevant independent variables that are hypothesized as being associated with the dependent variable. Nonexperimental descriptive studies can also be retrospective in that the data collected refer back to a prior point in time.

role analysis: A sociological technique based on the concept of a role as a patterned sequence of learned actions or deeds performed by a person in an interaction situation.

Rorschach test: A projective testing utilizing ten cards printed with inkblots to which the subject responds. The test is diagnostic of personality as a whole.

sampling: The process of selecting a fraction of the sampling units of a target population for inclusion in a study.

area sample: A probability sample in which the primary sampling units are households used in large-scale studies conducted by the U.S. Bureau of the Census and the National Center for Health Statistics of the U.S. Public Health Service. On a smaller scale, beds in a hospital can serve as the primary sampling unit, for example.

cluster sampling (multistage): Used in large-scale descriptive studies involving target populations with geographically dispersed sampling units. The cluster, or primary sampling unit, might represent a hospital or a block within a neighborhood. The elementary sampling unit on which measurements are desired might be the patients in the hospital or the residents of the block. Commonly used in epidemiological studies.

convenience sampling: Subjects are selected because they happen to be available for participation in the study at a certain time.

probability sampling: A method whereby each sampling unit in the target population has a known—greater than zero—probability of being selected in the sample. Neither the sampler nor the sampling unit has any conscious influence over the inclusion in the sample of a specific sampling unit, since the sampling units are selected by chance. Also known as random and scientific sampling. Distinguished from purposive sampling (convenience, quota, and purposive sampling) where the sampling units are deliberately selected according to certain criteria.

purposive sampling: A sample in which the sampling units are deliberately (nonrandomly) selected according to certain criteria that are known to be important and are considered to be representative of the target population. Purposive sampling is also known as judgment sampling.

quota sampling: Similar to a convenience sample, but in which the use of controls prevents overloading the sample with subjects having certain characteristics. The controls are established by determining the distribution of the sampling units according to those variables deemed to be important.

sequential sampling: The sampling units are taken into the study sequentially and the number to be included in the study is not fixed in advance. Useful in testing the effects of drugs on patients.

simple random sampling: Each sampling unit has an equal probability of being selected for the sample.

stratified random sample: The target population is subdivided into homogenous subpopulations. Then, a random sample or a sytematic sample is selected from each subpopulation.

systematic sampling: After a random start, every *n*th unit (name on a list, patient in a bed, house on block) in selected in the order in which the units are arranged.

sampling error (standard error): A measure of the extent to which the sample findings are different from what they would be if all the sampling units in the target population had been studied. For summary measures like the mean and percentage, the sampling error is the ratio of the variation (standard deviation) of the values of the measurements among the sampling units in the target population to the square root of the number of sampling units in the sample. This formula is modified according to the type of sampling design used. Measures of sampling error are also known as standard errors.

sampling units: The individual discrete members of a target population. Sampling units can consist of human beings, animals, plants, or inanimate objects.

scale: A device for determining the magnitude or quantity of the variable being measured possessed by the study subjects to whom it is applied (quantitative variables) or for determining the appropriate discrete class or category of the variable to which the study subject belongs (qualitative variables).

graphic rating scale: A scale in which the variable is qualitatively scaled along a continuum from one extreme to the other. A rater makes a direct rating on the scale.

Guttman-type scale: A scale in which the different items composing the scale have a cumulative property so that a person who responds a certain way to, say, the third item on a scale is almost certain to have responded the same way to the preceding two items.

interval scale: A quantitative scale in which the distance between the points is equal, so we can justifiably break the intervals down into finer subdivisions that will provide us with more refined distinctions among the study subjects we are measuring. An interval scale has no zero point (e.g., scale for body temperature) in contrast to a ratio scale (weight scale), which does.

Likert-type scale: An ordinal-type scale in which the variable is evaluated by a series of statements that when responded to by study subjects, according to, say, degree of favorableness or unfavorableness toward each statement, can provide a criterion measure of the variable.

nominal scale: A qualitative scale consisting of a number of discrete, mutually exclusive and exhaustive categories of a variable, each possessing a distinctive attribute in terms of the variable (e.g., sex: female-male; types of illnesses).

ordinal scale: A qualitative scale in which the different categories, included in the scale are related in terms of a graded order (e.g., excellent, very good, average, poor).

qualitative scale: A type of scale in which the subject is observed, and on the basis of the definition of the variable the subject is placed into one of its categories. The numerical data yielded by such a scale are called frequency data and show the number of subjects who are classified into each of the discrete categories of the scale.

Sometimes called enumeration scales. Nominal and ordinal scales are examples of qualitative scales.

ratio scale: A quantitative scale possessing a true zero point. A scale with an absolute zero point—the total absence of the variable—makes it possible to determine not only how much greater one measurement is from another as in an interval scale, but also how many times greater it is (e.g., a scale for the variable "time").

Thurstone-type scale: An ordinal scale useful in studying attitude-type variables in which an attempt is made to establish the quantitative distance between the categories included in the scale. Also known as the method of "equal-appearing intervals." A battery of statements, each with its own scale value, is presented to the rater, and he checks those statements which most closely represent his own position. An overall scale value is assigned on the basis of the average value of the items checked by the respondent.

science: A systematic method of describing and controlling the material world.

score: A quantitative value assigned to a scale, test, or other type of datagathering instrument to indicate the degree to which the respondent possesses the variable being measured.

serendipity: A situation in which a secondary discovery is more significant than the original objective of the research.

spurious correlation: This is said to occur when a direct cause and effect relationship is inferred between two variables when no such relationship actually exists. Instead, both variables are dependent upon a third variable that has not been controlled in the study.

statistical significance: To test whether two or more groups being compared in terms of a summary measure—a mean, a standard deviation, a percentage, or, nonparametrically, in terms of their rank order on a qualitative scale—could be considered to have come from the same target population or not (i.e., that they are essentially two independent samples from the same population).

statistics: Summary measures, such as percentages, means, medians, percentiles, and standard deviations, that are computed from measurements obtained from a sample of the total population. Estimates of population parameters.

stochastic process: A series of events for which the estimate of the probability of a certain outcome approaches the true probability as the number of events increases.

subjects in research: The persons or things from whom data are collected. Study subjects can be human beings, animals, plants, cells, or inanimate objects.

survey: Nonexperimental research conducted in a natural setting in which there is less control over the study subjects and the setting than in an experiment.

target population: The total membership of a defined set of subjects from which a sample for study is selected. Projection of data obtained in a study proceeds from the sample to the target population.

test of statistical significance: A statistical technique to test whether the summary measures being compared, after allowing for a sampling error, could be independent estimates of the same population parameter. If so, they can be considered as identical, and any differences among them can be attributed to sampling error.

nonparametric tests of statistical significance: Tests of significance, sometimes called order statistics. Many of these tests treat data in terms of ordinal rankings or comparisons, as in rank correlation and the sign test techniques as well as in the other nonparametric methods such as the runs tests, median test, and Mann-Whitney U test. Nonparametric tests, also known as distribution-free tests of statistical significance, make no assumptions about the nature of the distribution of the values of the measurements in the target population from which the sampling units were selected and require only that the sampling units be selected randomly and the measurements be independent.

parametric tests of statistical significance: Tests of parameters such as the mean and standard deviation that are based on random sampling distributions as the normal curve, the t distribution, and the F distribution. Parametric tests require that certain assumptions be met concerning the distribution of the values of the measurements in the target population from which the sampling units were selected. Parametric tests are useful in testing variables having quantitative scales, interval or ratio. Parametric tests are more sensitive than nonparametric tests.

power of a test of statistical significance: The probability of rejecting the null hypothesis when it is actually false. It is a measure of the sensitivity of the test—the extent to which it isolates real differences among the groups that were studied.

two-tailed test of statistical significance: The hypothesis to be tested states only that there is a difference between the summary measures for the groups studied, not that the difference is in any specific direction, i.e., higher or lower. A *one-tailed* test specifies the direction of the difference.

Type I error in a test of statistical significance: This error is incurred in a test of statistical significance when we reject the null hypothesis and accept the alternative hypothesis when in fact the null hypothesis is true. The level of significance selected in the test of significance (e.g., .05) is the risk of committing this error.

Type II error in a test of statistical significance: This error is incurred in a test of statistical significance when we accept the null hypothesis and reject the alternative hypothesis when the alternative hypothesis is actually true. Reducing the risk of Type I error increases the risk of committing a Type II error.

theory: Summarizes existing knowledge, provides an explanation for observed facts and relationships, and predicts the occurrence of as yet unobserved events and relationships on the basis of explanatory principles, embodied in the theory. Scientific theory is composed of definitions, postulates, and deductions.

thematic appreception test (TAT): A projective test in which a person is asked to tell a story suggested by a series of pictures.

t test: A parametric statistical test for small samples based on Student's *t* distribution. It can be used to test the significance of the difference in the values of summary measures for two samples. Significance is assessed by determining whether this difference exceeds the amount that could be attributed to random sampling. If it does not, the two sample summary measures can be considered to be independent estimates of the same population parameter and the two samples as having been randomly drawn from the same population. In a test of the differences between

two sample means, the t-test is in the form of the following ratio (under the null hypothesis the difference in population means is considered to be zero):

$$\frac{\text{Difference in sample means minus difference in population means}}{\text{Standard error of the difference in sample means}}$$

When the number of sampling units is large, the test is known as the T test and is based on the normal rather than the t distribution.

validity: A criterion for evaluating the quality of a measure or an instrument. A measure is valid if it actually measures what it is supposed to measure. Another term for validity is relevance. Validity is assessed by various concepts:

construct validity: The extent to which an instrument is consistent with and reflects the theory underlying it.

content validity: The extent to which an instrument adequately encompasses the pertinent range of subject matter.

face validity: Th extent to which a measure or an instrument appears as a logical and reasonable measure of what it is supposed to measure.

predictive validity: The extent to which a measure or an instrument is correlated with an objective criterion measure (e.g., job satisfaction with job turnover). This is the most important assessment of validity.

value: The individual's evaluation of the positive, neutral, or negative character of an object, someone's behavior, or a situation.

variable: The characteristic, property, trait, or attribute of the person or thing observed in a study. Variables must have a scale of measurement possessing at least two mutually exclusive values and must give rise to statistical data.

dependent variable: The variable that is observed to determine the effect of the manipulation of the independent variable. It can be called the criterion, effect, or response variable.

environmental variable: Relates to the many factors in the setting in which the individual is studied that can impinge on the individual (e.g., economic, anthropological, sociological, and physical factors).

extraneous variable: The variable (s) that are not of primary interest to the researcher but are present in large numbers in any study involving human beings. They include organismic and environmental variables. They may be controlled or uncontrolled.

independent variable: The variable that is changed or manipulated by the researcher. It may be called the experimental, treatment, causal, or stimulus variable.

organismic variable: Deals with all the many personal characteristics of human beings as individuals—physiological, psychological, and demographic.

weighted scoring: The value awarded for a response is not the same for all items in the instrument. In some cases, weighted scoring involves the assignment of different values for different responses to the same item.

Yule's coefficient of association: A technique to estimate the coefficient of correlation for qualitative variables, each having two categories.

$$\frac{ad - bc}{ad + bc}$$

where a, b, c, d are the four cells in a 2×2 table:

a	b
c	d

Bibliography

1. Aaron, H. J. and Schwartz, W. B., *The Painful Prescription. Rationing Hospital Care.* The Brookings Institution, Washington, DC, 1984.
2. Abdellah, F. G., *Overview of Nursing Research, 1955–1968.* National Center for Health Services Research and Development, Rockville, Md., 1971. Also see by the same author "Overview of Nursing Research, 1955–1968." *Nurs. Res.,* **19:**6–17, January-February 1970; **19:**157–62, March-April 1970; **19:**239–52, May-June, 1970; and "U.S. Public Health Service's Contribution to Nursing Research—Past, Present, Future." *Nurs. Res.,* **26:**244–49, July-August 1977.
3. Abdellah, F. G., "The Nature of Nursing Science. Conference on the Nature of Science in Nursing." *Nurs. Res.,* **18:**390–93, September-October 1969.
4. Abdellah. F. G., and Levine, E., *Appraising the Clinical Resources in Small Hospitals.* U.S. Public Health Service Monograph No. 24. Government Printing Office, Washington, DC, 1954.
5. Abdellah, F. G., "Criterion Measures in Nursing." *Nurs. Res.,* **10:**21–26, winter 1961.
6. Abdellah, F. G., and Levine, E., "Developing a Measure of Patient and Personnel Satisfaction with Nursing Care." *Nurs. Res.,* **5:**100–108, February 1957.
7. Abdellah, F. G., and Levine, E., *Effect of Nurse Staffing on Satisfactions with Nursing Care.* Hospital Monograph Series No. 4. American Hospital Association, Chicago, 1958.
8. Abdellah, F. G., and Levine, E., *Patients and Personnel Speak* (rev. ed.). U.S. Public Health Service Publication No. 527. Government Printing Office, Washington, DC, 1964.
9. Abdellah, F. G., Beland, I., Martin, A., and Matheney, R., *Patient-Centered Approaches to Nursing.* Macmillan Publishing Co., Inc., New York, 1960.
10. Abdellah, F. G., and Levine, E., "Work Sampling Applied to the Study of Nursing Personnel." *Nurs. Res.,* **3:**11–16, June 1954.
11. Abdellah, F. G., "The National Health Service Corps: Providing Settings for Nursing Practice," in Aiken, L. H. (ed.), *Health Policy and Nursing Practice,* American Academy of Nursing, Kansas City, MO, 1981.
12. Adam, E., "Frontiers of Nursing in the 21st

Century: Development of Models and Theories on the Concepts of Nursing." *J. Advanced Nurs.*, **8**(1):41–45, January 1983.

13. Aday, L. A., *The Utilization of Health Services: Indices and Correlates*. DHEW Publication No. (HSM) 73–3003. National Center for Health Services Research and Development, Hyattsville, MD, 1973.

14. Altman, S. H., *Present and Future Supply of Registered Nurses*. DHEW Publication No. (NIH) 73–134. U.S. Government Printing Office, Washington, DC, 1972.

15. American Academy of Nursing, *Models for Health Care Delivery: Now and the Future*. ANA, Kansas City, MO, January 20–21, 1975.

16. American Nurses' Association, *Facts About Nursing, 84–85* ANA, Kansas City, MO, 1985.

17. American Nurses' Association, Nursing. *A Social Policy Statement*. ANA, Kansas City, MO, 1980.

18. American Nurses' Association. *Human Rights Guidelines for Nurses in Clinical and Other Research*. ANA, Cabinet on Nursing Research, Kansas City, MO, 1985.

19. Anderson, E. T. *et al.*, *The Development and Implementation of a Curriculum Model for Community Nurse Practitioners*. U.S. Government Printing Office, Washington, DC, 1977.

20. Annas, G. J., "The Prostitute, the Playboy, and the Poet: Rationing Schemes for Organ Transplantation." *Am. J. Pub. Health*, **75**(2)187–189, February 1985.

21. Anscombe, F. J., "Sequential Medical Trials." *J. Am. Statistical Assoc.*, **58**:365–83, June 1963.

22. AORN Education, "An Introduction to Nursing Theories, Concepts, and Models." *AORN J.*, **32**(5):758, 760, 762, 764, November 1980.

23. Applied Management Sciences, *Review of Health Manpower Population Requirements Standards*. DHEW Publication No. (HRA) 77–22. Health Resources Administration, Hyattsville, MD, 1976.

25. Armitage, P., *Sequential Medical Trials*. John Wiley & Sons, Inc., New York, 1975.

26. Arnstein, M. G. (ed.), *International Conference on the Planning of Nursing Studies*. International Council of Nurses, Florence Nightingale Foundation, London, 1956.

27. Aspen Systems Corporation, *Selected Bibliographic References on Methodologies for Community Health Status Assessment*. DHEW Publication No. (HRA) 77–14550. Health Resources Administration, Hyattsville, MD, 1976.

28. Auger, J. A., and Dee, V., "Patient Classification System Based on the Behavioral System. Model of Nursing: Part 1." *J. Nursing Admin.*, **13**(4):38–43, April 1983.

29. Aydelotte, M. K., *Nurse Staffing Methodology: A Review and Critique of Selected Literature*.

DHEW Publication No. (NIH) 73–433. U.S. Government Printing Office, Washington, DC, 1973

30. Aydelotte, M. K., and Tener, M. E., *An Investigation of the Relation Between Nursing Activity and Patient Welfare*. State University of Iowa, Iowa City, 1960.

31. Babbie, E., *The Practice of Social Research* (3rd ed.). Wadsworth Publishing Co., Belmont, CA, 1983.

32. Bacon, F. "Advancement of Learning," in *Great Books of the Western World*. Encylopaedia Britannica, Inc., Chicago, 1952.

33. Bailey, J. T., "The Critical Incident Technique in Identifying Behavioral Criteria of Professional Nursing Effectiveness." *Nurs. Res.*, **5**:52–64, 1956.

34. Ball, M. J., and Hannah, K. J., *Using Computers in Nursing*. Reston Publishing Co., Inc., Reston, VA, 1984.

35. Barber, T. X., *Pitfalls in Human Research: Ten Pivotal Points*. Pergamon Press, Inc., New York, 1976.

36. Barzun, J., and Graff, H. P., *The Modern Researcher* (3rd ed.). Harcourt Brace Jovanovich, Inc., New York, 1977.

37. Batey, M. V. (ed.), *Communicating Nursing Research*: Vol. 4: *Is the Gap Being Bridged?* Western Interstate Commission for Higher Education, Boulder, CO., July 1971.

38. Batey, M. V. (ed.), *Communicating Nursing Research*: Vol. 7: *Critical Issues in Access to Data*. Western Interstate Commission for Higher Education. Boulder, CO., January 1975.

39. Batey, M. V. (ed.), *Communicating Nursing Research*, Vol. 8: *Nursing Research Priorities: Choice or Chance*. Western Interstate Commission for Higher Education, Boulder, CO., March 1977.

40. Batey, M. V. (ed.), *Communicating Nursing Research*, Vol. 9: *Nursing Research in the Bicentennial Year*. Western Interstate Commission for Higher Education, Boulder, CO., April 1977.

41. Batey, M. V. (ed.), *Communicating Nursing Research*, Vol. 10: *Optimizing Environments for Health: Nursing's Unique Perspective*. Western Interstate Commission for Higher Education, Boulder, CO., September 1977.

42. Battistella, R. M., and Weil, T. P., *Health Care Organization. Bibliography and Guidebook*. Association of University Programs in Hospital Administration, Washington, DC, 1971.

43. Baumann, A., and Bourbonnais, F., "Nursing Decision Making in Critical Care Areas." *J. Advanced Nurs.*, **7**(5):435–46, September 1982.

44. Benoliel, J. Q., "Ethics in Nursing Practice and Education." *Nurs. Outlook*, **31**(4):210–15, July-August 1983.

45. Bentkover, J. D., and Drew, P. G., *The Implications of Cost-Effectiveness Analysis of Medical Technology*, Case Study #14. Office of Technology Assessment, Washington, DC, September 1981.

46. Bergan, T., and Hirsch, G., *A National Model of Nurse Supply, Demand, and Distribution: Summary Report*. Western Interstate Commission on Higher Education, Boulder, CO., 1976.

47. Bermosk, L. S., and Mordam, M. J., *Interviewing in Nursing*. Macmillan Publishing Co., Inc., New York, 1973.

48. Berthold, J. S., Curran, M. A., and Barhyte, D. Y., *Educational Technology and the Teaching-Learning Process: A Selected Bibliography*. Division of Nursing, Bethesda, MD, 1970.

49. Beveridge, W. I. B., *The Art of Scientific Investigation* (rev. ed.). W. W. Norton and Co., New York, 1957.

50. Bircher, A. U., "On the Development and Classification of Diagnoses." *Nurs. Forum*, **14**:10–29, winter 1975.

51. Blalock, H. M., Jr., *Theory Construction*. Prentice-Hall, Englewood Cliffs, NJ, 1970.

52. Blalock, H. M., Jr. (ed.), *Causal Methods in the Social Sciences*. Aldine Publishing Co., Chicago, 1971.

53. Bloch, D., "Some Crucial Terms in Nursing: What Do They Really Mean?" *Nurs. Outlook*, **22**:689–94, November 1974.

54. Blumberg, M., and Drew, J. A., "Methods for Assessing Nursing Care Quality." *Hospitals, J.A.H.A.*, **37**:72–80, November 1, 1963.

55. Bohny, B. J., "Theory Development for a Nursing Science." *Nurs. Forum*, **12**(1):50–67, 1980.

56. Bolter, J. D., *Turing's Man. Western Culture in the Computer Age*. The University of North Carolina Press, Chapel Hill, NC, 1984.

57. Borger, R., and Cioffi, F., *Explanation in the Behavioral Sciences*. The University Press, Cambridge, 1970.

58. Braithwaite, R. B., *Scientific Explanation: A Study of the Functions of Theory, Probability and Law in Science*. Cambridge University, Cambridge, England, 1953.

59. Brink, P. J., and Wood, M. J., *Basic Steps in Planning Nursing Research: From Question to Proposal*. Duxbury Press, North Scituate, MA, 1978.

60. Brodt, D. E., "A Re-Examination of the Synergistic Theory of Nursing." *Nurs. Forum*, **19**(1):85–93, 1980.

61. Brook, R. H., *Quality of Care Assessment: A Comparison of Five Methods of Peer Review*. DHEW Publication No. (HRA) 74–3100. National Center for Health Services Research and Development, Hyattsville, MD, 1973.

62. Brown, E. L., *Newer Dimensions of Patient Care—Part I*. Russell Sage Foundation, New York, 1961.

63. Brown, E. L., *Newer Dimensions of Patient Care—Part II: Improving Staff Motivation and Competence in the General Hospital*. Russell Sage Foundation, New York, 1962.

64. Brown, M. (ed.), *Readings in Gerontology*. C. V. Mosby Co., St. Louis, 1978.

65. Burling, T., Lentz, E. M., and Wilson, R. N., *The Give and Take in Hospitals*. G.P. Putnam's Sons, New York, 1956.

66. Butterfield, S. E., "In Search of Commonalities: An Analysis of Two Theoretical Frameworks." *Int. J. Nurs. Studies*, **20**(1):15–22, 1983.

67. Cambridge Research Institute, *Trends Affecting the U.S. Health Care System*, DHEW Publication No. (HRA) 76–14503. U.S. Government Printing Office, Washington, DC, 1975.

68. Campbell, C., *Nursing Diagnosis and Intervention in Nursing Practice*. John Wiley & Sons, Inc., New York, 1978.

69. Carpenter, C. R., "Computer Use in Nursing Management." *J. Nurs. Admin.*, **13**(11):17–21, November, 1983.

70. Chapin, F. S., *Experimental Designs in Sociological Research*. Greenwood Press, Inc., Westport, CT, 1974.

71. Chapman, C. M., "The Paradox of Nursing." *J. Advanced Nurs.*, **8**(4):269–72, July 1983.

72. Chaska, N. L. (ed.), *The Nursing Profession. A Time to Speak*. McGraw-Hill Book Co., New York, 1983.

73. Chinn, P. L., *Advances in Nursing Theory Development*. Aspen Systems Corporation, Rockville, MD, 1983.

74. Chinn, P. L. (ed.), "Testing of Nursing Theory." *Advances Nurs. Sci.*, **6**(2): 1–89, January 1984.

75. Chinn, P. L., and Jacobs, M. K., *Theory and Nursing. A Systematic Approach*. The C. V. Mosby Co., St. Louis, 1983.

76. Christy, T. E., "The Methodology of Historical Research." *Nurs. Res.* **24**, 189–92, May/June 1975.

77. Clearinghouse on Health Indexes, *Cumulated Annotations, 1976*. DHEW Publication No (PHS) 78–1225. National Center for Health Statistics, Hyattsville, MD, 1978

78. Cochran, W. G., *Planning and Analysis of Observational Studies*. John Wiley & Sons, Inc., New York, 1983.

79. Cochran, W. G., *Sampling Techniques*. John Wiley & Sons, Inc., New York, 1977.

80. Cohen, J., and Cohen, P., *Applied Multiple Regression/Correlation Analysis for the Behavioral Sciences*. John Wiley & Sons, Inc., New York, 1975.

81. Colton, T., *Statistics in Medicine*. Little, Brown and Co., Boston, 1974.

82. Commission on Human Resources, National Research Council, *Personnel Needs and Training for Biomedical and Behavioral Research*,

Vols. I and II. National Academy of Sciences, Washington, DC, 1977.

83. Cox, D. R., and Snell, E. J., *Applied Statistics.* Chapman and Hall, New York, 1981.

84. Crawford, G., "The Concept of Pattern in Nursing: Conceptual Development and Measurement. *Advances Nurs. Sci.,* **5**(1):1–6, October 1982.

85. Cronbach, L., *Essentials of Psychological Testing* (3rd ed.). Harper and Row, New York, 1970.

86. Dawes, R. M., *Fundamentals of Attitude Measurement.* John Wiley & Sons, Inc., New York, 1972.

87. DeGeyndt, W., and Ross, K. B., *Evaluation of Health Programs: An Annotated Bibliography.* Systems Development Project, MN, 1968.

88. De la Cuesta, C., "The Nursing Process: From Development to Implementation," *J. Advanced Nurs.,* **8**(5):365–71, September 1983.

89. Delbecq, A. L., VandeVen, A. H., and Gustafson, D. H., *Group Techniques for Program Planning: A Guide to Nominal Group and Delphi Processes.* Scott, Foresman, Glencoe, IL., 1975.

90. DHEW/Public Health Service, *National Conference on Health Promotion Programs in Occupational Settings: The Proceedings.* DHEW Publication, Office of Health Information and Health Promotion, Washington, DC, January 17–19, 1979.

91. DHHS, *Health United States 1985,* DHHS Publication No. (PHS) 86-1232, DHHS PHS, National Center for Health Statistics, Hyattsville, Md, 1985.

91a. DHHS, *Alzheimer's Disease.* DHHS Publication No. (ADM) 84–1323.) U.S. Government Printing Office, Washington, DC, 1984.

91b. DHHS, *Health Technology Assessment Reports, 1983.* DHHS/PHS, DHHS Publication No. (PHS) 84–3372, Washington, DC, 1984.

91c. DHHS/PHS, *2nd National Conference on Computer Technology and Nursing.* NIH Publication No. 84–2623, Bethesda, MD, 1984.

91d. DHHS/PHS/NIH, *NIH Task Force on Nursing Research.* Report to the Director, National Institutes of Health, Bethesda, MD, December 1984.

91e. DHHS/PHS. *Proceedings of Prospects for a Healthier America:* Achieving the Nation's Health Promotion Objectives. DHHS, PHS, November 1984.

91f. DHHS/PHS. *Vision Research.* A National Plan 1983–1987. The 1983 Report of the National Advisory Eye Council. NIH Publication No. 83–2469, National Institutes of Health, 1983.

92. Dickson, G., and Lee-Villasenor, H., "Nursing Theory and Practice: A Self-Care Approach." *Advances Nurs. Sci.,* **5**(1):29–40, October 1982.

93. Dillon, W. R., and Goldstein, M., *Multivariate Analysis: Methods and Applications.* John Wiley & Sons, Inc., New York, 1984.

94. Division of Manpower Intelligence, *An Annotated Bibliography of Basic Documents Related to Health Manpower Programs.* DHEW Publication No. (HRA) 75–7. U.S. Government Printing Office, Washington, DC, 1974.

95. Division of Nursing, *Effectiveness and Efficiency of Nursing Programs.* DHEW Publication No. (HRA) 74–23. Health Resources Administration, Hyattsville, MD, 1973.

96. Division of Nursing, *First Report to the Congress, February 1, 1977. Nurse Training Act of 1975.* Report of the Secretary of Health, Education, and Welfare on the Supply and Distribution of the Requirements for Nurses as Required by Section 951, Nurse Training Act of 1975. Title IX, Public Law 94–63. DHEW Publication No. (HRA) 78–38. U.S. Government Printing Office, Washington, DC, 1978.

97. Division of Nursing, *Source Book: Nursing Personnel.* DHEW Publication No. (HRA) 81–21. U.S. Government Printing Office, Washington, DC, 1981.

98. Division of Nursing, *Survey of Registered Nurses Employed in Physicians' Offices.* DHEW Publication No. (HRA) 75–50. U.S. Government Printing Office, Washington, DC, 1975.

99. Donabedian, A., "Some Issues in Evaluating the Quality of Nursing Care." *Am. J. Pub. Health,* **59**:1833–36, October 1969.

100. Downs. F. S., and Newman, M. A., *A Source Book of Nursing Research.* F. A. Davis, Philadelphia, 1973.

101. Doyle, T. *et al., The Impact of Health System Changes on the Nation's Requirements for Registered Nurses.* DHEW Publication No. (HRA) 78–9. U.S. Government Printing Office, Washington, DC, 1978.

101a. Duespohl, T. A., *Nursing in Transition.* Aspen Systems Corporation, Rockville, MD, 1983.

102. Dunn, H. L., "The Biological Basis for High-Level Wellness." Council for High-Level Wellness, Washington, DC, October 1959.

103. Dunn, H. L., "Points of Attack for Raising the Levels of Wellness." *J. Nat. Med. Assoc.,* **49**:225–55, 1957.

104. Edmunds, L., "A Computer Assisted Quality Assurance Model." *J. Nurs. Admin.,* **13**(3):36–43, March 1983.

105. Edwards, A. L., *Experimental Design in Psychological Research* (4th ed.). Holt, Rinehart and Winston, New York, 1972.

106. Edwards, A. L., *Statistical Analysis* (4th ed.). Holt, Rinehart and Winston, New York, 1974.

107. Edwards, W. M., and Flynn, F., *Gerontology: A Core List of Significant Works.* Institute of Gerontology, The University of Michigan–Wayne State University, Ann Arbor, MI, 1978.

108. Ehrat, K. S., "A Model for Politically Astute Planning and Decision Making." *J. Nurs. Admin.*, **13**(9):29–35, September 1983.

109. Elliott, J. E., and Kearns, J. (eds.), *Analysis and Planning for Improved Distribution of Nursing Personnel and Services: Final Report.* DHEW Publication No. (HRA) 79–16, U.S. Government Printing Office, Washington, DC, 1979.

110. Ericksen, G. L., *Scientific Inquiry in the Behavioral Sciences.* Scott, Foresman and Co., Glenview IL, 1970.

111. Erickson, H. C. *et al., Modeling and Role-Modeling. A Theory and Paradigm for Nursing.* Prentice-Hall, Inc., Englewood Cliffs, NJ, 1983.

112. Evans, D. L. "Every Nurse as Researcher: An Argumentative Critique of Principles and Practice of Nursing." *Nurs. Forum,* **19**(4):335–39, 1980.

113. Fagerhaugh, S. *et al.,* "The Impact of Technology on Patients, Providers, and Care Patterns." *Nurs. Outlook,* **28**:666–72, November, 1980.

114. Farrand, L. L. *et al.,* "A Study of Construct Validity: Simulations as a Measure of Nurse Practitioners' Problem-Solving Skills." *Nurs. Res.,* **31**(1):37–42, January-February 1982.

115. Finney, D. J., *Experimental Design and Its Statistical Basis.* University of Chicago Press, Chicago, 1974.

116 Fisher, R. A., *The Design of Experiments* (2nd ed.). Oliver and Boyd, London, 1935. (See also 1974 edition with G. T. Prance).

117. Fitzpatrick, J. J., and Whall, A. L., *Conceptual Models of Nursing: Analysis and Application.* Robert J. Brady Co., Bowie, MD, 1983.

118. Flagle, C. D., "How to Allocate Progressive Patient Care Beds," in L. E. Weeks and J. R. Griffith (eds.), *Progressive Patient Care: An Anthology.* The University of Michigan, Ann Arbor, 1964, pp. 47–57.

119. Flagle, C. D., "Operational Research in the Health Services," in *Research Methodology and Potential in Community Health and Preventive Medicine. Ann. N.Y. Acad. Sci.,* **107**:748–59, May 23, 1963.

120. Flaskerud, J. H., "Utilizing a Nursing Conceptual Model in Basic Level Curriculum Development." *J. Nurs. Educ.,* **22**(6):224–227, June 1983.

121. Flook, E. E., and Sanazaro, P. J., (eds.), *Health Services Research and R&D in Perspective.* Health Administration Press, The University of Michigan, Ann Arbor, 1973.

122. Forrest, I., "Management Education and Training of Nurses: Research Study," *J. Advanced Nurs.,* **8**(2):139–145, March 1983.

123. Fortin, F., and Kerouac, S., "Validation of Questionnaires on Physical Function." *Nurs. Res.,* **26**:128–35, March-April 1977.

124. Friedman, L. M., Forberg, C. D., and DeMets, D. L., *Fundamentals of Clinical Trials.* John Wright, Littleton, MA, 1984.

125. Gebbie, K. M. (ed.), *Summary of the Second National Conference on Classification of Nursing Diagnoses.* National Group for the Classification of Nursing Diagnoses, St. Louis, 1976.

126. George, F. L., and Kuehn, R. P., *Patterns of Patient Care.* Macmillan Publishing Co., Inc., New York, 1955.

127. Georgopoulos, B. S. (ed.), *Organization Research on Health Institutions.* Institute for Social Research, The University of Michigan, Ann Arbor, 1972.

128. Gingras, P. (ed.), *National Conferences.* DHEW Publication No. (HRA) 77–3. U.S. Government Printing Office, Washington, DC, 1977.

129. Giovannetti, P., *Patient Classification Systems and Their Uses: A Description and Analysis.* DHEW Publication No. (HRA) 78–22, National Technical Information Service, Springfield, VA, 1978.

130. Goldfarb, M., "Methodological Approaches for Determining Health Manpower Planning Models." *Med. Care Rev.,* **32**:1–27, June 1975.

131. Gordon, M., *A First Course in Statistics.* Macmillan Publishing Co., Inc., New York, 1978.

132. Gortner, S. R., and Nahm, H., "An Overview of Nursing Research in the United States." *Nurs. Res.,* **26**:10–33, January-February 1977.

133. Gray, R., and Sauer, K., *Nursing Resources and Requirements: A Guide for State Level Planning.* Western Interstate Commission on Higher Education, Boulder, CO, 1978.

134. Greenberg, B. G., "The Philosophy and Methods of Research," in *Report on Nursing Research Conference,* H. H. Werley (ed.). Walter Reed Army Institute of Research, Washington, DC, 1962, pp. 1–100.

135. Grobe, Susan J., *Computer Primer and Resource Guide for Nurses.* J. B. Lippincott Co., Philadelphia, 1984.

136. Gulick, E. E., "Evaluating Research Requests: A Model for the Nursing Director." *J. Nurs. Admin.,* **11**(1):26–30, January 1981.

137. Gittentag, M., and Struening, E. L., *Handbook of Evaluation Research.* Sage Publications, Inc., Beverly Hills, CA, 1975.

138. Habenstein, R. W. (ed.), *Pathways to Data.* Aldine Publishing Co., New York, 1970.

139. Hadley, B. J. (ed.), *Methods for Studying Nurse Staffing in a Patient Unit.* DHEW Publication No. (HRA) 78–3, U.S. Government Printing Office, Washington, DC, 1978.

140. Hagen, E., and Wolff, L., *Nursing Leadership Behavior in General Hospitals.* Teachers College, Columbia University, New York, 1961.

141. Haldeman, J. C., and Abdellah, F. G., "Concepts of Progressive Patient Care." *Hospitals, J.A.H.A.,* **33**:38–42, 142, 144, 41–46, May 16 and June 1, 1959.

142. Hanchett, E. S., *The Problem Oriented System: A Literature Review*. DHEW Publication No. (HRA) 78–6. Health Resources Administration, Hyattsville, MD, 1977.

143. Hardy, L. K., "Nursing Models and Research—A Restricting View?" *J. Advanced Nurs.*, 7(5):447–451, September 1982.

144. Hardy, M. E., "Theories: Components, Development, Evaluation." *Nurs. Res.*, 23:100–107, March-April 1974.

145. Hardy, M. E., *Theoretical Foundations for Nursing*. MSS Information Corp., New York, 1973.

146. Harris, M. I., "Theory Building in Nursing." *Image*, 4:6–10, 1971.

147. Hasselmeyer, E. G., *Behavior Patterns of Premature Infants*. U.S. Public Health Service Publication No. 840. Government Printing Office, Washington, DC, 1961.

148. Haussmann, R. K. D., and Hegyvary, S. T., *Monitoring Quality of Nursing Care, Part III: Professional Review for Nursing: An Empirical Investigation*. DHEW Publication No. (HRA) 77–70. Health Resources Administration, Hyattsville, MD, 1977.

149. Haussmann, R. K. D., Hegyvary, S. T., and Newman, J. F., *Monitoring Quality of Nursing Care, Part II: Assessment and Study of Correlates*. DHEW Publication No. (HRA) 76–7. Health Resources Administration, Hyattsville, MD, 1976.

150. Hawkins, J. W., "A Nursing Model for Delivery of Primary Health Care for Women." American Nurses' Association Publication, G-14(7):22–28, 1980.

151. Health Resources Administration, *Conditions for Change in the Health Care System*. DHEW Publication No. (HRA) 78–642, U.S. Government Printing Office, Washington, DC, 1978.

152. Henderson, V., *Nursing Studies Index*, Vol. IV, *1957-1959*. J. B. Lippincott Co., Philadephia, 1963. See also Vol. III, *1950-1956* (1966); Vol. II, *1930-1949* (1970); and Vol. I, *1900-1929* (1972).

153. Henderson, V., "Research in Nursing Practice—When?" *Nurs. Res.*, 4:99, February 1956.

154. Henderson, V., *The Basic Principles of Nursing Care*. Cornwell Press, Ltd., London, 1958.

155. Henderson, V. A., "Preserving the Essence of Nursing in a Technological Age." *J. Advanced Nurs.*, 5:245–60, 1980.

156. Hess, I., Riedel, D. C., and Fitzpatrick, T. B., *Probability Sampling of Hospitals and Patients* (2nd ed.). Bureau of Hospital Administration, Research Series No. 1, University of Michigan, Ann Arbor, 1975.

157. Hiestand, D., and Ostow, M., *Health Manpower Information for Policy Guidance*. Ballinger Publishing Co., Cambridge, MA, 1976.

158. Hildebrand, D. K., Laing, J. D., and Rosenthal, H., *Prediction Analysis of Cross Classifications*. John Wiley & Sons, Inc., New York, 1977.

159. Hill, A. B., *Principles of Medical Statistics* (4th ed. rev.). Oxford University Press, New York, 1971.

160. Hodgman, E. C., "Research Policy for Nursing Services: Part I." *J. Nurs. Admin.*, 11(4):30–33, April 1981.

161. Hollander, M., and Wolfe, D. A., *Nonparametric Statistical Methods*. Wiley-Interscience, New York, 1973.

162. Hopkins, C. E., *et al.*, *Outcomes Conference I–II: Methodology of Identifying, Measuring and Evaluating Outcomes of Health Service Programs, Systems and Sub-systems*. National Technical Information Service, Springfield, VA, 1970. (Report No. HSRD 70–39.)

163. Horn, B. J., and Swain, M. A., *Criterion Measures of Nursing Care Quality*. DHEW Publication No. (PHS) 78–3187. National Center for Health Services Research, Hyattsville, MD, 1978.

164. Howland, D., "A Hospital System Model." *Nurs. Res.*, 12:232–36, fall 1963.

165. Howland, D., and McDowell, W. E., "The Measurement of Patient Care: A Conceptual Framework," *Nurs. Res.*, 13:4–7, winter 1964.

166. Hughes, E. C., Hughes, H. M., and Deutscher, I., *Twenty-Thousand Nurses Tell Their Story*. J. B. Lippincott Co., Philadelphia, 1958.

167. Institute of Medicine, *A Manpower Policy for Primary Health Care*. National Academy of Sciences, Washington, DC, 1978.

167a. Institute of Medicine, Div. of Health Sciences Policy, *Responding to Health Needs and Scientific Opportunity: The Organizational Structure of the National Institutes of Health*. National Academy Press, Washington, DC, 1984.

167b. Institute of Medicine, Div. of Health Care Services, *Nursing and Nursing Education: Public Policies and Private Actions*. National Academy Press, Washington, DC, 1983.

168. Jacox, A. and Prescott, P., "Determining a Study's Relevance for Clinical Practice." *Am. J. Nurs.*, 78:1882–89, November 1978.

169. Jelinek, R. C., and Dennis, L. C., *A Review and Evaluation of Nursing Productivity*. DHEW Publication No. (HRA) 77–15. U.S. Government Printing Office, Washington, DC, 1976.

170. Jelinek, R. C., Haussman, R. K. D., Hegyvary, S. T., and Newman, J. F., Jr., *A Methodology for Monitoring Quality of Nursing Care*. DHEW Publication No. (HRA) 76–25. U.S. Government Printing Office, Washington, DC, 1975.

171. Jennett, B., *High Technology Medicine. Benefits and Burdens*. The Nuffield Provincial Hospitals Trust, London, 1984.

172. Jessen, R. J., *Statistical Survey Techniques*.

John Wiley & Sons, Inc., New York, 1978.

173. Johns, E., and Pfefferkorn, B., *An Activity Analysis of Nursing*. Committee on the Grading of Nursing Schools, New York, 1934.

174. Johnson, M., "Some Aspects of the Relation Between Theory and Research in Nursing." *J. Advanced Nurs.*, **8**(1):21–28, January 1983.

175. Johnson, W. L., "Research Programs of the National League for Nursing." *Nurs. Res.*, **26**:172–76, May-June, 1977.

176. Johod, G., *Information Storage and Retrieval Systems for Individual Researchers*. Wiley-Interscience, New York, 1970.

177. Jones, D. C. *et al.*, *Trends in Registered Nurse Supply*. DHEW Publication No. (HRA) 76–15. U.S. Government Printing Office, Washington, DC, 1976.

178. Jones, P. E., and Jakob, D. F., *An Investigation of the Definition of Nursing Diagnoses*. University of Toronto, Toronto, 1977.

179. Jones, P. S., "An Adaptation Model for Nursing Practice." *Am. J. Nurs.*, **78**:1900–1906, November 1978.

180. Kalisch, P. A., and Kalisch, B. J., *Nursing Involvement in the Health Planning Process*. DHEW Publication No. (HRA) 78–25. (HRP-0500201.) National Technical Information Service, Springfield, VA, 1977.

181. Kalisch, P. A., and Kalisch, B. J., *The Advance of American Nursing*. Little Brown and Co., Boston, 1978.

182. Kane, R. A., and Kane, R. L., *Assessing the Elderly. A Practical Guide to Measurement*. Lexington Books, D. C. Heath and Co., Lexington, MA, 1981.

183. Kempthorne, O., *The Design and Analysis of Experiments*. Robert E. Krieger Publishing Co., New York, 1973.

184. Kendall, M. G., and Buckland, W. R., *A Dictionary of Statistical Terms* (3rd ed.). Longman Group Ltd., London, 1976.

185. Ketefian, S., (ed.). *Translation of Theory into Nursing Practice and Education*. Division of Nursing, School of Education, Health, Nursing and Arts Professions. New York University, New York, 1975.

186. Kim, H. S. *The Nature of Theoretical Thinking in Nursing*. Appleton-Century-Crofts, Norwalk, CT, 1983.

187. Kim, H. S., "Use of Roger's Conceptual System in Research: Comments." *Nurs. Res.*, **32**(2):89–91, March-April 1983.

188. King, I. M., *Toward a Theory for Nursing. General Concepts of Human Behavior*. John Wiley & Sons, Inc., New York, 1971.

189. Knapp, R. G., *Basic Statistics for Nurses*. John Wiley & Sons, Inc., New York, 1978.

190. Knopf, L., *From Student to Registered Nurse: A Report of the Nurse Career-Pattern Study.*

DHEW Publication No. 72–130. U.S. Government Printing Office, Washington, DC, 1972.

191. Knopf, L., *Registered Nurses One and Five Years After Graduation*. National League for Nursing, New York, 1975.

192. Knowlton, C. N., *et al*, "Systems Adaptation Model of Nursing for Families, Groups and Communities." *J. Nurs. Educ.*, **22**(3):128–131, March 1983.

193. Kodadek, S. (ed.). *Inventory of Innovations in Nursing*. DHEW Publication No. (HRA) 77–2. U.S. Government Printing Office, Washington, DC, 1976.

194. Krone, K. P., and Loomis, M. E., "Developing Practice—Relevant Research: A Model That Worked." *J. Nurs. Admin.*, **12**(4):38–41, April 1982.

195. Kruskal, W. H., and Tanur, J. M., *International Encyclopedia of Statistics*. The Free Press, New York, 1978.

196. Larson, E., "Health Policy and NIH: Implications for Nursing Research." *Nurs Res.*, **33**(6):352–56, November/December, 1984.

197. LeRoy, L., "Case Study #16: The Costs and Effectiveness of Nurse Practitioners," in *The Implications of Cost-Effectiveness Analysis of Medical Technology*, Office of Technology Assessment, Washington, DC, July 1981.

198. Levine, E., "Experimental Design in Nursing Research." *Nurs. Res.*, **9**:203–12, fall 1960.

199. Levine, E., "The A.B.C.'s of Statistics." *Am. J. Nurs.*, **59**:71–75, January 1959.

200. Levine, E., "What Do We Know About Nurse Practitioners?" *Am J. Nurs.*, **77**:1799–1803, November 1977.

201. Levine, E. (ed.), *Research on Nurse Staffing in Hospitals: Report of the Conference*. DHEW Publication No. (NIH) 73–434. U.S. Government Printing Office, Washington, DC, 1973.

202. Levine, E., and Wright, S., "New Ways to Measure Personnel Turnover." *Hospitals, J.A.H.A.*, **31**:38–42, August 1, 1957.

203. Levine, H. D., and Phillip, P. J., *Factors Affecting Staffing Levels and Patterns of Nursing Personnel*. DHEW Publication No. (HRA) 75–6. U.S. Government Printing Office, Washington, DC, 1975.

204. Light, R. J., and Pillemer, D. B., *Summing Up. The Science of Reviewing Research*. Harvard University Press, Cambridge, MA, 1984.

205. Little, A. D., Inc., *Computer-Based Patient Monitoring Systems*. DHEW Publication No. (HRA) 76–3143. National Center for Health Services Research, Hyattsville, MD, 1976.

206. Lum, J., and Leonhard, G. (eds.), *Report of the Panel of Expert Consultants*. Western Interstate Commission for Higher Education, Boulder, CO, 1978.

207. Maranell, G. M., *Scaling: A Source Book for Be-*

havioral Scientists. Aldine Publishing Co., Chicago, 1974.

208. Marascuilo, L. A., *Statistical Methods for Behavioral Science Research.* McGraw-Hill Book Co., New York, 1971.

209. Matek, S.J., *Accountability: Its Meaning and Its Relevance to the Health Care Field.* DHEW Publication No. (HRA) 77–72. (HRP-0500101.) National Technical Information Service, Springfield, VA, 1977.

210. Mayers, M. G., *A Systematic Approach to the Nursing Care Plan.* Appleton-Century-Crofts, New York, 1972.

211. McCormick, K. A., "Nursing in the Computer Revolution." *Computers in Nursing,* 2(2):4, 30, March/April 1984.

212. McFarlane, E. A., "Nursing Theory: The Comparison of Four Theoretical Proposals." *J. Advanced Nurs.,* 5(1):3–19, January 1980.

213. McKay, R., and Segall, M., "Methods and Models for the Aggregate." *Nurs. Outlook,* 31(6):328–334, November/December 1983.

214. McLaughlin, J. S., "Toward a Theoretical Model for Community Health Programs." *Adv. Nurs. Sci. Application of Theory,* 5(1):7–28, October 1982.

215. Mechanic, D., "Approaches to Controlling the Costs of Medical Care: Short-Range and Long-Range Alternatives." *N. Engl. J. Med.,* 298:249–54, Feb. 2, 1978.

216. Medicus Systems Corporation, *Effects of Nursing Education on Nursing Performance.* Prepared under contract No. HRA 231–77–0121 with Division of Nursing, HRA. Hyattsville, MD, 1979.

217. Melia, K. M., "Tell It As It Is—Qualitative Methodology and Nursing Research: Understanding the Student Nurse's World." *J. Advanced Nurs.,* 7(4):327–335, July 1982.

218. Melnyk, K. A. M., "The Process of Theory Analysis: An Examination of the Nursing Theory of Dorothea E. Orem." *Nurs. Res.,* 32(3):170–74, May-June 1983.

219. Menish, J., *et al., A Legislative Primer for Nurses.* Standing Committee on Government Affairs of the Emergency Dept. Nurses Association, Barbara Vanderkolk and Associates, Inc., 1982.

220. Meyer, B., and Heidgerken, L. E., *Research in Nursing.* J. B. Lippincott Co., Philadelphia, 1962.

221. Meyer, G. R., *Tenderness and Technique: Nursing Values in Transition.* Institute of Industrial Relations, University of California, Los Angeles, 1960.

222. Mill, J. S., *A System of Logic.* University of Toronto Press, Toronto, 1975.

223. Mosteller, F., Rourke, R. E. K., and Thomas, G. B., Jr., *Probability with Statistical Applications.* Addison-Wesley Publishing Co., Inc., Reading, MA, 1974.

224. Mosteller, F., and Tukey, J. W., *Data Analysis and Regression.* Addison-Wesley Publishing Co., Reading, MA, 1977.

225. Nash, P. M., *Evaluation of Employment Opportunities for Newly Licensed Nurses.* DHEW Publication No. (HRA) 75–12, U.S. Government Printing Office, Washington, DC, 1975.

226. Nathan, R. A., Associates, Inc., *Methodological Approaches for Determining Health Manpower Supply and Requirements.* Vol. 1. *Analytical Perspective.* Vol. 2. *Practical Planning Manual.* DHEW Publication No. (HRA) 76–14511 and DHEW Publication No. (HRA) 76–14512. National Technical Information Service, Springfield, VA, 1976.

227. National Center for Health Services Research, *Criterion Measures of Nursing Care Quality.* NCHSR Research Summary Series, DHEW Publication No. (PHS) 78–3187, Washington, DC, August 1978.

228. National Center for Health Services Research, *Recent Studies in Health Services Research.* DHEW Publication No. (HRA) 77–3162. National Center for Health Services Research, Hyattsville, MD, 1977.

229. National Center for Health Statistics, *Health United States, 1985.* DHEW Publication No. (PHS) 86–1232. U.S. Government Printing Office, Washington, DC, 1985.

230. National Commission for Manpower Policy, *Employment Impacts of Health Policy Developments.* Special Report No. 11. The Commission, Washington, DC, October 1976.

231. National League for Nursing, *Selected Management Information Systems for Public Health/Community Health Agencies.* National League for Nursing, New York, 1978.

232. National League for Nursing, *Nursing Data Book.* National League for Nursing, New York, 1984.

233. Newman, M., "What Differentiates Clinical Research?" *Image,* 14(3):86–91, October 1982.

234. Norbeck, J. S., "Social Support: A Model for Clinical Research and Application." *Adv. Nurs. Sci.,* 3(4):43–59, July 1981.

235. Notter, L., and Spector, A. F., *Nursing Research in the South: A Survey.* Southern Regional Education Board, Atlanta, 1974.

236. Office of Federal Statistical Policy and Standards, *Social Indicators, 1976.* U.S. Government Printing Office, Washington, DC, 1977.

237. Payne, L., "Health: A Basic Concept in Nursing Theory." *J. Adv. Nurs.,* 8(5):393–395, September 1983.

238. Peplau, H. E., *Interpersonal Relations in Nursing.* G. P. Putnam's Sons, New York, 1952.

239. Phillips, D. S., *Basic Statistics for Health Science Students.* W. H. Freeman and Co., San Francisco, 1978.

240. Phillips, T. P. (ed.), *The Doctorally Prepared Nurse. Report of Two Conferences on the De-*

mand for and Education of Nurses with Doctoral Degrees. DHEW Publication No. (HRA) 76–18. U.S. Government Printing Office, Washington, DC, 1976.

241. Polit, D., and Hungler, B., *Nursing Research: Principles and Methods, 2d edition,* J. B. Lippincott Co., Philadelphia, 1983.

242. Posavac, E. J., and Carey, R. G., *Program Evaluation. Methods and Case Studies.* Prentice-Hall, Inc., Englewood Cliffs, NJ, 1980.

243. Pratt, J., and Gibbons, J. D., *Concepts of Non-Parametric Theory.* Springer Verlag Inc., New York, 1981.

244. Reiser, S. J., and Anbar, M (eds.), *The Machine at the Bedside. Strategies for Using Technology in Patient Care.* Cambridge University Press, Cambridge, MA, 1984.

245. Reiter, F., and Kakosh, M. E., *Quality of Nursing Care. A Report of a Field Study to Establish Criteria, 1950–1954.* Institute of Research and Studies in Nursing Education, Division of Nursing Education, Teachers College, Columbia University, New York, 1963.

246. Rieken, H. W., and Ravich, R., "Informed Consent to Biomedical Research in Veterans Administration Hospitals." *JAMA,* 248(3)344–48, July 16, 1982.

247. Riehl, J. P., and Roy, Sister C., *Conceptual Models for Nursing Practice.* Appleton-Century-Crofts, New York, 1974.

248. Roberts, D. E., and Freeman, R. B. (eds.), *Redesigning Nursing Education for Public Health: Report of the Conference, May 23–25, 1973.* DHEW Publication No. (HRA) 75–75, Health Resources Administration, Hyattsville, MD, 1975.

249. Robinson, J., and Sachs, B., *Nursing Care Models for Adolescent Families.* American Nurses' Association, Kansas City, MO, 1984.

250. Rogers, M. E., "Some Comments on the Theoretical Basis of Nursing Practice." *Nurs. Sci.,* 1:11–13, 60–61, April-May 1963.

251. Rogers, M. E., *An Introduction to the Theoretical Basis of Nursing.* F. A. Davis Co., Philadelphia, 1970.

252. Roper, N., *et al., Using a Model for Nursing.* Churchill Livingstone, Inc., New York, 1983.

253. Rossi, P. H., Wright, J. D., and Anderson, A. B., *Handbook of Survey Research,* Academic Press, New York, 1983.

254. Rutman, L., *Evaluation Research Methods: A Basic Guide.* Sage Publications, Beverly Hills, CA, 1977.

255. Saba, V. K., and McCormick, K. A., *Essentials of Computers for Nurses.* J. B. Lippincott Co., New York, 1986.

256. Schlotfeldt, R. M., "The Significance of Empirical Research for Nursing." *Nurs. Res.,* 20:140–42, March-April 1971.

257. Schwartz, D., Henley, B., and Zeitz, L., *The Elderly Ambulatory Patient: Nursing and Psycho-* *social Needs.* Macmillan Publishing Co., Inc., New York, 1964.

258. Schwirian, P. M., *Prediction of Successful Nursing Performance, Part I and Part II.* DHEW Publication No. (HRA) 77–27. U.S. Government Printing Office, Washington, DC, 1977.

259. Schwirian, P. M., "Toward an Explanatory Model of Nursing Performance." *Nurs. Res.,* 30(4):247–253, July-August 1981.

260. See, E. M., "The American Nurses' Association and Research in Nursing." *Nurs. Res.,* 26:165–71, May-June 1977.

261. Segall, M., and Sauer, K., "Nurse Staffing in the Context of Institutional and State-Level Planning." *Nurs. Admin. Q.,* 2:39–50, fall 1977.

262. Selltiz, C., Jahoda, M., Deutsch, M., and Cook, S. W., *Research Methods in Social Relations,* (3rd ed.). Holt, Rinehart and Winston, New York, 1976.

263. Selye, H., *From Dream to Discovery: On Being A Scientist.* Arno, New York, 1975.

264. Shelly, G. B., and Cashman, T. J., *Computer Fundamentals for an Information Age.* Anaheim Publishing Co., Inc., Brea, CA, 1984.

265. Shock, N. W., *et al., Normal Human Aging.* DHHS, PHS, NIH Publication No. 84–2450, U.S. Government Printing Office, Washington, DC, 1984.

266. Shuman, L. S., Speas, R. D., Jr., and Young, J. P., *Operations Research in Health Care: A Critical Analysis.* The Johns Hopkins University Press, Baltimore, 1975.

267. Simmons, L. W., and Henderson, V., *Nursing Research: A Survey and Assessment.* Appleton-Century-Crofts, Inc., New York, 1964.

268. Sloan, F. A., *Equalizing Access to Nursing Services: The Geographic Dimension.* DHEW Publication No. (HRA) 78–51, U.S. Government Printing Office, Washington, DC, 1978.

269. Som, R. K., *A Manual of Sampling Techniques.* Crane, Russak and Co., Inc., New York, 1973.

270. Somers, A. R., *Health Care in Transition: Directions for the Future.* Hospital Research and Educational Trust, Chicago, 1971.

271. Stanford, E. D., and Kinsella, C. R., *Assessment of Nursing Services: Report of the Conference, June 1974.* DHEW Publication No. (HRA) 75–40. Health Resources Administration, Bethesda, MD, 1975.

272. Stevenson, J. S., *Issues and Crises During Middlescence.* Appleton-Century-Crofts, New York, 1977.

273. Strauss, A. L., "Patients' Work in the Technologized Hospital." *Nurs. Outlook,* 29(7):404–412, July 1981.

274. Stumpf, J. C., "Communication Abilities of Veterans Administration Nurses." Doctoral Dissertation, University of Utah, Salt Lake City, 1961.

275. Sudman, S., *Applied Sampling.* Academic Press, New York, 1976.

276. Sultz, H. A., Zielezny, M., and Kinyon, L., *Longitudinal Study of Nurse Practitioners—Phase 1.* DHEW Publication No. (HRA) 76-43. U.S. Government Printing Office, Washington, DC, 1976.

277. Surgeon General's Consultant Group on Nursing, *Toward Quality in Nursing: Needs and Goals.* Government Printing Office, Washington, DC, February 1963.

278. Sweeney, M. A., *The Nurse's Guide to Computers.* Macmillan Publishing Company Inc., New York, 1985.

279. Tai, S. W., *Social Science Statistics: Its Elements and Applications.* Goodyear Publishing Co., Santa Monica, CA, 1978.

280. Taylor, S. P., "Bibliography on Nursing Research, 1950–1974." *Nurs. Res.,* **24:**207–25, May-June 1975.

282. Thibodeau, J. A., *Nursing Models: Analysis and Evaluation.* Wadsworth Health Sciences Division, Monterey, CA, 1983.

283. Tippett, L. H. C., *Random Sampling Numbers.* Cambridge University Press, Cambridge, London, 1927.

284. U.S. Public Health Service, *Research in Nursing 1969–1972.* DHEW Publication No. (NIH) 73–489. Division of Nursing, Bethesda, MD, 1973. See also *Research in Nursing 1955–1968.* PHS Publication No. 1356. Division of Nursing, Bethesda, MD, 1970.

285. U.S. Public Health Service, Division of Hospital and Medical Facilities, *Elements of Progressive Patient Care.* U.S. Public Health Service Publication No. 930-C-1. Government Printing Office, Washington, DC, 1962.

286. U.S. Senate Special Committee on Aging in Conjunction with AARP, *Aging America. Trends and Projections.* Second Printing, U.S. Senate Special Committee on Aging, Washington, DC, 1984.

287. Van Den Berg, J. H., *Medical Ethics and Medical Power.* W. W. Norton and Co., New York, 1978.

288. Verhonick, P. J., *Descriptive Study Methods in Nursing.* Scientific Publication No. 219. Pan American Health Organization, Washington, DC, 1971.

289. Volicer, B. J., *Multivariate Statistics for Nursing Research.* Grune & Stratton, Inc., Orlando, FL, 1984.

290. Vreeland, E. M., "Nursing Research Programs of the Public Health Service." *Nurs. Res.,* **13:**148–58, spring 1964.

291. Vreeland, E. M., "The Nursing Research Grant and Fellowship Program in the Public Health Service." *Am. J. Nurs.,* **58:**1700–1702, December 1958.

292. Walker, L. O., and Avant, K. C., *Strategies for Theory Construction in Nursing.* Appleton-Century-Crofts, Norwalk, CT, 1983.

293. Walters, L., and Kahn, T. J. (eds.), *Bibliography of Bioethics, Vol. 10,* Kennedy Institute of Ethics, Georgetown University, Washington, DC, 1984.

294. Watson, B., and Mayers, G., *Assessment and Documentations: Nursing Theories in Action.* Charles 13, Slcak, Inc., NJ, 1981.

295. Weisberg, H. F., and Bowen, B. D., *An Introduction to Survey Research and Data Analysis.* W. H. Freeman and Co., San Francisco, 1977.

296. Werley, H., "Promoting the Research Dimension in the Practice of Nursing Through the Establishment and Development of a Department of Nursing in an Institute of Research." *Military Med.,* **127:**219–31, March 1962.

297. Werley, H., and Fitzpatrick, J. J. (eds.), *Annual Review of Nursing Research,* Vol. 2, Springer Publishing Co., New York, 1984.

298. White, C. M., *Sources of Information in the Social Sciences.* American Library Association, Chicago, 1973. .

299. Wieczorek, R. R. (ed.), *Power, Politics, and Policy in Nursing.* Springer Publishing Co., New York, 1985.

300. Williams, C. A. (ed.), *Nursing Research and Policy Formation. The Case for Prospective Payment.* American Academy of Nursing, Kansas City, MO, 1983.

301. Wong, J., and Mensah, L. L., "A Conceptual Approach to the Development of Motivational Strategies." *J. Adv. Nurs.,* **8**(2):111–16, March 1983.

302. Wooldridge, P. J., Leonard, R. C., and Skipper, J. K., Jr., *Methods of Clinical Experimentation to Improve Patient Care.* C. V. Mosby Co., St. Louis, 1978.

303. Wooldridge, P. J., *et al., Behavioral Science and Nursing Theory.* C. V. Mosby Co., St. Louis, 1983.

304. Yura, H., *Nursing Leadership Theory and Process* (2nd ed.). Appleton-Century-Crofts, New York, 1981.

305. Yura, H., Ozimek, D., and Walsh, M. B., *Nursing Leadership: Theory and Process.* Appleton-Century-Crofts, New York, 1976.

306. Yura, H., and Walsh, M. B., *The Nursing Process: Assessing, Planning, Implementing, Evaluating* (2nd ed.). Appleton-Century Crofts, New York, 1973.

307. Nicoll, L. H., *Perspectives on Nursing Theory.* Little Brown and Co., Boston, 1986.

Index

Abbreviations, selected standard, 302
Abdellah, Faye G., 3, 32, 33, 54, 359
"Absolute" research, *see* Descriptive
  research
Abstract journals, 97
Abstract physical representations, 110
Administrative problems in research,
  see Research tactics
Aggression, model for study of, 65–66
Algorithm, *382*
Alternative hypothesis, 282–284
American Academy of Nursing, 33
American Hospital Association, 21, 34,
  95, 201, 233
American Nurses' Association, 3, 21, 30,
  31, 33, 86, 88, 95, 159, 233
  clinical sessions (1962), 95
  Cabinet on Nursing Research, 34, 42,
    43

Commission on Nursing Research, 33,
  314
Council on Computer Applications, 34,
  378–379
Council of Nurse Researchers, 33
Inventory of Registered Nurses, 31
research conferences, 32
study of economic security by, 30
American Nurses' Foundation, 31, 94, 95
  establishment, 29
Analysis of covariance, 186, 266, *382*
Analysis of variance, 184, 189, 192, 262,
  265–266, 286, *382*
Anecdotal data, 130
Applied research, 9, 289
  decision making, 10
  developmental studies, 10
  evaluative research, 10–11
  problem solving, 10

Note: *Italicized* numbers refer to glossary definitions

Artificial relationships, 120–121
Associative relationships, 119–120, 200–201, *383*
Assumptions, 122, *383*
Attribute correlation, 133
Audimeter, 238
Audiovisuals, 97–98
Automation in nursing, 39, 40
Aydelotte, Myrtle, 157

Balanced design, 191
Balancing, 149, 185–186, *383*
Basic (pure) research, 9, 289
Bayesian statistics, 284, 287, *383*
Behavior
  child, *see* Child behavior
Behavioral sciences, *see* Social sciences
Bias
  controlling of, 81
  response error, 240, 243
  See also Hawthorne effect
Bibliographies, 98
Bibliographic developments affecting
  nursing, 94–97
Bimodal, *383*
Binary, *383*
Bivariate distribution, 263, 290
Boyle, Rena, 46
Bross, Irwin, 109
Brown report, 30
Budget for research, 343–347
Bunge, Helen, 31, 33
Burgess, May Ayres, 30

Calibration, *383*
Campbell, Donald, 179
Canonical correlation, *383*
"Carry-back" studies, *see*
  Nonexperimental research
"Carry-forward" studies, *see* Explanatory
  research
Case studies, 18, 129, *383*
  of descriptive studies, *see* Descriptive
    research
  of explanatory studies, *see* Explanatory
    research
  of methodological studies, *see*
    Methodological research

typology for nursing research, *see*
  Typology for nursing research
Causal relationships, 119–120, 171
Causal variable, *see* Independent variable
Causation, *383*
Cause and effect, 116–118, 165–167, *383*
  misinterpretation in statistical tables, 294
Central limit theorem, *383*
Central tendency (measures of), 254, 255–256, 294
Chapin, Stuart, 13, 165
Charts, flow, 111
Chi-square test, 199, 269–273, *383*
Child behavior,
  relationship between nursing care and
    behavior of premature infants,
    86–87, 138, 185, 197
Christy, Teresa, 204, 205
Class interval, *383*
Classification scales, *see* Qualitative scales
Classification schemes for research topics, 87
Clinical trials of drugs, 11, 16, 89
Cluster, 225, *383*
Cluster analysis, *383*
Cluster sampling, 224–226
Cochran, William, 147, 165, 185
Coding, 133, 140
Coefficient of association (Yule's), 268–269, *396*
Coefficient of correlation, 268–269, *383*
  rank correlation coefficient, 275–276
Cohen, Morris, 130, 167
Cohort studies, 80, 203, *384*
Columbia University, Teachers College, 31, 94, 205
Committee on the Cost of Medical Care, 30
Committee for the Study of Nursing
  Education, 29
Committee on the Grading of Nursing
  Schools, 30
Common sense as substitute for research, 23
Community health centers, hospitals as, 40
Community Studies, Inc., study of nursing
  care by, 157–158
Comparative experiments, 165, *384*

Comparative group, *see* Control group
"Comparative" research, *see* Explanatory research
Computer-assisted information retrieval, 101–103
Computers, 83, 243, 245–249, 376–377, *384*
  mainframe, 246
  microcomputer (personal computer), 83, 246
  minicomputer, 246
  nursing information system, 378
Conceptual framework, 47, *384*
Conceptualization, 107, *384*
Concomitant variation, 166–167, *384*
Confidence coefficient, 242, *384*
Confidence interval, 242, *384*
Consensual validation, *384*
Constellation, *384*
Construct, *384*
Consultants, 310, 421
Content analysis, *384*
Continuum, *384*
Contrast group, *see* Control group
Control, *384*
Control group, 183, *384*
  two-group design with, 182–188
Convenience samples, 227
Correlation coefficient, 263
  rank, 134
Costs of research projects, *see* Financial support for research
Co-twin control, 185
Covariance, analysis, 186, 266, *382*
Criterion measures, *see* Dependent variables
Cross-sectional design, 80, 201–202, 203, *385*
Cross-tabulation, 133, 173, 176, 186, 249
Cybernetics, *385*
Curn project, 42

Data
  analyzing, 261–277
  interpreting, 279–295
    in statistical tables, 290–295
  methods of collecting and processing, 82–83, 232–243
    direct collection of data, 235–239

enhancing precision, 240–241
importance of pretest, 239
mechanical collection, 238
preparing summary measures and tabulations of data, 249–251
processing data by hand, 249–250
processing data by computer, 247–249
sampling, *see* Sampling
selection, 239
use of existing data, 232–233
use of observer to collect data, 233–235
  primary data, 233
  secondary data, 232–233
  summarization, 251–259
DaVinci, Leonardo, 9
Databases on-line, 101–103
Decennial census, 240
Decision making, *385*
  applied research and, 10
Deduction, *385*
  as part of theory, 51
  See also Hypotheses
Definitions, as part of theory, 51
Degrees of freedom in chi-square test, 271
Delphi technique, *385*
Deming, W. Edwards, 240
Demography, *385*
Demonstration project, 122
Demonstrations, 11, *385*
Dependent variables (criterion measures), 116–117, 147–148, 252
  evaluating sufficiency and efficiency, 148–155
  multiple, 263
  role in nursing research, 155–160
  selection, 147–148
Descriptive research, 12, 81, 115, 200
  sampling error in, 262
Design, *see* Research design
Developmental research,
  applied research and, 10
Dewey, John, 50
Diagnostic process, 367
  See also Nursing diagnosis
Diagrams, 110–111
Diary method, 237
Dictated research, 77
Discriminant analysis, 276, *385*

Distribution-free (nonparametric) tests, 273–276
See also Chi-square test
Division of Hospitals, *see* U.S. Public Health Service, Division of Hospitals
Division of Nursing, *see* U.S. Public Health Service, Division of Nursing
Division of Research Grants, *see* U.S. Publio Health Service, Division of Research Grants
Donabedian, Avedis, 156
Double-blind technique, 187–188, *385*
DRGs (Diagnostic Related Groups), 246, 358–359, 369
Drug lists, 98–99
Drugs, clinical trials, 11, 16, 90
Dumas, Rhetaugh, 158
Dummy tables, 79, 249–250

Ecology, *385*
Education, nursing, *see* Nursing education
Educational institutions, research in, 21, 318, 341–342
See also specific educational institutions
Edwards, Allen, 192
Effect, *385*
See also Cause and effect
Effect variables, *see* Dependent variables
Emerson, Haven, 29
Emotional stress, model for study of, 66
Empirical, *385*
Empirical evidence as substitute for research, 23
Empirical law, *385*
Empirical test, *385*
Empiricism (scientific), *385*
Enumeration scales, 128, 133
See also Qualitative scales
Environmental variables, 119, 126, 172, 175, 182, 184, 225
Epistemology, *385*
Equal-appearing intervals method, 136, 140, *386*
Equipment, budget for, 343
ERIC, 96
Errors, *386*
  experimental, 183, 184
  observer, 243
  processing, 243

response, 243
sampling, 217, 219, 224, 225, 240, 241–242, 261–262, 280
  computing, 220, 223, 241
Types I and II errors, 283
Estimate, precision, 240–242
Evaluative research, 81
Ex post facto data, 176
Ex post facto hypothesis, 123
Ex post facto studies, *see* Nonexperimental research
Experience as substitute for research, 22
Experiment, how to conduct, 192–194, *386*
Experimental error, 182
Experimental field studies, 19
Experimental design, *see* Experimental research
Experimental group, 167–168, 176, *386*
Experimental research, 80–81, 164–200, *386*
  advantages and disadvantages, 168–170, 175
  barriers, 15–17
  cause and effect, 165
  comparison of nonexperimental, 13–15, 172–175
  descriptive studies, 164
  practical problems, 169, 194–198
  with random assignment, 182–192
  in studies of patient care, 198–200
  types, 80, 176–192
  variables in explanatory studies, 78, 172, 175–176
Explanatory experimental research, 167, 176–192, 209
Explanatory research, 12, 115, 125, 175, 200–201, *386*
Explanatory variables, 78, 118–119, 126, 147, 168
Exploratory study, *386*
Extraneous variables, 126, 179, 180, 209, 216, 294
Extrapolation, *386*

Facilities for research, securing of, 314
Fact, *386*
Factor, *386*
Factor analysis, 277, *386*

Factorial design, 190–192, 265, *386*
Factual questionnaires, 236–237
Faith as substitute for research, 23
Federal government
   role in furthering nursing research,
      318–322
   grants and fellowships, 325
   university research vs. federal research,
      318, 341–342
   U.S. Public Health Service, *see* U.S.
      Public Health Service
Federal Nursing Services, 207
Field surveys, 18, *386*
Financial support for research, 317
   budget determination, 343,
      345–347
   preparing research proposal,
      343–351
   responsibilities of universities and health
      agencies, 318, 341–342
   See also Federal government
Findings, *see* Research findings
Fisher, R. A., 160, 165, 190, 265
Fitzpatrick, M. Louise, 204–205
Flagle, Charles, 87
Flow charts, 111
Follow-up studies, *see* Prospective design
Frequency data, 128, 133
Frequency distribution, *386*
F-test, 194, 266, *386*
"Function" studies, 86, 88
Funds for research, *see* Financial support
   for research

Gantt chart, 111
Gaussian curve (normal curve), 254
GEMNAC, 34, 359
Generalization, 83, 216, *387*
General linear hypothesis, 83, 168, 266,
   387
Goldmark, Josephine, 29, 358
Gortner, Susan, 33
Grants for research, *see* Research grants
Graphic Rating Scale, 135, 237
Grouped data, 258–259
Guttman-type scale, 46, 138–139

Habit as substitute for research, 23
Hand processing of data,

Hasselmeyer, Eileen, 86–87, 138, 185,
   197
Hawthorne effect, 7, 17, 178, 179–180,
   182, 187, 194, 218, *387*
   sampling and, 218
   use of placebo to measure, 187
Health care assessment, 369
Health Care Financing Administration,
   326–329
Health policy, research in, 360–361
Hegyvary, Sue, 159
Henderson, Virginia, 31, 32, 56, 377
Hilbert, Hortense, 32, 33
Historical method, 204, *387*
Historical research, 81, 204–207, 358
Histories, 99–100
Hospitals
   as community health centers, 40
Human subjects, rights, 314–317,
   348–350
Hypotheses, 78, 114–124, 147, *387*
   alternative, 282–284
   assumptions and, 122
   examples, 115–116
   general linear, 83
   null, 121, 280–282
      overuse, 289
      Types I and II errors, 283
   as part of theory, 51
   from problem to, 123–124
   stating, 121–122
   types, 119
"Hypothetical universe," 216, 285

Independent variable, 116–117
   multiple comparison groups with
      multiple, 190–192
   multiple comparison groups with single,
      188–190
Indexes, 33, 100–101
Induction, *387*
Inference, *387*
Institute of Medicine, 34
Institute of Research and Service in
   Nursing Education, 31
Institutional review board, 315
Instruments to collect data, 148
   criteria for evaluating, 239–240
   mechanical, 238
   paper and pencil, 237–238

Interagency Conference on Nursing Statistics, 96
Interagency Council on Library Resources, 97
Interagency Council on Library Tools, 94–95
Interdisciplinary research, 310–311
International health research, 364–365
Interval scales, 140–145
Interviewing, 235, *387*
Investigation, *387*

Job satisfaction of nursing personnel, 137–138, 150
Johns, Ethel, 205
Johns Hopkins Hospital, 146
  Operations Research Division, 21
Joint method of agreement and difference, 166
Journals (nursing), 97
  Nursing Research, 31, 94, 97
Judgment samples, 227

Kempthorne, Oscar, 12
Kish, Leslie, 225
Krutch, Joseph Wood, 154
K-test, 265
Kolmogorov-Smirnov D test, *387*
Kuder-Richardson formula, 87

Lambertsen, Eleanor, 205
Landmark studies, 86
Lang, Norma, 160
Latin-square design, 189–190, 199, 265, *387*
Legal guides, 101
Lentz, Edith, 46
Level of significance, 282–284, *387*
Levine, Eugene, 359
Library of Congress, 207
Lifelike physical representations, 109–110
Likert-type scale, 137–138
Limitations on research, 122–123
Literary Digest poll, 217
Literature, review, 77, 94–105
  guidelines, 104–105

Longitudinal studies, *see* Prospective design; Retrospective design
Lysaught, Jerome, 33

Mann-Whitney U test, 276, *387*
Matching, 184–187, *387*
Mathematical models, 111, 249
McCormick, Kathleen, 40
McClure, Margaret, 5,
Mead, Margaret, 12
Mean, 242, 256
  test of significance of differences between two, 263-265
Meaningfulness of a measure, 154–155
Measurement scales, *see* Quantitative scales
Measures of central tendency, 255–256, *387*
Measures of variation, 256–258, *388*
Mechanical instruments to collect data, 151, 233, 238
Median, 256
Medicus Corporation, 358
MEDLARS, 96, 101, *388*
MEDLINE, 101, 207
Meltzer, Lawrence, 158
Merton, Robert, 51, 88
Meta Analysis, *388*
Method of agreement, 165, *388*
  joint method of difference and, 166
Method of difference, 165–166, 180, *388*
  joint method of agreement and, 166
Method of residues, 167, *388*
Mid-Atlantic Regional Nurses Association, 32
Midwest Alliance in Nursing, 32
Midwest Alliance in Nursing, 32
Mill's (John Stuart) five canons, 165, 166, 167, 180
Mode, 134, 255
Models, 52–70, 108–112, *388*
  clinical practice, 60
  nursing care, 52–53, 62–64
  nursing supply, requirements and distribution, 70
  reaction, 61–62
  as source of research topics, 87
  for study of aggression, 65–66
  for study of emotional stress, 66

for study of pain, 64–65
for study of role of public health nurse, 66–70
types, 109–112
  mathematical, 111
  physical, 110–111
  statistical, 111–112
Multiclinic trials of drugs, 7
Multiple regression, 262, 267
Multistage sampling, 224
Multivariate analysis, 197–198, 245, *388*
Multivariate analysis of variance, 266
Multivariate distribution, 291

Nagel, Ernest, 130, 167
Narrative data, 129–130
National Advisory Council on Nursing Training, 34, 318
National Committee for the Improvement of Nursing Services, 31
National Institute of Nursing, 34
National Institutes of Health, *see* U.S. Public Health Service
National League for Nursing, 21, 29, 32, 95, 206–207
National Nursing Accrediting Service, 31
National Organization for Public Health Nursing, 29, 30, 205
National Science Foundation, 44
National Technical Information Service, 95
Natural settings for research, 18–19
Need for research, 23–24, 38
New England Board of Higher Education, 32
New York Academy of Medicine, 29
Neyman-Pearson approach, 284, *388*
Nightingale, Florence, 3, 28, 54
Nite, Gladys, 157
Nominal scales, 133, 140
  developing quantitative scales from, 145–147
Nonexperimental research, 200–209
  advantages and disadvantages, 170–172, 175
  comparison of experimental and, 13–15, 172–175
  conducting, 207–209
  cross-sectional design, 201–202
  mixed designs, 203–204

prospective design, 202–203
retrospective design, 202
variations, 80–81
Nonparametric (distribution-free) tests, 263, 273–276
  See also Chi-square test
Nonparticipant observer, 233–234
Nonprobability samples, 227–228
Nonquantitative data, 129–130
Normal curve (Gaussian curve), 131, 242, 254, *388*
Norms, *389*
Notter, Lucille, 33
Null hypothesis, 280–282, *389*
  overuse, 289
  Types I and II errors and, 283
Nurses as researchers, 40–41, 313
Nursing archives at N.L.M., 206–207
Nursing care, *see* Nursing practice
Nursing care model, 62–64
Nursing, defined, 4, *389*
Nursing diagnosis, 47, *389*
Nursing education, 39
Nursing Research (journal), 8, 31, 32, 33, 94, *389*
Nursing science, 40, 47, *389*
  development of theories in, 363–364
Nursing Studies Index, 94
Nutting, Adelaide, 205

Observer, 233–235, *389*
  nonparticipant, 233–234
  participant, 234–235
Observer error, 151–152, 235
One-group, before-after design, 178–180
One-group design, 176–178
One-tailed vs. two-tailed tests, 282
Operational definition, 79, 126, 147, *389*
Optimum allocation, *389*
Order statistics, *see* Nonparametric tests
Ordinal scales, 133–135
  in social science research, 135–140
Orem, Dorothy, 57
Organismic variables, 119, 126, 172, 182, 185, 238

PACE (Patient Appraisal and Care Evaluation), 160, 369

Pain
  model for study, 64–65
Paired comparisons, 139–140
Pairing, 149, 184–185, *389*
Panel design, *390*
Parameters, 217, 263, *390*
Parametric tests, 263–270, 286
  F-test, 265–266
  t-test, 263, 264–265
  procedure for, 264
  for proportions, 269–270
  See also Nonparametric tests
Participant observer, 234–235
Path analysis, 276, *390*
Patient, 38–39
  criterion measures, 155–156
  classification, 145–147, 152
  development of methodology to
    evaluate, 62–64
  care, 138, 155–156, 361, 365–368,
    369
  measurable components, 155–156
  Progressive Patient Care, *see*
    Progressive Patient Care
  self-care, 40
  use of experimental approach in studies
    of, 198–200
  common medical and nursing needs, 39,
    64
Peer review of research grants, 322–324
Pencil and paper instruments to collect
  data, 150
Percentage, *390*
Percentile, 257–258, *390*
Pfefferkorn, Blanche, 30
Phenomenon, *390*
Physical models, 109–110
Physical sciences, use of concepts from,
  43–44
Pilot study, *390*
Placebo, 187, *390*
Pre-test, 76
Point estimate, 261
Poisson distribution, *390*
Population, *see* Sampling units; Target
  population
Postulates as part of theory, 51
Power of a test, 283–284
Practical significance, 153, 154

Prediction, 111, *390*
Predictive relationships, *see* Relationships,
  predictive
Premise, *390*
Presbyterial Hospital (Philadelphia)
Pretest, 76, *390*
  importance, 239
Preventive health care, 42–43, 370–372
Principal investigator, 342
Prior probabilities, 284
Privacy Act (1975), 316
Probability (random) sampling, 219–227
  cluster sampling, 224–226
  mixed sampling designs, 226
  sampling error in, 217, 219, 220
  sequential sampling, 226–227
  simple random samples, 219–222
  stratified random samples, 223–224
  systematic sampling, 222–223
Problem,
  formulation, 76–77, 87–89
  from problem to hypothesis, 123–124
"Problem finding," process of, 50–51
Problem solving, applied research and, 10
Processing error, 243
Product-moment method, 268, *390*
Professional salaries, budget for, 343,
  346–347
Progressive Patient Care, 110
Projective techniques, 238, *390*
Proportions, test of significance for,
  269–270
Prospective design, 14, 80, 202–203, *390*
PSRO (Professional Standards Review
  Organization), 160
Public health nurses,
  conceptual framework for study of role,
    66–70
Public Health Service Act of, 1944, 320
Publication of research findings,
  initial planning for, 299–300
  as motivation for research team,
    311–313
  preparation of final report, 300–301
Pure (basic) research, 9
Purposive samples, 227

Q-sort, 46, 139–140, *390*

Qualitative scales, 128, 131−140
  nominal, 133
    developing quantitative scales from,
      145−147
  ordinal, 133−135
    in social science research, 135−140
  summarization of data from, 251−255
  use by nonparticipant observer, 234
Qualitative variables
  tests of significance for, 269−276
    chi-square, 269−273
    distribution-free, 273−276
    for proportions, 269−270
  See also Qualitative scales
Quality of patient care, 358, 367
Quantification, 128−129, 130−131
Quantitative scales, 128−129, 131−132,
    140−145
  developed from nominal scales,
    145−147
  interval and ratio, 140−145
  measures of central tendency, 254,
    255−256, 294
  summarization of data from, 254−259
  use by nonparticipant observer, 233
Quantitative variables
  tests of significance for, 263−269
    analysis of variance, 265−266
    of difference between two means,
      263−265
    regression techniques, 266−268
  See also Quantitative scales
Quasi-experiments, 80
Questionnaires, factual, 236−237
Quota samples, 227−228

Random assignment, see also
    Randomization
  experimental designs with, 182−192
Random (probability) sampling, 219−227,
    391
  cluster sampling, 224−226
  mixed sampling designs, 226
  sampling error in, 217, 219, 220
  sequential sampling, 226−227
  simple random samples, 219−222
  stratified random samples, 223−224
  systematic sampling, 222−223

Random start, 222, 391
Randomization, 81, 149, 166, 167, 174,
    175, 182−184, 196−197, 200, 203,
    219, 261−262, 280, 391
Range, 257
Rank correlation method, 275−276
Rates, 242, 251−253, 269−270
  in vital statistics, 253
Ratio scales, 140−145
Reaction model, 61−62
Reference material for research in nursing,
    94−105
Regression analysis, 186, 266−268,
    391
Regression coefficient, 266
Reiter, Francis, 157
Relationships, 166−167
  interpersonal, in nursing, 45−46
  predictive, 111
    artificial, 166
    associative, 119−121, 166
    causal, 119−121, 166
    spurious, 120, 174
Relevance, in reaction model, 61
Reliability, 151−152, 391
  of data-collecting instruments, 239
  of dependent variables, 151−152
Repeated measures analysis of variance,
    266
Replication, 391
Reports, see Research findings
Research, 4, 391
Research climate, 5−7
Research content, see Subjects of research
Research design, 80−81, 392
  choice, 208−209
  determining, 80−81
  experimental, 167−168
    advantages and disadvantages,
      168−170, 175
    barriers, 15−17
    cause and effect in, 165
    comparison of nonexperimental and,
      13−15, 172−175
    practical problems in, 169
    in studies of patient care, 198−200
    types, 80, 176−192
    variables in explanatory studies, 78,
      172, 175−176

Research design (*continued*):
  nonexperimental, 170–172
    advantages and disadvantages of, 170–172, 175
    comparison of experimental and, 13–15, 172–175
    conducting, 207–209
    cross-sectional, 201–202
    mixed designs, 203–204
    prospective, 202–203
  retrospective, 202
  variations, 80–81
Research findings, 41–42
  analysis and interpretation, 261–295
    errors in use and interpretation of tests of significance, 284–290
    interpreting data in statistical tables, 290–295
    tests of significance for qualitative variables, 269–276
    tests of significance for quantitative variables, 263–269
  communication of, 298–305, 312–314
    initial planning for publication, 299–300
  evaluation, 303–305
Research grants, 317
  federal, 318–341
    nursing research grants and fellowships, 325–326
Research Grants Index, 95
Research institutes, 21
  See also specific research institutes
Research need, 355–358
Research on Aging Act, 372
Research personnel, *392*
Research, practice based, 5
Research priorities, 356–358
Research problem, 87–93, *392*
Research process,
  data in, *see* Data
  research design, *see* Research design
  research findings, *see* Research findings
  research tactics, *see* Research tactics
  steps in, 75–76
    define variables, 78–80
    delineate target population, 81
    determine how results will be interpreted, 83–84
    determine how variables will be quantified, 78–80
    determine method of communicating results, 84
    determine research design, 80–81
    formulate framework of theory, 77–78
    formulate hypotheses, 78
    formulate method for analyzing data, 83
    formulate problem, 76–77, 87–89
    review literature, 77
    select and develop method for collecting data, 82
  variables, *see* Variables
Research proposal, 75, *392*
  research substitutes, 21–23
Research tactics, 309–351
  financial support, 317
    budget determinations, 343–347
    preparing research proposal in applying for, 344–350
    responsibilities of universities and health agencies, 318, 341–342
    See also Federal government
  human rights, 314–317, 348–350
  major deterrents to research, 350
  motivating research team, 311–312
  nurse as researcher, 313
  research as organized activity, 309–310
  securing adequate staff, 310–311
  securing facilities to conduct research, 314
  sponsorship, 315
Research team
  motivation, 311–312
Research topics, 76–77
  source, 86–87
Research training, 318, 341
Response error, 326
Results
  communicating, 84, 298–305
  interpreting, 83, 290–295
Retrospective design, 14, 80, 81, 148, 180, 202
Roberts, Mary, 29, 205
Role analysis, 46, *392*
Rorschach test, 126, *392*

Saba, Virginia, 40
Sampling, 82, 217–228, *392*
  advantages, 218–219
  history, 217–218
  nonprobability samples, 219, 227–228
  probability (random), 219–226
    cluster sampling, 224–226
    mixed sampling designs, 226
    sequential sampling, 226–227
    simple random samples, 219–222
    stratified random samples, 223–224
    systematic samples, 222–223
  See also Sampling units
Sampling error, 217, 219, 224, 225, 240, 261–262, 280, *393*
  computing, 220, 223, 241
Sampling units (study population), 82, 215, *393*
  number, 195–196, 222, 223
  selection, 222
  size, 235
  See also Sampling
Scales, 79–80, 131–147, *393*
  qualitative, *see* Qualitative scales
  quantitative, *see* Quantitative scales
Scalogram analysis, *see* Guttman-type scale
Schematic diagrams, 110–111
Science, 7–8, *394*
  nursing as, 46–47
  social, *see* Social science
  scientific method, 8–9
Score, *394*
Secretary's Committee to Study Extended Roles for Nurses, 33
Self-care as form of therapy, 40
"Self-coded" questionnaires, 237
Sensitivity of a measure, 152–154
Sequential sampling, 226–227
Serendipity, *394*
Settings for research, 17–20
  choice, 195
  highly controlled, 17–18
  natural, 18–19, 182
  partially controlled, 19–20
  securing, 314
Sign test, 274
Significance, statistical, *see* Tests of significance
Simmons, Leo, 31, 32

Simple random samples, 219–222
Simulation, 249
Smith, Dorothy, 158
Social sciences, 44
  impact on nursing research, 44
    formulation of problems, 45–46
    research methodology, 46
  measuring instruments, 144–145
  ordinal scales, 135–140
  variables, 144–145
Sociogram, 46, 235
Sociometry, 234
Southern Regional Educational Board, 32
Spurious correlation, *394*
Spurious relationships, 120–121
Staff for research, 310–311
Standard deviation, 258–259
Statistical models, 111–112
Statistical packages for computers, 248
Statistical significance, 196, *394*
  meaning, 279–280
  tests, *see* Tests of significance
Statistical sources, 101
Statistical tables
  interpreting data in, 290–295
  skeleton layout of, 250–251
Statisticians, 91, 220
Statistics, 217, *394*
Stewart, Isabel, 205
Stimulus, *see* Independent variable
Stochastic process, *394*
"Stopping rules," 226
Stratified random samples, 223–224
Student's *t* distribution, see *t*-test
Subjects of research, 20–21, *394*
  number, 195–196
  selection, 214–217
  volunteers, 228
Surgeon General's Consultant Group on Nursing, 32
Surgeon General's Report on Health Promotion and Disease Prevention, 33
Surveys, 170–171, *394*
  See also Nonexperimental research
Symbolic models, 109
  mathematical, 111
  statistical, 111–112
Systematic sampling, 222–223

Tables, *see* Statistical tables
Tabulated data, 232–233
Target population, 194, 215–217, *394*
  delineating, 81–82, 215–217
  See also Sampling; Sampling units
Tate, Barbara, 33
Tax Equity and Fiscal Responsibility Act
    (1982), 327, 369
Taylor, Susan, 31–32
Teachers College, Columbia University,
    31, 94
Team research, *see* Research team
Technology, 377
Television, closed-circuit, study,
Tests of significance, 184, 263–276, 279,
    394
  errors in use and interpretation,
    284–290
  for qualitative variables, 252,
    269–276
    chi-square, 270–273
    distribution-free, 273–276
    for proportions, 269–270
  for quantitative variables, 263–269
    analysis of variance, 184
    of difference between two means,
      263–265
    regression techniques, 266–268
Thematic apperception test (T.A.T.), 126,
    395
Theory, 106–108, 363–364, *395*
  and models, 52, 108–112
  comparison of nursing theories, 54–59
  development, 107–108
  finding existing, 108
  role in research, 51–52, 106–107
  search in nursing for, 50–51
  as source of research topics, 87
  See also Hypotheses; Models
Thurstone-type scale, 135–137
Tippett, L. H. C., 218
Topics, *see* Research topics
Tradition as substitute for research, 23
Trial and error as substitute for research,
    22, 178
t-test, 194, 264, 265, *395*
  procedure, 264–265
  for small samples, 264–265
T-test, 265
Two-group, before-after design, 181–182

Two-group design, 180–181
  with control group, 182–188
Two-tailed vs. one-tailed tests, 282, 284
Type I error, 283–284
Type II error, 283–284
Typology for nursing research, 24, 87
  aims or research, 11–12
  classification by research content, 24
  classification by research design, 13

U.S. Bureau of Labor Statistics, 233
U.S. Bureau of the Census, 12, 115, 218,
    233, 240
U.S. Public Health Service, 30, 32, 95,
    201, 224, 233, 371
  Alcohol, Drug Abuse and Mental
    Health Administration, 329–331
  Center for Disease Control, 330–331
  Division of Nursing, 21, 28, 31, 94, 95,
    96, 222, 325–326
    Grants and Fellowships, 32
  Division of Research Grants, 95, 318,
    325
  Food and Drug Administration, 331
  Health Resources and Services
    Administration, 34, 331
  National Advisory Council on Nurse
    Training, 318
  National Center for Health Services
    Research, 332–333
  National Center for Health Statistics, 12
  National Center for Nursing Research,
    34
  National Health Planning Information
    Center, 96
  National Institutes of Health, 44,
    96–97, 228, 320–325, 333–341
  National Library of Medicine, 96,
    206–207, 340–341
Univariate distribution, 290
Universe, *see* Sampling units; Target
    population
Universities
  responsibilities on conducting research,
    318, 341–342
  university research vs. federal research,
    318
  See also specific universities
University of Minnesota, 30

Validity, 148 – 150, *395*
  content, 150 – 151, 233
  construct, 150 – 151
  face, 150
  of data-collecting instruments, 238, 239
  of dependent variables, 148 – 150
  predictive, 150
Value, *395*
  in reaction model, 61
Vanderbilt University, 30
Variables, 78 – 79, 125 – 162, 175, 182, 187, *395*
  in associative relationships, 117, 119 – 120
  dependent, 118 – 119, 127 – 128, 175, 182
    criteria for evaluating sufficiency and efficiency of, 148 – 155
    multiple, 197 – 198
    role in nursing research, 155 – 160
    selection, 147 – 148
  environmental, 119, 126, 172, 175, 182, 184, 225
  explanatory, 118 – 119, 148, 175
  in explanatory research, 175 – 176
  extraneous, 118 – 119, 149, 171, 173, 175 – 176, 179, 180, 181, 182, 183, 188, 190
  independent, 116 – 117, 118 – 119, 126 – 127, 175, 182, 183
    multiple comparison groups with multiple, 190 – 192
    multiple comparison groups with single, 188 – 190
  methods of collecting data and, 238
  organismic, 119, 126, 172, 182, 185, 238
  quantification, 79, 128 – 129
  scales, *see* Scales
  tests of significance for qualitative, 269 – 176
  tests of significance for quantitative, 263 – 269
Variance, analysis of, 184, 189, 192, 262, 265 – 266, 286
Variation (measures), 257 – 259
Verbal descriptive data, 129 – 130
Vital statistics, rates used, 253
Volunteers, 228

Walter Reed Army Institute of Research, 32
Wandelt, Mabel, 358
Weighted scoring, *396*
Wellness scale, 147
Western Council on Higher Education in Nursing, 32, 95, 96
Western Reserve University, 30, 206
Wilcox, Jane, 152
Working papers, use of, 84
Wright, Stuart, 137

Yale University, 30, 31, 94, 95
Yate's correction for continuity, 271
Yule's coefficient of association, 268 – 269, *396*

Z-test, 265